Introduction to Health Sciences Librarianship

THE HAWORTH PRESS
Titles of Related Interest

Computers in Libraries: An Introduction for Library Technicians by Katie Wilson

An Introduction to Reference Services in Academic Libraries edited by Elizabeth Connor

Handbook of Electronic and Digital Acquisitions edited by Thomas W. Leonhardt

New Directions in Reference edited by Byron Anderson and Paul T. Webb

Real-Life Marketing and Promotion Strategies in College Libraries edited by Barbara Whitney Petruzzelli

A Guide to Developing End User Education Programs in Medical Libraries by Elizabeth Connor

Planning, Renovating, Expanding, and Constructing Library Facilities in Hospitals, Academic Medical Centers, and Health Organizations by Elizabeth Connor

The Practical Library Trainer by Bruce E. Massis

The Practical Library Manager by Bruce E. Massis

E-Serials Collection Management: Transitions, Trends, and Technicalities edited by David C. Fowler

Introduction to Technical Services for Library Technicians by Mary L. Kao

Health Care Resources on the Internet: A Guide for Librarians and Health Care Consumers edited by M. Sandra Wood

Introduction to Health Sciences Librarianship

M. Sandra Wood, MLS, MBA, AHIP, FMLA
Editor

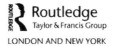
Routledge
Taylor & Francis Group

LONDON AND NEW YORK

First Published by

The Haworth Press, Taylor & Francis Group, 270 Madison Avenue, New York, NY 10016.

Transferred to Digital Printing 2008 by Routledge
270 Madison Ave, New York NY 10016
2 Park Square, Milton Park, Abingdon, Oxon, OX14 4RN

For more information on this book or to order, visit
http://www.haworthpress.com/store/product.asp?sku=6041

or call 1-800-HAWORTH (800-429-6784) in the United States and Canada
or (607) 722-5857 outside the United States and Canada

or contact orders@HaworthPress.com

PUBLISHER'S NOTE
The development, preparation, and publication of this work has been undertaken with great care. However, the Publisher, employees, editors, and agents of The Haworth Press are not responsible for any errors contained herein or for consequences that may ensue from use of materials or information contained in this work. The Haworth Press is committed to the dissemination of ideas and information according to the highest standards of intellectual freedom and the free exchange of ideas. Statements made and opinions expressed in this publication do not necessarily reflect the views of the Publisher, Directors, management, or staff of The Haworth Press, or an endorsement by them.

Cover design by Kerry E. Mack.

Library of Congress Cataloging-in-Publication Data

Introduction to health sciences librarianship / M. Sandra Wood, editor.
    p. cm.
  ISBN: 978-0-7890-3595-0 (hard : alk. paper)
  ISBN: 978-0-7890-3596-7 (soft : alk. paper)
  1. Medical librarianship. 2. Medical librarianship—United States. I. Wood, M. Sandra.

  Z675.M4I58 2007
  026'.61—dc22

                  2007047081

CONTENTS

About the Editor   xi

Contributors   xiii

Foreword   xxi
Joanne Gard Marshall

Preface   xxiii
M. Sandra Wood

Acknowledgments   xxvii

SECTION I: INTRODUCTION/OVERVIEW

Chapter 1. Overview of Health Sciences Libraries and Librarianship   3
Mary Moore

Introduction   3
The Profession of Health Sciences Librarianship   4
Health Sciences Libraries   10
The U.S. National Library of Medicine   17
Trends Affecting Health Sciences Librarianship   20
Conclusion   27

Chapter 2. The Health Care Environment   31
Logan Ludwig

Introduction   31
The Modern Health Care System   33
The Changing Federal Role in U.S. Health Care   36
Organizational Components of Academic Medicine   40
Medical Education   44
Health Sciences Research   48
The Future of Academic Medicine   51
Conclusion   57
Appendix 2.A. Selected Federal Legislation with Important Health Aspects,
Including Health Care Information Policy Legislation   58

SECTION II: TECHNICAL SERVICES

**Chapter 3. Journal Collection Development:
Challenges, Issues, and Strategies**   69
Laurie L. Thompson
Mori Lou Higa

Introduction   69
Selection   70

Online Licensing and Negotiation/Vendor Relations 82
Copyright 85
Open Access 87
Benchmarking/Evaluating Use of Resources 89
Digital Archives 92
Conclusion 94

Chapter 4. Monographic and Digital Resource Collection Development **97**
Esther Carrigan
Mori Lou Higa
Rajia Tobia

Introduction 97
Overview and Relationships 98
Monograph Selection and Collection Development Policies 100
Selection and Evaluation of Digital Resources 109
Preservation 119
Conclusion 123

Chapter 5. Organizing Resources for Information Access **127**
Maggie Wineburgh-Freed

Introduction 127
Brief History of Information Organization by Libraries 127
Overview: Current Methods 128
Current Cataloging Practices 131
Organizing Specific Materials 140
Glimpses of What's to Come 141
Appendix 5.A. Resource Bibliography for Organizing Information 142

SECTION III: PUBLIC SERVICES

Chapter 6. Access Issues **147**
Elizabeth R. Lorbeer
Cindy Scroggins

Introduction 147
Fundamentals of Access 148
Access Services 148
Physical Access 149
Electronic Access 152
Shades of Gray: Services Straddling The Physical and Electronic Divide 154
Wireless Network Access 156
Access for the Disabled 157
Conclusion 158

Chapter 7. Information Services in Health Sciences Libraries **161**
Elizabeth H. Wood

Introduction 161

Information in the High-Tech Environment   162
Types of Health Sciences Information Needs   163
Librarian-User Interaction   164
Virtual Reference   167
The Reference Interview   167
Single-Service Desks and Triaging Requests   168
Selected Information Services   169
Information Service Ethics   172
Conclusion   176

Chapter 8. Information Retrieval in the Health Sciences   **179**
        Elizabeth H. Wood

Introduction   179
Types of Literature in the Health Sciences   180
Databases in the Health Sciences   181
MEDLINE   182
Other Major Databases in the Health Sciences   187
Full-Text Databases   191
Providing Search Services   192
The Mediated Search Process   193
Evaluating and Delivering the Results of the Search   197
Conclusion   197

Chapter 9. Marketing, Public Relations, and Communication   **201**
        Patricia C. Higginbottom
        Lisa A. Ennis

Introduction   201
Marketing in Libraries   203
How Marketing Has Changed   203
Marketing in Health Sciences Libraries   204
Methods for Promoting Libraries   204
Print/Physical Materials   204
In-Person Events   207
The Virtual World   209
Communication   212
Funding Issues   214
Conclusion   215
Appendix 9.A. Additional Readings   215

Chapter 10. Information Literacy Education in Health Sciences Libraries **217**
        Stewart M. Brower

Introduction: What Is Information Literacy?   217
Information Literacy Standards and Objectives   218
Criticisms of Information Literacy   221
Learning Theories and Pedagogies   222
The Millennials   224
Planning an Information Literacy Program   225

Information Literacy Program Designs 227
IL Instruction Activities and Techniques 229
Information Literacy Assessment 236
The Future of Information Literacy 239

Chapter 11. Evidence-Based Practice **241**
Jonathan D. Eldredge

Introduction 241
Librarians' Roles in EBM 242
Evidence-Based Librarianship 252
Conclusion 265

Chapter 12. Health Informatics **271**
K. Ann McKibbon
Ellen Gay Detlefsen

Introduction 271
Definitions 272
History 272
Types of Data Used in Health Informatics 273
Formats of Health Information 274
Domains of Health Informatics 275
Bioinformatics 275
Imaging Informatics 276
Clinical Informatics 277
Public Health Informatics 281
Standards and Vocabulary 283
Information Retrieval and Automatic Classification 286
Privacy, Confidentiality, and Security 288
Education in Health Informatics 289
Future 290
Health Sciences Librarians and Health Informatics 290
Conclusion 291
Appendix 12.A. Health Informatics Associations and Journals 292

SECTION IV: ADMINISTRATION

Chapter 13. Management in Academic Health Sciences Libraries **301**
Francesca Allegri
Martha Bedard

Introduction 301
Managing in the Academic Health Sciences Environment 301
The Roles of Library Administrators 302
Managing Personnel 315
Managing Facilities 329
Conclusion 331
Appendix 13.A. Additional Readings 331

Appendix 13.B. Select List of Trend Reports   333

Appendix 13.C. The University of Tennessee Graduate School of Medicine,
    Preston Medical Library & Learning Resource Center   334

Appendix 13.D. Checklist for Librarian Recruitment
    (for permanent positions)   335

Chapter 14. Management of and Issues Specific to Hospital Libraries   **341**
    Dixie A. Jones

Introduction   341
Reporting Structure   342
Staffing   343
Standards/Accreditation   344
Populations Served   345
Services   346
Collection Development and Management   349
Networking and Visibility   352
Marketing and Proving Value of Services   353
Roles   354
Space and Library As Place   358
Legal/Ethical Issues   358
Time Management   359
Strategic Planning   360
Professional Development   360
Technology Issues   361
Security   362
Data Collection   363
Fiscal Management   365
Conclusion   365
Appendix 14.A. Additional Readings   366

Chapter 15. Library Space Planning   **369**
    Elizabeth Connor

Introduction   369
Background   369
Trends in Library Design   370
Predesign Planning   374
Site Visits, Research, and Readings   374
Library Standards   376
Hiring Consultants and Architects   377
Facility Planning As Part of Strategic Planning   377
Significance of Library 2.0 on Design   378
Advice for Newbies   379
Conclusion   383
Appendix 15.A. Suggested Readings   384

SECTION V: SPECIAL TOPICS

Chapter 16. Special Services Provided by Health Sciences Libraries   **397**
    Brenda L. Seago

    Introduction   397
    Personal Digital Assistants   398
    Course Management Systems   400
    Manikins/Simulators   402
    Audience Response Systems   404
    Videoconferencing   405
    Instructional Design   407
    Podcasting   408
    Streaming Video   409
    Conclusion   409

Chapter 17. Health Sciences Librarianship in Rare Book and Special Collections   **413**
    Stephen J. Greenberg
    Patricia E. Gallagher

    Introduction   413
    Collection Policies   415
    Reference Areas   418
    Reference Services   421
    Education and Training   421
    Reference Sources   422
    Technical Services   422
    Storage and Stack Security   423
    Conclusion   425

Chapter 18. Consumer Health Information   **429**
    Catherine Arnott Smith

    Introduction   429
    CHI in Libraries   430
    The National Library of Medicine and CHI   434
    CHI Seekers   437
    Challenges in CHI Provision   440
    Providing for CHI Services   444
    CHI Service Evaluation   451
    Collaboration   452
    Resources for Consumer Health Information Practice   454

Glossary   **459**

Index   **483**

ABOUT THE EDITOR

M. SANDRA WOOD, MLS, MBA, AHIP, FMLA, is Librarian Emerita, Pennsylvania State University. Previously, she was Librarian, Reference and Database Services, The George T. Harrell Library, The Milton S. Hershey Medical Center, The Pennsylvania State University College of Medicine, Hershey, Pennsylvania. At Hershey, she served in various capacities in the reference department, was promoted academically to Librarian, and was tenured. Ms. Wood holds an MLS from Indiana University (1970) and an MBA from the University of Maryland (1983). She retired in December 2005 with over thirty-five years of experience as a medical reference librarian; her experience and interests are in general reference, management of reference services, database and Internet searching, and user instruction. Ms. Wood has been widely published in the field of medical reference, is Editor of *Medical Reference Services Quarterly* and *Journal of Consumer Health on the Internet,* and is Co-Editor of the *Journal of Electronic Resources in Medical Libraries* (Haworth). She is author or editor of numerous books for The Haworth Press, including *Health Care Resources on the Internet: A Guide for Librarians and Health Care Consumers,* and was editor of *Reference and Information Services in Health Sciences Libraries,* Volume 1 of MLA's series, Current Practice in Health Sciences Librarianship. She has been an active member of the Medical Library Association (MLA) and the Special Libraries Association. Her activities in MLA include serving as Chairman and Section Council Representative of the Reference Services Section (now Public Services Section); serving on three National Program Committees and two MLA Nominating Committees; and serving on numerous national committees, including the Credentialing Committee. She has received MLA's Eliot Award and the Chapter Achievement Award from the Philadelphia Chapter/MLA. Ms. Wood was elected to MLA's Board of Directors (1991-1995) and served as MLA's Treasurer. Ms. Wood has been a Distinguished Member of the Academy of Health Information Professionals since 1990 and a Fellow of the Medical Library Association since 1998.

Introduction to Health Sciences Librarianship
© 2008 by The Haworth Press, Taylor & Francis Group. All rights reserved.
doi:10.1300/6041_a

CONTRIBUTORS

Francesca Allegri, MSLS, is Head of User Services, Health Sciences Library, University of North Carolina at Chapel Hill, Chapel Hill, North Carolina. As head of the public services department (twenty-two FTEs), Ms. Allegri is part of the library's senior management team at the University of North Carolina at Chapel Hill's Health Sciences Library. She is also a graduate of the National Library of Medicine/Association of Academic Health Sciences Libraries Leadership Fellows Program. Prior to that, she held two positions in the Health Sciences Library's administrative unit managing professional librarian recruitment, staff development, planning, and institutional data collection and reporting. She also served four years as Department Head of the education department at the Health Sciences Library and has had leadership experience in campus organizations, such as the University Managers Association. Earlier, Ms. Allegri served as Assistant Head at the University of Illinois Library of the Health Sciences in Urbana, Illinois. She holds an MSLS from the University of Illinois at Urbana-Champaign, Urbana, Illinois.

Martha Bedard, MSLS, AHIP, is Dean of the University of New Mexico Libraries, Albuquerque, New Mexico. Formerly, she was Associate Dean for Information and Collection Services, Texas A&M University Libraries, College Station, Texas. There, she had responsibility for the reference, instruction, educational media, collections, acquisitions, and cataloging operations at Texas A&M, the fifth largest public university in the United States. She also served as the Associate Dean and Director of the Texas A&M Medical Sciences Library, managing a budget of 3.5 million dollars and faculty and staff of thirty-five FTEs. She was a tenured Full Professor of Library Science at Texas A&M and holder of the Lila B. King endowed professorship. Prior to her leadership roles in Texas, she was the Associate Director for Library Services at the University of North Carolina Health Sciences Library, after directing hospital and medical center libraries in Massachusetts. Ms. Bedard is an Association of Research Libraries (ARL) Research Library Leadership Fellow, having completed an extensive two-year pilot leadership development program which aims to build leadership skills in current librarians who will be the next generation of deans and directors of large academic libraries. Ms. Bedard received an MSLS from Simmons Graduate School of Library Science, Boston, Massachusetts, and is active in local, state, and national professional organizations.

Stewart M. Brower, MLIS, AHIP, is Director of the University of Oklahoma–Tulsa Library. He is a Founder and Co-Editor of *Communications in Information Literacy,* an independent, peer-reviewed journal on library user education, and Co-Editor of the "Informatics Education" column in *Medical Reference Services Quarterly.* He has been an active member of the Medical Library Association for fourteen years, recently serving as Chair of the Public Services Section (2004-2005).

Esther Carrigan, MLS, AHIP, is Associate Dean and Director of the Medical Sciences Library, Texas A&M University, College Station, Texas. She manages a budget of 3.5 million dollars and a faculty and staff of thirty-five FTEs. Collection management responsibilities have been a key component of her positions for over twenty years, most recently as Associate Director for Collection Services and then as Deputy Director. She has presented papers, posters, and written articles on the management of information resources and on organizational change. Ms.

Introduction to Health Sciences Librarianship
© 2008 by The Haworth Press, Taylor & Francis Group. All rights reserved.
doi:10.1300/6041_b

Carrigan is a guest lecturer and WebCT instructor for a course on health sciences information management at the University of North Texas School of Library and Information Sciences, focusing on the management of information resources in health sciences libraries. Ms. Carrigan received her MLS from the State University of New York at Buffalo. She is a distinguished member of the Academy of Health Information Professionals and is active professionally at the state, regional, and national levels. Ms. Carrigan is the 2007 recipient of the Louise Darling Medal for Distinguished Achievement in Collection Development from the Medical Library Association. She currently serves as Chief Licensing Agent for the South Central Academic Medical Libraries Consortium (SCAMeL) and leads the SCAMeL Collection Development Interest Group.

Elizabeth Connor, MLS, AHIP, is Science Liaison and Associate Professor of Library Science at the Daniel Library of The Citadel, The Military College of South Carolina, in Charleston, South Carolina. Ms. Connor's recent publications include editing *A Guide to Developing End User Programs in Medical Libraries; Planning, Renovating, Expanding, and Constructing Library Facilities in Hospitals, Academic Medical Centers, and Health Organizations;* and *Evidence-Based Librarianship: Case Studies and Active Learning Exercises.* She is Co-Editor of *Journal of Electronic Resources in Medical Libraries.* Ms. Connor has planned several library building projects and worked as a predesign building consultant for several medical library clients.

Ellen Gay Detlefsen, MA, MS, DLS, MPhil, is Associate Professor, Program in Library & Information Science, School of Information Sciences, and Core Training Faculty, Department of Biomedical Informatics, School of Medicine, University of Pittsburgh, Pittsburgh, Pennsylvania. Dr. Detlefsen has been a faculty member in library and information science for thirty-five years. Her areas of expertise and teaching competence include biomedical and health sciences information, medical informatics, and resources and services for special populations, such as patients and health care consumers and the aging and their caregivers. She speaks frequently on the issues related to both formal and continuing education for the health information professions, on information behavior research, on consumer health care information, and on medical informatics. She is also the developer of, and regular instructor for, Internet workshops for the American College of Psychiatrists, the American Association for Geriatric Psychiatry, and the American Medical Association's Medical Communications Conference. Dr. Detlefsen holds an MS in Library Service (1969), an MA in American History (1973), a DLS in Library Science (1975), and an MPhil in American History (1978), all from Columbia University in New York City.

Jonathan D. Eldredge, MLS, PhD, is Associate Professor for the School of Medicine and the Health Sciences Library and Informatics Center at the University of New Mexico, Albuquerque, New Mexico. Dr. Eldredge has published twenty-one articles and five book chapters on evidence-based librarianship (EBL). He created the Medical Library Association's continuing education course on EBL in 1998 and has taught this course a total of twenty-one times in the United Kingdom, in Canada, and across the four time zones of the continental United States. During 2006 Jon created a forty-two-hour Web-based mentored version of this course for the Medical Library Association. He has been the principal investigator in four randomized controlled trials. He also served two terms of office as Chair of the MLA Research Section. He is Associate Editor for *BMC Biomedical Digital Libraries* and serves on the editorial boards of both *Hypothesis* and *Communications in Information Literacy.* Jon has been heavily involved in teaching medical students, physician assistant students, and primary care providers evidence-based medicine (EBM) skills for over a decade. He received his BA (cum laude) from Beloit

College, Beloit, Wisconsin, his MLS from the University of Michigan, Ann Arbor, Michigan; and a second MA and his PhD from the University of New Mexico, Albuquerque, New Mexico .

Lisa A. Ennis, MS, MA, is Systems Librarian at the Lister Hill Library of the Health Sciences, University of Alabama–Birmingham, Birmingham, Alabama. Ms. Ennis has a long history of public services librarianship, including government documents, instruction, and reference. She has published several articles on numerous library topics, including digital reference, management, and technostress. Her new book *Government Documents Librarianship: A Guide for the Neo-Depository Era* was published in June 2007 by Info Today, Inc. Lisa received her MS in information sciences from the University of Tennessee (1997), Knoxville, Tennessee, and an MA in history from Georgia College & State University (1994), Milledgeville, Georgia.

Patricia E. Gallagher, MLS, MA, AHIP, is currently Acting Head of Public Services at the New York Academy of Medicine; previously she worked as Librarian in the Helene Fuld School of Nursing, and Assistant Director and Archivist at the Phillips Library of Beth Israel Medical Center, both in New York City. She is the author of many articles on consumer health and evidence-based medicine. In addition, she is Co-Author (with Stephen J. Greenberg) of the Medical Library Association's *BibKit: History of the Health Sciences,* now in its second edition. Ms. Gallagher is active in both the New York–New Jersey Chapter and the History of the Health Sciences Section of MLA, is a Distinguished Member of the Academy of Health Information Professionals, and is Managing Editor of NOAH: New York Online Access to Health, <http://www.noah-health.org>. Ms. Gallagher received her MLS from Queens College, CUNY, Queens, New York, and her MA from Hunter College, CUNY, in New York City.

Stephen J. Greenberg, MSLS, PhD, received his doctorate in early modern history from Fordham University, in New York City, with a dissertation on early printing and publishing. After teaching for several years, he returned to school and earned his library degree from Columbia University, also in New York City, specializing in rare books. Since 1992, he has worked in the History of Medicine Division at the National Library of Medicine, where he is currently Coordinator of Public Services. His papers and publications span a number of fields, including the history of printing and publishing, medicine and surgery in early modern Europe, and the history of medical librarianship. In 1996, he was awarded MLA's Murray Gottlieb Prize. He has taught many continuing education courses to both national and regional audiences, and he is Co-Author (with Patricia E. Gallagher) of the MLA's *BibKit: History of the Health Sciences,* now in its second edition. He is also Adjunct Professor at the College of Library and Information Studies at the University of Maryland, College Park, Maryland, where he lectures on the history of the book.

Mori Lou Higa, MLS, AHIP, is Manager of the Collection Development Department at the University of Texas Southwestern Medical Center Library in Dallas, Texas. She holds an MLS from San José State University, San José, California. Ms. Higa joined UT Southwestern Medical Center Library in 1993 as Information Services Librarian. Since then, she has managed the new North Campus branch library, led the library's strategic planning activities, and established the library's first Digital Infrastructure Research and Development (DIRD) Department. Ms. Higa led the implementation efforts for the library's link resolver and federated search engine, participated in the assessment and planning for a major staff reallocation, and played an integral role in the first redesign of the library's Web site. Ms. Higa presently manages the library's collection development activities and a staff of two FTEs. She has presented papers and posters relating to various library activities and has also authored articles on the use of focus groups in the strategic planning process and in the redesign of a library's organizational structure.

Patricia C. Higginbottom, MLS, AHIP, is Associate Director for Public Services at the Lister Hill Library of the Health Sciences at the University of Alabama, Birmingham, Alabama. She has worked in various positions there since 1993. She's an active member of MLA and has served as Chair of the Leadership and Management Section. In 2002-2003, she was selected as a Fellow in the NLM/AAHSL Leadership Fellows Program, which focuses on preparing emerging leaders for director positions in academic health center libraries. Pat received an MLIS from the University of Alabama, Birmingham, Alabama.

Dixie A. Jones, MLS, AHIP, is Librarian, Overton Brooks VA Medical Center, Shreveport, Louisiana. Ms. Jones holds an MLS from Louisiana State University, Baton Rouge, Louisiana. She has over thirty years of experience in health sciences libraries. After retiring from LSU Health Sciences Center Library in Shreveport as an associate professor, she returned to service in a hospital setting at the Overton Brooks VA Medical Center Library. She has served as President of the Health Sciences Library Association of Louisiana, as well as the South Central Chapter of the Medical Library Association. Ms. Jones served as Chair of MLA's Hospital Libraries Section and, prior to that, as Chair of its Standards Committee. A distinguished member of the Academy of Health Information Professionals, she recently completed a term as Treasurer and member of the Board of Directors of the Medical Library Association. She has authored and edited numerous publications and is currently the "Specialty of the House" column editor for the *Journal of Hospital Librarianship.*

Elizabeth R. Lorbeer, MLS, EdM, is Associate Director for Content Management at the University of Alabama, Birmingham, Alabama. Her primary responsibilities include the successful planning, organization, and direction of the library sections which support the collections. She is a member of her campus's Scholarly Communications Task Force to educate faculty and students on open access issues. Ms. Lorbeer is engaged in a variety of professional activities, including Chair of the Collection Development Section of the Medical Library Association, Advisory Board Member to the American Medical Association and *New England Journal of Medicine,* and a popular invited speaker at national and regional conferences. One of her many contributions at the association level is her presentations on licensing of library resources. Considered an expert in her specialty, she was invited to participate in two national teleconferences on licensing electronic journals. Her other research interests include usage statistics as an economic factor in scholarly communications. Her latest article "COUNTER Data: Expanding Horizons for Librarians and Users" was published in *What Counts and What Doesn't: An Insider's Guide to Usage Reports.* To view her research interests and publications go to <http://myprofile.cos.com/elorbeer>. Ms. Lorbeer has an MLS from SUNY Buffalo, Buffalo, New York, and an EdM in higher education administration from Boston University, Boston, Massachusetts.

Logan Ludwig, MLS, PhD, AHIP, holds a BS from Southern Illinois University, in Carbondale; an MLS from the University of Missouri, in Columbia; and a PhD from St. Louis University. He is currently Associate Dean for Library & Telehealth Services, Health Sciences Library, Loyola University Stritch School of Medicine, Maywood, Illinois. In addition to managing the Health Sciences Library, Dr. Ludwig provides leadership for Loyola's international telemedicine projects, the Illinois Rural Telehealth Alliance, and the Loyola University Health System E-Learning Project. He is Adjunct Professor of Library and Information Science at Dominican University, River Forest, Illinois; has held numerous leadership roles in a number of professional associations, including presidency for two international health communications associations; is Past President for the Association of Academic Health Sciences Libraries (AAHSL); has served as Midwest Medical Library Association (MLA) Chapter President; and is Library Buildings Editor for the *Journal of the Medical Library Association.* He is a Distinguished Member of the MLA Academy of Health Information Professionals and has received several professional association distinguished service awards. He also serves as a grant review panelist for the NIH Center for Scientific Review and as a member of the Association of American Medical Colleges (AAMC) Council of Academic Societies. He has served on the American Library Association's (ALA) Intellectual Freedom Principles for Libraries in a Networked World Task Force and the Distance Education and Copyright Committee. As a past Chair of the MLA Governmental Relations Committee, he has testified before the U.S. House Appropriations Subcommittee on Labor, Health and Human Services, Education, and Related Agencies regarding NLM funding, telemedicine, electronic publishing, and intellectual property rights. He is a well-known author and speaker, having published over fifty articles and given numerous presentations on information management and technology, library design, telemedicine, copyright, and intellectual property rights.

Joanne Gard Marshall, MLS, MHSc, PhD, is Alumni Distinguished Professor at the School of Information & Library Science at the University of North Carolina, Chapel Hill, North Carolina, where she served as Dean from 1999 to 2004. Prior to 1999, Dr. Marshall was a faculty member at the University of Toronto where she taught courses in health sciences information resources, management of corporate and other specialized information centers, research methods, and online information retrieval. In addition to her PhD in public health, Dr. Marshall holds an MHSc from McMaster University, Hamilton, Ontario, and an MLS from McGill University, Montreal, Quebec. In 2005 she received a DLitt from McGill University in recognition of her contribution to improving research and practice in health library and information science. Before assuming her faculty appointment at the University of Toronto, Dr. Marshall worked for fifteen years as a librarian in various academic and health sciences libraries. During 2004-2005 she served as President of the Medical Library Association (MLA). Dr. Marshall has received a number of awards, including a doctoral fellowship and the MLA Eliot Prize for the most significant research in medical librarianship for 1982 and 1992. She received the Award of Outstanding Achievement from the Canadian Health Libraries Association in 1992 as well as several awards from the Special Libraries Association (SLA), including the H. W. Wilson Award in 1997, the John Cotton Dana Award in 1998, and the Factiva National Leadership Award in 2004. She is a Fellow of both the Medical Library Association and the Special Libraries Association. Her research interests include information needs and uses of health care providers and consumers; evidence-based information practice; and workforce issues in library and information science.

K(athleen) Ann McKibbon, MLS, PhD, is Associate Professor, Health Information Research Unit, Clinical Epidemiology and Biostatistics, Faculty of Health Sciences, McMaster University, Hamilton, Ontario, Canada. She holds an MLS from the University of Western Ontario (1972), London, Ontario, and a PhD in medical informatics from the University of Pittsburgh (2005), Pittsburgh, Pennsylvania. Dr. McKibbon worked in academic science and technology and special libraries before coming to McMaster University Faculty of Health Sciences in the late 1970s. Her research has always been concerned with how clinicians use information. Research projects included early studies of clinicians using MEDLINE® in clinical care. She also worked with the group that produced the Clinical Queries in PubMed®. She has been associated with the developers of evidence-based medicine since its inception and has written a book for librarians who are interested in searching for information using evidence-based practice methods and techniques. She is currently developing an MSc program in eHealth at McMaster University.

Mary Moore, MA, PhD, is Executive Director of the Louis Calder Memorial Library and Biomedical Communications at the Leonard M. Miller School of Medicine, University of Miami.

She previously served as Head of Reference and Customer Service for the National Library of Medicine and also worked in the private sector in market research and competitive intelligence. In 2004, her library was the first health sciences library to receive the Institute of Museum and Library Services (IMLS) National Award, the nation's highest honor for excellence in public service by museums and libraries, from First Lady Laura Bush. She was named Alumna of the Year at the School of Information at the University of Texas in Austin. She has received funding and awards from AT&T, Frost Bank, ISI, the National Library of Medicine, SBC, and Rittenhouse for research and projects in knowledge management and health informatics. Dr. Moore holds an MA from the University of Missouri at Columbia and a PhD from the University of Texas at Austin.

Cindy Scroggins, MLS, has served as Director of the Baylor Health Sciences Library in Dallas, Texas, since 1995. She holds an MLS from Texas Woman's University, Denton, Texas. She authored the chapter on library management in Priscilla K. Shontz's *The Librarian's Career Guidebook* (Scarecrow Press, 2004). Ms. Scroggins is also the recipient of several grants, including a National Library of Medicine information systems grant of over $270,000.

Brenda L. Seago, MLS, MA, AHIP, is Associate Professor and Director of the Computer Based Instruction Lab in the School of Medicine at Virginia Commonwealth University, Richmond, Virginia. She also serves as Administrative Director of the Center for Human Simulation and Patient Safety, a joint undertaking of the Medical College of Virginia Hospitals and the School of Medicine. Ms. Seago holds an MA from Virginia Polytechnic Institute and State University (1983), Blacksburg, Virginia, and an MLS from the University of Maryland (1986), College Park, Maryland. She is currently in the dissertation phase of her doctoral program in public policy and administration, with a focus on health policy, at Virginia Commonwealth University. Ms. Seago has been an active member of the Medical Library Association (MLA) for more than twenty years, serving as a member of the Publications Committee, the Continuing Education Committee, the *Bulletin* Editorial Board, *JAMA* Journal Reviews Editor, and, most recently, Chair of the Educational Media and Technologies Section (2006-2007) of MLA. She is a distinguished member of the Academy of Health Information Professionals. She has also served as Column Editor for *Medical Reference Services Quarterly.*

Catherine Arnott Smith, MA, AMLS, MSIS, PhD, is Assistant Professor, School of Library and Information Studies, University of Wisconsin, Madison, Wisconsin. She has an MA in American history/administration of archives and an AMLS (library science), both from the University of Michigan (1992), Ann Arbor, Michigan; and an MSIS in information science/medical informatics (2000) and PhD in library and information science/medical informatics (2002), both from the University of Pittsburgh, Pittsburgh, Pennsylvania. Dr. Smith was formerly a medical librarian at the Galter Health Sciences Library, Northwestern University, Chicago, Illinois, and a medical information systems specialist at Lincoln National Reinsurance Companies, Fort Wayne, Indiana. She held a National Library of Medicine medical informatics predoctoral fellowship between 1997 and 2002 at the Center for Biomedical Informatics, University of Pittsburgh, and was the first recipient of the Donald A. B. Lindberg Research Fellowship from the Medical Library Association in 2003. Her research has additionally been supported by IBM's Center for Healthcare Management and the National Historic and Public Records Commission; her research interests include consumer health vocabularies, alternative medical vocabularies, and the content and structure of medical records.

Laurie L. Thompson, MLS, AHIP, joined the staff of the University of Texas Southwestern Medical Center Library in Dallas, Texas, as Director of Libraries in 2003; she is currently Assistant Vice President for Library Services at UT Southwestern. Prior to that, she was Director of

Libraries at the Health Sciences Library, State University of New York Upstate Medical University, Syracuse, New York, for five years. She has also held positions at the Himmelfarb Health Sciences Library at the George Washington University Medical Center, in Washington, DC; the National Library of Medicine, Bethesda, Maryland; and Hawaii Medical Library at the Queen's Medical Center, in Honolulu, Hawaii. Ms. Thompson holds an MLS from the University of Hawaii. Ms. Thompson co-developed with an attorney at the Medical Library Association, a continuing education course on licensing electronic resources. She has taught the course to librarians throughout the country since 1997. She has lectured on copyright issues in libraries and higher education and was privileged to attend several working group sessions of CONFU: The Conference on Fair Use in Washington, DC.

Rajia Tobia, AMLS, AHIP, is Associate Library Director for Collection Development at the University of Texas Health Science Center at San Antonio Library, where she has held a number of positions in public and technical services. She began her career as Serials Librarian and Medical Center Librarian at the University of South Alabama Biomedical Library in Mobile, Alabama. She is a Distinguished Member of the Academy of Health Information Professionals and has served on a number of committees within the Medical Library Association and its regional chapter. She is a member of the Editorial Board of the *Journal of Electronic Resources in Medical Libraries* and has contributed articles to a number of journals during her career in health sciences librarianship. Ms. Tobia has participated in developing and implementing several National Library of Medicine grants and contracts aimed at outreach to health professionals and public librarians in the south Texas region. She received an MLS from the University of Michigan, Ann Arbor, Michigan.

Maggie Wineburgh-Freed, MSLS, AHIP, is Associate Director for Collection Resources at the University of Southern California Norris Medical Library, Los Angeles, California. She holds an MSLS from Simmons College, Boston, Massachusetts, and is a Distinguished Member of the Academy of Health Information Professionals. She began her career in medical librarianship as an intern in the catalog department at Harvard University's Countway Library of Medicine, Boston, Massachusetts. She served as an information specialist at the Countway's Vision Information Center and participated in four months of MEDLARS indexing and search training at the National Library of Medicine, including an intensive study of NLM's Medical Subject Headings. She performed indexing and searching at the University of California's Brain Information Service, and then headed the Women's Hospital Library at Los Angeles County + University of Southern California Medical Center before coming to USC to head the Norris Medical Library catalog section. For a number of years she taught the continuing education class MeSH and NLM Classification for Catalogers. She is an active member and past Chair of the Medical Library Association Technical Services Section.

Elizabeth H. Wood, MA, MSLS, AHIP, retired recently after twenty-seven years in health sciences librarianship. At the University of Southern California Norris Medical Library (1979-1995), Los Angeles, California, she was Head of Acquisitions/Serials, Computer Services Librarian, and Head of Reference. She received tenure at USC. At Oregon Health & Science University (1995-2000), Portland, Oregon, she was Head of Research & Reference Services and Customer Support. In 2000-2001 she was awarded a Fellowship in Medical Informatics from the National Library of Medicine. From 2001-2006 she was Director of Lee Graff Library at City of Hope National Medical Center & Beckman Research Institute, Duarte, California. In all of these positions she acted as liaison and served on committees in Schools of Medicine, Pharmacy, Nursing, and Allied Health. Her degrees include an MA in musicology from California State University, Los Angeles (1978), and an MSLS in library science from the University of Southern California (1980), Los Angeles; she has been a Distinguished Member of the Academy of Health Information Professionals since 1992. Ms. Wood has been very active in the Medical Library Association. She chaired Sections: Public Services, Pharmacy & Drug Information, and Library Research (including six years as editor of the newsletter *Hypothesis*). She taught continuing education courses in Information Resources in Clinical Medicine, The Internet: Access and Resources, Introduction to Health Informatics (her own authorship), Using and Understanding Medical Terminology, Drug and Pharmaceutical Information Resources, and Introduction to Reference Services in the Health Sciences. She served twice on the editorial board of the *Bulletin/Journal of the Medical Library Association (JMLA),* and on the National Nominating Committee. She served on and chaired the Books Panel. Other committees include Section Council, numerous prize juries, and liaison to other organizations. She worked for many years indexing allied health journals for *CINAHL (Cumulative Index for Nursing and Allied Health Literature)* and exhibiting for them at professional conferences. Among her publications are articles in *JMLA, Medical Reference Services Quarterly, Journal of Electronic Resources in Medical Libraries, Journal of Consumer Health on the Internet, Journal of the American Medical Informatics Association,* and *Journal of the American Society for Information Science.* In retirement, Ms. Wood continues to write, edit, and index.

Foreword

Above all else, the strength of a profession depends on the richness of its knowledge base. Not only does the knowledge base have to exist, it also has to be recorded and shared in an organized and coherent manner. In this book, M. Sandra Wood has brought together twenty-four authors who are experts in their respective areas within health sciences librarianship. Her selection of authors and topics and her organization of the content in a single volume have resulted in a valuable resource that will serve us now and well into the future. The content is suitable for use by a wide range of audiences, including students, educators, associations, library and information service managers, practitioners, and the myriad of for-profit and not-for-profit organizations whose products and services are essential to the work of health sciences librarians.

The publication of this comprehensive text is particularly timely because we are entering a period of major change in the age structure of the library and information services workforce. The first of the baby boomers, a group born between 1946 and 1964, turned sixty in 2006, and the next two decades will be characterized by increasing numbers of retirements. Librarianship will likely be affected even more by this demographic shift than other professions due to the high proportion of second career entrants to the field and the reduced hiring in libraries during the 1970s and 1980s. Never has there been a more important time for us to attend closely to issues of recruitment of new entrants to the field, retention of experienced librarians, succession planning, and the recording and sharing of our knowledge base. If we are to maintain the strength of our workforce, professional education will have to take place in multiple contexts. We need to strengthen the range of not only educational activities in our schools of library and information science but also continuing education offerings in our professional associations and in the workplace itself. Creating educational opportunities for new entrants to the field as well as for experienced health sciences librarians will be keys to our future success.

Health sciences libraries have always held a special appeal for those of us who have been fortunate enough to work in them. Health is a vital resource for everyday life for all human beings, and quality information services are important components of the broad infrastructure needed to support health. In addition to supporting research and educational programs in the health sciences, libraries also serve a vital function in providing up-to-date information to support patient care locally and globally. Libraries are also increasing their support of areas such as health care administration, health policy, public health, and specialized areas such as bioinformatics. In recent years, the patient care support function of libraries has broadened beyond the provision of information services to health care providers to include patients and their families and the general public. All of these trends illustrate the ever growing importance of library and information services to the health field.

This book begins with an introductory chapter on the field and a chapter on the health care environment that looks at the context of our practice. As special librarians working in the health field, our role demands that we be ever mindful of, and responsive to, the changing milieu in which we work. Given that health care continues to be one of the most volatile and changing sectors of the economy, we have shown tremendous ability to morph and move with the times and we must continue to do so. The chapter on health informatics that appears later in the book re-

Introduction to Health Sciences Librarianship
doi:10.1300/6041_c

minds us of the second major trend that is affecting our work as health sciences librarians: changing information technologies. The combination of the ongoing challenges created by the changing health care system as well as changing technologies will ensure that our jobs will never be dull!

Regardless of who our users are and what information formats are being employed to deliver information, the basic functions of libraries continue to be at the center of our practice. The book is well stocked with chapters on these key functions, including collection development; information access; information retrieval; and the management of information services. The management area is further developed in chapters on special services related to media, such as podcasting and course management systems, planning, communications, and marketing. Librarians are increasingly playing an instructional role with their users, as reflected in the chapter on information literacy. The book includes a look at the complementary roles played by academic and hospital libraries in the network of health information provision and the importance of the work done by libraries in both collecting and preserving unique special collections.

Trends suggest that the need for health information in all formats, especially in electronic form, will continue to grow in the future. Health care providers look to libraries and librarians as trusted sources of information, a role that is highly dependent on our own knowledge base and its application to practice. In the health sciences, we have participated in the development of evidence-based health care by providing information services that support health care professionals who are applying the best available evidence from the research literature to patient care. While service to others will continue to be one of our major roles for the future, the time has now come for the library profession to further develop, codify, and implement on a large scale its own version of evidence-based practice as library and information professionals. All librarians need to consciously seek out and use the best available evidence from their own literature and from demonstrated best practices in the field to continuously improve their services. The chapter on evidence-based practice and the contents of this book as a whole provide an excellent guide for us to use as we strive to meet the challenges of the present and the future.

Joanne Gard Marshall, PhD, FMLA
Alumni Distinguished Professor
School of Information and Library Science
University of North Carolina at Chapel Hill

Preface

When I retired in December 2005 after more than thirty-five years as a medical librarian and over twenty-five years as an editor of a professional journal *(Medical Reference Services Quarterly),* I had no idea that a short time later, I would begin to work on a textbook for health sciences librarianship. However, with retirement, came the time to reflect on the need for such a book, and the time to actually devote to the project. Thus began the concept of a single volume that would reflect current and future trends in health sciences librarianship, a volume that could be used in both graduate library schools for beginning librarians and also for practicing health sciences librarians, and a volume that would be "fast-tracked" through the writing and publication process so that it would not be outdated immediately upon publication. Little did I know that it would consume much of my time for more than a year and would involve twenty-four authors and multiple volume and chapter reviewers. In the end, hopefully, the profession will benefit from the content that so many talented health sciences librarians have shared with both their colleagues and those new to the profession.

To keep content current and relevant, authors were asked to write their chapters within a six-month time period, with several months for editing, and a shortened production time. An ambitious eighteen-month cycle was established at the outset. Most authors were "on board" fairly early in the project, although there were some changes in chapter authors along the way. Ultimately, I believe that the volume has assembled one of the finest groups of authors representing all aspects of the profession of health sciences librarianship.

Authors were informed that the textbook would be used in graduate library schools, by beginning and practicing medical librarians, and by experienced librarians catching up on newer developments in the field. The intent was that the work would capture current practice along with an indication of where the field of health sciences librarianship is going. Emphasis was to be placed on the last five to six years, the current status of the field, and the near-term future. It was noted that some areas would require historical background, although, with some exceptions, this was not the focus.

As the volume progressed, chapter authors had many questions, among which was the question of standardized terminology. "What do we call the users of health sciences libraries?" Also, would we use "medical libraries" or "health sciences libraries"? Being a democratic person, I put these questions to a vote among the chapter authors. Authors were asked to vote on their preference for "clients," "patrons," or "users" to describe persons served by libraries. The vote was literally evenly split; therefore, chapter authors have been allowed to use their preferred terminology. While this makes for inconsistency in the volume, it meant that authors felt more comfortable using the terminology that they preferred. With the question of health sciences versus medical libraries, the vote favored health sciences libraries, but authors have been allowed to use either health sciences or medical, as they preferred.

Authors were also asked to vote on the title of the book. From a selection of about eight potential titles, the one selected was *Introduction to Health Sciences Librarianship,* a reflection of the content of the volume. The more general "health sciences" enlarges the scope of the content to apply not just to medical libraries but to libraries in biomedical, nursing, allied health, phar-

doi:10.1300/6041_d

macy, and veterinary settings, and more. "Introduction" was chosen over words such as "Handbook" and "Principles" as reflecting the intent of the content—that it would provide all of the information necessary to introduce a new librarian to the state of the art of the profession.

Determining the order of chapters themselves proved to be more difficult than I anticipated. Ultimately, chapters in the book fall into five sections:

> *Section I: Introduction/Overview*—Chapter 1, "Overview of Health Sciences Libraries," and Chapter 2, "The Health Care Environment"
>
> *Section II: Technical Services*—Chapter 3, "Journal Collection Development"; Chapter 4, "Monographic and Digital Resource Collection Development"; and Chapter 5, "Organizing Resources for Information Access"
>
> *Section III: Public Services*—Chapter 6, "Access Issues"; Chapter 7, "Information Services in Health Sciences Libraries"; Chapter 8, "Information Retrieval in the Health Sciences"; Chapter 9, "Marketing, Public Relations, and Communication"; Chapter 10, "Information Literacy Education in Health Sciences Libraries"; Chapter 11, "Evidence-Based Practice"; and Chapter 12, "Health Informatics"
>
> *Section IV: Administration*—Chapter 13, "Management in Academic Health Sciences Libraries"; Chapter 14, "Management of and Issues Specific to Hospital Libraries"; and Chapter 15, "Library Space Planning"
>
> *Section V: Special Topics*—Chapter 16, "Special Services Provided by Health Sciences Libraries"; Chapter 17, "Health Sciences Librarianship in Rare Book and Special Collections"; and Chapter 18, "Consumer Health Information"

As part of the overall writing and editing process, chapters in the book were reviewed by several librarians, including Lynda Baker, Associate Professor of Library Science at Wayne State University, who served as overall reviewer of the volume. Individual chapters were reviewed by other colleagues. A list of reviewers appears in the acknowledgments.

While the textbook is intended as an introduction, some topics, of necessity, may be more advanced than others. For example, evidence-based librarianship is a fairly advanced concept that is new even to many practicing librarians, but is important enough to be included in the textbook. Health informatics is another topic that may be advanced for a beginning librarian, but it's important for health sciences librarians to be aware of this related field. These chapters were placed further back in the volume so that the reader could gain a background in the overall field of health sciences librarianship before being exposed to these topics.

In several of the chapters readers will find features called "A Day in the Life of . . ." These are intended to introduce new librarians to specific types of jobs, and what to expect in a typical day. Practicing health sciences librarians contributed a summary of a single day, or of a composite day, to create these "scenarios."

Throughout the book, you will notice bolded terms. These are the glossary words chosen by each chapter author. Usually, first use of the word in a chapter, excluding use in the summary or a section heading, is bolded. If a glossary word was used in one chapter but not designated as a glossary term by the author of another chapter, it will not be bolded; thus, there will be some inconsistency among chapters. The editor has merged definitions provided by authors, where applicable. Outside sources of definitions are acknowledged in the glossary.

Also throughout the book, readers will note the frequent mention of many organizations, but three stand out: the Medical Library Association (MLA), the Association of Academic Health Sciences Libraries (AAHSL), and the U.S. National Library of Medicine (NLM). This reflects the major influence that these organizations play in the practice of health sciences librarianship. Two are professional organizations; one is a government library.

All of the chapters address topics that are important for beginning and practicing health sciences librarians to be knowledgeable about. Taken together, they provide a sound foundation for all levels of health sciences librarians—students through experienced librarians—to gain both practical and theoretical knowledge about the profession. I am pleased to note that many of the chapters are reflective of librarianship in general, so that librarians in academic, public, and special libraries will also benefit from this book.

As I finished editing this volume, it occurred to me how ironic a situation this was. I was retiring at a time when health sciences librarianship—in fact librarianship in general—was in the midst of significant technological change that would open up exciting new roles for librarians. How I wish that I might be starting all over again—at the beginning of a new, thirty-five-year career as a health sciences librarian. What a wonderful time for a new librarian to be entering the profession!

M. Sandra Wood
Librarian Emerita
Penn State University Libraries

Acknowledgments

I would first like to acknowledge the dedication and hard work of all of the authors and contributors to this textbook. Each author brought unique talents and expertise to the book; I am indebted to them for their valuable contributions. Their knowledge and attention to detail is evident in the quality of each chapter. Throughout the writing and editing, several authors helped to maintain my good spirits and to keep me focused with their great sense of humor.

I am also grateful to the many individuals, including practicing health sciences librarians, library school faculty, and library school students, who have reviewed the chapters in this text. Their comments have resulted in revision and editing that has improved the overall quality of this textbook.

I especially would like to acknowledge the time and effort of Lynda M. Baker, PhD, Associate Professor, Library & Information Science Program, Wayne State University, who took on the role of reviewing the entire content of this volume; her wide-ranging knowledge was invaluable. Lynda's efforts were tireless, as she provided immediate, constructive feedback to help keep the textbook on track.

I am appreciative also of the foreword written by Joanne Gard Marshall, one of the most respected librarians in the field, a former president of the Medical Library Association, and a well-known library educator.

The following individuals also need to be acknowledged for reviewing specific chapters of the book; some reviewed multiple chapters; others reviewed just one chapter. All comments contributed to and improved the final content of the book.

Lynda M. Baker, PhD: All chapters
Cheryl R. Dee, PhD: Chapters 3 and 13
Jon Eldredge, PhD: Chapters 3, 9, 10, and 12
Jean Estrada: Chapter 13
Marie Fitzsimmons: Chapters 7 and 8, with special thanks for graphics support
Carole M. Gilbert: Chapter 14
Gale G. Hannigan, PhD: Chapter 13
Crystal Helcel: Chapter 13
Carol G. Jenkins: Chapter 13
Mellanye Lackey: Chapter 13
K. Ann McKibbon, PhD: Chapter 11
Michelynn McKnight, PhD, and students in her Louisiana State University School of Library and Information Science Course: Approximately half the chapters, and especially Chapters 1 and 2
Students of the School of Information and Library Science, University of North Carolina at Chapel Hill: Chapter 13

SECTION I:
INTRODUCTION/OVERVIEW

Chapter 1

Overview of Health Sciences Libraries and Librarianship

Mary Moore

SUMMARY. Similar in many aspects to other librarians, health sciences librarians are distinctive in their professional values, training, and in the nature of the work they perform. Professional organizations assist health sciences librarians by offering opportunities for continuing education, communication, and advocacy. Most health sciences librarians work in libraries that are located in academic health science centers, hospitals, corporations, associations and societies, the government, and other settings. These libraries are diverse in their mission and goals, collections, facilities, clients, and services offered. With the largest health sciences library collection in the world, the U.S. National Library of Medicine is central to health sciences library services, providing leadership and direction, and producing comprehensive services and products. Among the many trends and issues influencing health sciences librarianship, the impact of technology is probably the largest. Information technologies pervade every aspect of health sciences librarianship and provide new career opportunities for health sciences librarians. Librarians must be alert to changes in health care, education, information technologies, communications, and research, as these are likely to impact the future of health sciences librarianship.

INTRODUCTION

Libraries are in the most rapid period of transformation in their history, facing revolutionizing technologies, an overabundance of information, and a magnitude of transformations in the environment. In the not too distant past, people came to the library when they needed information. Now information is everywhere, and this radically redefines what a library is and what it does. Library mission and goals statements, organizational structures, and physical facilities are being redesigned for increased relevance to client needs. Libraries face more competition than in the past, and librarians must find and communicate the unique competitive advantages of libraries in comparison to bookstores or Google. Most people would agree that libraries have a unique advantage in that they offer the highly qualified, professional services of librarians. Librarians organize and find information, teach others how to use information, and have taken on new roles in making existing information more useful (value-added services and products).

Health sciences libraries are similar in many ways to other libraries. The most important distinctions in health sciences libraries are shown in Figure 1.1 and described as follows:

- *The **profession** of health sciences librarianship.* These libraries have specialized health sciences librarians and informationists,[1, 2] who are trained to deliver services for clients

Introduction to Health Sciences Librarianship
doi:10.1300/6041_01

who specifically need biosciences information. Professional organizations support health sciences librarians.

- *The nature of the library collection.* Generally, health sciences libraries have digital and print resources, such as books, journals, and multimedia materials, on topics in the biosciences. Electronic resources are especially useful, and the collections of some health sciences libraries are almost entirely online. In addition, these libraries often provide access to value-added databases. These databases consolidate and synthesize information from research studies or journal articles to help with patient care decisions.
- *The nature of the organizations served, their mission, and goals.* Health sciences libraries may serve universities, medical center complexes, hospitals, government organizations, corporations, associations, and more. Library facilities in these organizations may vary in support of their missions. One particular library, the U.S. **National Library of Medicine (NLM),** provides leadership, products, and support for health sciences libraries and those they serve.
- *The services provided.* Health sciences librarians help health professionals and students access and use the information they will need to provide patient care and conduct research. Health care professionals may need education and training on how to use complex health sciences information resources. They may need specific answers to health care questions. They often need accurate, current information, delivered quickly. Health sciences librarians deliver all of these services.
- *Specific trends.* These trends may affect health care, education, information technologies, communication, and research, as well as library and information sciences.

This chapter provides an introduction to these topics, many of which will be covered more thoroughly in the following chapters.

THE PROFESSION OF HEALTH SCIENCES LIBRARIANSHIP

Professions can be characterized as having common philosophies or values, a knowledge base that provides context, advanced education, competencies and skills, guidelines for ethical behavior, professional organizations, admission requirements (such as licensing, certification, or credentialing), and continuing education.[3] Health sciences librarianship meets the criteria for a profession. Aspects of the profession will be touched upon throughout this chapter, and elaborated upon throughout this book.

Values

Health sciences librarians share common values. Some examples follow:

1. Libraries are important, and information found in libraries can improve the quality and reduce the costs of health care.
2. Clients have a right to privacy. Requests for health sciences information must be confidential.
3. Health care information should not be censored or withheld because it presents a particular point of view that is unpopular with one group or another.
4. People should have access to information that is needed for them to make informed health decisions. Within the guidelines of fair use and intellectual property rights, health sciences and research information should be shared.

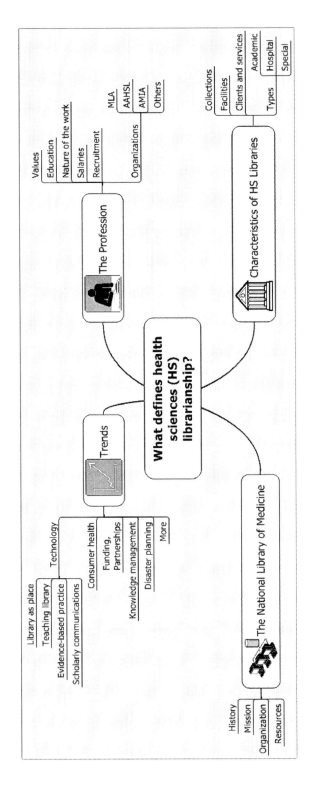

FIGURE 1.1. What Defines Health Sciences Librarianship?

In 1994, the *Code of Ethics for Health Sciences Librarianship*[4] was approved by the membership of the **Medical Library Association (MLA),** the major professional organization of health sciences librarians. This code guides the behavior of health sciences librarians and is discussed in detail in Chapter 7 under the topic Information Service Ethics.

Knowledge Base and Education for Health Sciences Librarianship

Preparation for work as a health sciences librarian generally requires a master's degree in library or information science from an American Library Association accredited program, as well as coursework specific to health sciences librarianship. Coursework could cover the health sciences environment, health sciences information resources, health informatics, or a practicum in a health sciences library. Some specialized librarians or informationists[1] may need additional graduate or professional degrees in the biosciences. An informationist is an expert in finding and retrieving literature to support informed decisions in research or health care. In addition to searching databases, informationists can read, interpret, and evaluate information, and then synthesize results. They may create products from what they have learned, such as flowcharts, databases, or white papers (authoritative written reports) for the research or health care team they serve.

The Medical Library Association, described later in this chapter, is the foremost professional organization for health sciences librarianship. MLA publishes a statement of the competencies, knowledge, and skills needed for health information professionals.[5] This policy statement provides guidance for the educational programs that prepare students for careers in health sciences librarianship. The statement also helps health sciences librarians identify additional skills and competencies they need to further their training.

In 1991, MLA first drafted an educational policy statement, called the *Platform for Change*.[6] Sixteen years later, the organization is revising the original document. The revision is called *The Platform for Lifelong Learning and Professional Success*.[7] Some competencies and examples of knowledge and skills are included in Table 1.1.

Nature of the Work

Health sciences librarians may provide services for clients (often called public services); services related to obtaining, organizing, and making library collections available (often called technical services); information technology services (often related to library systems, Web services, or personal computer support); administrative services to manage the library; outreach services (for the community or unaffiliated health care providers); services to manage the knowledge generated by the parent organization or institution (**knowledge management**); and more. Table 1.2 provides more details, with examples of the work that might be performed. In an academic library, an individual might perform activities in just one column. In a one-person library, an individual might perform some activities from every category.

In larger academic or government libraries, health sciences librarians are more likely to specialize, while in smaller libraries, duties may be more diverse. Health sciences librarians are often called upon to do things out of the ordinary because they have shown success in dealing with clients' questions. Some librarians take on duties in creating databases, organizing continuing education for health professionals, coordinating telemedicine, training others to deliver distance education, managing institutional records, and more.

TABLE 1.1. MLA Competencies and Skills for Health Sciences Librarianship

Competency	Examples of Skills
Practice-related competencies	• Goal-setting and outcomes assessment • Anticipation of trends • Management of the change process
Personal characteristics	• Commitment to lifelong learning • Ethical behavior • Self-motivation
Knowledge of health sciences and skills	• The health care environment • Information technologies and policies • Trends of organizations and government agencies
Leadership and management	• Planning • Staff development and mentoring • Demonstrating the relevance of the profession to institutional goals
Health sciences information services	• Assessing and understanding client needs • Forging and maintaining alliances • Managing electronic resources
Health sciences resource management	• Selection and acquisition of resources • Negotiation of purchase and licensing • Copyright, privacy, and intellectual property issues
Information systems and technology	• Principles of automated systems, databases, networks, and IT security • Informatics applications • Integration of systems and technologies
Curricular design and instruction	• Adult learning theory • Instructional development • Educational needs assessment
Research, analysis, and interpretation	• Ability to formulate a research question • Knowledge of research methodologies • Ability to communicate results

Source: Adapted from Medical Library Association. MLANET. *Platform for Lifelong Learning and Professional Success.* The Educational Policy Statement of the Medical Library Association. Revised Edition. Rev. Draft April 13, 2006. Available: <http://www.mlanet.org/pdf/ce/mlplatprof success26.pdf>. Accessed: March 5, 2007.

Salaries

Mean salaries for librarians working in colleges and universities and for federal government librarians are listed in the *Occupational Outlook Handbook,* available online.[8] As described later in the chapter, the **Association of Academic Health Sciences Libraries (AAHSL)** is the

TABLE 1.2. Examples of Duties of Health Sciences Librarians

Public Services	Outreach	Technical Services	Information Technology and Multimedia Services	Knowledge Management	Administration
• Teaching clients about health sciences resources • Reference desk duties • Attending clinical rounds • Developing content for online education • Conducting in-depth searches of the biomedical literature • Attending institutional review boards (IRBs)	• Writing plans and proposals for services to unaffiliated health professionals or the community • Exhibiting on library services at professional conventions • Exhibiting and training at community health fairs • Working with school nurses, teachers, public librarians, senior centers, public health workers, emergency operations centers, etc. • Conducting evaluations and writing reports	• Selecting library materials • Processing materials for the collection • Reviewing or developing contracts for library resources • Negotiating to purchase electronic resources • Working with consortia to jointly purchase or share resources • Managing acquisitions • Making materials available by cataloging or assigning metadata	• Managing library systems and desktop support • Developing Web sites • Conducting usability studies • Collection development for nonprint and multimedia materials • Developing services, such as podcasting, RSS feeds, streaming media	• Managing institutional archives • Developing institutional repositories (usually collections of materials developed locally that are digitized and organized using special software) • Developing databases • Analyzing data, articles, or reports • Synthesizing information from numerous sources and creating white papers • Managing institutional records • Training about options in scholarly communications	• Strategic planning • Assuring needs of multiple constituents are met • Gathering information and analyzing trends • Personnel management • Budget management • Identification of alternative funding options • Creating and coordinating accreditation or other reports • Promotion of value of library • Officially representing the library

foremost organization for academic and university health sciences center libraries. Each year the organization gathers and publishes key statistical measures to help its members evaluate their own performance. The AAHSL *Annual Statistics* reports mean salaries for health sciences librarians working in academic libraries.[9] In the 2007 AAHSL salary survey, the median starting salary was $40,966, the mean was $41,522 and the standard deviation was $8,552. Information on hospital and other medical librarian salaries is also available through the Medical Library Association. MLA collects salary data from its membership approximately every three to four years. In the 2005 MLA survey, the median starting salary was just under $40,000, and the average salary was $57,952.[10]

Recruitment for Librarianship

In the past, it was not uncommon for librarian supply and demand to have been uneven.[11] Now it appears those leading many health sciences libraries may be nearing retirement, and there may not be enough new librarians entering the field to meet demand in the future. The *Occupational Opportunity Handbook* estimates that three of five librarians age forty-five or older will be retiring in the next ten years, providing good opportunities for those in the field.[8] The Medical Library Association's Salary Survey also confirmed the aging of the profession.[10] Recruiting new librarians into the profession is a priority for MLA and AAHSL. However, some trends show librarians are working later in life and postponing retirement, so it is difficult to know how imminent the crisis is.

Health sciences librarianship could be strengthened with increased diversity in race, ethnicity, age, and gender. There appear to be salary gaps based on gender and race that need to be addressed.[10, 12]

Professional Organizations and Associations

Professional organizations are important to the work of all health sciences librarians, providing opportunities for continuing development, communication, and advocacy. Some of the relevant organizations, including MLA and AAHSL, are described in this section.

The Medical Library Association

The Medical Library Association,[13] the major association for health sciences librarians, was founded over a hundred years ago by four librarians and four physicians, including eminent physicians John Shaw Billings and William Osler. A comprehensive history of the organization, *Guardians of Medical Knowledge,* reveals details of how the association was established, including how physicians of the day perceived the role of medical libraries in promoting gentility and culture, and how it took the leadership of MLA many years to allow women librarians to lead the organization.[14]

Now MLA has grown to include 1,200 institutions and 3,800 health information professionals, primarily in the United States and Canada, but also worldwide. Regular, institutional, international, affiliate, and student memberships are available.

The organization provides various programs to meet the needs of its members, including meetings, publications, career information resources, professional credentialing, honors and awards, scholarships, advocacy for the profession, and more. Each year the participating libraries in the MLA Exchange offer thousands of surplus volumes of journals to other libraries. MLA hosts an annual meeting with continuing education, a conference program, business meetings, committee meetings, and exhibits. The Web site <http://www.**mlanet**.org> lists the MLA sections on special topics and geographic groups, or chapters. These chapters, affiliated with the MLA, also meet regionally each year.

Among MLA's publications are a professional journal, a newsletter, books, booklets, and published hospital library standards. The *Journal of the Medical Library Association* is the profession's premier peer-reviewed journal in the field and is available as an **open access** journal through **PubMed Central**.[15] In addition, the *MLA News* provides current information, as does MEDLIB-L, an e-mail discussion list. Many items, including the membership directory, are published online.

The association is well-known for its active focus on professional development. MLA's educational policy statement, described previously in this chapter, has been widely distributed, and is the basis for educational programs for health information specialists. MLA continuing education programs are available at the annual meeting, chapter meetings, and locally, as well as online. Courses to help information professionals gain knowledge, skills, and competencies are available at the annual meeting, regional meetings, online, or by teleconference.[16] MLA's **Academy of Health Information Professionals (AHIP)** recognizes librarian achievement in academic preparation, professional experience, and professional accomplishment.[17] MLA is the only professional library association with a comprehensive credentialing program.

Table 1.3 provides information on other organizations and how they support the profession of health sciences librarianship.

More International Organizations

There are organizations to support health sciences libraries and librarians in many countries, as well as organizations supporting health information management that may be of interest to librarians. Many of the organizations listed in Table 1.3 maintain links to additional relevant associations on their Web sites.

HEALTH SCIENCES LIBRARIES

Health sciences libraries differ from many other libraries in the content of collections, aspects of the facilities, clients served, types of libraries, and the emphasis placed on certain services. One particular library, the U.S. National Library of Medicine, is especially noteworthy. It provides leadership and services for other health sciences libraries and clients around the world.

Collections

Clients of health sciences libraries need the most current and comprehensive health information. Because of this, a larger percentage of the library collection may be devoted to journals. Most health sciences libraries strive to provide as much of the collection as possible through electronic materials, but not all resources are available electronically. Some specialty areas lag behind others in providing electronic access.

In addition, clients need help sifting through the huge volume of information that is available. Therefore, health sciences libraries may provide access to online databases to support clinical diagnosis and treatment decisions. They may also provide multimedia materials. Examples might include videos on dissection of the human body, or how to perform physical examinations or medical procedures. Many health sciences libraries also provide materials for health consumers. In addition, health sciences libraries may also have special collections of rare, unique, or historical materials, sometimes including the archives and records of the organizations they serve.

TABLE 1.3. Other Organizations Supporting the Profession of Health Sciences Librarianship (in alphabetical order)

Organization	How the Organization Supports Health Sciences Librarianship
American Medical Informatics Association (AMIA) <http://www.amia.org>	Supports the use of health information and technology for patient care, teaching, research and health information. Working groups on clinical information systems, genomics, knowledge discovery, open source and public health informatics. Special working group for student members. Each group has an online discussion group. Publishes the *Journal of the American Medical Informatics Association.*
The Association of Academic Health Sciences Libraries (AAHSL) <http://www.aahsl.org/>	Founded by medical school library directors in 1978. Promotes cooperation among academic health sciences libraries and with the Association of American Medical Colleges. Membership includes directors of medical school and osteopathic libraries in the United States and Canada. Publishes the *Annual Statistics of Medical School Libraries in the United States and Canada,* which reports comparative data about academic health sciences library collections, budgets, personnel, and services. More than 100 libraries submit data annually.
Canadian Health Libraries Association/ Association des bibliothèques de la santé du Canada (CHLA/ABSC) <http://www.chla-absc.ca/>	Seeks to improve health and health care by promoting excellence in access to information. Began in 1976, growing from the Canadian Group of the MLA and the Canadian Association of Special Libraries and Information Services. Represents about 400 members. Has chapters and interest groups and provides conferences, continuing education, and awards. *The Journal of the Canadian Health Sciences Libraries Association* is available in open access at <http://pubs.nrc-cnrc.gc.ca/jchla/jchla.html>.
European Association for Health Information and Libraries (EAHIL) <http://www.eahil.net>	Established in 1984, the membership represents about thirty European countries. EAHIL seeks to unite and motivate those working in European health and medical libraries. Provides professional development, interlibrary cooperation, and professional exchanges of librarians. Publishes the *Journal of the European Association for Health Information and Libraries.*
International Federation of Library Associations (IFLA) <www.ifla.org>	IFLA seeks to promote high standards in the delivery of library and information services and encourage widespread understanding of the value of good library services throughout the world. Membership includes 1,700 individuals, associations, and institutions in 150 countries. Health sciences librarians may join the Section of Health and Biosciences Libraries in the Division of Special Libraries. The International Congress of Medical Librarianship meets under the auspices of IFLA approximately every five years. IFLA publishes the *IFLA Journal.*
International Medical Informatics Association (IMIA) <http://www.imia.org>	IMIA works to promote informatics in health care and research and to further international cooperation. Represents medical and health informatics in its close ties with the World Health Organization. Membership is available to national, institutional, and affiliate members and to fellows. IMIA hosts a World Congress on Medical and Health Informatics.
Special Libraries Association (SLA) <http://www.sla.org>	The Medical Section of the Biomedical and Life Science Division is for members in the biomedical and health sciences. SLA offers a discussion group, meets annually, has a strong continuing education program, and publishes *Information Outlook.*

Facilities

Library facilities can range from large (more than 100,000 square feet) to almost completely online, with a small staff. Because health care decisions depend on the most current and accurate information, health sciences libraries need to assure that this information is available anytime, anywhere. The library facility therefore may become less important to some researchers and clinicians. However, the health sciences library may continue to be a home away from home for medical students, residents, and graduate students, who may spend many hours reading and studying.

New buildings, additions, and renovations are listed in the December issue of *Library Journal,* usually called the "Architectural Issue" or "The Year in Architecture." The list includes libraries, the status of the project, the cost, the gross area, and the square foot cost, as well as seating capacity and book capacity. For example, in 2006-2007, the Biomedical Library at the University of California in San Diego was building an addition and renovating the existing library, with a project cost of $40 million.[18]

Clients

Libraries must consider all constituent groups in providing services and developing policies and procedures. Since it is useful to compare and contrast different groups of users, basic comparative information is provided in this section, and more information is provided in Chapter 7, "Information Services in Health Sciences Libraries."

Almost all clients can be categorized according to their role in the organization. The main roles in health care organizations are education, research, patient care, community service, and administrative support. Some of these clients also can be further categorized according to whether they work in the **basic sciences** or **clinical sciences.** These distinctions may become confusing, however, because there is often overlap among groups, and one individual may have multiple roles or affiliations with several institutions.

Basic Sciences and Clinical Sciences

Clients can include those working in basic sciences and those working in the clinical sciences. Basic scientists might include anatomists, biochemists, cell biologists, immunologists, microbiologists, molecular biologists, geneticists, pharmacologists, or physiologists, among others. Basic scientists often hold PhD degrees, and they often work in laboratories. In many medical schools, students spend the first two years studying the basic sciences so they can apply this fundamental knowledge to learning clinical concepts and skills in the second two years.

The clinical sciences are concerned with patient care. For instance, the departments of family medicine, internal medicine, obstetrics and gynecology, pediatrics, psychiatry, and surgery would be considered clinical sciences departments. Clinical sciences faculty often hold MD degrees and may also include individuals with other degrees.

Education

Those working in educational services and programs include students and faculty. Students in the educational programs for each of the health sciences disciplines will have different needs. Students in undergraduate programs (for example, the biosciences, premedical, undergraduate nursing, or allied health programs) may have more in common with other university students than with health care researchers. They may look to the library for a place to study, benefit from education and training programs on how to use its resources, and use monographs for broad overviews on various topics. They will use the library to write papers, and they will begin to learn how to use the library for patient care.

Graduate students might be enrolled in master's or doctoral programs in the biosciences, nursing, or allied health. Graduate students in the biosciences are more likely to use journal articles to find the latest information. Those pursuing advanced degrees may need library resources to complete theses and dissertations.

Medical and dental students have first completed a bachelor's degree. Postbaccalaureate students beginning studies in medicine or dentistry may use the library in ways that are similar to undergraduate students. In programs where students have primarily didactic (teaching classroom) experiences in the first two years, they may spend longer periods of time studying in the library. When they reach the clinical years, they may be more interested in journal articles and databases that help them understand treatment protocols.

Teaching faculty may include basic scientists, clinical scientists, physicians, nurses with advanced degrees, allied health practitioners, and more. Teaching faculty primarily use the library to support their educational activities, often looking for illustrations of principles and procedures and video to demonstrate processes. Librarians are often teaching partners with faculty members, helping to bring an understanding of information resources into the classroom. Many libraries are adding online repositories of materials locally developed (such as lecture notes, PowerPoint slides, and test questions) to support teaching and learning. Some librarians work with teaching faculty to select and acquire materials to help students become more successful learners.

Patient Care

Those working in patient care include practitioners who treat patients and support staff. Clinical practitioners or health practitioners might include physicians, nurses, dentists, allied health practitioners, pharmacists, and students studying in these fields.

Physicians generally complete a four-year medical degree, followed by residency training, and sometimes postgraduate fellowships. They can be generalists, specialists, and subspecialists. Physicians' information needs are often for patient care and are sometimes urgent; physicians are often interested in information that helps identify a course of action, rather than everything that has ever been published on a topic. Some physicians conduct research and publish review articles, examining the state-of-practice on a particular topic. Physician information behavior has been well studied, but because information technology is changing behavior so rapidly, it is difficult to predict physician information needs by past studies.

Residents are physicians who have completed medical school, are in a residency program, and are receiving specialized advanced training. They were once called house staff because they virtually lived at the hospital, and although that is no longer true, the name persists. Residents are continuing their education, and so may request comprehensive information on a patient care situation encountered. They may be assigned to use library resources as part of learning activities.

Nurses may have different levels of education, postdegree training, specialties, or certification. Nurses are often the information providers for many on the health care team. They may learn to search databases as part of undergraduate programs and to perfect those searching skills in graduate programs. Competency statements on developing skills in nursing evidence-based practice[19] mean nurses will become more involved in obtaining and producing needed literature for patient care.

Allied health professionals can include physician extenders or physician assistants, physical therapists, occupational therapists, dental hygienists, medical records professionals, and more. Their information needs vary according to the competencies required for their individual professions. Each career generally has at least one professional journal for the specialty.

Evidence-based information (see Chapter 11, "Evidence-Based Practice") is especially relevant to health practitioners. Databases that serve as clinical decision support tools may be particularly needed by this client group.

Research

Researchers can be categorized as basic science researchers or clinical researchers. Clinical researchers often work on what are called **clinical trials** of new procedures or drug treatments.

Many researchers are completely supported by grant funding. They create grant proposals, conduct research, and report the results to the funding agency. Results are also reported to the public through publications or open access on the Web. In general, researchers need extremely thorough, accurate, and current information to support research and teaching. They often want immediate access to that information from their laboratories, offices, or homes. They especially need information to support writing grant proposals, and the resulting publications. Researchers are often very knowledgeable about the impact of changes in scholarly communications.

Community Service

Community clients can include patients, family, friends, or just interested individuals, such as schoolchildren. Patient libraries date back to the early 1900s.[20, 21] However, those libraries were to exclude "morbid, gruesome and unwholesome" materials.[22] Where once it was believed that the value of treatment depended on a completely trusting relationship with one's physician,[23] the current perspective is more likely to be that an informed patient is a valued participant in the health care delivery team. Most health sciences libraries provide the same services to consumers that they do to health care professionals, although some private and corporate libraries are closed to the public. There are specific works developed using plain language and more general terminology, but consumers may also want technical materials, as well.

The term "unaffiliated health professionals" is generally for those practicing health care services in a community who are not faculty or employees of the parent organization of the library. These individuals may request access to academic health sciences library collections as a free community service or as a paid membership.

Administrative Support

Administrators may need the library to help them make informed decisions quickly. Librarians can help administrators research what other health science centers or hospitals are doing (called "benchmarking," comparing the institution to a peer organization, or **competitive intelligence,** identifying the services and strengths of rival institutions) or construct databases of best practices in certain activities. Librarians can research the comparative advantages of one software package over another, or create databases of area donors.

Types of Health Sciences Libraries

Health sciences libraries can be located at academic health sciences centers (which include universities with health sciences degree programs), hospitals, health research companies, insurance agencies, medical publishers, health academies, government agencies with health missions, and more. Within health sciences librarianship, most libraries fit into the categories of academic health sciences libraries, hospital libraries, and special (corporate, association, or government) libraries.

Academic Health Sciences Libraries

Academic health sciences libraries support the mission and goals of the parent organization. In general, these libraries provide information resources and services to support the educational, research, clinical care, and community service missions of their health sciences universities.

Description and duties. Each year, AAHSL describes a composite library, constructed from the means and medians of various responses. The 2005-2006 composite health sciences library is compiled from data from 125 academic medical libraries in the United States and Canada.[12] Table 1.4 draws data from the 2005-2006 composite academic health sciences library.

Working in a large university environment often means the librarian has a more specialized job. Mean salaries are reported to be higher than in hospitals (however, not as high as some federal librarian positions).[10] Opportunities for advancement may be more obvious in academic health sciences libraries with large numbers of librarians.

Accreditation. The library is part of the accreditation process of the professional schools of the university. For example, the Liaison Committee on Medical Education (LCME)[24] may review a university's health sciences library as part of the accreditation review of the university's medical school. In addition, there may be a regional accreditation of the university as a whole. For instance, a health sciences university in Chicago might undergo the accreditation process of the Higher Learning Commission of the North Central Association of Colleges and Schools,[25] and the library would be reviewed in this process. Health sciences libraries are generally evaluated in terms of their abilities to support the mission and goals of the professional program or university undergoing accreditation, and on having qualified library staff, appropriate resources, and training for faculty and students available.

Growth. The number of academic health sciences libraries has grown only slightly over many years. An analysis of academic library statistics in the United States and Canada by Byrd and Shedlock in 2003[26] found that, when controlled for inflation, the total expenditures of these libraries had remained level over a twenty-five-year period. Over time, there have been declines in circulation, interlibrary loan, and on-site use. There has been steady growth over time in size of collections, number of library staff, reference questions, and service hours. Recently, sizable increases in electronic resources, Web use, and teaching activities have been measured.

TABLE 1.4. Composite Academic Health Sciences Library

Measure	Mean Values	Trend from 2004-2005
Hours the library is open weekly	98	No change
Professional staff	12.4	No change
Total staff	34	−1.5%
Total print monograph volumes	192,989	−9.1%
Health sciences electronic serials	4,009	+5.8%
Health sciences databases	110	+11%
Total annual expenditures	$3,583,397	+9%
Collection expenditures	$1,622,438	+11.5%
Gate count	243,926	−2.6%
Circulation of print materials	72,484	−19.7%
Reference questions	15,894	−10%
Education sessions taught	310	+17%
Libray home page views (median)	1,831,676	Not available

Source: Adapted from 2005-2006 AAHSL *Annual Statistics.*

Hospital Libraries

The goals of hospital libraries reflect the goals of their parent hospitals and health sciences centers. The main purpose of the hospital is to provide effective patient care, while protecting patient safety and constraining costs. Hospital libraries provide the resources and services so hospital employees can accomplish those goals.

Description and duties. Although there can be large, complex hospital libraries, work in many hospital libraries may have much in common with special libraries. Many hospital libraries are staffed by just one librarian. Hospital libraries generally focus on providing access to materials rather than owning large collections. Hospital libraries may have a small core collection and request other needed materials from large academic health sciences libraries. The emphasis is on relevance of the collection and on quick and expert customer service. Because there may be fewer clients, the librarian often knows client needs well and anticipates needs before they arise. In this environment, librarians may take on responsibilities beyond those commonly associated with library work. They may be asked to apply their organizational or problem-solving skills to manage other services, possibly including education, electronic health records, or more. They are often asked to serve on hospital-wide committees, such as continuing education, patient education, information technology, research, ethics, and more. In a survey of hospital committee participation in 2006, the authors found that 94.5 percent of responding hospital librarians participated in hospital committees.[27]

Accreditation. No specific standards are enforced for accrediting hospital libraries, but the Joint Commission on Accreditation of Healthcare Organizations (Joint Commission, formerly JCAHO)[28] has several standards, rationales, and elements on management of information, information planning, and information-based decision making. Hospitals must provide information services for the purpose of improved patient outcomes, patient safety, and health practice. Medical Library Association Standards for Hospital Libraries help to define the Joint Commission standards.[29] This will be further discussed in Chapter 14, "Management of and Issues Specific to Hospital Libraries."

Growth. The expansion in numbers of large teaching hospitals in the late 1960s and 1970s probably led to the increase in hospital libraries. In 1962, there were 3,192 hospitals that had professional libraries, but few had professional librarians. The **American Hospital Association (AHA)** survey in 1989 found 2,167 hospital libraries that had organized collections, trained staff, schedules of services, and facilities.[30]

The Medical Library Association has an active Hospital Libraries Section (HLS), with a newsletter, online discussion list, and blog.[31] In 2003, the HLS had 1,388 members.[32] At the end of 2006, it had 1,132 members,[33] which seems like a substantial decline. However, another measure, the number of hospital libraries that are members of the National Network of Libraries of Medicine (NN/LM) of the National Library of Medicine shows only a slight decline (see Table 1.5).

TABLE 1.5. Change in Numbers of Hospital Libraries Between 2004 and 2007

Hospital Libraries	April 2004*	December 2007**	Percent Change
Full network members	1929	1911	−1 percent
Total network members	2911	2887	−1 percent

Source: *Dudden, R. F.; Corcoran, K.; Kaplan, J.; Magourik, J.; Rand, D.C.; and Todd Smith, B. "The Medical Library Association Benchmarking Network: Development and Implementation." *Journal of the Medical Library Association* 94(April 2006):107-17. **NN/LM Members Directory Advanced Search. Available: <http://nnlm.gov/members/adv.html>. Accessed: December 29, 2006.

The NN/LM is a program of the National Library of Medicine, which is described later in this chapter. The NN/LM was originally designed to establish a network of medical libraries, especially for resource sharing and interlibrary loan. To be a full network member, a library is required to have a library or information center that is fully staffed, have an Internet connection, have a collection, lend materials in that collection, and provide services such as collection sharing and reference. Libraries or information resources that do not meet the requirements for full members may become affiliated network members.

Special Health Sciences Libraries

The category of special libraries often includes corporate libraries and association or society libraries. Sometimes it includes government libraries. To make things even more confusing, some people would place all medical or health sciences libraries into a particular group under the general category of special libraries.

Mission and goals. Like other health sciences libraries, the missions and goals of special libraries are reflective of the missions of the parent organizations. For example, corporations are likely to be in the business of making profits, and a corporate health sciences library would therefore support this endeavor. Librarians must prove they are cost-effective and could face downsizing if they are not. Likewise, they sometimes share the earnings when the company is profitable.

Description and duties. Special libraries can include corporate libraries, and also professional association libraries and government libraries, such as the National Library of Medicine. Some health sciences librarians are employed in the private sector, working for research organizations; in companies with pharmaceutical, health technology, or insurance services; or at health care associations. Others are privately employed as health information consultants, sometimes gathering or analyzing information for U.S. and international companies. Still others work in government libraries, dealing with health sciences issues, such as the U.S. Food and Drug Administration.

Accreditation. Special libraries are not generally accredited.

Growth. No current studies report on the prevalence of corporate health sciences librarians. The Corporate Information Section of the Medical Library Association has around seventy members.[34] The Special Libraries Association (SLA) has a section devoted to biosciences and health sciences librarians. SLA also has established competencies for special librarians, available at <http://www.sla.org/content/learn/comp2003/index.cfm>.

In corporate libraries, librarians are more likely to be able to follow through on the answer to a question from start to finish. They may write white papers on the background of legislation on a particular topic or explore the feasibility of providing a product to a new market segment. They may use the Internet or other tools to conduct corporate intelligence, finding information on competitors. Corporate decisions are sometimes based on the librarian's research.

Special health sciences libraries also include government libraries, such as the library at the Centers for Disease Control or the Food and Drug Administration Library. The largest of these government health sciences libraries is the National Library of Medicine. It influences the practice of health sciences librarianship worldwide.

THE U.S. NATIONAL LIBRARY OF MEDICINE

History

The National Institutes of Health (NIH),[35] a part of the U.S. Department of Health and Human Services, began in 1887 as a one-room laboratory at the Marine Hospital in New York. Now the NIH in Bethesda, Maryland, funds more medical research than any other organization in the world, with a budget in 2005 of $28 billion. The NIH has supported research that resulted in awards of more than eighty Nobel Prizes. Its primary mission is to pursue knowledge about living systems and to apply that knowledge to extend healthy life, reducing the burdens of illness and disability. The NIH includes twenty-seven institutes and centers, such as the National Cancer Institute; the National Heart, Lung and Blood Institute; and the National Human Genome Research Institute.[36]

The U.S. National Library of Medicine[37] began as a small collection of books and journals in the U.S. Army's Office of the Surgeon General in 1836.[38] NLM became part of NIH in 1956. In 1962, it moved to its current location on the National Institutes of Health campus in Bethesda, Maryland.

Almost twenty years in the making, Wyndham Miles's book, *A History of the National Library of Medicine,* provides colorful details, photos, and illustrations.[38] Miles elaborates on the significant skill of founder John Shaw Billings for talking people out of their collections of rare medical books, but he also tells how a library clerk who spoke ten languages was denied a promotion because he was "too valuable to the library" and describes various idiosyncrasies of the early NLM librarians. Eminent heart surgeon Michael DeBakey also published a personal perspective on the National Library of Medicine in 1991.[39]

Mission

The mission of NLM is to collect, organize, and make available biomedical information for scientists, educators, health practitioners, and the public. It carries out programs to strengthen and develop health sciences library services in the United States. NLM's Web products include **PubMed®,** a massive online index to biosciences literature, and MedlinePlus, which provides consumer health information as a benefit to people around the world. Other services include research in biomedical communications; resources in molecular biology, biotechnology, toxicology, and environmental health; and supportive funding for research, training, bioinformatics product development, and more.

The NLM building, itself, serves as a symbol of how important health sciences information is to the nation and how important it is to preserve that information. Built during the Cold War in 1962, the library's walls are made from thick stone. The roof is designed to collapse in case of physical disaster, protecting the collections that lie underground in fifty miles of shelving.

Today, NLM serves in a leadership role for other health sciences libraries, setting the tone for nationwide priorities. For example, in the past, NLM primarily provided services for health care practitioners. When NLM expanded its mission in 1997 to include Web site services for health consumers, most academic libraries followed suit.

Organization

NLM is composed of seven divisions: Library Operations, the **National Center for Biotechnology Information (NCBI), Lister Hill National Center for Biomedical Communications (LHNCBC), Specialized Information Services (SIS),** the Office of Health Information Programs Development (OHIPD), the Office of Computer and Communications Systems (OCCS), and the Extramural Grants Program.

Library Operations provides services for other biomedical libraries and the public. It acquires, organizes, and preserves materials included in the largest collection of health sciences resources in the world. It also provides technical processing (indexing and cataloging) for these materials; reference and customer services for all NLM products and services; the **MEDLINE®** database, including the **Medical Subject Headings (MeSH)** thesaurus and a database with indexing for most of the health science journal articles in the world; the historical collections and services; and the National Network of Libraries of Medicine.

NN/LM[40] has the mission of advancing medicine and improving public health by providing all U.S. health professionals with access to biomedical information. NN/LM also seeks to help the public make informed health decisions by improving its access to health information. This mission is administered through a national network of health sciences libraries. Figure 1.2 depicts the regions of the NN/LM.

There are eight Regional Medical Libraries, around 160 Resource Libraries (primarily at medical schools), and almost 6,000 total network members in the NN/LM. The network promotes NLM products and services and teaches people how to use those resources, as well as coordinating services, such as an interlibrary loan network. Programs target underserved health professionals in rural or inner-city areas. NN/LM promotes projects to reduce health disparities by increasing access to information.

LHNCBC supports research and development in areas of knowledge management, data visualization, medical imagery, medical language processing, and more. NCBI focuses on molecular biology and genetic information and tools. SIS provides a minority outreach program, as well as databases on drug reactions and chemical structures. OHIPD plans, develops, and evaluates nationwide outreach and consumer health, and conducts international programs. OCCS provides computer support for all NLM programs and services, and the Extramural Program provides grants, contracts, and fellowships to support research and services related to the NLM programs.

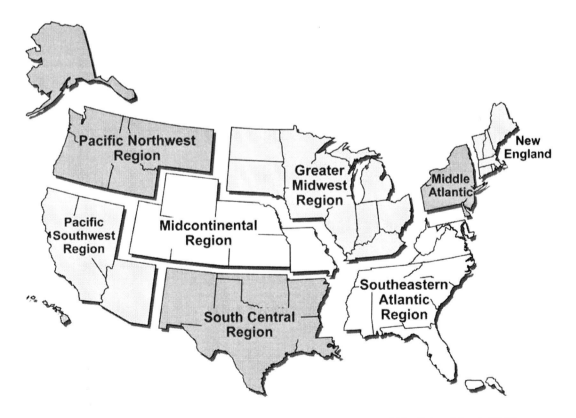

FIGURE 1.2. Regions in the National Network of Libraries of Medicine, March 2007

NLM Resources and Tools

NLM's electronic resources that are available worldwide through the Web include these and more:

- PubMed:[41] 15 million references to articles in 5,000 peer-reviewed biomedical journals.
- MedlinePlus:[42] Consumer health information on thousands of health topics from primarily government sources, drug information, a medical encyclopedia and dictionary, illustrations, tutorials, and directories of health providers, facilities, and support groups. MedlinePlus en español is the Spanish version.
- **ClinicalTrials.gov:**[43] Information on thousands of research trials on drugs and medical treatment that are sponsored by NIH, including information on the purpose of the study, criteria for participation, location of the study, and contact information.
- Entrez:[44] The search system for biomedical and molecular biology databases, including PubMed, Nucleotide and Protein Sequences, Protein Structures, Complete Genomes, Taxonomy, and others.
- **TOXNET:**[45] A collection of databases on toxicology, toxic chemicals, and environmental health. The TOXNET databases include **Toxline,** a database of bibliographic information; HSDB, the Hazardous Substances Data Bank; Gene-Tox, containing information about genetic toxicology; and CCRIS, the Chemical Carcinogenesis Research Information System. NLM also provides Haz-Map, an occupational health database; AltBib, a list of references about alternatives to animal testing; and links to related Internet sites. To explore TOXNET and other NLM databases, link to <http://toxnet.nlm.nih.gov>.
- **PubMed Central:**[46] PubMed Central is a service maintained by the NLM that provides free online access by the public to health information. It is committed to long-term preservation of materials. In 2005, NIH enacted a policy on **public access.** This policy asked scientists who received NIH funding to place full-text copies of the results of the studies on PubMed Central, where the information could be available to the public. However, almost a year later, the rate of compliance was reported to be very low, fewer than 4 percent.

NLM has multiple publications, electronic mailing lists, and opportunities for training and professional development. The **Associate Fellowship Program** is a year-long competitive program developed for new graduates with leadership potential to learn in depth about NLM programs and services. Other programs provide opportunities to focus on informatics. NLM supports funding for fellowships in medical informatics and medical librarianship, as well as training on specific databases and resources. More information is available from the *Fact Sheet on Opportunities for Training and Education Sponsored by the National Library of Medicine.*[47]

TRENDS AFFECTING HEALTH SCIENCES LIBRARIANSHIP

A brief discussion of trends affecting health sciences librarianship is presented here to give the reader a broad understanding of the issues that may have a significant impact on the profession. The chapters that follow will focus on the specifics of health sciences librarianship and will expand on many of the topics. Figure 1.3 diagrams the trends discussed here.

The Impact of Technology

Beginning with library automation in the early 1960s, librarians were among the first professionals to see the practical value of information technology. Now information technology per-

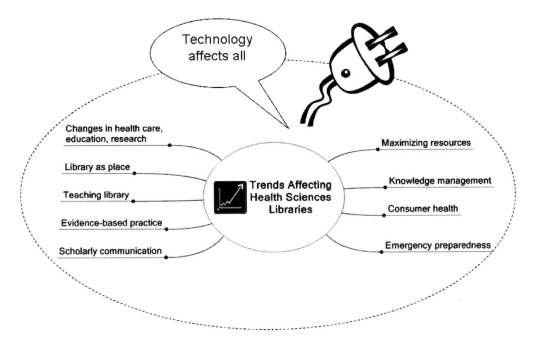

FIGURE 1.3. Trends Affecting Health Sciences Librarianship

vades everything health sciences librarians do. Technology is no longer a trend but has become the norm. Technology has an impact on library collections, personnel, services, and space, as described in Table 1.6.

Technology has spawned an expectation for immediate gratification in users. A wait of three days for an interlibrary loan or two hours for a remotely stored item is too long. Health sciences libraries provide access to their collections through the Internet, as well as providing access to resources through portable or handheld devices that could be used at patients' bedsides or in clinics. Many librarians help keep health professionals aware of how information technology can be used to provide immediate access to health sciences information.[48]

In 2004, President George W. Bush announced the intention to develop a national electronic health record.[49] This initiative is called the Nationwide Health Information Network. He established a National Coordinator for Health Information Technology within the Department of Health and Human Services to lead the effort. The impact of this effort would be significant if these systems of health records could be connected and then researched. State and regional health information exchanges would present a step toward the nationwide network. Libraries continue to strive toward the integration of health information resources with the electronic health care record.[50] This topic is more fully described in Chapter 12, "Health Informatics."

Concern has grown about what some have called a "digital apocalypse" where the Internet, or even electricity, would become unavailable. This might be caused by events such as terrorism, power overloads and outages, or natural disasters. Of course, challenges to how information is distributed freely on the Web can also come from laws and policies that restrict access, corporate decisions to charge for information, or the limitations placed on Web use in some nations. As health sciences libraries become increasingly dependent on technology to provide services, interruption of electricity or Internet services could have a disastrous impact on information used for patient care.

TABLE 1.6. Impact of Technology and Implications for Health Sciences Libraries

Impact of Technology	Possible Implications for Health Sciences Libraries
Information anywhere, anyplace	Less need to come to the library. Changes in why clients do come to the library (to focus, use superior technology, or obtain expert training or assistance, rather than to use print collections). Librarians can work outside the library more easily. Need for real-time services, like virtual reference.
The information blastoma: too much information, too many choices	Too much to read, too many places to look for information. Valuable information can be overlooked. Much information is useless. "Satisficing": settling for the first answer, rather than finding complete solutions. Time wasted trying to find unfamiliar or lost information. Difficulty making decisions on what is relevant.
Anyone can publish; anyone has access to information	Changes in scholarly publishing patterns from traditional published journals to more immediate or informal possibilities. Opportunity for others to filter information for quality, or for online peer review of information. Opportunity for value-added, synthesizing products. Opportunities for health sciences Wikipedias. Opportunities to teach people to evaluate quality of information.
Immediate gratification; no need to wait for answers	Less patience and more complaints about waiting for interlibrary loan delivery. Less patience to read through lists of results, or entire articles. Need for value-added products that help save time. Need for creative approaches to save time, like the related articles algorithm in PubMed.
Disintermediation: the loss of respect and need for experts (People are not required to be journalists to blog, or librarians to search PubMed.)	The decline of expert searching. Changes in how the reference desk is staffed. Assumption that anyone who works in a library can help. Possible loss of job satisfaction if expert skills are less appreciated.
Expectation that all information is free because most information is free on the Web (PubMed and MedlinePlus are free.)	Lack of understanding that other online resources, like many online journals, have charges. Unwillingness to pay for anything—photocopying, printing, document delivery, library fees. Less income leads to cost cutting in libraries.
More complex information	More opportunities for training.
When the lights go out . . .	Libraries must implement robust disaster plans.

The Library As Place

In the 1930s, Andrew Keogh, Yale Librarian, joked about what should be engraved above the door to the Sterling Memorial Library, by saying, "This is not the Yale library. That is inside." (What was actually carved by the entrance was, "The library is the heart of the university."[51]) If this story were rephrased for today for a health sciences library, Keogh might have said, "This is not the library. That is online." Because health sciences clients need accurate, current, and relevant information, as quickly as possible, librarians seek to place more and more resources online.

Many libraries were built before information technologies became ubiquitous. Eventually, it becomes necessary to rethink library space and how it has been assigned. It may become readily apparent that expansive shelves for print journals will not be needed as much as computer stations or study space.

All libraries—university, research, public, school, and health sciences—face challenges with space and design. Leighton and Weber, in their comprehensive update of Keyes Metcalf's work, *Planning Academic and Research Library Buildings,*[52] reiterate that a library building must first reflect the purpose of the library and the mission of the university. Demas and Scherer list trends that help make libraries more useful, distinctive, and attractive places:[53]

1. Reading and study spaces
2. Collaborative workspaces for group study, tutoring, and conversations
3. Spaces for group gatherings
4. Learning and teaching spaces
5. Technology-free zones
6. Archives, special collections, and exhibit spaces
7. "What's new" spaces
8. Cultural events spaces
9. Age-specific (or in the case of health sciences libraries, client-specific) spaces
10. Shared spaces (multiuse spaces—libraries paired with senior centers, for example)
11. Art spaces
12. Nature, natural light, and landscapes
13. Interior design trends (such as creating spaces that resemble living rooms)

Two opposing perspectives of the future of the library have emerged. In one, administrators with a limited view of libraries might think the ubiquity of information on the Web means they can convert library space into needed staff offices or patient services, but this might be premature, as library facilities have continued to be needed long past the time a completely virtual library was originally visualized. Presenting a progressive alternative, some university libraries have been reconceptualized as the academic heart of the organization. Rather than storehouses for books and journals, libraries become multipurpose shared spaces to support education and research.

So what aspects of this discussion are unique to health sciences libraries? The answer comes back to the mission of the institution and the distinct needs of the clients that it serves. The National Library of Medicine and the Association of Academic Health Sciences Libraries held a symposium in 2003,[54] and a consensus of experts on the future of the **library as place (Delphi study)** was developed.[55] Here are some expert opinions for the future (2010-2025):

- Libraries will have chief responsibility for obtaining, providing access to, and teaching how to use genomic and other databases, and image repositories.
- Libraries will collect and make accessible faculty lectures, institutional archives, and other locally developed resources.
- Libraries will support information needs of remote users.
- The electronic article, rather than the book or journal issue, will be the chief unit for scholarly information.
- Remote storage will become more practical, and stacks will decrease.
- Libraries will support knowledge management and clinical trials.
- Clients will use the library for time-saving or value-added information services.
- Library space will be less consistent and more tailored to institutional needs.

Those clients who come to study in a health sciences library, come to stay, and so require conveniences that may be seen as luxuries in other libraries. Temporary cubicle space or individual study rooms (called "hotelling") may be assigned for conducting library research or studying. These spaces may include whiteboards, footstools, seat cushions, or accommodations for food and drink.

Planning manuals from the 1970s (the latest such manuals are available) recommend medical libraries should allow seats in the library for 20 percent of undergraduate students and 25 percent of graduate students in the life sciences.[56] Library planning literature prior to the popularity of the Internet underestimates the need for access to information technology services. Because advanced technology is crucial to their missions, health sciences libraries include computer laboratories, information and learning commons, multimedia development pods, or **collaboratories.** The term "collaboratory" originally meant online laboratories where researchers could work, interact, use instrumentation, share data, and use digital libraries,[57] but it has now evolved to also include physical spaces that are equipped with state-of-the-art technologies. The purpose of collaboratories is to promote computer-supported cooperative work. With new initiatives, library staff space may need to be renovated to support things such as knowledge management, offices for scholarly communication, or research and development. More information is provided in Chapter 15, "Library Space Planning."

The Teaching Library

As information resources become more numerous and complex, clients must learn how to become skilled in using those resources. Guskin writes, "A **teaching library** [emphasis added] is a library that is more than a support unit for academic programs and research. It is a library that is actively and directly involved in advancing all aspects of the mission and instructions of higher education: teaching, research and community service."[58]

Some academic librarians serve on curriculum committees for the professional schools they serve. Hospital libraries have an increased role in teaching residents, physicians, and nurses about things such as evidence-based resources, described in the next section and in Chapter 11 on evidence-based practice. Library renovations generally now include increased numbers and size of classrooms and seminar rooms within the library. See Chapter 10, "Information Literacy Education in Health Services Libraries," for more information on the educational role of the library.

Evidence-Based Practice

Evidence-based practice takes into account both the clinical expertise of the practitioner and the best available evidence from research studies. Health practitioners should use both to make decisions about an individual patient's care. Librarians at health sciences universities can teach students, faculty, staff, and researchers techniques to evaluate the literature and determine the strength of the evidence behind written reports. In addition, librarians at some health centers have systematically reviewed published literature and evaluated and summarized the quality of the evidence presented.[59] This topic is covered in Chapter 11.

Scholarly Communications

When scholars find, use, and create information, the end product is called "scholarly communications."[60] Scholarly communications might be informal or formal. Early studies of informal communications coined the phrase **invisible colleges** and encouraged sociological research on how scientists communicate.[61-64] Now informal scholarly communications might include e-mail or blogs intended for a small group of specialists. Formal scholarly communications (also called scholarly publishing) are often more permanent and include journal articles, books, multimedia, software, and databases. The Web and electronic publishers have influenced significant changes to scholarly publishing, as more and more materials move from print to electronic formats.

This change has had a large impact on libraries, in terms of how to manage journal subscriptions and make materials available to users. Libraries may have hundreds of licenses with various publishers providing electronic resources. Libraries must determine how to best make resources available to clients within the restrictions of the licenses.

Many health sciences libraries also encourage researchers to make research results available to the public as quickly as possible, in accordance with recommendations from the U.S. federal government. New methods for scholarly communications have arisen, including open access resources, provisions for increased public access to research results, and local publishing opportunities, including institutional repositories. In May 2005, the National Institutes of Health issued a policy encouraging researchers to submit electronic versions of manuscripts resulting from NIH funded research to PubMed Central.[65] This policy is called the National Institutes of Health Policy on Enhancing Public Access Resulting from NIH-Funded Research, commonly referred to as the "Public Access Policy." Authors submit to PubMed Central the final versions of manuscripts when they are accepted for publication. Other proposed legislation would strengthen this recommendation and extend it to other U.S. federal government agencies. More information on the important topic of how scholarly communication is changing appears in Chapter 3, "Journal Collection Development."

Consumer Health

Although many libraries have missions that included outreach, libraries were given an important tool in 1998, when the U.S. National Library of Medicine introduced MedlinePlus,[42] one of the most comprehensive Web tools for consumer health information. MedlinePlus includes hundreds of health topics, a health dictionary, an encyclopedia, drug information, tutorials, and more, all provided free and without advertising. This resource, plus the supportive funding for outreach projects available through the National Network of Libraries of Medicine, described earlier, meant the majority of health sciences libraries were able to provide some services for the general public, if this is supported by their missions. The **Go Local** project took this a step further. Go Local Web sites are developed by local or state organizations or institutions. These sites link databases of local health care providers, facilities, and support groups with health care topics in MedlinePlus. So, while MedlinePlus provides authoritative information on diseases, conditions, and wellness, Go Local provides links to community services. More information on consumer health is provided in Chapter 18, "Consumer Health Information."

Maximizing Resources

Health sciences libraries have struggled to maintain adequate funding over the years. Problems often have been related to annual increases in the cost of research journals that have outpaced the cost of inflation. The result has been that libraries repeatedly had to reduce the number of journal subscriptions in their collections. With the movement to electronic journals, if a library has budget problems, it is now more likely it will have to consider reducing journal packages of many titles, rather than individual subscriptions.

The American Library Association has reported, "Right now, America's libraries are facing the deepest budget cuts in history. Across the country, libraries are reducing their hours, cutting staff or closing their doors—drastic measures that were not taken even during the Great Depression."[66]

Some hospital libraries are affected by budget reductions and even closures, but the budgets of academic health sciences libraries have remained steady, even when accounting for inflation, according to AAHSL.[26] Nonetheless, some academic libraries are hiring experienced development officers and increasing usage fees to raise funds for innovative services.

Health sciences libraries have become especially successful in developing partnerships to increase access to materials and stretch their funding, sometimes saving their institutions millions of dollars. For many years, health sciences libraries have joined with one another in **consortia** and created group agreements for document delivery, collection development, or collective purchasing. Participating libraries may agree to charge reduced rates, or even no fees, for interlibrary loan. They may agree that each participating library would concentrate on specialized areas and develop stronger collections in those areas. Perhaps the most consequential partnerships have been those in which libraries cooperate to negotiate reduced prices for journal packages and databases. Consortia also provide forums for libraries to share information on best practices.

A consortium may be composed of libraries in a particular city, state, or region, or a particular type of library (for example, a consortium of cancer libraries). Described previously, the U.S. National Network of Libraries of Medicine might be the largest consortium of health sciences libraries in the world.

Knowledge Management

In 2003, AAHSL issued the document *Building on Success:* **Charting the Future** *of Knowledge Management Within the Academic Health Center.*[67] This important work, written for leaders of key U.S. health institutions, alerts them to new roles health sciences libraries could play that would have a positive impact on the quality and cost of education, clinical care, research, and community outreach. These roles are related to documenting and making available the institution's most important asset, the knowledge of its people.

Knowledge management has to do with acquiring, storing, analyzing, and making available for use the results of human knowledge. This could include publications, but it could also involve capturing successful processes in achieving a certain outcome, for example, what works best in delivering library outreach services to a community. Knowledge management is more fully described in Chapter 14 on hospital libraries.

Health Sciences Research

Two events have helped strengthen the role of the health sciences librarian in supporting research:

1. In 2001, Ellen Roche, a twenty-four-year-old volunteer in an asthma research trial at one of the nation's most prestigious institutions died during the study. The death could have been prevented with a comprehensive literature search, as the drug being studied had been shown to be dangerous thirty-five years previously.[68] In some universities and hospitals, this event led to the appointment of librarians on institutional review boards, to confirm that comprehensive literature searches have been conducted before research trials were conducted.[69, 70]
2. In 2005, Dr. Elias Zerhouni of the U.S. National Institutes of Health, reported that the United States had invested more money in health research per person than any other nation in the world; however, the quality of health in the United States was lower than other nations, according to health outcomes rankings.[71] In an effort to make research more relevant to patient care and health, NIH reconfigured its support of health research. The term "translational science" relates to how well research results can translate into improved patient care and health. Funding for this initiative comes from clinical and translational science awards (CTSAs) available to U.S. academic health sciences institutions. These awards encourage innovative training programs for new researchers, and collaborations and partnerships among health care organizations and the communities they serve. The CTSA initiative could elevate the role played by informatics and libraries. This is described further in Chapter 2, "The Health Care Environment." Several health sciences libraries are playing key roles in their institutions' CTSA initiatives.

Emergency Preparedness and Disaster Planning

After Hurricane Katrina, the United States realized what might happen when a major population center is struck by a serious disaster. Katrina clarified that, in times of emergency, a nation needed health information, not just immediately for those health practitioners providing emergency services, but also for health facilities and providers attempting to continue to provide health care services after the emergency. Networks of libraries came together to provide services for libraries that had been incapacitated, including reference, document delivery, and services for displaced students. Katrina emphasized the value of planning ahead for disaster, and emergency and disaster planning is a high priority for NLM. Katrina also helped librarians understand how accustomed people had become to having health care information readily available online. In 2005, the National Library of Medicine sponsored a symposium on the Role of Information Services for **Emergency Preparedness** and Response.[72] In 2006, the National Library of Medicine and the Medical Library Association convened an Emergency Access Initiative. The purpose was to provide full-text access to key medical or scientific journals from participating publishers in the event of an emergency.

These are only a few of the trends having an impact on how the profession of health sciences librarianship is changing. Health sciences librarians should be especially aware of trends in information technology, health care, education, research, and communications, as these have a significant impact on the future of the profession.

CONCLUSION

This chapter has provided a brief introduction to the profession of health sciences librarianship; a description of health sciences libraries; an introduction to the National Library of Medicine, the largest health sciences library in the world; and a discussion of some trends that are having an impact on health sciences librarianship. The following chapters will elaborate on many of the topics presented here. In particular, the next chapter will describe the health sciences environment, which is essential in understanding how health sciences libraries have evolved.

REFERENCES

1. Davidoff, F., and Florance, V. "The Informationist: A New Health Profession?" *Annals of Internal Medicine* 132(June 20, 2000): 996-8.

2. Plutchak, T.S. "The Informationist—Two Years Later." *Journal of the Medical Library Association* 90(October 2002): 367-9.

3. Abbott, A. *The Systems of Professions: An Essay on the Division of Expert Labor.* Chicago: The University of Chicago Press, 1988.

4. Medical Library Association. *Code of Ethics for Health Sciences Librarianship.* Available: <http://www.mlanet.org/about/ethics.html>. Accessed: February 21, 2007.

5. Medical Library Association. "Educational Policy of the Medical Library Association." Available: <http://www.mlanet.org/education/>. Accessed: December 29, 2006.

6. Medical Library Association. *Platform for Change.* Available: <http://www.mlanet.org/education/platform/>. Accessed: March 5, 2007.

7. Medical Library Association. *Platform for Lifelong Learning and Professional Success.* Available: <http://www.mlanet.org/pdf/ce/mlplatprofsuccess26.pdf>. Accessed: March 5, 2007.

8. U.S. Department of Labor. Bureau of Labor Statistics. *Occupational Outlook Handbook, 2006-7.* Available: <http://www.bls.gov/oco/ocos068.htm>. Accessed: December 29, 2006.

9. Association of Academic Health Sciences Libraries. "About the Annual Statistics." Available: <http://www.aahsl.org/new/display_page.cfm?file_id=78>. Accessed: December 29, 2006.

10. Medical Library Association. *Hay Group/MLA 2005 Salary Survey.* Available: http://www.mlanet.org/publications/hay_mla_05ss.html>. Accessed: February 15, 2007.

11. Lipscomb, C.E. "Librarian Supply and Demand." *Journal of the Medical Library Association* 91, no. 1 (January 2003): 7-9.

12. Byrd, G. ed. *Annual Statistics of Medical School Libraries in the United States and Canada, 2005-2006.* 29th ed. Seattle, WA: The Association of Academic Health Sciences Library Directors, 2007.

13. Medical Library Association. Available: <http://www.mlanet.org/>. Accessed: December 29, 2006.

14. Connor, J. *Guardians of Medical Knowledge: The Genesis of the Medical Library Association.* Lantham, MD: Rowman & Littlefield, 2000.

15. PubMed Central. Archive of the *Journal of the Medical Library Association.* Available: <http://www.pubmedcentral.nih.gov/tocrender.fcgi?journal=93&action=archive>. Accessed: March 5, 2007.

16. Medical Library Association. "Education." Available: <http://www.mlanet.org/education/index.html>. Accessed: December 29, 2006.

17. Medical Library Association. "The Academy of Health Information Professionals." Available: <http://mlanet.org/academy/>. Accessed: December 27, 2006.

18. Fox, B.L. "Betwixt and Be Teen: Library Buildings 2006." *Library Journal* 131, no. 20 (December 2006): 45.

19. Academic Center for Evidence-Based Practice in Nursing. Available: <http://www.acestar.uthscsa.edu/Competencies.htm>. Accessed: March 5, 2007.

20. Perryman, C. "Medicus Deus: A Review of Factors Affecting Hospital Library Services to Patients between 1790-1950." *Journal of the Medical Library Association* 94(July 2006): 263-9.

21. Beausejour, M.M. "How the Hospital Serves the Community." *Michigan Library Bulletin* (1923): 117-20.

22. Jones, E.K. "The Growth of Hospital Libraries." *Modern Hospital* 18(May 1922): 452-4.

23. Bartlett, E.E. "Historical Glimpses of Patient Education in the United States." *Patient Education and Counseling* 8(1986): 135.

24. Liaison Committee on Medical Education. Available: <http://www.lcme.org>. Accessed: December 29, 2006.

25. The Higher Learning Commission. Available: <http://www.ncahlc.org/>. Accessed: December 29, 2006.

26. Byrd, G.D., and Shedlock, J. "The Association of Academic Health Sciences Libraries: An Exploratory Twenty-Five-Year Trend Analysis." *Journal of the Medical Library Association* 91(April 2003): 186-202. Available: <http://www.pubmedcentral.nih.gov/picrender.fcgi?artid=153160&blobtype=pdf>. Accessed: December 29, 2006.

27. Birr, R.A.; Zeblisky, K.A.; and Mathieson, K.M. "From Artsy to Zany: Hospital Library Committee Participation." Western MLA Chapters 2006 Annual Meeting, October 14-17, Seattle, WA. Available: <http://depts.washing.edu/pncmla/pncmla2006/posters.html>. Accessed: February 19, 2007.

28. Medical Library Association. "Librarians Guide to a JCAHO Survey." Available: <http://www.mlanet.org/resources/jcaho.html>. Accessed: December 29, 2006.

29. Medical Library Association. Hospital Libraries Section. "Standards." Available: <http://www.hls.mlanet.org/otherresources/standards.html>. Accessed: December 29, 2006.

30. American Hospital Association. *Survey of Health Sciences Libraries in Hospitals—1989.* Chicago: American Hospital Association, 1991.

31. Medical Library Association. Hospital Libraries Section. Available: <http://www.hls.mlanet.org>. Accessed: December 5, 2006.

32. Dudden, R.F.; Cocoran, K.; Kaplan, J.; Magourik, J.; Rand, D.C.; and Todd Smith, B. "The Medical Library Association Benchmarking Network: Development and Implementation." *Journal of the Medical Library Association* 94(April 2006): 107-17.

33. Kate Corcoran, e-mail message to Jonquil Feldman, December 28, 2006.

34. Kate Corcoran, telephone conversation with author, December 28, 2006.

35. National Institutes of Health. Available: <http://www.nih.gov/>. Accessed: December 29, 2006.

36. National Institutes of Health. "About NIH." Available: <http://www.nih.gov/about/>. Accessed: December 29, 2006.

37. National Library of Medicine. "About the National Library of Medicine." Available: <http://www.nlm.nih.gov/about/index.html>. Accessed: December 29, 2006.

38. Miles, W.D. *A History of the National Library of Medicine: The Nation's Treasury of Medical Knowledge.* Washington, DC: Government Printing Office, 1982.

39. DeBakey, M.E. "The National Library of Medicine. Evolution of a Premier Information Center." *JAMA; Journal of the American Medical Association* 266(September 4, 1991): 1252-8.

40. National Library of Medicine. *Fact Sheet: National Network of Libraries of Medicine®.* Available: <http://www.nlm.nih.gov/pubs/factsheets/nnlm.html>. Accessed: December 29, 2006.

41. National Center for Biotechnology Information. Available: <http://www.ncbi.nlm.nih.gov/>. Accessed: December 29, 2006.

42. MedlinePlus. Available: <http://medlineplus.gov>. Accessed: December 29, 2006.

43. ClinicalTrials.gov. Available: <http://clinicaltrials.gov/>. Accessed: December 29, 2006.

44. Entrez. Available: <http://www.ncbi.nlm.nih.gov/Database/index.html>. Accessed: December 29, 2006.

45. National Library of Medicine. "NLM Databases and Electronic Resources." Available: <http://www.nlm.nih.gov/databases/>. Accessed: December 29, 2006.

46. PubMed Central. Available: <http://www.pubmedcentral.nih.gov/>. Accessed: December 29, 2006.

47. National Library of Medicine. *Fact Sheet: Opportunities for Training and Education Sponsored by the National Library of Medicine.* Available: http://www.nlm.nih.gov/pubs/factsheets/trainedu.html>. Accessed: December 29, 2006.

48. Giustini, D. "How Web 2.0 is Changing Medicine." *BMJ; British Medical Journal* 333(December 23, 2006): 1283-4. doi:10.1136/bmj.39062.555405.80. Available: <http://www.bmj.com/cgi/content/extract/333/7582/1283>. Accessed: December 29, 2006.

49. The White House. "Transforming Health Care. The President's Health Information Technology Plan." Available: <http://www.whitehouse.gov/infocus/technology/economic_policy200404/chap3.html>. Accessed: December 29, 2006.

50. Humphreys, B.L. "Electronic Health Record Meets Digital Library: A New Environment for Achieving an Old Goal." *Journal of the American Medical Informatics Association* 7(2000): 444-52.

51. Schiff, J.A. "The Heart of Yale: Celebrating the 75th Anniversary of Sterling Memorial Library, 1930-2005." *Nota Bene. News from the Yale Library* 18(Fall 2005): 1.

52. Leighton, R.D., and Weber, D.C. *Planning Academic and Research Library Buildings.* 3rd ed. Chicago: American Library Association, 2000.

53. Demas, S., and Scherer, J.A. "Library Design Trends." In *The Whole Library Handbook.* 4th ed., edited by G.M. Eberhart, 55-9. Chicago: American Library Association, 2006.

54. Symposium on Building and Revitalizing Health Sciences Libraries in the Digital Age. The Library As Place [electronic resource]. National Library of Medicine and the Association of Academic Health Sciences Libraries, November 5-6, 2003 [2004].

55. Ludwig, L., and Starr, S. "Library As Place: Results of a Delphi Study." *Journal of the Medical Library Association* 93, no. 3 (July 2005): 315-26.

56. The Planning and Management Systems Division of the Western Interstate Commission for Higher Education and the American Association of Collegiate Registrars and Admissions Officers. *Manual 4,* on academic support facilities (tables B.20-B.23), as cited in Leighton and Weber, *Planning Academic and Research Library Buildings,* 728-39.

57. Wulf, W. "The National Collaboratory." In *Toward a National Collaboratory. Report of the National Science Foundation Workshop,* Rockefeller University, New York, March 1989.

58. Guskin, A.E.; Stoffle, C.J.; and Boisse, J.A. "The Academic Library As a Teaching Library." *Library Trends* 28, no. 2 (Fall 1979): 283.

59. McMaster University. Health Information Research Unit. "Evidence-Based Health Informatics." Available: <http://hiru.mcmaster.ca/>. Accessed: December 29, 2006.

60. Association of Research Libraries. "Scholarly Communication." Available: <http://www.arl.org/osc/index.html>. Accessed: December 29, 2006.

61. Price, D.J. *Little Science, Big Science.* New York: Columbia University Press, 1963.

62. Kuhn, T.S. *The Structure of Scientific Revolutions.* Chicago: University of Chicago Press, 1970.

63. Crane, D. *Invisible Colleges: Diffusion of Knowledge in Scientific Communities.* Chicago: University of Chicago Press, 1972.

64. Merton, R.K. *The Sociology of Science: Theoretical and Empirical Investigations.* Chicago: University of Chicago Press, 1973.

65. National Institutes of Health. Office of Extramural Research. "NIH Public Access Policy." Available: <http://publicaccess.nih.gov/policy.htm>. Accessed: December 29, 2006.

66. American Library Association. "The Campaign to Save America's Libraries." Available: <http://www.ala.org/ala/issues/campaignsal.htm>. Accessed: December 29, 2006.

67. Association of Academic Health Sciences Libraries. *Building on Success: Charting the Future of Knowledge Management Within the Academic Health Center.* Available: <http://www.aahsl.org/document/Charting_the_Future_viewable.pdf?CFID=692989&CFTOKEN=97790818>. Accessed: December 29, 2006.

68. Steinbrook, R. "Protecting Research Subjects: The Crisis at Johns Hopkins." *New England Journal of Medicine* 346(February 28, 2002): 716-720. Available: <http://content.nejm.org/cgi/content/full/346/9/716>. Accessed: March 5, 2007.

69. Robinson, J.G.; Gehle, J; and Lipscomb, C. "Medical Research and the Institutional Review Board: The Librarian's Role in Human Subject Testing." *Reference Services Review* 33, no.1 (2005): 20-4.

70. Tomlin, A. "Hospital Librarians and the Johns Hopkins Tragedy." *Journal of Hospital Librarianship* 2, no. 4 (2002): 89-96. Available: <http://www.haworthpress.com/store/ArticleAbstract.asp?ID=19725>. Accessed: March 5, 2007.

71. Zerhouni, E.A. "Translational and Clinical Science: Time for a New Vision." *New England Journal of Medicine* 353(October 13, 2005): 1621-3. Available: <http://content.nejm.org/cgi/content/full/353/15/1621>. Accessed: December 29, 2006.

72. "Partners in Information Access for the Public Health Workforce. The Role of Information Services in Emergency Preparedness and Response." MLA CE 800, May 15, 2005. Available: <http://phpartners.org/mlace800 agenda.html>. Accessed: February 20, 2007.

Chapter 2

The Health Care Environment

Logan Ludwig

SUMMARY. Health care today is an enterprise of multilayer, multitasking organizations, associations, and institutions—medical, nursing, and health professions schools; academic and community hospitals; private practices; medical research centers; professional associations; private industry—that share common missions, champion the application of new knowledge, provide professional education , conduct research, and provide quality care. This overview of health care examines fundamental questions about health care, significant milestones in health care, the impact of governmental legislation, the current environment of U.S. academic medicine and biomedical research, and future scenarios for academic medicine and their possible impact on health care and health sciences librarianship.

INTRODUCTION

Health care today is an enterprise of multilayer, multitasking organizations, associations, and institutions—medical, nursing, and health professions schools; academic and community hospitals; private practices; medical research centers; professional associations; private industry—that share common missions. They champion the application of new knowledge in the alleviation of suffering, rehabilitation of injury, and prevention of disease and premature death; provide general professional education and specialized graduate training for future health care professionals; conduct biomedical, behavioral, clinical, and **health services research;** and provide quality care for millions. Together, these institutions also play a significant role in society's obligations to provide health care to its poorest population.

Worldwide, there are a multitude of different approaches for providing health care services to a nation. A full exploration of each of these approaches is not possible here, but it is important to examine how our society has answered some fundamental questions about health care and to note significant events that have brought health care to where it is today. This chapter begins with a review of a few fundamental questions about health care and an overview of health care today, primarily in the United States. It discusses the impact of governmental legislation on health care. It then explores important events in medical education and the current environment of U.S. **academic medicine** and biomedical research. It concludes with a review of potential future scenarios for health care and their possible impact on health care and health sciences libraries.

Fundamental Questions

Before nations can discuss the particulars of health care delivery and funding, it is necessary for them to decide how they want to answer three fundamental questions: (1) Is health care a so-

Introduction to Health Sciences Librarianship
doi:10.1300/6041_02

cietal priority? (2) Is health care a right or a privilege? (3) What role should government play in the provision of health care services? How a nation responds to these fundamental questions often determines how a nation will develop its health care system.

In nations where health care is considered a right rather than a privilege, a national health care plan supported by taxes is more often the norm than not. In nations where society decides there is not a basic, fundamental right to access to health care services, health care is usually treated as a commodity not unlike many others, and access to services is based solely on ability to pay. Currently, U.S. society appears to be divided in its view of health care as a right versus a privilege. The United States is one of a few nations without a national health care plan and, on one hand, has often been chastised as spending more of its gross national product (GNP) on health care than does any other nation (16 percent in 2004).[1] On the other hand, in a country where health care is viewed as a societal priority if not a right, one should not automatically assume more health care spending is necessarily bad.

Origins of Modern Health Care

In most nations, modern health care has come a long way from very humble beginnings. In the more medically advanced countries of the United States and Canada and in Europe, health care technology was virtually nonexistent in the 1800s. There was no real measure of quality of health care delivery, and there were few effective diagnostic and/or treatment modalities to offer patients. Most hospitals in the United States were for mental patients. Existing allopathic hospitals often separated the charity wards from the wards with paying patients, and physicians worked both areas of these hospitals in a nonregulated environment. As a rule, physicians were solo practitioners functioning in a fee-for-service environment. They were free to bill patients whatever they felt appropriate, frequently "overcharging" the paying patients to subsidize their charity cases.

Medical Education in the Nineteenth Century

During the nineteenth century, the status of medical education was a major problem. Originally, medical "students" merely spent some time with a practitioner to learn the art, without much formal education or data on what worked and what did not. Numerous proprietary medical colleges sprang up, but many provided substandard education, in part because they had no hospital affiliation. The earliest American medical schools were founded at the University of Pennsylvania (1765), the College of Physicians and Surgeons at Columbia University (1767), and Harvard University (1782).[2]

However, in the late nineteenth century, a growing science-based reform movement in U.S. medicine, advanced by such schools as Harvard University, the University of Pennsylvania, and the University of Michigan, saw the development of medical schools that added rigorous laboratory-based training and scientific faculty. In 1910 the Carnegie Foundation, in cooperation with the American Medical Association (AMA) Council on Medical Education, funded the landmark report *Medical Education in the United States and Canada*.[3] Flexner seems to have used the Johns Hopkins University Medical School as his ideal model; Hopkins' fledgling program began in 1893 and emphasized a rigorous, scientific basis for research and clinical training and dictated that its medical students obtain supervised experience working with hospital patients. Flexner's report recommended that over half of the medical schools in the United States and Canada close because they didn't meet standards.

The **Flexner Report** surely changed the face of medicine and medical education in the United States and Canada and solidified the preeminence of the university-based medical school and **teaching hospital** model. After the Flexner Report, the number of medical schools in the

United States and Canada fell from 155 in 1910 to 85 in 1920; medical schools remained few in number until after World War II.[4] However, three postwar factors have radically changed the then quaint nature of medicine: investment in biomedical and behavioral research, government regulations of health care, and health care consumer and workforce changes.

Beginnings of Biomedical and Behavioral Research

Investment in biomedical and behavioral research, especially by the federal government, transformed academic health sciences centers into complex enterprises encompassing hospitals, schools, and large-scale research institutions. Following World War II, a visionary national science policy called for significant investment in basic science, including health-related research, by the federal government. Vannevar Bush's landmark report, *Science—The Endless Frontier,*[5] promulgated the "social contract" between the federal government, which would invest in the development of scientific knowledge and training of scientific investigators, and universities that would be the principal loci of this research and educational activity. The **National Institutes of Health (NIH)** became the primary federal agency responsible for implementation of this social contract for health-related research. Today, academic health sciences centers almost invariably describe their mission in terms of clinical, teaching, and research objectives and are beginning to add a fourth leg to this traditional "three-legged stool," that of community service.

THE MODERN HEALTH CARE SYSTEM

U.S. health care at the end of the twentieth century occupies a completely different place in the economy, in the mind of the public, and in its impact on the government at all levels than it did 100 years ago, at the beginning of the twentieth century, or at the beginning of the country in the late 1700s, when the U.S. Constitution was adopted. Citizens view health care as essential to their lives and as a societal privilege. It is an unusual day when no articles in major national newspapers relate to some aspect of health.

Many experts now agree that U.S. health care has had great success, especially in the area of technology which is generally available to affluent and middle-class consumers of health care services. Despite many advances in modern health care and important advances in medical technology, much of the general public does not view the U.S. health care system as perfect or as nonproblematic. In fact, public perception of health care overall and the role of government in health care is fraught with recognition of diverse problems, such as barriers to care, lack of health insurance for many people, and discussions of a "crisis" in health care.

To understand the changing views of the public, changes in health professions education and research, and the changing role of federal governmental involvement in health care, it is helpful to cover some major aspects of the U.S. health care system, including the levels of health care, the costs of health care, and providers of health care.

Levels of Care

Primary, Secondary, and Tertiary Care Levels

One classic distinction between health care in the United States and health care in other countries is the distinction among primary, secondary, and tertiary levels of care. **Primary care** involves treatment of the most common problems, as well as preventive care, such as treatment of sore throats, vaccinating babies, and hypertension screening. **Secondary care** is health care provided for more specialized problems and includes setting a broken leg, or care for older patients with acute renal failure. **Tertiary care** is reserved for the most specialized and unusual health care problems, like open heart surgery and lung transplants. It is not the type of care provided by most community hospitals. In a large urban area, there may be one or several hospitals that provide a few or the complete range of levels of care, while in a rural area, it is likely that tertiary care may not be available at the local hospital.

Regionalized versus Dispersed Care

Another distinction in health care delivery systems is that between a *regionalized* and a *dispersed* model of care. In a regionalized system, personnel and facilities will be differently assigned to tiers of care that correspond to the primary-secondary-tertiary care structure, and patients will flow across the levels of care as needs dictate. The regionalized model closely resembles that used by the British National Health Services, many other countries like Scandinavia, and some of the developing Latin American nations. The U.S. health care model does not tend to be a regionalized system.[6]

At a more community-based level, the dispersed model is applied by some U.S. **health maintenance organizations (HMOs),** especially those that operate with a closed panel of physicians who work full-time for a plan in a group practice approach. In these plans, patients must obtain their care from physicians within the closed plan, and they generally begin with a generalist physician who provides primary care and perhaps some secondary care. Tertiary care is provided by physicians within the plan or, in some cases, by outside physicians who contract with the group.

The dispersed model of health care generally gives greater choice to patients and caregivers at the national and local levels. In the dispersed model, there is no explicit regionalization, so one community may have five or six different facilities providing highly specialized care, in contrast to a regionalized model where a community is likely to have only one or two such centers. In a dispersed model, if a community could generate enough funds to attract the appropriate physician, a small town might still have available more advanced cardiac services. This model, in which patients are not required to have a primary care physician, is a better description of the current operation of the U.S. health care system overall, although it embodies elements of both the regionalized and dispersed models.

Health Care Costs

Most health care financial analysts describe four categories of health care: how much money is spent, where the money comes from (direct out-of-pocket, private insurance, government), what it is spent on (fees to individual providers, fees to hospitals, costs of pharmaceuticals or medically related supplies), and how it is paid out to providers (per unit of service, per item of care, per hospital discharge, per day of long-term care services).

Rising health care costs have been an important factor in the U.S. health care system since the 1940s, and today concerns about costs are increasing. National health care costs have grown at a rate substantially outpacing the GNP in most years since 1940. Prior to World War II only about 4 percent of the GNP was spent on health care.[7] By 1960, this figure had increased to 5.3 percent, by 1994 it had increased to 11 percent, and by 2004 it had increased to 16 percent.[8]

The sources of the nation's health care dollars over time are shown in Figure 2.1, and where those dollars went is shown in Figure 2.2. These figures also show the changing influence of government. Only $0.24 out of every 1960 health care dollar came from government programs; by 1994 this had risen to $0.45 out of each health care dollar,[8] and by 2004 the figure had changed to $0.33.[8] Where health care dollars actually went remained remarkably similar until the last ten years, as the importance of hospital care within the overall continuum of care has declined. In 2004, prescription drug spending accounted for 15 percent of personal health care

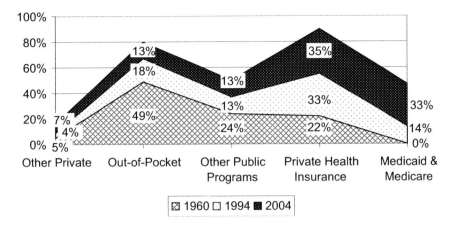

FIGURE 2.1. Health Care Spending: Where the Dollars Came From. *Source:* Centers for Medicare & Medicaid Services, Office of the Actuary, National Health Statistics Group. *Note: Other Public* includes programs such as workers' compensation, public health activity, Department of Defense, Department of Veterans Affairs, Indian Health Service, state and local hospital subsidies, and school health. *Other Private* includes industrial in-plant, privately funded construction, and nonpatient revenues, including philanthropy.

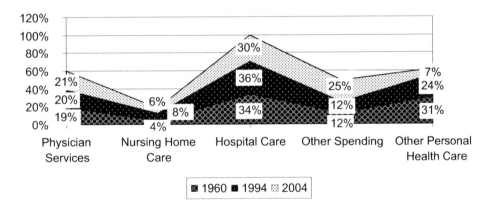

FIGURE 2.2. Health Care Spending: Where the Dollars Went. *Source:* Centers for Medicare & Medicaid Services, Offices of the Actuary, National Health Statistics Group. *Note: Other Spending* includes dentist services, other professional services, home health, durable medical products, over-the-counter medicines and sundries, public health, other personal health care, research, and structures and equipment.

spending but has been slowing in recent years due to lower-priced generic drugs, increased over-the-counter use of antiulcerants and antihistamines, a shift toward greater mail order dispensing, and reduced consumption of certain drugs due to safety concerns.

Most hospital care today is financed by insurance or government programs and accounts for nearly one-third of the total national health care expenditures. The most rapidly growing category of health care expenditures is for home health care and stems in part from rapid growth in home-based hospice care. These shifts in the growth of health care costs can be attributed to several factors, including government influence, inflation rates, population growth, increased rates of health care usage, increases in the proportion of the elderly population, and increases in the intensity of services provided.

Providers of Care

A major piece of today's health care delivery system is providers of care, whether that means physicians, nurses, technicians, and aides or institutional providers of care, such as hospitals, ambulatory surgery centers, or nursing homes. The number of different types of health care professionals and the number of people employed in the health care system have increased dramatically in the twentieth century. In 1910, only 1.3 percent of all employed people were in the health care sector. By 1950 this figure had almost doubled to 2.5 percent and it doubled again in the next thirty years; today the health care industry is the largest single employer of all industries monitored by the Department of Labor.[9] Not only have the numbers of people employed in health care increased, but the types of jobs have changed and the numbers of different categories of health care workers have increased. There are now over 700 different job categories in the health care industry.

In addition to changes in who provides health care, changes have occurred in where the care is provided. More and more services, such as outpatient surgery and advanced types of diagnostic procedures, are being provided in ambulatory care settings. In the past, ambulatory care was provided in doctors' offices or in a few outpatient settings, such as hospital clinics; today, sites are more varied and can include special facilities for outpatient surgeries; emergency care and walk-in clinics; group care settings, such as health maintenance organizations (HMOs); as well as the doctor's office.

The hospital has played a central role in health care delivery, training of personnel, and conduct and dissemination of health-related research. There have really been two traditions of hospital services in the United States—one in the private sector, especially nonprofit hospitals, and one in the public sector. Hospital care for the poor was concentrated in county or municipal hospitals until the introduction of the **Medicaid** program in 1965. The private sector consisted of voluntary hospitals, including typical community hospitals, those affiliated with religious associations, and other types of nonprofit facilities. In 1900, half of the hospitals were for-profit, but by 1970 only 13 percent of the hospitals were for-profit.[10]

This change from for-profit to nonprofit status was influenced greatly by changes in how patients pay for health care services. Up until World War II, most hospital care for middle-class people was paid for through savings. The Depression caused major problems for hospital incomes; their financial solvency was threatened, which led to the idea of voluntary group hospitalization plans, especially through Blue Cross. Private insurance for health care grew rapidly, so that by 1965 most of the working population had third-party health insurance. With the introduction of **Medicare** for the elderly and Medicaid for the poor, important groups of people who did not previously have money or insurance for care received other options. Later, the introduction of the **diagnosis-related groups (DRGs)** reimbursement plan as a part of the Tax Equity and Fiscal Responsibility Act of 1982[11] converted the way Medicare paid for hospital care from a cost-based reimbursement system to a prospective per-case system, with over 460 different diagnosis-related payment categories based on the diagnosis of the patient.

THE CHANGING FEDERAL ROLE IN U.S. HEALTH CARE

Medicare, Medicaid, and DRGs are examples of direct political attempts and involvement to influence the way health care is delivered. This process has produced significant legislation directly affecting health care, and health care experts believe that in the near future five areas of health care are likely to be most affected by governmental legislation: health care coverage, taxation as it relates to Employee Retirement and Income Security Act (ERISA) policy, Medicaid, Medicare, and managed care. Factors such as the nature and history of existing institutions, the general climate of opinion, ritualized methods for dealing with social conflict, and general goals and values of a society each play a role in the formulation of health care policy. Within this somewhat circular and ongoing process almost all decisions are subject to subsequent modifications. Rising health care costs often set off concerns among insurance programs and employers that force them to attempt to contain health care expenditures. These factors in turn have an impact upon the providers of health care—especially hospitals and physicians. Providers then try to take actions that directly affect consumers of care—individual patients, communities, and employers in the workforce.

Federal Legislation

Early 1900s

Involvement of the U.S. federal government in health care is not a recent phenomenon (see Appendix 2.A). It began almost as soon as the nation secured its independence but became prominent in the 1900s when political parties in the United States began to run on platforms supporting national health care. The Socialist Party became the first political party in the United States to endorse national health insurance shortly after a national health care plan was initiated in Europe in 1883 by German Chancellor Otto Von Bismarck. Theodore Roosevelt's Progressive Party ticket also fought unsuccessfully for national health insurance in 1902.[12]

In 1929, 1,500 Texas schoolteachers negotiated with Baylor University Hospital to provide up to twenty-one days of inpatient hospital care per year for its members for a fee of $0.50 per month. This program laid the foundation for what would eventually become the Blue Cross Plan.[13] A similar concept, prepaid medical service, was developed by Dr. Sidney Garfield in the early 1930s. His plan, which originated in the Mojave Desert, was expanded during construction of the Grand Coulee Dam under the direction of Henry J. Kaiser. This program, which was extended to Kaiser's employees at his steel mills and shipyards in the 1940s, was the beginning of the Kaiser Permanente organization.[14] In 1932, the Committee on the Cost of Medical Care,[15] a privately funded organization, called for American health care to move toward group practice and group payment and made recommendations to improve efficiency in health care and help curb the upward spiral in health care costs. Also in 1932, with Franklin Roosevelt's election, national health insurance came into the national spotlight. However, with the Depression at its height, FDR gave priority to Social Security.[13]

1940s and 1950s

Several pieces of Truman-era legislation also had profound effects on the course of the U.S. health care system. In 1946, the **Hill-Burton Act** provided a huge amount of federal money for hospital construction.[16] From 1946 until the early 1970s, Hill-Burton money helped construct over 400,000 hospital beds (and many health sciences libraries), and another congressional act, the GI Bill, financed higher education for veterans. Many used this opportunity to study medicine. Based on the War Labor Board's 1942 decision that fringe benefits were not restricted by wage/price freezes, and buttressed by the Supreme Court's Inland Steel decision in the late 1940s, health benefits became standard conditions of employment that unions sought to negotiate with employers.[17] These circumstances set the historical precedent for employer-provided health care benefits—the most common way that working Americans obtain health care coverage today.

In 1947, the **Taft-Hartley Act** restricted labor unions in many ways.[18] Although Britain adopted a national health service in 1948, weaker unions in the United States were unable to mobilize enough support to introduce a national health system. However, what the unions lacked in political clout in the late 1940s and early 1950s they made up for on a local level by being able to negotiate with employers for health insurance benefits. Responding to the market this created, the commercial insurance industry offered health insurance policies that employers could provide to workers. During 1950-1965, supported by an increasing base of private health insurance, the average annual rate of increase in real national health expenditures was 6.3 percent.[7] One can see from a supply-and-demand perspective how this 6.3 percent increase occurred: through Hill-Burton, federal money built hospital beds (the supply side); because of political and legal changes in the late 1940s and early 1950s, wage earners had insurance plans to cover health care services (the demand side).

1960s and 1970s

By 1965, under the Lyndon Johnson administration, 5.9 percent of the GNP was being spent on health care.[19] In keeping with his Great Society plan, on July 30, 1965, in Independence, Missouri, in honor of Harry Truman, LBJ signed into law Title 18 and Title 19 of the Social Security Act. These historic acts created the Medicare and Medicaid programs to provide health care benefits for elderly and poor Americans. Medical societies threatened to strike when the programs went into effect, again fighting governmental intrusion into health care, but when the smoke cleared, Medicare and Medicaid turned out to be a windfall for both hospitals and physicians, since hospitals and doctors were reimbursed for whatever they charged. There were no incentives to be cost conscious, since as long as the charges were "reasonable," the government would pay the bill. This partially explains why, during 1967-1970 when overall inflation was 5.2 percent, Medicare hospital expenditures increased at an average annual rate of 18.1 percent.[20]

In 1969, Nixon administration officials met with Paul Ellwood, MD, who advocated prepaid, not-for-profit plans he called health maintenance organizations.[21] The AMA opposed HMOs and backed a national health care plan (Medicredit) that would provide tax credits to buy private health insurance. There was such concern over health care costs because the average annual rate of real national health care expenditure increases from 1966 to 1971 was 7.6 percent. Responding to this concern in 1971, Nixon called for a 6 percent ceiling on the price increases to Medicare for hospitals and a 2.5 percent ceiling on increases in doctors' fees during the general wage/price freeze then in effect. This concern over health care costs prompted Gerald Ford in 1974 to withdraw his support for a national health care plan because of fears that it would worsen inflation. Similarly, Jimmy Carter backed a voluntary effort by hospitals and physicians to control rising health care costs.[22] The health care industry wanted to prove to the Carter administration that costs could be controlled without governmental intervention. As a result, during 1978-1979, hospital costs per patient day did not increase at all in real terms, a monumental feat considering the upward trends in health care expenditures in the previous years.

1980s and 1990s

In his report to Congress in December of 1982, Secretary of Health and Human Services Richard Schweiker outlined a plan to control rising health care costs.[23] As mandated by the Tax Equity and Fiscal Responsibility Act (TEFRA) in 1982, the government would put into place, in 1983, a reimbursement plan for Medicare patients. With a fixed reimbursement per Medicare patient, hospital length of stay decreased dramatically, not only for the over-sixty-five population but also for the general population. Although hospitals were now faced with fixed reimbursement for Medicare patients, there was no similar incentive for physicians, and physician fees continued to rise faster than the consumer price index.

Under the Medicare prospective payment system, attention focused on hospital cost per case rather than on cost plus margin. Charges became meaningless: a hospital could charge whatever it wanted, but these charges would no longer be reimbursed; only a flat fee would be paid for services rendered. Hospital financial officers soon realized that Medicare payments for hospital services were inadequate to cover the cost of those services provided. At that time, indemnity insurance plans were still reimbursing at rates well above hospital costs. In order to remain financially solvent, charges were increased to indemnity patients in order to partially pay for the services provided to Medicare patients. Consequently, an era of cost shifting began. However, the advent of HMOs and other managed care plans in the 1980s and 1990s significantly limited hospitals' abilities to shift costs, and the prospective payment system of 1983 began to reward cost-conscious provision of health care services.[24]

In 1996, during his first term as president, Clinton did see the passage of the Kennedy-Kassebaum Bill. This legislation ensures improved access to care for individuals changing jobs and for those with pre-existing conditions, and it provides tax relief for nursing home/long-term care patients, among other provisions.[25] Passage of this bill, in the wake of the defeat of Clinton's Health Security Act, confirms that legislative changes in health care will most likely occur in an incremental fashion and will focus on aspects of health care important to society at the moment, such as rising costs, privacy of patient information, and quality of health care, rather than through a comprehensive, overriding governmental plan.

2000

President George W. Bush's administration has focused on three key health care reform components. The first component focuses on ensuring that every American can afford a health care plan through health credits, association health plans, long-term care, and tax exemptions for caregivers. The second component proposes improving the quality of health care by passage of a Patient's Bill of Rights, prohibiting genetic discrimination, and providing effective privacy protections for medical records. The third component seeks to increase biomedical research by improving public health systems, funding community health centers, and supporting the National Health Service Corps.[26]

Influence of Professional Library Associations

In many cases the aforementioned legislation has been monitored, influenced, or driven by several key health care professional associations, including those mentioned in other chapters. Professional health sciences library associations, especially the **Association of Academic Health Sciences Libraries (AAHSL)** and the **Medical Library Association (MLA),** are primarily concerned with legislation affecting national health information policy, health care and public health information resources, health research information resources, health education information resources, and the development and use of health information technologies.

National Health Information Policy

For health sciences libraries, national health information policy deals with such issues as **National Library of Medicine (NLM)** fiscal funding and reauthorization, which directly impact the NLM and other NIH institutes. This policy area also includes issues related to the **Institute of Museum and Library Services (IMLS)** budget, which provides funding to many state libraries that, in turn, use these funds to support local library programs. This legislative area also includes NLM services like **PubMed Central** and focuses on intellectual property and copyright law, which in recent legislative history has included the **Digital Millennium Copyright Act (DMCA),** DMCA anticircumvention rulemaking, the Digital Media Consumers' Rights Act of 2002, distance education, database protection, the Public Domain Enhancement Act of 2003, and licensing agreements.

Health Care and Public Health Information Resources

These issues include telemedicine and telehealth, patient privacy, access to government information, and consumer and patient health information. Patient privacy, especially medical records privacy, became a greater concern with the passage of the **Health Insurance Portability and Accountability Act (HIPAA)** in 1996 and the **USA PATRIOT Act** in 2001, and as health sciences libraries became more involved in linking scholarly communications information to the electronic patient record. In the last decade, concerns about access to government information have grown as many federally produced and owned information resources have been privatized and/or as federal agency libraries have been dismantled. Legislation dealing with PubSCIENCE, public access to scientific information, the depository library program, and the National Technical Information Services had become important priorities for all health sciences library associations.

Health Research and Health Education Information Resources

Both health research information resources and health education information resources legislation impact medical research, distance education, and graduate medical education. These issues may have less direct impact on health sciences libraries than the other areas of legislative concern mentioned earlier, but they affect the libraries' constituency and, in turn, affect the programs and services offered by the libraries.

Information Technologies

Legislation affecting the development of health information technologies impacts the health sciences library in many fundamental ways. In today's networked world, technology legislation impacts the library's ability to link people to people, people to business, people to information, and people to culture. This interconnected world encompasses an ever-expanding communications network via traditional telecommunications and computing systems. It also employs new frameworks that move data, audio, and video via increased bandwidth, wireless technologies, and systems not yet imagined. Crucial themes, like *privacy* (the freedom to choose the degree to which personal information is monitored, collected, disclosed, and distributed), *intellectual freedom* (the right to express ideas and receive information), and *equitable access* (user-centered, barrier-free, and format-independent access to information that achieves an open flow of ideas in a global, networked society) take center stage in our efforts to maintain the free flow of information in a democratic society.

ORGANIZATIONAL COMPONENTS OF ACADEMIC MEDICINE

Although there is little agreement on the definition of academic medicine, it has been defined as the capacity within medicine to think, study, research, discover, evaluate, innovate, teach, learn, and improve.[27] For librarians, it is probably more appropriately defined as a medical practice within some sort of institution of higher learning; is the alternative to private practice; and is the environment in which most health sciences librarians are employed. It may or may not involve some sort of research or teaching and is composed of four major organizational components: medical schools, teaching hospitals, health systems, and faculty practice organizations, which are interrelated but often are legally separated. The resulting configurations, which can also include other health professions schools (e.g., nursing, dentistry, or allied health) may be labeled academic medical centers, academic health centers, or academic health science centers. These terms can also identify teaching hospitals independent of a medical school but with large investments in graduate medical education programs.[28]

The organizational arrangements among the components of academic medicine (medical schools, teaching hospitals, health systems, and faculty practice plans) vary considerably, and the relationships can differ between medical schools and physicians (Is the faculty practice plan part of the university or is it a separate organization?), the medical school and the primary teaching hospital (Do they have common ownership or limited partners?), and among teaching hospital affiliates (Are they a part of or separate from the same health system?). At some institutions, these components are arranged in a "single ownership" model where the parent university has legal and financial control over the medical school, the primary teaching hospital, and the faculty practice plan. At the other extreme, the medical school may be a "limited partner" in the clinical delivery system. Many variations exist between these two extremes, and these variations will often influence reporting lines for the academic health sciences librarian, who may report to a medical school dean, a vice president, or a university dean, or for a teaching hospital librarian or a librarian employed by a hospital with an educational mission, both of whom may report to a medical education director or a systems director.

Teaching Hospitals

The term "teaching hospital" refers both to individual hospitals and to health systems and networks that contain hospitals and other components of the health care delivery system committed to educational activities in the health professions. Teaching hospitals are the primary sites for clinical education of medical students and **residents,** postgraduate fellowship training programs, and a significant proportion of other health professions education programs. Teaching hospitals are also distinguished by their programs of clinical research: testing and development of drugs, medical devices, and treatment methods.

U.S. teaching hospitals primarily developed in response to the medical education reform movement in the early twentieth century. Today, approximately 1,100 hospitals are involved in medical school education; the bulk of research and training, including three-fourths of all residency training, is concentrated in the approximately 400 hospitals and health systems that are members of the **Association of American Medical Colleges (AAMC) Council of Teaching Hospitals and Health Systems (COTH).**[28] In addition to short-term, nonfederal teaching hospitals, there are sixty-four Veterans Administration (VA) medical centers. About 70 percent of VA physicians hold joint faculty appointments at an affiliated medical school. In 2003, 85 percent of U.S. medical schools were involved in such affiliations. The VA maintains approximately 8,800 full-time residency positions (9 percent of all residents) and is the nation's largest provider of graduate medical education.[29]

While teaching hospitals, health systems, academic health sciences centers, and academic physicians provide the full range of patient care services, they also offer intensive specialized services at the cutting edge of medical innovation and technology. Of the nearly 400 members of COTH, the 281 short-term, nonfederal member hospitals comprise only 6 percent of all such U.S. hospitals; however, they account for 19 percent of beds, 21 percent of admissions, 22 percent of outpatient visits, 20 percent of surgeries, 16 percent of emergency room visits, and 20 percent of births.[28] In addition, teaching hospitals provide a disproportionate amount of care to the poor and medically indigent patient populations and those with the most severe and complex cases of disease and disability. In the process of delivering care, they train future physicians, nurses, and allied health professionals and foster an environment necessary for clinical and health services research to grow and flourish.

Medical Schools

At the turn of the twentieth century, as many as 160 medical schools operated in the United States, many of marginal or poor quality. With the elevated standards prompted by the Flexner Report, many of these institutions met their demise and few new schools were inaugurated. By 1960, only eighty-six U.S. medical schools were accredited by the **Liaison Committee on Medical Education (LCME)** of AAMC, the primary accrediting body for U.S. medical schools. Since 1980 to the present, the number of medical schools has remained fairly stable and in 2004 totaled 125 U.S. schools and seventeen Canadian schools. The number of medical school graduates has also remained steady at about 16,000 per year. In addition, twenty medical schools are accredited by the Bureau of Professional Education of the **American Osteopathic Association (AOA).** These schools graduate approximately 2,700 physicians each year with the degree of Doctor of Osteopathy (DO).[29] Forty-four states, the District of Columbia, and Puerto Rico each have at least one medical school, and the six states without medical schools have negotiated arrangements for their residents to receive training at schools in neighboring states. Fifty medical schools (40 percent) are private, although thirty-three of these schools receive financial appropriations from their state governments.

Medical schools share many purposes and objectives, but they are also quite diverse. While most are part of a comprehensive public or private university, twenty medical schools (six public and four private) are part of independent and freestanding health sciences universities.[28] Traditionally, medical schools were built, or affiliated with, major teaching hospitals and recruited full-time academic faculty. However, many of those founded in the 1970s were planned with community hospitals as the venue for teaching and community physicians as the teaching faculty. In many cases, these "community-based" schools were created because of the desire to produce primary care physicians who could practice in rural areas and other communities underserved by physicians. Three schools (Howard University, Morehouse College, and Meharry Medical College) were created in association with historically black institutions of higher education and have a special mission to educate minority physicians. One federally owned school (Uniformed Services University of the Health Sciences) trains physicians for the uniformed services. Five medical schools (Wright State University, University of South Carolina, East Tennessee State University, Texas A&M University, and Marshall University) trace their development to a special partnership between the VA and state governments.

Medical School Financing

Perhaps no measures better demonstrate the complexity of the modern medical school than do financial indices. Total revenues of $56 billion supported the operations of medical schools in 2002-2003, an average of $452 million per school.[29] Nationally, the 125 U.S. medical schools account for about 16 percent of total revenues among all higher education institutions and employ about 17 percent of all full-time faculties, even though they enroll only about 1 percent of all full-time students.

Medical schools also vary greatly in their level of financing. Research-intensive medical schools had medium revenues of $926 million to support their activities, while community-based medical schools had median revenues of $106 million.[30] Trends in the growth of financial resources for medical schools since 1960 are best understood in terms of distinct periods. The first distinct period (1960s-1970s) witnessed a fivefold increase in full-time faculty and a doubling of the number of medical students. In the second period (the 1980s), both the number of medical schools and student enrollment remained steady, but revenue continued to increase due to the sustained expansion of research programs and clinical services. In the third period (1990s into the twenty-first century), growth in medical school revenues has continued but at a more modest annual rate (5.5 percent adjusted for inflation).[28] The largest single source of revenue for medical schools is patient care reimbursement for physician services (about 36 percent in 2003). In the early 1970s, medical schools developed faculty practice plans (formal practice organizations for billing and collection). Payment for patient care services formerly made directly to the individual faculty physician began to flow into the faculty practice plan and to be recognized as revenue to the school.

Another significant source of funding for medical schools (24 percent in 2003) comes from the federal government in the form of grants and contracts for teaching, research, and service programs, including recovery facilities and administrative costs (i.e., indirect costs). Federal research funds totaling $111 billion in fiscal year 2005[31] represent the major component of federal support to medical schools. Revenue from affiliated teaching hospitals (12 percent) and state and local appropriations (6.5 percent) represent the next two largest sources of revenue for medical schools.

Student tuition and fees are often cited as sources of funding for higher education institutions; however, in the medical school arena, tuition and fees have always been a small but relatively stable component of revenues, about 3 percent to 4 percent, since the 1960s. Other sources of revenue include industry-sponsored support, foundation grants, gifts, and endowment income.

Medical School Faculty

Medical school faculty members are of two types: clinical faculty and basic science faculty. Traditionally, clinical faculties were MDs, physicians whose responsibilities included treating patients, conducting clinically oriented research, and instructing medical students in clinical rotations. Basic science faculty were typically PhD and MD research faculty who conducted research in the basic sciences (e.g., anatomy, physiology, pharmacology) and trained graduate students. In modern academic medicine, many of these traditional distinctions are not as clear as they once were. For example, many PhD researchers have appointments in clinical departments. Generally speaking, however, the historical distinction between clinical and basic science faculty still applies.[32]

Medical school faculty members differ from their colleagues in the arts and sciences and other university divisions in the extent to which they are able to generate revenues to support their salaries. This difference is particularly true of clinical faculty members, many of whom receive only modest support from medical school funds. Their compensation comes largely through clinical income, which underwrites time spent in teaching and research. Basic science faculty members can be self-supporting to a lesser degree through research grants and contracts. Most medical schools have created a variety of faculty appointment arrangements, with distinctive promotion criteria, to accommodate the differential roles of their faculty members. The majority of clinical faculty with primary responsibilities in patient care and teaching, for example, are now appointed to non-tenure-eligible clinician-educator tracks. Many schools have also introduced an incentive and pay-for-performance compensation structure that ties a portion of compensation to success in revenue-generating patient care activities.

Medical school faculty diversity has also changed as the proportion of full-time female faculty members has grown slowly but steadily, from 15 percent in 1975 to 30 percent in 2003. Women continue to lag behind men in occupying senior academic and administrative ranks at medical schools, comprising in 2003 only 17 percent of tenured faculty, 14 percent of full professors, 10 percent of department chairs, and 10 percent of medical school deans. Progress in increasing the number of minorities in medical school faculties is even less evident than is the case with women. In 2003, only 8 percent of full-time faculty identified themselves as Native American, African American, Hispanic, or multiracial.[28]

Faculty Practice Organizations

With the passage of Medicare and Medicaid and the growth in private health care insurance in the 1960s, the size of clinical faculty in medical schools involved in patient care activities grew rapidly. This growth spawned the development of academic faculty practice plans (arrangements for billing, collecting, and distributing professional fee income generated from the patient care services provided by faculty physicians) within or associated with medical schools. Faculty practice systems have also joined with hospitals and health systems in marketing services and contracting directly with large-scale purchasers of care. Of these plans, 43 percent are entities within the medical school or university structure, while another 40 percent are separate and independent not-for-profit corporations or foundations.[33] Public medical schools are more likely than private schools to have practice plans organized as separate legal entities because separate incorporation gives the faculty in public schools independence and flexibility that may not be possible within the rigidities of state personnel and administrative systems.

Initially, many medical schools created faculty practice plans that were departmentally based; however, with the transition to organized care systems, independent departmental practice plans rapidly became obsolete. The vast majority of schools now have plans that are, at minimum, federated in character—that is, department-based practices with shared management systems and some limited common governance, which allows for joint planning and contracting.

MEDICAL EDUCATION

Medical schools and teaching hospitals teach medical students and also train medical residents during the three- to seven-year period following the MD degree that leads to eligibility for licensure and board certification. They are also involved in continuing medical education programs that allow physicians to stay current with the fast-moving advances in diagnostic capability and therapeutic techniques and with the expanding knowledge on medical intervention outcomes. Medical schools are also committed to the education of biomedical scientists through PhD training programs.

Undergraduate Medical Education

All medical schools retain the prerogative to select their students and thereby are assured that the number of enrolling students matches available resources. Medical school admissions committees use broad-based selection criteria in the admission process, including prior academic achievement, assessments of the candidate's academic abilities and personal qualities by college faculty and advisors, and evidence of values and attitudes commensurate with a career of service. All medical schools conduct interviews to assess the personal qualities, values, and attitudes of applicants—a less common practice in business, law, and other professional schools.

Class Attributes

Historically, the total number of medical school applications has cycled between rather wide extremes (from a low of 26,702 in 1966 to a high in 1996 of 46,965). During the last fifteen years, medical school enrollment has remained remarkably stable. In 2003, women applicants to medical schools outnumbered men (17,672 versus 17,114) for the first time.[28] Racial and ethnic minority groups have not achieved the same success as women in entering the medical profession. Medical student diversity is important to ensure better educational experiences for all students. This diversity also provides exposure to fellow students and faculty from different backgrounds. Patient-physician race concordance can yield greater patient satisfaction and a more diverse physician workforce may result in improved health outcomes. Additionally, a more diverse research workforce can focus attention on problems disproportionately affecting minorities, and diverse management teams outperform those with more homogeneous ones.[34]

As a matter of principle, medical schools accept the most worthy candidates for admission, regardless of ability to pay. Tuition and fees, however, are rising and vary greatly among schools from approximately $5,000 per year for state residents at one public institution to more than $40,000 per year at one private institution. In 2003-2004, median annual tuition and fees at public medical schools totaled $16,332 for state residents and $32,662 for nonresidents; at private medical schools, tuition and fees amounted to $32,028 for residents and $33,100 for nonresidents.[28] A major consequence of rising tuition and fees, coupled with the limited availability of scholarships and caps on subsidized loans, is the growing indebtedness of medical school graduates. Four of every five members of the class of 2004 graduated with some educational debt. The median debt for indebted graduates of private medical schools was $140,000, and for public school graduates, $105,000, and more than 28 percent of those indebted graduates had debt exceeding $150,000.[35]

Student Curriculum

Although the myth lingers that the state of medical education today is virtually identical to that of fifty years ago, the medical curricula have undergone significant changes in how they are organized and the content that is taught. Today, most medical schools have centralized the governance of the curriculum in a school-wide executive committee with oversight responsibilities for all aspects of the curriculum. Various information management skills are integrated into course syllabi, textbooks, class notes, histology slides, and patient cases, and thus it has become increasingly advisable that the health sciences library director interacts with or serves as a member of the curriculum committee. Faculty and students recognize that medical school libraries help them stay abreast of the ever-expanding literature of medical knowledge and applications and that storage, retrieval, and management of information are increasingly essential functions of medical problem solving and decision-making.

Recent undergraduate medical education reforms include several major components (what students learn, how students learn, and how students are assessed), and much medical care focuses on chronic conditions, as increasingly physicians treat problems of aging, such as Alzheimer's disease, chronic neurodegenerative diseases, heart and circulatory failure, and bone and joint disorders. Therefore, educators have interwoven topics such as geriatrics and end-of-life care into medical school curricula. Issues such as cultural competence, nutrition, and family violence and abuse are also important components of undergraduate medical education, as is an enlarging focus on disease prevention, health promotion, and population-based approaches to health care.

Further, advances in molecular and cell biology and genetics in the last thirty years have expanded physicians' treatment options and challenge schools to integrate these concepts and their associated technologies into basic and clinical science instruction. Because physicians can no longer ignore the financial consequences of diagnostic tests and treatment decisions, medical decision-making and medical ethics have also been added to the curriculum. As medical care has become more complex, medical technologies have proliferated. Those seeking care have become more racially and ethnically diverse, and patients have become more knowledgeable and well informed. Thus, medical communication skills have also become an important part of the medical school curriculum.

While no two medical schools' curricula are the same, three basic approaches to undergraduate medical education exist:

1. *Classic 2 + 2 curriculum* adapts the traditional medical education structure of the twenty-first century by teaching the biomedical principles of anatomy, biochemistry, physiology, microbiology, and other basic science areas using a variety of instructional methods (e.g., lectures, discussion).
2. *Organ system approaches* to medical student learning organize the curriculum around components of the human body and each of its major organ systems at the macroscopic, microscopic, and molecular levels.
3. **Problem-based learning (PBL)** refers to student-centered, small-group instruction in which basic and clinical science topics are introduced within the context of case studies of patient problems. PBL aims to enhance skills in hypothesis development and deductive reasoning and to foster group communications skills required of health care professionals working within teams.[36]

The ways in which students are assessed for medical know-how and its application to patients also have undergone significant change. Today, medical schools routinely use standardized patients (laypeople carefully selected and trained to accurately simulate the motional and physical complaints of actual patients) to teach and assess physical examination skills and history taking. The vast majority of schools use the **Objective Structured Clinical Examination (OSCE)** for assessing students' performance in specific clinical tasks and use standardized patients to conduct OSCEs. All new physicians in the United States are required to pass the **National Board of Medical Examiners (NBME)** examination.[37] As part of its three-step examination for medical licensure, potential future physicians must take a one-day clinical skills test that mirrors a physician's typical workday in a clinic. In twelve interactions with standardized patients, examinees are expected to establish rapport, elicit pertinent historical information, perform focused physical examinations, communicate effectively, and document findings and diagnostic impressions.

The ways in which medical students learn to interact with, diagnose, and treat patients have undergone radical transformations also because of both educational advancements and changes to the health care delivery system. Experience in clinical settings occurs early in students' medical education. Some first-year medical students being to see patients immediately; others are assigned a patient or family in their first year and follow those patients throughout their four years. Medical schools still use teaching hospitals for inpatient services training; however, technological advances and the financial incentives inherent in managed health care systems have narrowed the scope of medical conditions for which patients are hospitalized. Today's medical schools rely on more than 1,000 community hospitals as inpatient sites for one or more required clerkships, some at great distance from the main medical school campus. A smaller subset—about thirty—have formally designated "clinical campuses," geographically distant from the main site, where a portion of the third- and fourth-year class receive clinical training.

Graduate Medical Education

Graduate medical education comprises the second phase of the formal education process that prepares doctors for medical practice. All medical school graduates who seek full licensure and board certification in a medical specialty or subspecialty must complete a period of residency training. Residency programs vary in length depending upon specialty, but, generally, it takes three to five years for initial board certification (see Table 2.1). Subspecialty training may last as long as eleven years. Residency as a component of medical education began at Johns Hopkins Hospital in the 1890s.[28] Residents were called "**house officers**" because they literally lived in the hospital. Even today, residents are sometimes referred to as "house officers" or "house staff."

Residents are expected to demonstrate competence in six domains of knowledge, skills, and attitudes deemed necessary to be effective and compassionate physicians:

1. Patient care that is compassionate, appropriate, and effective
2. Medical knowledge about established and evolving biomedical, clinical, epidemiological, and social-**behavioral sciences** and the application of this knowledge to patient care
3. Practice-based learning and improvement that involves investigation and evaluation of their own patient care appraisal and assimilation of scientific evidence
4. Interpersonal and communication skills with patients, their families, and other health professionals
5. Professionalism, that is, the commitment to fulfilling professional responsibilities, adherence to ethical principles, and sensitivity to diverse populations
6. Systems-based practice, the awareness of and responsiveness to the larger context and system of health care, and the ability to effectively marshal system resources

The **National Residency Matching Program (NRMP),** a not-for-profit corporation, was created in 1952 to provide a fair and impartial process for applying to, and obtaining, residency positions. The "match" links the preferences of applicants for residency positions with the preferences of residency programs for applicants. **Match Day** occurs in March each year, and in 2004, 14,609 fourth-year students at U.S. medical schools sought graduate training through the NRMP, with 93 percent successfully matched to a program of their choice.[38]

TABLE 2.1. Selected GME Training Requirements for Specialty Board Certification

SPECIALTY	# of Years of GME Required
Anesthesiology	4
Emergency medicine	3
Family practice	3
Internal medicine	3
Obstetrics/gynecology	4
Pathology	4
Pediatrics	3
Psychiatry	4
Radiology	5
Surgery	5

Source: ACGME (Accreditation Council for Graduate Medical Education).

HEALTH SCIENCES RESEARCH

How Health Sciences Research Is Financed

The success of the American biomedical research enterprise emerged to a great extent from a partnership between academic institutions and the federal government during World War II. The National Institutes of Health became the primary federal agency responsible for implementing the **social contract for health-related research** proposed in Bush's *Science—The Endless Frontier*. Today, NIH comprises twenty-seven institutes and centers, each focusing on a particular disease (e.g., National Cancer Institute), organ (e.g., National Eye Institute), stage of human development (e.g., National Institute on Aging), or cross-cutting mission (e.g., NLM). At its Bethesda, Maryland, campus, NIH also runs an intramural research program and houses supporting laboratories and a major clinical center.[39]

NIH devotes over 80 percent of its budget to extramural research (research conducted by scientists outside of NIH at universities, medical schools, hospitals, state and local governments, independent research organizations, and private industry). Medical schools and teaching hospitals receive approximately 55 percent to 60 percent of that extramural support. In 2003, NIH developed a "roadmap" initiative to define future strategic priorities for biomedical research. The roadmap centers on strengthening clinical research capacity by building cross-disciplinary and interdisciplinary research teams, developing "new pathways to discover" (e.g., molecular imaging, small-molecular libraries, bioinformatics, nanomedicine, and structural medicine), and creating new regional and national networks of physicians who conduct and participate in clinical trials.

Although small in comparison to NIH budget ($18.6 billion), the VA research program, which budgeted $406 million in 2004, makes an important contribution to biomedical, behavioral, and health services research.[40] Nearly 80 percent of the VA-funded scientists are clinical investigators, and 70 percent of VA research funding goes to clinical research. The VA research program funds more than 2,000 physicians and basic scientists nationwide, most of whom are faculty members at medical schools affiliated with VA medical centers.

Private industry sponsors a sizable portion of the total U.S. health-related research, but its support of research projects in academic medicine is relatively small. Such research tends to be largely directed to clinical drug trials sponsored by pharmaceutical and biotechnology companies. For many years, the federal government and industry traditionally maintained relatively distinct foci: industry tended to focus on applications and the development of health-related technology, especially with commercial laboratories and clinical trials; the federal government sponsored basic, clinical, and public health research, and some private research institutes. Today, these distinctions are not so clear.

How Biomedical Scientists Are Trained

Postbaccalaureate preparation for biomedical research consists of two stages.[28] First is the PhD program itself. Graduate programs in medical and health professions schools train over half of the nearly 6,000 PhDs awarded annually in biomedical-related disciplines. Approximately 27,000 students are currently enrolled in U.S. biomedical science graduate programs. The average time to earn a biological science degree is approximately 6.9 years. Dual-degree (MD/PhD) programs in medical schools account for a small but important percentage of PhD degrees. PhD graduate training is supported through a variety of sources: institutional funds, research assistantships funded through federal research grants, and NIH-funded research training. Typically, the second component of career preparation for biomedical scientists is postdoctoral training. A **postdoc** is an MD or a PhD scientist who received additional training in an established investigator's laboratory prior to launching an independent career.

How Biomedical Research Is Conducted

Biomedical research includes both studies designed primarily to increase the scientific base of information about normal or abnormal physiology and development and studies primarily intended to evaluate the safety, effectiveness, or usefulness of a medical product, procedure, or intervention. The terms "behavioral research" or "the behavioral sciences" may be used to refer either to studies of the behavior of individuals or to studies of the behavior of aggregates, such as groups, organizations, or societies. The broad objective of the behavioral and social sciences is similar to that of the biomedical sciences: to establish a body of demonstrable, replicable facts and theory that contributes to knowledge and to the amelioration of human problems. In academic medicine, most biomedical research is reviewed by the institution's **institutional review board (IRB);** NIH federally funded research involving human subjects requires IRB review.

Biomedical and Behavioral Research

It is neither possible nor necessary to draw a clean line between biomedical and behavioral research.[41] Some biomedical research pertains to behavior (e.g., in psychiatry, neurology, or epidemiology), and many of the methods used in behavioral research, such as observation and the questioning of subjects, are also used in biomedical research. Research may be designed to evaluate the behavioral changes that result from a biomedical intervention (e.g., lessening of depression after taking a particular medication or changes in psychiatric disorders following hemodialysis) or to examine physiological responses to behavioral interventions (e.g., lowering of blood pressure through biofeedback or weight loss through hypnosis). Some studies involve functions that are not easily defined as either behavioral or physiological (e.g., sleep, exercise, or diet). Thus, although it is sometimes useful to refer to biomedical or behavioral and social research as if they involve distinct activities, there is considerable overlap among the three areas.

Biomedical research also employs many methods and research designs. Studies designed to evaluate the safety, effectiveness, or usefulness of an intervention include research on therapies (e.g., drugs, diet, exercise, surgical interventions, or medical devices), diagnostic procedures (e.g., CAT scans or prenatal diagnosis through amniocentesis, chronic villi testing, and fetoscopy), and preventive measures (e.g., vaccines, diet, or fluoridated toothpaste). Research on normal human functioning and development can include studies of the human body while exercising, fasting, feeding, sleeping, or learning, or responding to such things as stress or sensory stimulation.

Some studies compare the functioning of a particular physiological system at different stages of development (e.g., infancy, childhood, adolescence, adulthood, or old age). Others are directed at defining normal childhood development so that deviations from normal can be identified. Sometimes research, particularly records research, is used to develop and refine hypotheses. Research on specific disease processes is often needed before improved methods of prevention, diagnosis, and treatment can be developed (e.g., research on the biochemical changes associated with AIDS or schizophrenia, or the neurological changes associated with senile dementia of the Alzheimer's type). Research on the human genome and genetic markers is expected to create new avenues for understanding disease processes and their eventual control.

Participants of some biomedical studies engage in ordinary tasks (e.g., exercise, learning a series of words, or responding to various sensory stimuli) as measurements of physiological and bodily functions are made. Although many procedures used in biomedical research are similar to those used in routine physical examinations, at times more invasive procedures (e.g., "spinal taps," skin or muscle biopsies, or X-rays used in conjunction with contrast dyes) must be used if a desired measurement is to be made. Although research designed to generate information about normal physiology or a disease process is not concerned with evaluating a medical intervention, it may still require the use of invasive procedures. When the research deals with subjects whose condition is not normal, the research can have either therapeutic or nontherapeutic purposes.

Clinical and Health Services Research

Clinical research and health services research are two specialized areas of biomedical research. Clinical research is the disease-oriented, often patient-centered, component of biomedical research; it aims to understand human disease, prevent and treat illness, and promote health. All basic biomedical advances must flow through this "neck of the scientific bottle" in order to have real world benefit for the public. New discoveries in genetics, bioengineering, neuroscience, and molecular and structural biology cannot be demonstrated to have practical benefit unless clinical researchers translate this science into new and effective medical practices and products (hence, the term **"translational research"**). Clinical research follows the general process outlined in Figure 2.3.

Health services research refers to studies conducted with access to, and consumption of, health care services; it focuses on utilization, costs, quality, delivery, organization, financing, and outcomes. It is a multidisciplinary field of inquiry that draws on researchers from biostatistics, epidemiology, health economics, nursing, operations research, psychology, medical sociology, and medicine.

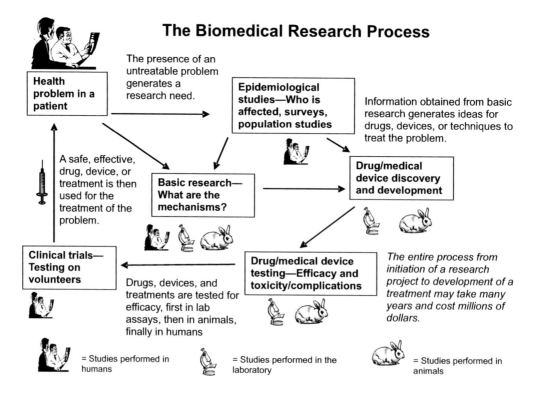

FIGURE 2.3. The Biomedical Research Process. *Source:* "The Process of Biomedical Research." Available at <www.ahc.umn.edu/rar/MNAALAS/Research_overview.pdf>.

The spectacular research accomplishments of the past half century have created tremendous scientific and medical advances, but they have also given rise to the potential for conflicts of interest (situations in which financial or other personal considerations have the potential to compromise the professional judgment of faculty conducting research). The Blue Ridge Academic Health Group has identified six categories of faculty relationships that give rise to conflicts of interest: research, consulting, licensing, equity, training, and gift relationships.[42] All of these relationships can make sense in the context of a particular situation or transaction, yet each carries varying degrees of secondary interest implications that need to be known and in many cases managed or prohibited.

Compliance and Regulatory Issues

The federal government and industry have traditionally maintained relatively distinct foci. Industry has tended to concentrate on applications and development of health-related technology, with the bulk of its investments spent in commercial laboratories and clinical trials. The federal government, on the other hand, has been the chief sponsor of basic, clinical, and public health research, conducted primarily by academic institutions, federal laboratories, and some private research institutions and organizations. Today these distinctions are becoming blurred and present tremendous implications for health care financing, quality of care, intellectual property rights, and medical ethics. The research agenda for the biotechnology industry, for example, extensively overlaps that of academe, is the domain of much collaborative research, and also the source of many questions about intellectual property rights ownership, scholarly communications, public trust, and conflicts of interest. Biomedical research tended to have little commercial value in an earlier era, but today, such research can provide the immediate foundation for lucrative commercial ventures.

Patient privacy was also of marginal concern in the days before large computer databases and the **electronic medical record (EMR).** This changed in 2001 when the Department of Health and Human Services, in response to a mandate written into the 1996 Health Insurance Portability and Accountability Act (HIPAA), issued the **Privacy Rule** to protect the privacy and confidentiality of individuals' personal health information and to give patients increased access to their medical records.[43] The Privacy Rule, which included requirements for burdensome patient forms and accounting requirements, encompassed nearly all medical records. The saga of the Privacy Rule, its subsequent revisions, and its effects are illustrative of the challenge faced by society in balancing individual privacy and promoting public health.

Although infrequent, violations of patient privacy and instances of scientific fraud and misconduct are serious threats to the integrity of science and undermine public trust and confidence. The health care community has a duty to uphold the core components of the responsible conduct of research: proper use of data acquisition, management, sharing, and ownership; ethical authorship and publication practices; reliance on peer review and integrity in collaborative research; ethical treatment of human subjects and research involving animals; proper procedures for assessing allegations of research misconduct; and policies addressing conflicts of interest and commitment.

THE FUTURE OF ACADEMIC MEDICINE

Indeed, the contribution of medicine to human health over the last century has been extraordinary. New genetic technologies, rapid advances in cell and molecular biology, and imaging technologies promise even more innovation and progress. Recent investments in academic medicine, most notably in the United States and the United Kingdom, are unparalleled. However, several national reports suggest that the prospect for medicine to lead the way into the twenty-first century may be in doubt,[36, 44-50] and critics are becoming increasingly concerned that medicine, particularly academic medicine whose value is not self-evident, is in crisis around the world.[51-56] Indeed, the lack of basic infrastructure in many countries has meant that academic medicine is floundering, if not absent. Even the current funding in industrialized countries may be wasted if structural changes are not made to allow academic medicine to capitalize on new investments and realize its global social responsibility.[49, 57, 58]

There is a fair amount of agreement about the threats and opportunities facing academic medicine; primarily these are as follows:

1. Rapid scientific development, particularly in genetics and information technology
2. Emergent diseases
3. Climate change
4. Health systems' failure to operate optimally in the areas of safety, quality, access, responsiveness, affordability
5. Increasing health burden
6. Aging of populations
7. A lack of capacity in translational research
8. A substantial gap between what actually happens in medical practice and what evidence suggests should happen

There is widespread, even universal, agreement that things are not right, but little agreement on the exact nature of the problem. Forums that have discussed this topic, mostly in the United States, United Kingdom, and Canada, report that academic medicine is in decline or is at least unprepared for future demands.[36, 44, 47, 49] However, this diagnosis is neither entirely clear nor consistent across settings (see Table 2.2), and the treatment is unknown. The stated reasons for this decline vary but include both internal factors (increasing pressures on clinical academic staff, the absence of a clear and flexible career structure for young doctors, and uncertainty about future job prospects and security) and external factors (globalization, loss of faith in expert knowledge, increased public accountability, aging populations, and fiscal restraint). Many people even in wealthier countries like the United States and the United Kingdom worry that the recent surge of funding will be wasted if structural changes are not made to allow academic medicine to capitalize on the new investments, such as creating more attractive and flexible career paths.[49, 57, 58]

Challenges to Academic Medicine

One of the biggest challenges facing academic medicine is the lack of capacity for translational research. What brings innovations directly to patients has impeded the translation of basic science discoveries into clinical studies and of clinical studies into medical practice and health decisions.[59] Those factors contributing to poor translation of research include the following: high costs, slow results, lack of funding, regulatory burdens, fragmented infrastructure, incompatible databases, a shortage of qualified investigators and willing participants, the lack of research funding for clinical trials, inadequate facilities to undertake patient-oriented clinical research, limited numbers of clinical academics, increasingly complex legal and ethical governance issues, and failings in health services.[46]

A second challenge facing academic medicine is the "know-do" gap between what is known about diseases and what is done to prevent and treat them. Studies in the United States and the Netherlands suggest that 30 percent to 40 percent of patients do not receive care commensurate with current scientific evidence, and that 20 percent to 25 percent of the care that is provided is

TABLE 2.2. Reports and Recommendations of Major National Academic Medicine Organizations

Country	Organization	Publication	Major Challenges Identified
United Kingdom	Academy of Medical Sciences	*Clinical Medicine in Jeopardy: Recommendations for Change* (June 2002)	Prolonged training
			Early financial distinctions
			Tensions between the responsibilities of teaching, research, and clinical service
			Need to promote academic medicine and make it once more an attractive career
	Academy of Medical Sciences	*Strengthening Clinical Research* (October 2003)	Clinical research not keeping pace with advances in basic scientific discovery, putting patients at a disadvantage
	Royal College of Physicians Academy of Medical Royal Colleges	*Clinical Academic Medicine: The Way Forward* (November 2004)	How to address the need to recruit more clinical staff
			How to make the academic career path more attractive and achievable
	Nuffield Trust Association of Academic Health Centers Association of Canadian Medical Colleges	*The Challenge to Academic Medicine: Leading or Following?* (January 2005)	Need for academic health sciences centers to get their own houses in order
			Transparency and accountability for handling funds
			Value of work to individuals, populations, and the economy
United States	Commonwealth Fund Task Force on Academic Health Centers	*Envisioning the Future of Academic Health Centers* (February 2003)	How to increase the efficiencies, organization, and infrastructure of existing academic health centers
	Institute of Medicine of the National Academies	*Academic Health Centers: Leading Change in the 21st Century* (July 2003)	How to make academic health centers less independent and more interdependent and complementary
	Association of Academic Medical Colleges	*Education Doctors to Provide High Quality Medicine: A Vision for Medical Education in the United States* (July 2004)	How to remedy shortcomings in the way physicians are educated

not needed or could be harmful.[60] Health sciences librarians can help lessen this gap by providing access to the best evidence-based medicine information. Further, the demand for more effective "working alliances" at many levels (between managed care organizations and health sciences centers, between clinicians and researchers, and between librarians and library users) remains and contradicts the goals of providing high-quality health care.[61]

A third challenge is the increasing difficulty for a person to be competent simultaneously in practice, research, and teaching. Because of the enormous time pressures and competing demands of research, teaching, and clinical practice, many people believe that the traditional triad has become untenable. As the chief medical officer in England argued, "In the past, clinical academics were required to fulfill multiple roles—researcher, teacher, administrator, professional leader—but the growing demands in all these areas means that today's 'jack of all trades' will be master of none."[55]

The lack of appropriate measures for assessing the contribution that teaching makes to medicine is a fourth major challenge. Traditional research assessment exercises often overemphasize the value of basic research, underemphasize the importance of applied research, and may distort the integrated approach to clinical practice, teaching, and research. This tends to discourage those wholly funded by research and/or physicians from teaching.

A fifth challenge at the heart of current challenges to academic medicine is the absence of a clear career path that is complicated by the lack of flexible training opportunities, insufficient mentoring, difficulties in obtaining research funding, and indebtedness. In the United States, 50 percent fewer of the current medical students have expressed interest in a research career.[62] An article by Goldacre and his colleagues regarding junior doctors in the United Kingdom suggests that even though the intellectual challenge of academic medicine is appealing, the difficulties in obtaining solid research funding and uncertainty regarding pay parity with clinical colleagues are significant disincentives.[63] Some evidence also indicates that indebtedness reduces the likelihood that doctors will choose academic medicine as their primary activity. In most countries, those doctors who pursue a career in research are likely to earn much less than those who spend at least some time in private practice. A recent American study found that 98 percent of its respondents cited the lack of mentoring as the first or second greatest obstacle to a successful career,[64] and a growing body of research suggests that women ascend the ranks of academic medicine more slowly, to lower levels, and with less pay than do their male colleagues.[65-67]

These challenges are compounded in a global context by what is referred to as the **10:90 gap** (10 percent of global spending for health research is allocated to the health problems of 90 percent of the population). As an example, diseases for which there is little market value for drug development have been particularly neglected. Additionally, critics of academic medicine also believe that undergraduate, graduate, and continuing medical education have not kept pace with patients' needs, public expectations, technological advances, and changing organizational requirements and financing. Nor is medical education in sync with the goal of bringing high-quality health care into the twenty-first century. Thus far it has failed to be adequately patient-centered, team-oriented, and evidence-based.[68, 69]

The incursion of the marketplace into academic medicine is a sixth challenge and is worrisome for fear that academic values are being lost and that medical education is compromised by commercial interests. However, academic medicine must rely on private funding, especially in developing countries where there is a lack of basic infrastructure and few formal medical organizations. This challenge is made more difficult by the fact that academic medicine leadership is sometimes inadequate and misses opportunities to lead efforts in the innovation, early application, and dissemination of new knowledge.

Academic medicine leadership fails too often to engage with the wider health community and local interests and fails to spend enough time interacting with citizen and patient groups and practitioners, despite the importance of ensuring that the agenda of academic medicine properly reflects the concerns of populations.[70] Other people believe that academic medicine has failed to position itself adequately as part of global health human resources and as part of a health sciences profession that includes nursing, public health, social work, and other stakeholders.[61]

Drivers of the Future

Much of what will determine the future of academic medicine lies outside the control of the medical academics themselves. As the world changes around them, they must follow. But change will come from inside academic medicine, and its leaders must be prepared to face the drivers of the future. A report by the International Campaign to Revitalise Academic Medicine (ICRAM)[71] and three similar and simultaneous publications about current challenges to, and alternative futures for, academic medicine have identified twenty drivers of change in academic medicine:

1. New science and technology, particularly genetics and information technology
2. The rise of sophisticated consumers
3. The feminization of medicine
4. Globalization
5. Emergent diseases
6. The increasing gap between rich and poor
7. The unimportance of distance (i.e., no longer means being remote)
8. The demand for more from health care by "big hungry buyers"
9. The spread of the Internet and digitalization
10. Managerialism
11. Increasing anxieties about security
12. The expanding gap between what can be done and what can be afforded in health care
13. The lack of agreement on where "health" begins and ends; continuum of care
14. The aging of society
15. The increasing accountability of all institutions
16. The loss of respect for experts
17. The rise of self-care
18. The rise of ethical issues, including conflicts of interest
19. The 24/7 society
20. The economic and political rise of China and India

Future Scenarios for Academic Medicine

The ICRAM group also suggested five future scenarios for academic medicine given the current instabilities and the driving forces noted previously. The scenarios span a period of twenty years, although some of their scenarios are more futuristic than others. They are not predictions, but a range of plausible stories about the future.

Scenario 1: Academic, Inc.

The first scenario was that research and teaching will move increasingly into the private sector. Big globally successful medical schools will swallow smaller schools. Competition among schools for most talented staff will become intense. Governments will continue to buy places in medical schools, but it's still mostly in the private sector. The way to survive would *not* be to try to compete head-on with comprehensive, top-ranked schools, but actually to do something in a niche, such as surgery or rural health. Research will go on mostly in the private sector, and in a very wide range of organizations, big and small. Perhaps because it will be necessary to produce a return on investment on this research, it will become increasingly relevant, addressing the problem that a lot of research at the moment isn't as relevant as should be.

In this scenario, this author sees many implications for health sciences librarians and libraries. It may mean that librarians will assume a greater role in assisting in niche training. Most libraries will have an information commons and will rely more heavily on data to justify their existence. Less federal funding will be available for libraries, and library foundation grants will become a larger source of supplemental income for them. Libraries may employ more customer satisfaction surveys with emphasis on outcomes measurements, and concerns about patient safety may permeate the library community in the sense of leaders and administrators seeing librarians as having a crucial role in improving safety.

Scenario 2: Reformation

The reformation scenario envisaged the end of medical schools, that teaching, learning, research, and quality improvement will take place in the practice setting and will be everybody's business. It would be a return in many ways to the kind of apprenticeship that existed before medical schools were established—very much a team enterprise. Although people will work in teams, nobody will be expected to be competent in all aspects of what's needed to research and teach, so there will be highly professional teachers and researchers in the team, but they'll be very directly related to practice. Much of the teaching will be done by patients. Research will grow directly out of questions arising from practice, addressing this problem of relevance. Leadership in this world will come not from medical schools or universities, but increasingly from specialist societies. Learning will be essentially by doing.

Should this scenario come to pass, this author believes it is more likely that more and more knowledge-based information databases will need to be made available, and existing libraries will survive by offering specialized or "boutique" services. Advanced learning and communications technologies, often supported by the virtual library, will encourage a team approach frequently led by an informationist. A national question-answering service will provide evidence-based responses to research questions that come from interactions between professionals and patients, but few librarians with specialized skills will be involved in the service. Fewer library associations will exist, especially at local and regional levels. The library will play a critical role in teaching students to first learn how to learn and then learn by doing. Difficulty in achieving consensus and stability among teams will create a need for changing and diverse library services, and where today there are thousands of journals sold on subscriptions, there will be thousands of editorially intensive databases also sold on subscriptions, many of them probably sold by existing science publishers.

Scenario 3: In the Public Eye

The third scenario is almost Orwell's Big Brother world, so success in this academic world comes from delighting patients and the public, using the media very effectively. The most successful academics are those who are very responsive to patients and the public. Some medical academics will become as well-known as film and rock stars and be feted by politicians. All academic institutions will become dominated by public citizens and patients, and the public and media relations department will be the most important department in any institution. Money will follow the public interest, much of the medical training again will be done by expert patients, and the competition for celebrity teachers will be very intense.

Here, libraries will focus on outreach services. Their role in training will diminish. The form and size of the library, and the parent institution, will range widely; some institutions will have a physical library, but most will not. Librarians will become more anxious about their job security and ability to succeed. Health information will become essentially unregulated, and information vendors will employ massive public relations campaigns to combat negative perceptions of their products and to hype, often with unfounded evidence, their superiority over other products.

Scenario 4: Global Academic Partnership

The fourth scenario foresaw a world where closing the global poverty gap is the most important thing on the agenda. This is a world where academic medicine takes a lead in this whole enterprise, and where money, prestige, and excitement lie with global health, rather than in doing drug trials on hypertension. Academic institutions form north-south partnerships; it becomes absolutely essential to be linked with an institution in the south. The brain drain is reversed; instead of smart people coming from south Asia to Britain or the United States, they begin to go the other way because that's where the action is, that's where the money is, that's where the problems are.

For health sciences librarians and libraries this could mean that a global network of libraries of medicine will become increasingly essential as information is cataloged and organized in disparate locations. Library collections may include several languages and/or the library will assist in providing electronic translation services. It will become increasingly difficult to distinguish public, academic, and health sciences libraries from one another.

Scenario 5: Fully Engaged

The last scenario may be the one nearest to current experience: academics recognize that it's very important to reach out energetically to the public, practitioners, and politicians. Faculty can't sit in an ivory tower and hope people will appreciate how wonderful they are; they've got to go out and market and promote themselves. Gowns will be out and focus groups will be in, trying to work out what it is that the world wants. Academies will be transformed into modern politically and media savvy organizations, often led by nonacademics who will recognize that they often don't have those skills that are essential for survival in this world. Medical students will become the drivers of medical education. Academic institutions will become the center of a vibrant community of patients, members of the public, practitioners of all stripes, policymakers, members of the media, marketing experts, and politicians, all of whom are interested in learning, studying, researching, and thinking about health care.

In this scenario, library, information technology, and medical professional associations will merge. Some form of library radio outreach show may return, probably in an Internet podcast version. The medical departmental library will go the way of the dodo bird, as electronic knowledge-based information resources become even more "user-friendly" but not necessarily more reliable as a search tool. Information professionals will have interesting opportunities to define their roles and contributions.

CONCLUSION

At no time in the history of medicine has the growth in knowledge and technologies been so profound, and the opportunities for health sciences libraries to build positive relationships with health care providers have never been greater. Since the first contemporary randomized controlled trial was conducted more than fifty years ago, the number of trials conducted has grown to nearly 10,000 annually.[72] The budget for NIH has doubled within the last five years to over $16 billion, and the investment by pharmaceutical firms in research and development has increased from $12 billion to $24 billion.[39] Genomics and other new technologies on the horizon offer the promise of further increasing longevity, improving health and functioning, and alleviating pain and suffering. Advances in rehabilitation, cell restoration, and prosthetic devices hold potential for improving health and functioning of many with disabilities.

However, the health care delivery system has not always been able to provide consistently high-quality health care or to keep pace with the rapid advances in medical science and technology. Research on the quality of care also reveals that today's health care systems often fall short in their ability to translate knowledge into practice, and to apply new technology safely and appropriately. The performance of health care systems varies considerably; the U.S. health care system may be exemplary, but many millions of Americans still fail to receive effective care. Aging populations and increased demands for new services, technologies, and drugs are increasing health care expenditures. Although improving, the health care delivery system remains highly fragmented and lacks sufficient interoperable clinical information systems. Mergers, acquisitions, and affiliations have been commonplace within health plans, hospitals, and physician practices. Physician groups, hospitals, and other health care organizations often operate as silos, providing care without the benefit of complete information about the patient's condition, medical history, services provided in other settings, or medications prescribed by other clinicians.[73] Fixing existing deficiencies in our health care delivery systems is not easy. It requires (1) applying evidence to health care delivery, (2) using information technology, (3) aligning payment policies with quality improvement, and (4) preparing the workforce.

Within this setting the health sciences library is affecting and being affected by a host of changes, including these:

1. A more diverse faculty and student body
2. The globalization and internationalization of institutional missions and outreach
3. The ability to deliver quality content to users' desktops
4. The shift from print-based collections to digitized collections
5. Rapidly emerging copyright and intellectual property issues
6. Contractual and organizational issues around shared storage and nonduplication of resources
7. The necessity for reorganizing and/or creating new physical workspaces for new forms of work[74, 75]

Health sciences libraries and librarians also share an increasingly important role in ensuring that patients receive care based on the best available scientific knowledge, and in promoting information transparency so that information is available to patients and health care providers to allow them to make more informed decisions. Librarians also have an enormous potential to transform health care by forming new partnerships with their constituents, by creating cooperative learning information centers, and by participating in the development and use of information technology applications in such areas as consumer health, professional education, public health, clinical care, and biomedical and health services research. Taking advantage of new information technologies will be an important catalyst to moving health care beyond where it is today and improving librarians' consultative and teaching roles.

For health sciences libraries and librarians, preparing the workforce will be among the most critical challenges. Issues related to library staffing, recruitment and retention, staff development and training, career paths, culture, leadership, organization, changing constituencies or communities, innovation and collaboration, and globalization are highly related to changes in the health care system. The ability of the profession to attract younger people is a growing concern, and there are a number of primary barriers to supporting currency in staff knowledge and skills. Yet, there are opportunities to deliver training and learning as well as opportunities for professional and support staff to advance and/or pursue related careers. The desirable characteristics of the library organization are likely to change as it responds to a changing environment, continuing changes in primary clients, and new developments in scholarly communications.

APPENDIX 2.A. SELECTED FEDERAL LEGISLATION
WITH IMPORTANT HEALTH ASPECTS,
INCLUDING HEALTH CARE INFORMATION POLICY LEGISLATION
(IN CHRONOLOGICAL ORDER)

The COPYRIGHT ACT OF 1790 was the first federal copyright act to be instituted in the United States, though most of the states had passed various legislation securing copyrights in the years immediately following the Revolutionary War. The stated object of the act was the "encouragement of learning," and it achieved this by securing authors the "sole right and liberty of printing, reprinting, publishing and vending" the copies of their "maps, charts, and books" for a term of fourteen years, with the right to renew for one additional fourteen-year term should the copyright holder still be alive.

The MERCHANT MARINE SERVICES ACT OF 1798 provided health services to U.S. seamen by taxing the employers of merchant seamen; the act funded the arrangements for their health care through the Marine Hospital Services.

The GENERAL IMMIGRATION LAWS OF 1882 included the first medical excludability provisions affecting those who wished to immigrate to the United States. It authorized state officials to board arriving ships to examine the condition of passengers.

The INTERNATIONAL COPYRIGHT ACT is the first U.S. congressional act that extended limited protection to foreign copyright holders from select nations. Formally known as the "International Copyright Act of 1891," but more commonly referred to as the "Chace Act" after Senator Jonathan Chace of Rhode Island, the act went into effect on July 1, 1891. On July 3, 1891, the first foreign work, a play called Saints and Sinners by British author Henry Arthur Jones, was registered under the act.

The BIOLOGICS CONTROL ACT was passed in the United States on July 1, 1902, after two incidents involving the deaths of children caused by contaminated vaccines. The act established the Center for Biologics Evaluation and Research (CBER), which was placed under the authority of the NIH by the Public Health Service Act of 1944, and became one of the centers of the Food and Drug Administration (FDA) in 1972. Although it was signed with much less fanfare than the Pure Food and Drug Act, the Biologics Control Act set a precedent for federal regulation of biological products.

The PURE FOOD AND DRUG ACT OF 1906 provided for federal inspection of meat products and forbade the manufacture, sale, or transportation of adulterated food products or poisonous patent medicines. The act arose due to public education and propaganda from people such as authors Upton Sinclair and Samuel Hopkins Adams, researcher Harvey W. Wiley, and President Theodore Roosevelt.

The COPYRIGHT ACT OF 1909 was a landmark statute in U.S. statutory copyright law. The act was superseded by the Copyright Act of 1976, but it remains effective for copyrighted works created before the 1976 act went into effect in 1978. It allowed for works to be copyrighted for a period of twenty-eight years from the date of publication, renewable once for a second twenty-eight-year term. As in the preceding Copyright Act of 1790, the copyrighted work could be extended for a second term of equal value. Under the 1909 act, federal statutory copyright protection attached to original works only when those works were (1) published and (2) had a notice of copyright affixed. Thus, state copyright law governed protection for unpublished works, but published works, whether containing a notice of copyright or not, were governed exclusively by federal law. If no notice of copyright was affixed to a work and the work was "published" in a legal sense, the 1909 act provided no copyright protection and the work became part of the public domain. The 1976 act changed this result, providing that copyright protection attaches to works that are original and fixed in a tangible medium of expression, regardless of publication or affixation of notice.

The SNYDER ACT OF 1920 was the first federal legislation to deal with health care for Native Americans.

The RANDSDELL ACT OF 1930 created the National Institutes of Health from the Hygienic Laboratory.

The FEDERAL FOOD, DRUG, AND COSMETIC ACT (FD&C) is a set of laws passed by Congress in 1938 giving authority to the Food and Drug Administration to oversee the safety of food, drugs, and cosmetics. In 1968, the Electronic Product Radiation Control provisions were added to the FD&C. Also in that year the FDA formed the Drug Efficacy Study Implementation (DESI) to incorporate into FD&C regulations the recommendations from a National Academy of Sciences investigation of effectiveness of previously marketed drugs. The act was amended by the FDA Modernization Act of 1997.

The HOSPITAL SURVEY AND CONSTRUCTION ACT, also known as the HILL-BURTON ACT, was passed in 1946. This act responded to the first of Truman's proposals and was designed to provide federal grants and guaranteed loans to improve the physical plans of the nation's hospital system. Money was designated to the states to achieve 4.5 beds per 1,000 people. The states allocated the available money to their various municipalities, but the law provided for a rotation mechanism, so that an area that received funding moved to the bottom of the list for further funding. Hill-Burton was set to expire in June 1973, but it was extended for one year in the last hour. In 1975, the act was amended and became Title 16 of the Public Health Service Act.

The PUBLIC HEALTH SERVICE ACT OF 1944 specified a role for the U.S. Public Health Service (PHS) in working with state and local health departments; revised and consolidated into one place all existing legislation pertaining to the PHS; provided for the organization, staffing, and functions and activities of the PHS; and allowed use of quarantines and inspections for the control of communicable diseases.

The INVENTION SECRECY ACT OF 1951 is a body of U.S. federal law designed to prevent disclosure of new inventions and technologies that, in the opinion of selected federal agencies, present a possible threat to the "national security" of the United States.

The FEDERAL EMPLOYEES HEALTH BENEFIT ACT OF 1959 permitted Blue Cross to negotiate a contract with the Civil Service Commission to provide health care coverage for federal employees.

The HEALTH PROFESSION EDUCATION ASSISTANCE ACT OF 1963 (an amendment to the Public Health Service Act) provided construction grants for facilities that train physicians, nurses, dentists, podiatrists, pharmacists, and public health professionals.

The NURSE TRAINING ACT OF 1964 added a new title, Title 8, to the Public Health Service Act; the act authorized separate funding in construction grants for schools of nursing.

The SOCIAL SECURITY ACT OF 1965 established Medicare and Medicaid. It did so by "liberating" the Social Security Trust Fund, changing its funding from a forced savings type of an account into a "pay as you go" type of fund. This system has caused concerns about its long-term stability.

The MEDICAL LIBRARY ASSISTANCE ACT (MLAA) was passed in 1965 to correct the imbalance between medical library resources and information needs of the health professional and to enable the NLM to (1) initiate programs to assist the nation's medical libraries and (2) develop a medical library network with the establishment of regional medical libraries to link the NLM with local institutions.

The CIGARETTE LABELING AND ADVERTISING ACT OF 1965 is a comprehensive act designed to provide a set of national standards for cigarette packaging, including the label "Caution: Cigarette Smoking May Be Hazardous to Your Health."

The COMMUNITY HEALTH SERVICES AND FACILITIES ACT, one of the important factors of the 1965 Community Health Centers Act, mandated appropriate mental health services for the younger population.

The NOISE CONTROL ACT OF 1972 continued government efforts to rid the environment of harmful influences on human health.

The CONSUMER PRODUCT SAFETY ACT OF 1972 created the Consumer Product Safety Commission to develop safety standards for consumer products.

The HEALTH MAINTENANCE ORGANIZATION ACT OF 1973, also known as the HMO ACT OF 1973, provided grants and loans to provide, start, or expand an HMO; removed certain state restrictions for federally qualified HMOs; and required employers with twenty-five or more employees to offer federally certified HMO options alongside traditional indemnity insurance upon request.

The OLDER AMERICANS ACT OF 1973 established the National Clearinghouse for Information on Aging and created the Federal Council on Aging.

The NATIONAL HEALTH PLANNING AND RESOURCES DEVELOPMENT ACT, or PUBLIC LAW 93-641, was passed in 1974. The act consolidated three distinct existing programs: *Hill-Burton Act, Regional Medical Programs,* and *Comprehensive Health Planning Act.* Congress realized that the provision of federal funds for the construction of new health care facilities was contributing to increasing health care costs by generating duplication of facilities. The intent of Congress in passing this act was to create, throughout the United States, a strengthened and improved federal-, state-, and area-wide system of health planning and resources development that would help provide solutions to several identified problems.

The COPYRIGHT ACT OF 1976 is a landmark statute in U.S. copyright legislation and remains the primary basis of copyright law in the United States. The act spelled out the basic rights of copyright holders, codified the doctrine of "fair use," and converted the term of copyrights from a fixed period requiring renewal to an extended period based on the date of the creator's death.

The ORPHAN DRUG ACT OF 1982 provided financial incentives for the development and marketing of orphan drugs which are products that treat a rare disease affecting fewer than 200,000 Americans. Since the act was passed, over 100 orphan drugs and biological products have been brought to market.

The NATIONAL ORGAN TRANSPLANT ACT OF 1984 made it illegal to acquire, receive, or transfer any human organ for valuable consideration for use in human transplantation if it involved interstate commerce.

The COMPREHENSIVE SMOKING EDUCATION ACT OF 1984 (also known as the ROTATIONAL WARNING ACT) is an act of the Congress of the United States. It was put in place by the Federal Trade Commission in order to regulate the size, wording, and implementation of warning requirements on tobacco products in the United States.

The DRUG PRICE COMPETITION AND PATENT TERM RESTORATION ACT, informally known as the "Hatch-Waxman Act," is a 1984 U.S. federal law which established the modern system of generic drugs. The informal name comes from the act's two sponsors, Representative Henry Waxman of California and Senator Orrin Hatch of Utah.

The NATIONAL CHILDHOOD VACCINE INJURY ACT (NCVIA) OF 1986 was enacted to reduce the potential financial liability of vaccine makers due to vaccine injury claims. The legislation was aimed at ensuring a stable market supply and providing cost-effective arbitration for vaccine injury claims.

The EMERGENCY MEDICAL TREATMENT AND ACTIVE LABOR ACT passed in 1986 as part of the Consolidated Omnibus Budget Reconciliation Act. It requires hospitals and ambulance services to provide care to anyone needing emergency treatment regardless of citizenship, legal status, or ability to pay. There are no reimbursement provisions; as a result of the act, patients needing emergency treatment can be discharged only under their own informed consent or when their condition requires transfer to a hospital better equipped to administer the treatment.

The AMERICANS WITH DISABILITIES ACT (ADA) OF 1990 provided a broad range of protections for the disabled and thus combined former legislation from the Civil Rights Act of 1964, the Rehabilitation Act of 1973, and the Civil Rights Restoration Act of 1988.

The RADIATION EXPOSURE COMPENSATION ACT (RECA) OF 1990 provides for the monetary compensation of people who contracted cancer and a number of other specified diseases as a direct result of their exposure to atmospheric nuclear testing, undertaken by the United States during the Cold War, or their exposure to high levels of radon while working in uranium mines.

The PATIENT SELF-DETERMINATION ACT passed in 1990 requires most hospitals to give patients information on state laws regarding advance directives, such as living wills.

AUDIO HOME RECORDING ACT (AHRA) OF 1992 amended the U.S. Copyright Act by adding Chapter 10, "Digital Audio Recording Devices and Media." The act was prompted by the release of the Sony Digital Audio Tape (DAT). The Recording Industry Association of America (RIAA), concerned that consumers' ability to make perfect digital copies of music would destroy the market for audio recordings, had lobbied Congress to pass the legislation.

The FREEDOM OF ACCESS TO CLINIC ENTRANCES ACT (FACE or the ACCESS ACT), passed in 1994, prohibits the use of intimidation or physical force to prevent or discourage persons from (1) gaining access to a reproductive health care facility (which most notably includes abortion clinics) or (2) exercising freedom to worship at a religious facility. The law also creates specific penalties for the destruction of, or damage to, a reproductive health care facility or place of religious worship.

The NEWBORNS' AND MOTHERS' HEALTH PROTECTION ACT OF 1996 requires plans that offer maternity coverage to pay for at least a forty-eight-hour hospital stay following childbirth (ninety-six-hour stay in the case of a cesarean section).

The MENTAL HEALTH PARITY ACT (MHPA) is legislation of 1996 and requires that annual or lifetime dollar limits on mental health benefits be no lower than any such dollar limits for medical and surgical benefits offered by a group health plan or health insurance issuer offering coverage in connection with a group health plan.

The HEALTH CENTER CONSOLIDATION ACT OF 1996 in the United States is commonly also called SECTION 330. The act brings together various funding mechanisms for the country's community health facilities, such as migrant/seasonal farmworker health centers, health care for the homeless, and health centers for residents of public housing. Previously, each of these organizations was provided grants under numerous other mechanisms.

The HEALTH INSURANCE PORTABILITY AND ACCOUNTABILITY ACT (HIPAA) was enacted in 1996. According to the Centers for Medicare and Medicaid Services' (CMS) Web site, Title 1 of HIPAA protects health insurance coverage for workers and their families when they change or lose their jobs. Title 2 of HIPAA, the Administrative Simplification (AS) provisions, requires the establishment of national standards for electronic health care transactions and national identifiers for providers, health insurance plans, and employers. The AS provisions also address the security and privacy of health data. The standards are meant to improve the efficiency and effectiveness of the nation's health care system by encouraging the widespread use of electronic data interchange in the U.S. health care system.

The NO ELECTRONIC THEFT ACT (NET ACT), a federal law passed in 1997, provides for criminal prosecution of individuals who engage in copyright infringement, even when there is no monetary profit or commercial benefit from the infringement. Maximum penalties can be five years in prison and up to $250,000 in fines. The NET Act also raised statutory damages by 50 percent.

The BALANCED BUDGET ACT OF 1997 was signed into law on August 5, 1997. It was an omnibus legislative package enacted using the budget reconciliation process and designed to balance the federal budget by 2002. Among many other things, the act contained major Medicare reforms.

The DIGITAL MILLENNIUM COPYRIGHT ACT (DMCA) OF 1998 criminalizes production and dissemination of technology that can circumvent measures taken to protect copyright, not merely infringement of copyright itself, and heightens the penalties for copyright infringement on the Internet. The DMCA amended Title 17 of the U.S. Code to extend the reach of copyright, while limiting the liability of online providers from copyright infringement by their users.

The WIPO COPYRIGHT AND PERFORMANCES AND PHONOGRAMS TREATIES IMPLEMENTATION ACT, a part of the Digital Millennium Copyright Act, was passed in 1998 and has two major portions, Section 102, which implements the requirements of the WIPO Copyright Treaty, and Section 103, which provides strong protection against the circumvention of copyright protection systems, with narrow exceptions, and prohibits the removal of copyright management information.

The COPYRIGHT TERM EXTENSION ACT OF 1998—alternatively known as the SONNY BONO COPYRIGHT TERM EXTENSION ACT or pejoratively as the MICKEY MOUSE PROTECTION ACT—extended copyright terms in the United States by twenty years. Before the act (under the Copyright Act of 1976), copyright would last for the life of the author plus fifty years, or seventy-five years for a work of corporate authorship; the act extended these terms to life of the author plus seventy years and ninety-five years, respectively. The act also affected copyright terms for copyrighted works published prior to January 1, 1978, increasing their term of protection by twenty years as well.

The WOMEN'S HEALTH AND CANCER RIGHTS ACT (WHCRA), passed in 1998, contains protections for patients who elect breast reconstruction in connection with a mastectomy. For plan participants and beneficiaries receiving benefits in connection with a mastectomy, plans offering coverage for a mastectomy must also cover reconstructive surgery and other benefits related to a mastectomy.

The PATRIOT ACT (UNITING AND STRENGTHENING AMERICA BY PROVIDING APPROPRIATE TOOLS REQUIRED TO INTERCEPT AND OBSTRUCT TERRORISM ACT) was signed into law in 2001. Among laws the U.S. PATRIOT Act amended are immigration laws, banking laws, and money laundering laws. It also amends the Foreign Intelligence Surveillance Act (FISA).

The TEACH ACT (TECHNOLOGY, EDUCATION AND COPYRIGHT HARMONIZATION ACT) was signed into law in 2002. Long anticipated by educators and librarians, TEACH redefines the terms and conditions on which accredited, nonprofit educational institutions throughout the United States may use copyright-protected materials in distance education—including on Web sites and by other digital means—without permission from the copyright owner and without payment of royalties.

The MEDICARE PRESCRIPTION DRUG, IMPROVEMENT, AND MODERNIZATION ACT (also called "MMA legislation") was enacted in 2003. It produced the largest overhaul of Medicare in its thirty-eight-year history.

The PARTIAL-BIRTH ABORTION BAN ACT (OR "PBA BAN") OF 2003 prohibits intact dilation and extraction, commonly known as "partial-birth abortion." Any person or physician found guilty of violating this law shall be fined or imprisoned not more than two years, or both. The bill "does not apply to a partial-birth abortion that is necessary to save the life of a mother whose life is endangered by a physical disorder, physical illness, or physical injury, including a life-endangering physical condition caused by or arising from the pregnancy itself."

The PENSION PROTECTION ACT OF 2006, the first major overhaul of the nation's pension laws since the Employee Retirement Income Security Act was enacted in 1974 includes provisions that would change the funding requirements for defined benefit plans and the way plan sponsors calculate their pension fund liabilities.

REFERENCES

1. Schuster, M.; McGlynn, E.; and Brook, H.R. "How Good Is the Quality of Health Care in the United States?" *Milbank Quarterly* 76, no. 4 (1998): 517-63.

2. Starr, P. *The Social Transformation of American Medicine.* New York: Basic Books, Inc., 1982.

3. Flexner, A. *Medical Education in the United States and Canada.* New York: Carnegie Foundation for the Advancement of Science, 1910.

4. Raffel, M.W. *The U.S. Health System, Origins and Functions.* 2nd ed. New York: John Wiley & Sons, Inc., 1984.

5. Bush, V. *Science—The Endless Frontier.* Washington, DC: U.S. Office of Scientific Research and Development, 1945.

6. Grumbach, K., and Bodenheimer, T. "The Organization of Health Care." *JAMA; Journal of the American Medical Association* 273, no. 2 (January 11, 1995): 160-7.

7. Levit, K.R.; Lazenby, H.C.; Sivarajan, L.; et al. "National Health Expenditures, 1994." *Health Care Financing Review* 17, no. 3 (Spring 1996b): 205-42.

8. Centers for Medicare & Medicaid Services, Office of the Actuary, National Health Statistics Group, 2007. Available: <http://www.cms.hhs.gov/>. Accessed: March 22, 2007.

9. Moscovice, I. "Health Care Professionals." Chapter 14 in *Introduction to Health Services,* edited by S.J. Williams and R.R. Torrens. New York: John Wiley and Sons, Inc., 1988.

10. Kronenfeld, J.J., and Whicker, M.L. *Captive Populations: Caring for the Young, the Sick, the Imprisoned, and the Elderly.* New York: Praeger, 1990.

11. Edwards, W.O., and Fisher, C.R. "Medicare Physician and Hospital Utilization and Expenditure Trends." *Health Care Financing Review* 11, no. 2 (Winter 1989): 111-6.

12. Lee, P.R., and Benjamin, A.E. "Health Policy and the Politics of Health Care." Chapter 15 in *Introduction to Health Services,* 4th ed., edited by S.J. Williams and P.R. Torrens. Albany, NY: Delmar, 1993.

13. Reagan, M.D. *The New Federalism.* New York: Oxford University Press, 1972.

14. Chelf, C.P. *Public Policymaking in America: Difficult Choices, Limited Solutions.* Santa Monica, CA: Goodyear, 1981.

15. Ross, J.S. "The Committee on the Costs of Medical Care and the History of Health Insurance in the United States." *Einstein Quarterly Journal of Biological Medicine* 19(2002): 129-34.

16. Mantone, J. "The Big Bang: The Hill-Burton Act Put Hospitals in Thousands of Communities and Launched Today's Continuing Healthcare Building Boom." *Modern Healthcare* 35, no. 33 (August 15, 2005): 6-7, 16.

17. Starr, P. *The Logic of Health Care Reform.* [Knoxville, KY]: The Grand Rounds Press, 1992.

18. Abraham, S.E. "The Impact of the Taft-Hartley Act on the Balance of Power in Industrial Relations." *American Business Law Journal* 33, no. 3 (Spring 1996): 341-71.

19. Brown, E.R., and Wyn, R. "Public Policies to Extend Health Care Coverage." Chapter 4 in *Changing the U.S. Health Care Delivery System,* edited by R.M. Anderson, T.H. Rice, and G.F. Kominski. San Francisco, CA: Jossey Bass Publishers, 1996.

20. Martin, P.P., and Weaver, D.A. "Social Security: A Program and Policy History." *Social Security Bulletin* 66, no. 1 (September 2005): 1-15.

21. Kress, J.R. *HMO Handbook: A Guide for Development of Prepaid Group Practice Health Maintenance Organizations.* Rockville, MD: Aspen Systems Corp., 1975.

22. Longest, B.B., Jr. *Health Policy Making in the United States.* Ann Arbor, MI: AUPHA Press, 1994.

23. Russel, C.C., Jr. *Revolution: The New Health Care System Takes Shape.* [Knoxville, KY]: The Grand Rounds Press, 1993.

24. DeParle, N.A. "Celebrating 35 Years of Medicare and Medicaid." *Health Care Financing Review* 22, no. 1 (Fall 2000): 1-7.

25. Beldon, R.J.; Brodie, M.; and Benson, J. "What Happened to Americans' Support for the Clinton Health Plan?" *Health Affairs* 14, no. 2 (Summer 1995): 7-23.

26. Moffitt, R.E. *An Examination of the Bush Health Care Agenda. The Heritage Foundation.* Available: <http://www.heritage.org/Research/HealthCare/bg1804.cfm>. Accessed: September 11, 2006.

27. Clark, J. "Five Futures for Academic Medicine: The ICRAM scenarios." *BMJ; British Medical Journal* 331(July 9, 2005): 101-4.

28. Association of American Medical Colleges. *The Handbook of Academic Medicine.* Washington, DC: AAMC, 2004.

29. Association of American Medical Colleges. *AAMC Data Book: Medical Schools and Teaching Hospitals by the Numbers.* Washington, DC: AAMC, 2006.

30. Mallon, W.T., and Bunton, S.A. *Characteristics of Research Centers and Institutes at U.S. Medical Schools and Universities.* Washington, DC: AAMC, 2005.

31. Research!America. *2005 Investment in U.S. Research.* Alexandria, VA: Research!America, 2006.

32. Liu, M., and Mallon, W.T. "Tenure in Transition: Trends in Basic Science Faculty Appointment Policies at U.S. Medical Schools." *Academic Medicine* 79, no. 3 (March 2004): 205-13.

33. The University Health System Consortium—AAMC Faculty Practice Solutions Center (FPSC). *Faculty Practice Solutions Center (FPSC) Annual Report,* Volume I: *An Emerging Clinical Imperative.* Washington, DC: AAMC, 2006.

34. Van Der Vegt, G.S.; Bunderson, S.J.; and Oosterhof, A. "Expertness Diversity and Interpersonal Helping in Teams: Why Those Who Need the Most Help End Up Getting the Least." *Academy of Management Journal* 49, no. 5 (October 2006): 877-93.

35. Association of American Medical Colleges. *Medical Education Costs and Student Debt: A Working Group Report to the AAMC Governance.* Washington, DC: AAMC, 2005.

36. Association of American Medical Colleges. *Educating Doctors to Provide High Quality Medical Care: A Vision for Medical Education in the United States. Report of the Ad Hoc Committee of Dean*s. Washington, DC: AAMC Institute for Improving Education, 2005.

37. National Board of Medical Examiners. *Subject Examinations: Content Outlines and Sample Items.* NBME, 2003. Available: <http://www.nbme.org/about/publications.asp>. Accessed: November 30, 2006.

38. National Residency Matching Program. Available: <http://www.nrmp.org/>. Accessed: November 29, 2006.

39. National Institutes of Health. Available: <http://www.nih.gov/>. Accessed: December 1, 2006.

40. Veterans Health Administration. Office of Research and Development. Department of Veterans Affairs. *2003 Annual Report: VA Research—Serving Our Nation's Veterans.* Available: <http://www1.va.gov/resdev/>. Accessed: November 15, 2006.

41. NIH. Protecting Human Research Subjects: Institutional Review Board Guidebook. *NIH Guide* 22, no. 29 (August 13, 1993). Available: <http://grants.nih.gov/grants/guide/notice-files/not93-209.html>. Accessed: October 17, 2006.

42. The Blue Ridge Academic Health Group. *Managing Conflict of Interests in AHCs to Assure Healthy Industrial and Societal Relationships.* Report 10, September 2006. Atlanta, GA: Emery University, 2006.

43. Wilson, J.F. "Health Insurance Portability and Accountability Act Privacy Rule Causes Ongoing Concerns Among Clinicians and Researchers." *Annals of Internal Medicine* 145, no. 4 (August 15, 2006): 313-6.

44. Academy of Medical Sciences. "The Tenure Track Clinician Scientist: A New Career Pathway to Promote Recruitment in Clinical Academic Medicine." *The Savill Report.* London: Academy of Medical Sciences, 2000.

45. Academy of Medical Sciences. *Clinical Academic Medicine in Jeopardy: Recommendations for Change.* London: Academy of Medical Sciences, 2002.

46. Academy of Medical Sciences. *From Laboratory to Clinic—Translating Medical Science into Patient Benefit.* London: Academy of Medical Sciences, 2003.

47. Academy of Medical Sciences. *Strengthening Clinical Research.* London: Academy of Medical Sciences, 2003.

48. Commonwealth Fund Task Force on Academic Heath Centers. *Envisioning the Future of Academic Health Centers,* Final Report. New York: Commonwealth Fund, February 2003.

49. Institute of Medicine of the National Academies. *Academic Health Centers: Leading Change in the 21st Century.* Washington, DC: Institute of Medicine of the National Academies, 2003.

50. Strategic Learning and Research Committee, Department of Health. *Developing and Sustaining a World Class Workforce of Educators and Researchers in Health and Social Care, 9–20.* London: Department of Health, 2004.

51. Clark, J., and Smith, R. "Academic Medicine: Resuscitation in Progress." *CMAJ; Canadian Medical Association Journal* 170, no. 3 (February 3, 2004): 309-11.

52. Bhutta, Z.A. "Practising Just Medicine in an Unjust World." *BMJ; British Medical Journal* 327, no. 7422 (November 1, 2003):1000-1.

53. Rottingen, J.A.; Thorsby, P.; Seem, J.; and Gautvik, K.M. "Medical Research at Norwegian Universities" (in Norwegian). *Tidsskrift for Den Norske Laegeforening* 118, no. 15 (1998): 2339-43.

54. Clark, J., and Tugwell, P. "Who Cares About Academic Medicine?" *BMJ; British Medical Journal* 329, no. 7469 (October 2, 2004): 751-2.

55. Donaldson, L. *On the State of the Public Health, Annual Report of the Chief Medical Officer, 36-43.* London: Department of Health, 2003). Available: <http://www.publications.doh.gov.uk/cmo/annualreport2003/focus.htm>. Accessed: November 29, 2006.

56. Royal College of Physicians and Academy of Medical Royal Colleges. *Clinical Academic Medicine: The Way Forward—A Report from the Forum on Academic Medicine.* London: Royal College of Physicians, 2004.

57. Peters, K. "Exceptional Matters." *Lancet* 364, no. 9451 (December 11-17, 2004): 2142-51.

58. Whitcomb, M.E. "Sustaining Biomedical Research: A Challenge for Academic Health Centers." *Academic Medicine* 80, no. 3 (March 2005): 203-4.

59. Institute of Medicine . *Crossing the Quality Chasm: A New Health System for the 21st Century.* Washington, DC: National Academy Press, 2001.

60. Grol, R. "Successes and Failures in the Implementation of Evidence-Based Guidelines for Clinical Practice." *Medical Care* 39, no. 8 (Suppl. 2, August 2001): II46-54.

61. Moses, H.; Thier, S.O.; and Matheson, D.H.M. "Why Have Academic Medical Centers Survived?" *JAMA; Journal of the American Medical Association* 293, no. 12 (March 23, 2005): 1495-500.

62. Andreoli, T.E. "The Undermining of Academic Medicine." *Academe Online* 85, no. 6 (November-December 1999). Available: <http://www.aaup.org/publications/Academe/1999/99nd/ND99Andr.htm>. Accessed: November 1, 2006.

63. Goldacre, M.; Stear, S.; Richards, R.; and Sidebottom, E. "Junior Doctors' Views About Careers in Academic Medicine." *Medical Education* 33, no. 5 (May 1999): 318-26.

64. Jackson, V.A.; Palepu, A.; Szalacha, L.; Caswell, C.; Carr, P.L.; and Inui, T. "'?Having the Right Chemistry': A Qualitative Study of Mentoring in Academic Medicine." *Academic Medicine* 78, no. 3 (March 2003): 328-34.

65. Anonymous. "Keeping Women in Hospital and Academic Medicine." *Lancet* 358, no. 9276 (July 14, 2001): 83.

66. Laine, C., and Turner, B.J. "Unequal Pay for Equal Work: The Gender Gap in Academic Medicine." *Annals of Internal Medicine* 141, no. 3 (August 3, 2004): 238-40.

67. Bickel, J.; Wara, D.; and Atkinson, B.F. "Increasing Women's Leadership in Academic Medicine: Report of the AAMC Project Implementation Committee." *Academic Medicine* 77, no. 10 (October 2002): 1043-61.

68. Association of Academic Health Centers. *Through a Prism: Perspectives on a Cross Professions Skill Set, Proceedings of the 11th Congress of Health Professions Educators.* Washington, DC: AAHC, 2004.

69. Frank, J.R., and Tugwell, P. "CanMEDS 2000." *Medical Teacher* 22, no. 6 (2000): 549-54.

70. Association of Academic Health Centers and Association of Canadian Medical Colleges. *The Challenge to Academic Medicine: Leading or Following? Proceedings of the Fifth Trilateral Conference.* London: Nuffield Trust, 2005. Available: <http://www.nuffieldtrust.org.uk/ecomm/files/11102challenge.pdf>. Accessed: November 29, 2006.

71. Chassin, M.R.; Galvin, R.W.; and the National Roundtable on Health Care Quality. "The Urgent Need to Improve Health Care Quality." *JAMA; Journal of the American Medical Association* 280, no. 11 (September 16, 1998): 1000-5.

72. Colby, D.C. "Doctors and Their Discontents." *Health Affairs* 16, no. 6 (November-December 1997): 112-4.

73. Picker Institute and American Hospital Association. *Eye on Patients Reports.* Chicago, IL: AHA, 1996.

74. Lincoln, Y.S, and Lechuga, V. *Research Libraries As Knowledge Producers: Final Technical Report to the Task Force on New Ways of Measuring Collections.* Washington, DC: Association of Research Libraries, 2006.

75. Ludwig, L.T., and Starr, S. "Library As Place: Results of a Delphi Study." *JMLA; Journal of the Medical Library Association* 93, no. 23 (July 2005): 315-26.

SECTION II:
TECHNICAL SERVICES

Chapter 3

Journal Collection Development:
Challenges, Issues, and Strategies

Laurie L. Thompson
Mori Lou Higa

SUMMARY. This chapter provides an overview of the major, current issues associated with journal collection development, with a particular emphasis on the challenges raised by electronic journals. It shares practical tools and information to help libraries survive and thrive with their journal collection development efforts. Specific journal selection criteria is the first of six main areas that will be addressed in this chapter. Standard considerations for print selection are expanded to include unique considerations for the electronic format. The now critical aspects of online license negotiation and effective negotiation practices are addressed in section two. The third section covers the basic principles of copyright, fair use, and key digital copyright concerns. Section four delves into the open access movement, providing background information, definitions, models of provision, and funding models. Benchmarking and journal evaluation strategies are discussed in the fifth section, and section six concludes with an overview of digital archives, covering the current environment, key players, and initiatives.

INTRODUCTION

Major changes in health sciences journal collection development can be traced back to 1992 with the release of the first peer-reviewed electronic scientific journal, *The Online Journal of Current Clinical Trials (OJCCT)*.[1] With the arrival of *OJCCT* and the subsequent proliferation of electronic journals, journal collection development began its whirlwind evolution. Setting aside high inflation and fluctuating exchange rates, the process of journal collection development up to that point had been relatively predictable and stable, focusing solely on print journals within a single institution's walls. With the arrival and growth of electronic journals, collection development activities expanded exponentially, as content providers and libraries began experimenting with and introducing new electronic publishing options, varied pricing models, and multiple delivery mechanisms. At the same time, new licensing options, collaborative purchasing arrangements, and methods to ensure perpetual digital access became critical considerations. The added complexities of the process increasingly require more time, effort, and information to make informed decisions and stay abreast of current developments.

Although most academic health sciences libraries and many hospital libraries have shifted collections support from print to electronic journals, most libraries continue to straddle an environment containing both print and electronic journals. The need to support two formats is likely to continue indefinitely for a number of reasons. First, not all content providers offer their journals in electronic format. Some are still in the process of converting, while others continue to

Introduction to Health Sciences Librarianship
doi:10.1300/6041_03

link online availability to the retention of print subscriptions. Additionally, to convert entire print collections to the electronic format would require additional time and effort, not to mention increased funding. Electronic options, licensing requirements, cost implications, and past and future need would have to be investigated and evaluated before any mass format conversion could take place. Many concerns also remain about the security and long-term reliability of digital journal archives. Print **backfiles** remain the standard, although electronic backfiles continue to grow. Last, while health sciences patrons appear to have voted overwhelmingly for electronic access with their fingertips, doubts remain about the electronic journal being the optimal choice for all user needs.

SELECTION

Traditional journal selection criteria continue to be applicable in today's mixed environment, but increased choices introduced by the electronic format and the dynamic publication environment require a much broader approach to journal selection. This section addresses both traditional elements and additional electronic selection considerations that can help librarians make educated journal decisions.

Internal Environment

Collection Policies

A formal **collection development policy** is the standard tool that defines and guides a library's overall collection approach. Walton et al. provide the rationale for developing and documenting a library's collection development policy:[2]

1. To provide a rational basis for selection and deselection decisions
2. To demonstrate that collections are developed to support specific institutional programs
3. To establish a framework for budget allocations and to lend legitimacy to those allocations
4. To communicate to users and other institutions the nature and limits of the collection
5. To promote consistency in collection development decision making and to minimize the effects of personal bias
6. To articulate criteria that govern collection development

At a minimum, standard collection policies define the library environment, its patrons, the purpose of the collection, and the subject areas to be collected. Effective policy statements can be a few pages in length or many-page efforts. Regardless of length, policies serve only as a framework for collection development; they do not define *how* to select or reject particular titles.[3]

Given the impact of electronic resources, some librarians have begun to define specific criteria for electronic journals in their policies. *MLA DocKit #3, Collection Development and Management for Electronic, Audiovisual, and Print Resources in Health Sciences Libraries,* Second Revised Edition, provides many useful, sample collection policies for a variety of medical libraries.[2]

Selection Committees

Librarians may establish committees to help capture and define patron journal needs and assist with journal evaluation. This approach is generally more applicable to academic or large hospital settings. These groups can vary in composition and can include library staff (e.g., reference librarians, outreach liaisons, education librarians, electronic resources librarians, and collection development representatives) and faculty, physicians, and students. Some groups are composed solely of library employees, while others have mixed membership. Groups may meet once a year, more frequently, or even virtually depending on the desired level of committee formality. Basic selection considerations should be gathered for each subscription under consideration and shared with committee members to provide a mechanism for objective assessment. It may not always be possible or practical to use selection committees, but they can provide valuable input in some environments.

Patron Recommendations

Individual patron recommendations provide immediate collection feedback and should always be given thoughtful consideration. Both print and electronic suggestion forms (see Figures 3.1 and 3.2) as well as in-person communication through individual interactions, focus groups, classes, surveys, and other mechanisms can be used to solicit feedback. Request forms can specify information required, such as the title, publisher, Web site URL, and justification of need. Forms can also be used to communicate the selection criteria that govern how decisions are made.

Interlibrary Loan Requests

A final approach to capture information about an institution's needs is to periodically review interlibrary loan requests from its patrons. A threshold based on the frequency of interlibrary loan requests can be established, automatically alerting those responsible for collection development. Consideration should be given to the status, number, and diversity of patrons making the requests. Multiple requests from a single individual or from temporary, visiting patrons are unlikely to represent broad institutional, long-term collection needs.

Basic Selection Considerations

Once potential journals are identified for consideration, a number of elements can help assess a journal's value for an institution. Standard selection criteria include journal quality, patron need, institutional relevance, cost, and electronic format considerations.

Journal Quality

1. *Is the journal considered to be a scholarly publication?* An editorial peer review process ensures that journal articles meet certain quality standards for methodology, accuracy, and analysis. Generally the peer review process will be highlighted in the journal's description. If there is no explicit statement of an external review process, inquiries can be made to the publisher to determine how article quality is assured. Quality editing will also guarantee a varied publication record of authors representing multiple views for appropriate content balance. It should be noted, however, that variations in editorial peer review practices do exist, and these have been documented in a number of excellent articles and studies.[4, 5]

2. *What types of articles are included?* Original scientific and clinical research articles report the results of research studies using acceptable research guidelines. Review articles summarize and analyze information on particular topics based on an examination of the published literature, saving readers time and effort by identifying and cumulating dispersed primary information appearing in multiple journals. Systematic review articles offer increased accuracy and reli-

HealthLinks
University of Washington

| PubMed | eJournals | Reference | How-To | Library Services |

off-campus access (log in)

Ask us!

| BioResearcher | Care Provider | Grant Seeker | MyHealth | Public Health | Social Worker | Student |

HealthLinks > HSL > Forms > HSL Purchase Recommendation Form

Search [HealthLinks ▼] [_____] [Go] ⓘ

Purchase Recommendation

The Health Sciences Libraries welcome collection recommendations from UW faculty, students and staff for purchases for the Health Sciences Library, the K. K. Sherwood Library at Harborview Medical Center, and the Social Work Library. Consider making a gift to support the collections.

Relevance to curriculum, research, and clinical practice will be considered. Before submitting a recommendation, please check the UW Libraries Catalog to see if the material is already owned in the UW Libraries. You may also recommend items by sending email to the HealthLinks Comments form. Reserve requests must be submitted using the reserve request form.

Name:	[_____]
Department:	[_____]
UW Affiliation:	[Faculty ▼]
Title:	[_____]
Author:	[_____]
Publisher, Date, Price:	[_____]
Format:	☐ Journal ☐ Book ☐ Electronic
Additional information:	[_____]
Reasons to Purchase:	☐ Curriculum ☐ Research ☐ Clinical Practice
What other departments or faculty might use this journal?	[_____]
Can you recommend a journal that might be canceled to offset the cost of this journal?	[_____]
Urgent Request?	[No ▼]
Not needed after:	[_____]

If you wish to be notified when the items arrives, you must supply your email address and library barcode.

Email Address:	[_____]
Library Patron Barcode Number:	[29352_____]
Notification:	[Notify me when the item becomes available. ▼]

[Submit Form] [Clear Form]

FIGURE 3.1. University of Washington, Health Sciences Libraries, Purchase Recommendation Form. Available at <https://healthlinks.washington.edu/hsl/forms/purchase.html>.

Harvey Cushing/John Hay Whitney Medical Library
Yale University School of Medicine

Email | Directories | Search | Ask a Librarian | Home

E-Journals | E-Books | Orbis | Databases | Request Articles & Books | Citation Matcher | More...

Home | Journals & Books | Request Articles & Books | Library Collection Journal Recommendation

Library Collection Journal Recommendation

- Please use a separate form for each item requested.
- Items in red are required fields.
- Journal subscriptions are reviewed on a regular basis for both additions and cancellations.

Journal Recommendation

Journal Title: [_____]

Publisher: [_____]

Price: $ [_____] annually

Comments: *(eg. Are there other important titles in the same discipline? What is the importance or impact of this journal? Are there other journals currently received which could be cancelled if we received this journal?)*

[_____]

Patron Information

Name: [_____]

Campus Address: [_____]

Dept: [_____]

Telephone: [_____]

E-mail address: [_____]

Would you like us to contact you regarding this recommendation? ○ Yes ◉ No

[Send Recommendation]

Historical | Nursing | Public Health | Yale University | Yale Library | YSMInfo | Medical Center | Y-Axis

Questions/Comments? Ask a Librarian | Webmaster | Last Updated: Monday, 10-Oct-2005 16:58:49 EDT. (MG)
© Copyright 2006. Yale University. All rights reserved.
XHTML, CSS, Section 508 Compliance.

Text Only | 🖶 Printer-Friendly Version

FIGURE 3.2. Yale University, Cushing/Whitney Medical Library, Journal Collection Recommendation Form. Available at <http://www.med.yale.edu/library/collections/cdjrnl.html>.

ability by providing an overview of primary studies with explicit and reproducible methods. Case studies or reports focus on the etiology, diagnosis, and management of individual cases. All articles provide scholarly value, and journals can contain a mixture of different types of articles or a single article type, such as those included in review journals.[6]

3. *Does a quality scientific, technical, medical (STM) publisher, a scholarly society or association, or one with some type of reputable pedigree publish the journal?* While it is somewhat subjective to define what may be considered "quality" commercial publishers, highly cited articles are generally indicative of credible publications with solid reputations. Citation indexes such as Thomson Scientific's *Science Citation Index* and *Social Sciences Citation Index* can help identify such articles by capturing cited article references. In addition to commercial publishers, most scholarly societies, professional associations, and university presses will offer quality journal content.

4. *What is the quality of the editorial representatives and article contributors?* Institution affiliations should be listed for both editors and authors. One can review individual publication records of contributors and editors to help assess authoritativeness.

5. *Has the journal followed some type of regular publication schedule?* Delays can indicate a variety of problems, such as insufficient amounts of acceptable content, editorial issues, or funding concerns. Publication delays can also disrupt a library's annual subscription fees and budget planning.

6. *How many years has the journal been in existence?* Longevity is generally an indicator of stability and scholarly need. However, journals with a limited publication life should not be ignored since these often provide forums for new areas of research.

7. *What sources index the journal's contents?* Indexing by traditional indexing and abstracting services, such as MEDLINE, BIOSIS, and CINAHL (*Cumulative Index to Nursing and Allied Health Literature*), or citation indexes, such as *Science Citation Index,* indicates that the journal has met certain standards, such as quality of content, quality of editorial work, production quality, and audience relevance. Inclusion in newer citation databases, such as Elsevier's Scopus <http://www.info.scopus.com/>, and current literature tools, such as the Faculty of 1000 options from Biology Reports Ltd. and Medicine Reports Ltd. <http://www.sciencenavigation.com/default.asp>, should also be considered.

8. *Is a journal review available?* In the not too distant past, individual journal reviews were published with some regularity in journals such as *JAMA*. Due to the increased speed of publication of electronic journals and relative ease of obtaining free or complimentary online access, individual published journal evaluations are far less prevalent. One source that includes reviews of online journal collections is *The Charleston Advisor* <http://www.charlestonco.com/>. An at-a-glance rating system based on content, searchability, pricing options, and contract options is highlighted along with rigorous evaluations.

9. *What is the journal's **impact factor**?* Thomson Scientific (parent company for the Institute for Scientific Information or ISI) produces *Journal Citation Reports (JCR)* <http://scientific.thomson.com/products/jcr/>, which can help assess a journal's usefulness through scholarly acceptance and utilization. The annual *JCR* uses a quantitative approach to evaluate and compare journals based on an impact factor covering thousands of international science and social science journals. The ISI impact factor measures the frequency that an "average article" in a journal has been cited for a particular year. This impact factor, when combined with other selection criteria, helps provide a broad approximation of a journal's prestige, identifies core journals in a particular subject category, and allows comparisons with other journals in similar subject specialties. Much has been written about the potential for misinterpretation and misuse of a journal's impact factor, and Eugene Garfield, the co-creator of the impact factor, has always cautioned that this tool be used with discretion.[7, 8]

10. *Can local feedback be obtained from specialists in the subjects addressed by the journal?* If time allows, opinions of journal content and local need can be solicited from faculty or other health care professionals.

Patron Need, Collection Relevance, and Balance

As part of the journal's assessment, the extent of institutional need and collection "fit" should be considered. Patrons must remain in the forefront of any decision-making about new journals. Occasionally, only a small percentage of an institution's patrons may need a particular journal, but this should not diminish the fact that they represent a clientele that must be supported. Several questions can help define local patron need and relevance:

1. Have affiliated patrons recommended the journal?
2. Has the library received multiple recommendations from diverse users for the same journal?
3. Has the library received requests for articles regularly and from diverse users of the journal via interlibrary loan?
4. Is the journal aligned with subjects defined in the library's collection development policy?
5. Does the journal support the overall mission and goals of the parent institution?
6. Would the journal expand support for existing programs or serve new institutional departments, programs, or research needs?
7. Has the journal experienced large cost increases over time?
8. Does the library's current collection already provide sufficient support in the journal's subject area?
9. How many journals or total budget amount is already devoted to the subject?
10. How much usage have other journals in the same subject received, and what has been their value for cost?
11. Is the institution experiencing growth or expansion in the areas addressed by the journal?

Journal Cost and Fiscal Realities

The library's budget will have a large influence on journal decisions. Since journal subscriptions generally require a long-term commitment of funds, the selector must consider the journal's current cost, the impact of inflation, and the library's ability to sustain the subscription given its current and future budget outlook.

Additional Electronic Selection Criteria

Many selection issues involving electronic journals have overlapping implications, particularly when it comes to licensing. Rather than attempt to artificially separate **license** terms from selection criteria, some concepts will be merged in this section. Other, broader licensing concerns will be addressed in the Online Licensing and Negotiation/Vendor Relations section, which appears later in this chapter.

When considering new subscriptions or format changes for existing subscriptions, selectors should determine whether a license will be required for electronic access. This varies by publisher and vendor. Licenses and their level of acceptability can influence the selection assessment process and have a large impact on the amount of time and effort involved to acquire new subscriptions.

Format

1. In what format is the subscription offered?
2. If an electronic subscription is available, is the electronic journal sold separately or must libraries buy a print subscription that includes online access? While the number of bundled subscriptions combining print with online access has lessened, some publishers continue to require this combination approach.
3. What is the library's preferred format option for journal subscriptions?

Access and User Considerations

1. How is electronic access controlled? Most publishers offer IP (Internet protocol) authentication to restrict access. Another common option is to manage access with a username and password. To determine the best approach for the library, give broad consideration to the amount of staff time that will be required to manage access, any difficulties the library might experience with compliance, and the patron's ease of access.
2. Is access limited to a defined group of workstations?
3. Can patrons access the journal from remote locations, such as offices, labs, or home locales?
4. Is walk-in access permitted within the library for all library visitors?
5. Is access permitted for all desired patron groups? If not, the significance of those who will be excluded should be assessed. The stated scope of acceptable use and limitations on fair use in the license must be adequate for all users.
6. Are there any limitations on the use of the product, such as printing for personal use only?
7. If a patron has access problems, is the library positioned to provide support, and what support might the publisher offer?

Budget Considerations

1. What is the cost basis for institutional access? Common institutional pricing models are increasingly based on "tiers," which reflect the institution's type (hospital, academic) and/or size (number of total full-time equivalents [FTEs], number of students or faculty, bed counts, single site versus multisite or consortia). Another factor that influences subscription costs may be the actual content coverage. For example, there may be one price for the current year's subscription with additional costs for legacy content or backfiles.
2. Is the journal sold separately or is it sold as part of a package? While many journals are sold as individual institutional subscriptions, other options exist. Some may be sold as part of a full-text database or aggregation such as CINAHL Full Text or MDConsult. Other journals may be grouped as part of a publisher's journal package, such as the American Association for Cancer Research's (AACR) suite of five AACR journals. It may be more cost-effective to consider a package purchase over an individual subscription.
3. Is there an option for electronic-only access that is sufficient to eliminate other formats? At this time, many libraries are shifting existing print subscriptions to the electronic format. The elimination of duplicate formats can provide cost reductions and eliminate ongoing costs for shelving and binding print journals.
4. Can the scope of use, number of users, or categories of users be adjusted downward to reduce the subscription costs? If vendors factor in use and users, determine if there is any pricing flexibility based on the number of anticipated users. Additional users, such as alumni, may affect the price.

5. What are the costs for the different access methods? Access by single ID and password is usually intended for limited users and will be priced less than site licenses aimed at a broader user population (e.g., site license by IP address recognition, site licenses for a specified number of concurrent users, site licenses for a single geographic location, and site licenses for multiple locations).
6. Are there technical infrastructure and staff support costs that need to be considered? Patron authentication requirements may impose additional costs. A proxy server may be required to validate legitimate users and provide remote access, and institutional network firewalls can cause problems that could be costly to solve.
7. Does the license contain restrictions on charging for patron use beyond reasonable administrative costs?
8. If a library charges for its services, are its policies and practices in alignment with the terms of the contract?
9. If a consortia purchase, are there any hidden costs, such as restricted access, limited product assistance, or inability to request customization?

Acquisitions Process

1. Can the library's **subscription agent** address all aspects of the purchasing process? For example, the agent may be able to bill for consortia purchases, but library staff may need to address pricing and title verification, licensing negotiations, and serve as the intermediary between the consortium and the agent.
2. Does the publisher offer a commission to the subscription agent? If agent commissions are not provided, the library may need to pay an agent surcharge, which increases costs.
3. Can the library initiate payment in advance of the completion of the license? In some cases, journal access may not be possible until completion of the license or receipt of payment.

Content Considerations

1. *Interlibrary loan.* Some licenses restrict or prohibit interlibrary loan. Are the restrictions acceptable to the library? How will the library staff control interlibrary loan use if necessary?
2. *Archival access.* If a library chooses to end its subscription after a few years, the license should specify whether the library retains archival access rights to the years subscribed. The vendor may offer a means to acquire access to subscribed content even after cancellation.
3. *Content stability.* Content, especially for large journal packages, may change frequently, with journals added or removed with little notice to the library or the users. Shifts of journals between publishers can easily result in the loss of electronic access. A process for changes should be clearly defined in the license.
4. *Duplication.* Electronic journals may be narrower or broader in scope than their print counterparts. The online product may add enhancements such as linked databases, special graphics, or video clips. The online product may also eliminate some elements of the print product, such as commercial or classified advertisements or editorial comments.
5. *Reserves.* If electronic reserves are not permitted, the license may permit use for print reserves. There may be special authentication requirements for electronic reserves use.
6. *Content selection.* Some journals may be obtained as part of a package, with some content elements adding little value to the library's collection. How will the extra material be handled? If elements may be omitted, how will they be chosen?

Consortia Opportunities

Libraries should determine if any consortia purchasing arrangements are available. Various entities, including libraries, library associations, regional networks, cooperative support organizations, and state and university systems, have joined forces, allowing them to leverage their buying power. Group or consortia purchases can broaden collection access, provide discounted fees, and reduce administrative effort to negotiate with vendors. To ensure adequate consortia benefit, most group purchases will involve groups of journals.

Compromise, however, is a necessary component of consortia purchases, which include benefits and drawbacks. A library may not be allowed to cancel subscriptions that are part of a consortia purchase, access may include low-priority journals, and the purchasing process may be time-consuming. In consortia arrangements, each library will need to determine an acceptable cost benefit for their participation and the journal access obtained.

Coverage

The selector should determine if there is any type of **embargo** on current access. Some publishers will restrict access by controlling the time frame when access is offered. For example, a six-month embargo means the most current six months will not be available. If currency is critical, libraries should avoid options that delay access to current content.

The library should also ascertain the number of years that will be included with current subscriptions. Some electronic subscriptions will automatically include a number of back years, while others may limit access to only the current subscription year and future years as long as a subscription is retained. Backfiles offer additional value for a library's subscription. Freely available backfiles, such as those offered on PubMed Central, should also be considered since these can help supplement the value of subscriptions.

Vendor Use Statistics

An increasing number of publishers and vendors are providing **COUNTER (Counting Online Usage of NeTworked Electronic Resources)** compliant patron use statistics. Launched in 2002, COUNTER is an international initiative to define and achieve consistency with the usage measurement for electronic information resources.[9] Libraries should determine if COUNTER statistics are supplied for future subscription evaluation and encourage and educate vendors who are not aware of this effort to standardize online usage data.

Librarians should also familiarize themselves with **SUSHI (Standardized Usage Statistics Harvesting Initiative),** a companion effort to COUNTER that began in 2005. Considerable time and effort are required to consolidate COUNTER data into a usable format. The SUSHI protocol is aimed at automatically integrating statistical data into electronic repositories and may ultimately become a standard for new electronic resource management (ERM) systems.[10-12]

Useful Resources

Core Lists

Preselected lists can help identify core recommended journals. Such lists have been created by others who have already performed the background work by assessing journal quality, relevance, subject, and patron need. Core lists can help identify high-priority journals, build new collections, and provide guidance for budget reductions. A few prominent core lists are included in the following list. Additional subject-oriented resource lists for both journals and books can be located at the Medical Library Association's Collection Development and other section Web sites.[13-15]

1. *Abridged Index Medicus (AIM)*. *AIM* began in 1970 as a way to "afford rapid access to selected biomedical journal literature of immediate interest to the practicing physician."[16] It offers a subset of 100+ core clinical journals indexed for *Index Medicus*. Although *AIM*'s print format ceased in 1997, *AIM* remains a useful core list and continues to be accessible through PubMed and other MEDLINE providers as a journal subset.[17]
2. *Brandon/Hill Selected Lists*. Begun in the 1960s by Alfred N. Brandon, *Selected List of Books and Journals for the Small Medical Library* became a standard selection guide geared toward hospitals and small medical libraries. Starting in the 1970s, Dorothy R. Hill joined Alfred Brandon in maintaining and expanding the original recommendations with two additional lists for nursing and allied health. Although these lists focused on print resources only and updates ceased as of 2004, these recommendations continue to provide valuable collection development guidance for core book and journal resources.[18]
3. *ACP* (American College of Physicians) *Journal Club*. More than 100 journals are reviewed to "select from the biomedical literature articles that report original studies and systematic reviews that warrant immediate attention by physicians attempting to keep pace with important advances in internal medicine."[19] *ACP Journal Club* has been published on a bimonthly basis since 1991, and the listing of journals reviewed is freely available on the American College of Physicians' Web site.
4. *AACP* (American Association of Colleges of Pharmacy) *Core Journals List*. A companion to *AACP Basic Resources for Pharmaceutical Education*, the free *Core Journals List* is compiled from holdings of representative libraries that serve schools and colleges of pharmacy. The latest list, Second Edition, 2003, includes a core list of 109 journal titles. The complete "Master List" of all 628 journals held by the representative libraries can be obtained upon request.[20]
5. InfoPOEMs. Since 1996, the POEMs (Patient-Oriented Evidence that Matters) database has continuously reviewed and synthesized evidence-based research applicable to clinical practice from more than 100+ international medical journals. POEMs journal articles are required to meet three criteria: address questions clinicians face; measure outcomes relating to symptoms, morbidity, quality of life, and mortality; and have the potential to change practices.[21] The journals reviewed for InfoPOEMs supply a quality core clinical collection with an emphasis on evidence-based medicine. InfoPOEMs maintains and freely distributes the current listing of the reviewed journals on its Web site.
6. Customized core lists. Libraries may also want to consider the holdings of other libraries with similar missions. By combining these data with local faculty and curriculum input, customized core lists can be developed, such as the approach taken by the Florida State University College of Medicine Medical Library.[22]

WorldCat and Open WorldCat (from OCLC)

WorldCat <http://www.oclc.org/worldcat/default.htm> and Open WorldCat <http://www.oclc.org/worldcat/open/> can be used to search library holdings information for over 9,000 institutions, which is especially helpful when seeking benchmarking data. WorldCat, a subscription-based service from OCLC: Online Computer Library Center, is the world's largest computerized library catalog that includes item descriptions and library locations for institutions of all sizes and types. Open WorldCat, meanwhile, offers selected, abridged WorldCat records from participating OCLC member libraries available at no cost through common search engines, such as Google, Yahoo! Search, and other outlets.

Journal Citation Reports

The ISI impact factor measures how often articles are cited in a specific journal. Citation data for more than 7,500 journals is summarized annually in Thomson Scientific's *Journal Citation Reports* <http://scientific.thomson.com/products/jcr/>. ISI's impact factor should be used cautiously and only in conjunction with other selection criteria.[7, 8] Many elements can affect a journal's impact factor, including the inclusion of review articles and letters, self-citations, the number of previously published articles in a particular journal, journal title changes, and variations between disciplines.

Subscription Agents

Subscription agents serve as intermediaries between librarians and publishers. They save librarians time and effort by handling journal acquisition and renewal processes, resolving subscription problems such as nonreceipt, and maintaining the libraries' subscription information and history. Agents also provide a wealth of centralized data, containing specific information about individual journals, such as available formats, pricing options, package opportunities, and indexing. Both the librarian's and subscription agent's roles have evolved with the introduction of electronic journals. Since many consortia and individual libraries are now dealing directly with publishers and vendors, the number of subscription agents has declined over the past ten years and the agent's role continues to be redefined. Agents are currently exploring new opportunities to add value for libraries and publishers, such as assisting with consortia billing, handling electronic journal packages, and facilitating online activation for electronic subscriptions. As with librarians, the agent's role continues to evolve.[23]

Indexing

1. List of MEDLINE journals—MEDLINE, the **National Library of Medicine**'s principal bibliographic citation database, indexes over 5,000 international biomedical journals.[24] Before journals can be included in MEDLINE, they must undergo a thorough review process based on consideration of "scientific policy and scientific quality."[25]
2. Other major quality indexing sources, such as BIOSIS, CINAHL, PsycINFO, EMBASE, *Chemical Abstracts,* and *Science Citation Index,* should be considered. The quantity and accessibility of indexing sources can help serve as indicators of potential patron use.

Serials Information Sources

Serials directories, NLM's online catalog, and publishers' Web sites can provide useful starting points for basic journal information. Although inaccuracies with certain data elements in serials directories have been documented, these sources can help verify title and publication information quickly.[26] Maintaining currency and accuracy of information with the influx of electronic journals and evolving formats is challenging at best. Locating current pricing information in particular is often like searching for a needle in a haystack. Whenever in doubt, publishers' Web sites, direct publisher contact, or requests via subscription agents tend to provide the most useful methods to verify critical information. The following list identifies some useful sources that can serve as a starting point for locating basic journal information:

1. *Ulrich's Periodicals Directory* (Bowker, 45th ed., 2007) and Ulrichsweb.com (CSA) <http://www.ulrichsweb.com/ulrichsweb/>
2. *Standard Periodical Directory* (Oxbridge Communications, 2006 edition)

3. *Librarian's Handbook* (EBSCO)
4. NLM LocatorPlus <http://locatorplus.gov/>

Future Journal Pricing Predictions

Annual price surveys can help estimate potential price increases for both new subscriptions and renewals. *Library Journal* publishes an annual periodicals price survey that provides annual cost predictions by broad subject, the average cost per title, and the percent of change.[27] EBSCO Information Services also provides annual serials price projections on its Web site that incorporate world currency impacts.[28] In addition to broad subject-oriented price predictions, some publishers will offer individual annual inflation rates for their particular journals, usually through newsletters, e-mail, or Web sites.

Selected Discussion Lists

A number of discussion lists focus on collection development issues and can be useful for monitoring trends and obtaining feedback as specific questions arise; these include the following:

1. Collection Development Section (Medical Library Association) <http://colldev.mlanet .org/newsletter/discussion_list.html>: Forum for various collection development issues, including policies, consortia, and licensing
2. ERIL-L (Electronic Resources in Libraries) <http://listserv.binghamton.edu/cgi-bin/wa .exe>: Discussion forum for those dealing with the practical aspects of managing electronic resources in libraries
3. LIBLICENSE-L <http://www.library.yale.edu/~llicense/mailing-list.shtml>: Discussion of issues related to licensing of digital information by academic and research libraries
4. NewJour (New Journal and Newsletter Announcement) <http://gort.ucsd.edu/newjour/ NewJourWel.html>: Announcements of new electronic journals and newsletters

Selected Conferences

Interaction with colleagues who may have different perspectives or expertise can help broaden any librarian's understanding of current issues, identify new trends, and help one plan proactively for the future. The following are good venues:

1. Acquisitions Institute at Timberline Lodge <http://www.libweb.uoregon.edu/events/aitl/ index.html>: Annual gathering of librarians, vendors, and publishers to discuss acquisitions issues
2. Charleston Conference: Issues in Book and Serials Acquisitions <http://www.katina .info/conference/>: Fall meeting of librarians, publishers, and vendors offering varied viewpoints on acquisitions issues
3. Medical Library Association Conference (MLA) <http://mlanet.org/am/index.html>: Annual meeting of an educational organization consisting of more than 1,100 institutions and 3,600 individual members in the health sciences field; includes a Collection Development Section that sponsors programs specific to varied collection development issues
4. North American Serials Interest Group (NASIG) <http://www.nasig.org/index.htm>: Independent organization that promotes communication and ideas related to serials publications

ONLINE LICENSING AND NEGOTIATION/VENDOR RELATIONS

Analyzing and negotiating licenses have become essential tasks for the acquisition of electronic products. The products are often expensive and collectively consume large amounts of a library's budget. Their licenses or contracts must be analyzed to determine what the vendor requires of a library that purchases its product. The license will state the standard terms under which the library is expected to offer the product, including definitions of authorized users, equipment requirements, scope of authorized use, and circumstances that would constitute a breach of the contract.

Due to the overlapping elements involving selection criteria, readers should refer to the separate Additional Electronic Selection Criteria section earlier in this chapter for additional licensing considerations.

Who Needs to Be Involved?

A library with a large enough staff can assemble a team that can help clarify many of the issues that will arise with the acquisition and licensing of electronic products. Each team member has a role to play in the decision-making process, with questions to ask and information to gather. Members may ask similar questions, but the answers will reflect each team member's unique perspective. The team should have members who represent the budget, information systems, the product's users and their educational needs, the library's collections, the library's consortium memberships, and legal concerns. If possible, the person who will be conducting the negotiations should also be part of the team. If the library is not large enough for a representative for each role, one or two librarians may have to play several roles or enlist colleagues from outside the library to help. While nonlibrary colleagues may be unfamiliar with library operations, they can often provide valuable expertise.

Information Systems

Librarians should consider technical impact and support needs when selecting journals and vendors. The information systems (IS) department, either in the library or elsewhere in the institution, will be responsible for any installation, implementation, and maintenance that may be required. This may include configuring hardware and software, network access, Web page design or URL entry and maintenance, or database design and maintenance.

Additional Hardware or Software

Both present and near future needs should be assessed honestly. Insufficient hardware or software will result in poor product delivery and dissatisfied users.

Compatibility with Existing Software and Delivery Systems

Institutional network firewalls can cause difficulty in the delivery of, or access to, products outside of the institution's network. Some products require a specific Web browser that the institution may not support.

Archival Data

If archival data are acquired when a license expires, they will need to be supported for the foreseeable future. The library will need to maintain the proper hardware, software, and operating system to access the data or be able to convert the data to newer formats as the need arises.

System Restrictions or Monitoring

The license may require the library to monitor for fair use violations or to prohibit access by certain user groups. The IS department would need to develop a means to meet these license obligations. For more information, see Chapter 6, "Access Issues."

Security and Authentication

All authentication and security requirements should be clearly defined within local capabilities. Information about individual authentication with an ID and password will need to be maintained by the library, the IS department, or the vendor. Firewalls and proxy servers can cause complications that should be solved before the contract is signed.

System Upgrades or Migrations

If the library upgrades its hardware, software, operating system, or network, the product must still remain accessible.

New Operating Platforms

If the vendor has plans to migrate the product to new or different operating platforms, the library may not be able to change its configuration to continue using the product and might lose access.

Negotiations, Final Signature, and Consortium Considerations

Before entering into any licensing negotiations, it is important to determine who has the authority to sign a contract that legally binds the library and its parent institution to specific terms. The library director may have that authority. In a U.S. public (or state-owned) college or university, the final signatory authority may reside in a campus or state contracts, purchasing, or legal office. In a hospital, the chief executive officer, chief financial officer, or legal counsel may be the only one who can sign an agreement. The final signatory may not wish to participate as a team member in the evaluation and negotiation process but should be kept informed of progress and complications.

Once the library has decided to purchase an electronic product and evaluated the license, one person should assume responsibility for negotiating with the product's vendor. The negotiator may be from the library, the contracts or purchasing office, or the legal counsel's office but should be well-versed in negotiating strategies. If the negotiator does not participate in the license analysis team, he or she should be kept informed on all aspects of the analysis. After negotiations have begun, other contact with vendor sales or technical representatives should cease.

It is important to be aware of institutional requirements for purchasing electronic materials. There may be specific rules for "sole-source" purchases or institutional reviews required for acquisitions that exceed a certain price.

If a product is being purchased through a consortium, it may be difficult to learn the terms of a license before it has been signed. If possible, the library should be represented in some way on the consortium's governing board or product evaluation team. Once an agreement is reached and the product is available to consortium members, a copy of the license should be requested and analyzed for the library's ability to comply. If the library is unable to comply with already negotiated terms, it may have to cancel the subscribed product.

Legal Considerations

The library's parent institution has access to legal advice, either from an in-house attorney or a private law firm. The institution may also have a contracts administrator. A cordial relationship should be established between the library and the legal representatives, as they can provide invaluable assistance with license agreements. However, it may be difficult to communicate with them effectively without some advance preparation.

A relationship should be established *before* there is a license to sign. During an initial conversation the library's needs should be outlined and a mutual communication strategy developed. The most efficient way to communicate should be established, either by telephone, e-mail, fax, or memo, as well as how to differentiate urgent questions from routine matters. Issues or problems that *require* communication between the library and the legal counsel should be clearly defined. The legal representative should explain how best to ask questions. The license could be copied with questionable clauses circled, or a memo with the pertinent points highlighted might be preferred.

It is the librarian's responsibility to educate the attorney or contracts administrator about the library, electronic licensing, and copyright. Most health science administrators or attorneys will be more experienced with personnel or malpractice issues than licensing. A license may appear perfectly acceptable from a legal standpoint, but not meet the library's needs. Licensing and copyright have changed dramatically in the past few years, so it is likely that the legal representative will not be current. The most effective way to provide education is to offer some selected background reading or a few good licensing Web sites, such as the LibLicense Web site <http://www.library.yale.edu/~llicense/index.shtml>.

Know the Library's Users

It is essential to know the library's core and peripheral clientele, as well as where they are located and how they use the library's electronic products. Lists of all possible user information, such as user categories, locations, and desired scope of use, prepared before a license is analyzed will make the task easier. Every license will define authorized users, use locations, and scope of authorized use in its own terms. It is much easier to spot problems in the definitions or user categories if they are compared to a list of definitions used by the library. It could be difficult and possibly expensive to add a new authorized user group or location, or to change the scope of use after the license has been signed.

Users of a health sciences library might include students (full-time, part-time, extension, consortium, and distance-learning students); faculty (full-time, part-time, clinical, adjunct, volunteer, visiting, emeritus, and preceptors); academic and research staff (full-time, part-time, temporary, and floating staff); visitors (sponsored visitors, alumni, general public); hospital employees (physicians, residents and interns, nurses, and staff); patients and families; contractors; affiliates or consortium members (hospitals, libraries, universities); and others.

The library will need to determine what scope of use is desired for each electronic product and then verify that the use is permitted under the terms of the license. Provisions for downloading, e-mailing, and printing information must be considered. Use of online journal articles for print or electronic reserves, institutional course packs, or for interlibrary loan may be needed. Articles may be needed in the classroom or distributed to distance education students.

Reviewing the License

A good license analysis team will help uncover potential problems with the product that can be addressed in the final license. However, the license itself may pose problems. A vendor's standard license agreement can seem quite intimidating, with clauses and appendices and legal definitions to decipher. The license should be read and analyzed carefully with minimum distraction. The analysis should include scenarios for what might go wrong if the product is purchased with the vendor's form license.

A license clause that does not make sense should be highlighted and clarification sought from the vendor, contract officer, or legal counsel. Assumptions should not be made based on previous agreements. Some license clauses are perfectly clear but present unreasonable terms. The offending clause should be removed if possible, or an alternate clause that is more acceptable be developed. It is important to take comprehensive notes during all discussions with the vendor's representatives. These notes should be shared with the license evaluation team, which should be vigilant for inconsistencies. All license definitions should conform to the library's definitions. The terms of a signed license supersede existing law, so use restrictions should be compared to copyright law and fair use provisions and the comparison used to justify license changes.

From the beginning of the selection process through the final license negotiation, it is important to keep all information related to the product and license together in one place for ease of use. Final contracts should be kept in a single location that can be accessed easily by both collection development staff as well as the library's administration. Each license folder should include information about the vendor, location, representatives, e-mail addresses, and phone and fax numbers. It is useful to include a summary of terms, including any use restrictions, in an easy-to-access place. An online, networked file or database, such as those included in an ERM system can be useful for maintaining pertinent information.[29]

COPYRIGHT

Copyright is rooted in the Constitution of the United States. Article 1, Section 8, states, "The Congress shall have power . . . [t]o promote the progress of science and useful arts, by securing for limited times to authors and inventors the exclusive right to their respective writings and discoveries." This purpose, to promote the progress of science and useful arts, parallels the missions of medicine and research that are supported in health sciences libraries. The first Copyright Act was passed in 1790. Major revisions followed in 1831, 1879, and 1909 in response to changes in technology, such as recorded sounds, visual images, and photocopies.

Copyright, a form of intellectual property law, protects original works of authorship, including literary, dramatic, musical, and artistic works such as poetry, novels, movies, songs, computer software, and architecture. It is intended to provide a balance between individual property rights and the betterment of society. It gives authors and creators the right to reproduce, distribute, perform, display, and license (or transfer) their works. These rights can be divided, distributed, and unbundled. In order to be copyrighted, a work must be an "original expression" in a "tangible medium." Copyright does not protect facts, ideas, systems, or methods of operation, although it may protect the way these things are expressed. Works produced by U.S. government agencies are also not eligible for copyright protection.

If the owner of a copyrighted work sells a copy of that work, the ownership of the copy transfers to the purchaser under the "first sale doctrine." Publishers sell copies of books to libraries, which then own the books and may do with them what they wish. This makes services such as lending and borrowing possible.

The current Copyright Act (Title 17 of the U.S. Code) was enacted as public law on October 19, 1976, and has been amended several times since then (see the act including all its amendments at <http://lcweb.loc.gov/copyright/title17/>). Section 106 states that only the copyright holder has the right to copy, distribute, make derivative works, perform, display, or broadcast a copyrighted work. However, the Copyright Act also recognizes the concept of "fair use" for educational purposes. Section 107 states that "fair use of a copyrighted work, including such use by reproduction in copies . . . for purposes such as . . . teaching (including multiple copies for classroom use), scholarship, or research, is not an infringement of copyright." The act then describes four conditions to be considered for determination of fair use: (1) the *purpose* and character of the use, including whether such use is of a commercial nature or is for nonprofit educational purposes; (2) the *nature* of the copyrighted work; (3) the *amount* and substantiality of the portion used in relation to the copyrighted work as a whole; and (4) the *effect* of the use upon the potential market for or value of the copyrighted work.

U.S. Copyright Office Circular 21, *Reproduction of Copyrighted Works by Educators and Librarians,* provides guidance for fair use copies made for classroom use:

1. The copies meet tests of brevity and spontaneity:
   a. Brevity: no more than a complete article, or 10 percent of a work, or one illustration, etc., per article.
   b. Spontaneity: the decision to use the work did not leave enough time to obtain permission to copy.
2. No more than three articles from the same volume.
3. The copies do not create or substitute for anthologies or collected works.
4. The copies do not substitute for the purchase of the materials from the publisher.
5. The copies are made for one semester only.
6. The copies include a notice of copyright.[30]

Circular 21 also summarizes the *National Commission on New Technological Uses of Copyrighted Works (CONTU) Guidelines on Photocopying and Interlibrary Arrangements.*[30] These guidelines were developed by librarians, publishers, and educators to help librarians provide legal, fair use copies for interlibrary loan. Section 108 of the Copyright Act prohibits systematic photocopying of copyrighted materials but permits interlibrary arrangements as long as they do not do so in amounts that would substitute for a subscription.

There have been no official guidelines to address digital reproductions, although serious attempts have been made. From May 1994 until September 1997, ninety-three organizations representing for-profit and nonprofit publishers, the software industry, government agencies, scholarly societies, authors, artists, photographers and musicians, the movie industry, public television, licensing collectives, libraries, museums, universities, and colleges met for a Conference on Fair Use, or CONFU, to develop guidelines for fair use copying of digital works. Discussions covering twenty areas of concern were eventually reduced to four topics: distance learning, digital image collections, electronic reserves, and multimedia. However, the participants could come to no consensus and CONFU disbanded.[31]

The failure of CONFU to develop new guidelines has left libraries still puzzling over how to apply the 1976 Copyright Act to new digital technologies. Because digital works are so easily copied and distributed, the owner of a copyright to digital materials is likely concerned about preventing unauthorized downstream uses as well as protecting or enhancing revenues. A vendor's license terms for a digital work may be written to ensure that there is no damage to potential sales of the material or loss of potential revenue. For example, many licenses for library resources will limit access only to registered students, faculty, and staff; or only from a particular machine or machines; or only in a particular place, such as the library; or only from a particular domain. The license may not allow the library to keep a copy of the work when the license is terminated or expires. Finally, the license may attempt to limit users' copies and transmissions of the work. The library must work to negotiate the best possible terms for each license to preserve fair use of the material at a reasonable cost and to make users aware of any restrictions that may exist. If possible, the material use guidelines should be kept technology neutral and should give local and remote users equal access.

Even though CONFU failed, many libraries and universities use the draft guidelines to determine fair use for copyrighted material being posted in digital format:

1. Short items (an article from a journal or a chapter from a book or conference proceedings) or excerpts from longer items may be used.
2. The instructor, the library, or another unit of the educational institution must possess a lawfully obtained copy of the work.
3. The total amount of material included for a specific course should be a small proportion of the total assigned reading for that course.
4. Any copyright statement from the original work should be displayed on a preliminary or introductory screen: "The work from which this copy is made includes this notice: [restate the copyright notice: e.g., Copyright 1996, XXX Corp.]." The notice should also caution against further electronic distribution of the digital work.
5. Appropriate citations or attributions to the source should be included.
6. Access should be limited to students registered in the course, and to instructors and staff responsible for the course or the electronic system. Methods for limiting access could include individual passwords; passwords for each class; retrieval of works by course number or instructor name, but not by author or title of the work; or access limited to workstations that are ordinarily used by, or are accessible to, only enrolled students or appropriate staff or faculty.
7. Permission from the copyright holder is required if the item is to be reused in a subsequent academic term for the same course offered by the same instructor, or if the item is a standard assigned or optional reading for an individual course taught in multiple sections by many instructors.
8. Material may be retained in electronic form while permission is being sought or until the next academic term in which the material might be used, but in no event for more than three calendar years, including the year in which the materials are last used.

Where to Learn More

1. U.S. Copyright Office <http://lcweb.loc.gov/copyright/>
2. Copyright and Fair Use, Stanford University <http://fairuse.stanford.edu/>
3. The University of Texas Crash Course in Copyright <http://www.utsystem.edu/OGC/IntellectualProperty/cprtindx.htm>
4. Copyright Management Center, Indiana University–Purdue University, Indianapolis <http://www.iupui.edu/~copyinfo/home.html>

OPEN ACCESS

Traditional scholarly journal publishing follows a simple model. Authors submit their work to a particular journal for review. If the work is accepted for publication, the author signs an agreement with the publisher to publish the work, usually assigning all copyright for the work to the publisher. The publisher then prints and distributes the work in the journal. Libraries buy the journals through subscriptions and make the content available to their users. Unless the author negotiates to keep copyright, the rights to the content of the journal belong to the publisher. The vast majority of electronic scholarly publishing follows the same model.

STM journal prices have consistently risen at rates that exceed the U.S. Consumer Price Index since at least the mid-1970s.[32-34] Libraries have responded in numerous ways: canceling journal subscriptions, reducing other acquisitions, consortia purchasing, and interlibrary loan.

The library has long been embedded in the scholarly communications process. Libraries purchase and make available the literature necessary for academic research. Researchers use the literature to further their own work, which they publish in books and journals that are purchased by the library. Academic researchers are often under pressure to "publish or perish," meaning that they must publish a certain amount in order to obtain academic tenure. The quantity of publications and the quality of the journals in which the researcher publishes are both considerations in tenure decisions.

Open access publishing has evolved as one response to the increasing prices and decreasing availability of commercial scholarly publishing. It dates nearly to the beginning of the Internet, with the free distribution of the online journal *New Horizons in Adult Education* first published by Syracuse University in 1987.[35] The Budapest Open Access Initiative (BOAI) <http://www.soros.org/openaccess/>, issued in February 2002, is the first major statement on open access. BOAI includes a definition of open access, background information, a list of frequently asked questions, and a list of signatories. Two other important statements followed: the Bethesda Statement on Open Access Publishing <http://www.earlham.edu/~peters/fos/bethesda.htm> in June 2003 and the Berlin Declaration on Open Access to Knowledge in the Sciences and Humanities <http://oa.mpg.de/openaccess-berlin/berlindeclaration.html> in October 2003.

Open access publishing has come to mean online information that is available to anyone without barriers, particularly cost. There are many variations on open access, including articles that are free of copyright or license restrictions. Some publishers impose embargoes on articles before they are offered as open access. For example, PubMed Central, a repository for open access materials in the biomedical and related sciences, permits contributing publishers to withhold free access to journal articles published within the previous three, four, six, twelve, or up to thirty-six months. After the embargo, the articles are freely available.[36]

Open access journals are just one method of open access publishing. Institutional repositories have become another way for researchers and authors to make their research available. These repositories can include previously unpublished articles, pictures and other media, teaching objects, and other scholarly material, as well as legal copies of peer-reviewed published articles as permitted by the publisher or copyright owner. The SHERPA/RoMEO Web site maintains a list of publishers' republishing policies <http://www.sherpa.ac.uk/romeo.php> that can help authors determine the legality of the copies they wish to post. Authors and researchers may also choose to self-publish or self-archive their work on individual Web sites.

Open access journals are funded differently from traditional journals. Instead of subscriptions, the acquisition of funding resources is "redirected," usually to the author or the author's institution. Thus, an author will pay a fee to have his work published. This fee may be offset if the author's institution is a member of the organization that is publishing the journal. Authors are also encouraged to incorporate funding for open access publishing into their research grant proposals.

Two sources of information about open access journal titles are as follows:

1. Directory of Open Access Journals (DOAJ)—This service, available at <http://www.doaj.org>, lists free, full-text, quality-controlled scientific and scholarly journals with the goal to cover all subjects and languages.
2. PubMed Central (PMC)—PMC <http://www.pubmedcentral.nih.gov/> is a free archive of biomedical and life sciences journals. PMC also has the author manuscripts of articles pub-

lished by NIH-funded researchers in various non-PMC journals. Similar manuscripts from researchers funded by the Wellcome Trust are available in PMC as well.

Open access publishing is a rapidly growing and changing field. Some resources to use to stay current include these:

1. BOAI Forum—A low-traffic moderated discussion list to support the Budapest Open Access Initiative, the forum announces new BOAI funding programs, publications, and news and collects the open access wisdom of the worldwide network of BOAI supporters. It is available at <http://www.soros.org/openaccess/forum.shtml>.
2. SCHOLCOMM Discussion List—Sponsored by the Association of College and Research Libraries (ACRL), this forum is for the examination and analysis of topics such as open access to scholarly information, new models of scholarly publishing, increasing journal prices, copyright law and policy, related technologies, and federal information law and policies that impact the access of scholars, students, and the general public to scholarly information. It can be accessed at <http://www.ala.org/ala/acrl/acrlissues/scholarlycomm/scholcommdiscussion.htm>.
3, SPARC Open Access Forum—Sponsored by the Association of Research Libraries (ARL), this forum is for discussion of news and analysis of the open access movement to disseminate scientific and scholarly research literature online, free of charge, and free of unnecessary licensing restrictions. It is available at <http://www.arl.org/sparc/soa/index.html#forum>.

BENCHMARKING/EVALUATING USE OF RESOURCES

Evaluation is a necessary component of collection development, and there are a number of strategies for deciding whether to cancel or retain subscriptions. Similar strategies can help a library decide when or whether to switch print subscriptions to the electronic format. Many factors have overlapping elements, and consideration is rarely given to one isolated facet of information. There is no single approach to evaluation since there are many different reasons to initiate specific or conduct ongoing evaluation efforts.[6] Evaluation also includes personal judgment based on expertise and knowledge of the library's patrons and parent institution, and of publishing environments. Additionally, the use of benchmarking operates under the assumption that rigorous validation was used to establish the standards or bases for benchmarks used by other institutions, which may or may not be the case. Included in this section are some initial considerations to factor into the evaluation efforts of any library.

Cost-Effectiveness

One of the most common methods to evaluate the value of a library's journals is to look at the cost per use and compare this with other journals in the collection. The simplest approach is to divide the annual subscription cost by the number of actual uses a journal has received during the subscription year: *annual subscription cost / annual uses = journal cost per use*. This approach works most effectively with individual subscriptions that are not purchased as part of a package. At this time, manual reshelving counts of print journals, site clicks for journal access points, and vendor-supplied usage data are typical methods for gathering journal use data. Each usage count has its faults. Patrons may reshelve print journals; they may access electronic journals directly, bypassing library-provided access points; and vendor data may be unavailable or provided in a nonstandardized format.

When subscriptions are purchased as part of an electronic journal package, the value of the package as a whole should be evaluated. In this case, the annual cost of the package would be divided by total uses of all journals: *annual e-journal package cost / total annual uses of journals contained within the package = package cost per use.* While this approach does not take into consideration individual journal use, the overall package value needs to be considered, at a minimum, if that is how a library obtains it.

For cost-per-use data to be used effectively, a library must understand its range of cost-per-use data and what the library's budget can sustain. An analysis of individual journal data may show that a library's annual cost per use ranges from a few cents per use to over $100.00 per use. Once the range is determined, a library can then identify an acceptable cost-per-use threshold for its individual journals. If a library can provide journal articles through interlibrary loan at a lower fee, the evaluator may consider cancellation of particular subscriptions. Additionally, in cases of budget reductions, a cost-per-use threshold can be used to identify potential journals for cancellation objectively and systematically.

Generally, a library should have multiple years' worth of local use data before relying solely on a cost-per-use approach to analyze journal need. One year's worth of use data is unlikely to be representative of long-term institutional need. Trend or multiple years' statistics should be considered to see if the journal use is increasing, declining, or remaining stable. Over time, continued high or low use can serve as a solid indicator of journal need or declining need.

Environmental Trends

While libraries must focus on their individual institution's trends to make effective journal decisions, it is useful to stay abreast of environmental trends and view an institution's local data in the context of broader information patterns. At this point, journal collection development is responding and adapting to changing patron behavior and a changing publication environment. Comparing local data to larger environmental trends is always a good reality check as well as a useful tool to plan proactively for future collection development strategies.

Two recent studies illustrate both expected and unexpected usage behavior. Carol Tenopir, Donald W. King, and Amy Bush recently examined the medical school faculty's use of print and electronic journals at the University of Tennessee Health Science Center.[37] As with many other patron groups, it might be expected that the evidence would show clear support for the electronic options, but this was not the case. Medical faculty continued to rely on print journals more heavily than electronic journals, which could be attributed in part to the faculty's continued reliance on, and number of, personal print subscriptions.

In an earlier study at the Library of the Health Sciences–Peoria, University of Illinois, Chicago, the introduction of 104 core electronic medical journals resulted in a more predictable, though not necessarily desirable, trend.[38] There was a marked decrease in overall usage of print journals, even those available only in print. The authors speculate that the desire and convenience for electronic access was more important to patrons than actual journal quality.

Academic facilities have clearly shifted the majority of funding to support the electronic format. Studies continue to monitor shifting usage patterns in the health sciences field and new publication options, such as open access initiatives, continue to evolve. It is likely that libraries and library patrons will remain in a state of transition for at least the next few years. Keeping an eye on environmental trends helps libraries evaluate their current situation and plan more effectively for the future.

Core Titles

Core lists, discussed earlier in this chapter in the first section on selection, can also provide guidance when evaluating current subscriptions. A library may choose to retain core titles regardless of other factors. Core titles may be related to an institution's accreditation status or regarded as high-priority subscriptions that would be eliminated only as a last resort in the case of forced budget reductions. A library might also require that a reasonably stable electronic alternative, such as PubMed Central, must exist before core title subscriptions would be considered for cancellation.

Consortia Packages

Given the increased interinstitutional sharing of costs, consortia packages should be assessed regularly to ensure that the library is getting the best possible value for its journal investment. As noted previously, consortia purchases contain risks that must be taken into consideration when evaluating journal subscriptions for possible elimination. If a license is in place for a consortia package, the license will inevitably contain some restrictions to protect the vendor or publisher from loss of revenue. Individual title cancellations may not be possible, despite low use, if a library wishes to continue its participation in the consortia purchase. Title swapping may be possible if the value of the swapped title remains the same. Assuming the library is receiving adequate benefit for the overall cost of the package, a library should consider the percentage of individual titles that do receive acceptable use. If the cost per use of the package as a whole is acceptable but use of multiple titles is limited, a library may want to consider if better value could be obtained by individually licensing those titles that do receive use or swapping titles to expand collection access.

Multiple Collection Overlap

Libraries are often presented with multiple subscriptions for electronic access to identical titles. While overlap is not sought deliberately, this has become a common occurrence due to consortia packages, journal aggregators such as EBSCO*host,* and free or open access journals.

When evaluating the value of a library's journal collection, libraries should consider the value their patrons are receiving from overlapping electronic access options and if they have the option to eliminate the overlap. In some cases, multiple access points may be warranted. Increased security for long-term accessibility and stability is more likely through a publisher's subscription than a journal aggregator or free site. Extended coverage may be provided by some, while others offer only embargoed access. The ease of access may also be simplified through IP authentication as opposed to sites requiring some type of registration or usernames and passwords.

Archival Policies

When evaluating electronic journals, a library must take into consideration the archival implications of canceling its electronic subscriptions. Unless there is a guarantee of continued access to the subscribed years, the library may be at risk for losing archival online access. Some repositories, such as PubMed Central, JSTOR, and BioOne, offer acceptable alternative archival solutions with reasonably sound perpetual access policies. Alternatively, some libraries have initiated local agreements to guarantee some type of archival print retention within certain geographic areas.

Serials Analysis Tools

Some subscription agents offer a variety of standardized reports (e.g., historical price analysis and online availability) to help evaluate and assess a library's current subscriptions. A growing number of additional, third-party tools have been developed that automate some of the processes involved with journal evaluation. These products can also provide more granular views of the value of a library's journal collection and provide varied views of current subscriptions, complete holdings, or subscriptions based on a particular format. Some selected tools from major vendors follow:

- *Journal Use Reports (JUR)* (Thomson Scientific)—Launched in Spring 2006, *JUR* <http://scientific.thomson.com/webofknowledge/jur-cust.html> combines COUNTER compliant journal usage data, journal citation metrics from *Journal Citation Reports*, institutional publication data, and article citation data from Web of Science. By examining individual faculty publication records and journal citation data alongside use and cost, *JUR* intends to provide a more complete picture of journal performance and institutional research activity.
- Ulrich's Serials Analysis System (CSA)—This system, available at <http://www.ulrichsweb.com/ulrichsweb/analysis/>, is intended to "identify, analyze, evaluate, and create reports about a library's print and electronic serials holdings." Internal data about a library's print and electronic serials collection is compared against Ulrichsweb.com that contains Ulrich's database of serials titles, publisher information, and electronic journal availability data.
- WorldCat Collection Analysis Tool (OCLC)—Released in 2005, WCA <http://www.oclc.org/collectionanalysis/default.htm> allows libraries to "compare their collections with those of peer libraries, and compare, as a group, the level of overlap or uniqueness of their collections." It is sold on a subscription basis to any library with holdings in WorldCat. Some predefined peer groups are readily available, including one for the top nursing schools based on rankings by *U.S. News & World Report*.
- ScholarlyStats (MPS Technologies)—This product, available at <http://www.scholarlystats.com/>, serves as a single portal for a library's vendor usage statistics. It is intended to decrease the amount of administrative staff effort spent on gathering and organizing usage data and help libraries more effectively demonstrate the value of their online content by actively using their statistics. Consolidated reports include the total number of journals accessed, total use by platform, average use by platform, and most and least used journals.

DIGITAL ARCHIVES

As the number of electronic journals and the number of researchers relying on electronic journals grows, concerns with the fragility of digital information also increases. One of the essential challenges still to be resolved is how best to address and guarantee that electronic content will be preserved for future generations. In the past, librarians confidently relied upon multiple paper copies to provide a permanent historical record. Digital information is far less secure, with increased opportunities for alteration and removal of data. Unlike physical libraries, newer retention sources are viewed as being less trustworthy. Ongoing discussions are focused on what needs to be archived, who should be responsible, and the best methods and repositories to ensure secure archival access. This section summarizes current concerns, identifies essential players and initiatives, and includes suggested strategies to address the preservation issue.

Much of this information is synthesized from Kate O'Dohonue's thoughtful 2005 dissertation, "The Accessing and Archiving of Electronic Journals: Challenges and Implications Within the Library World."[39] Her excellent treatise on this topic highlights many of the problems associated with digital e-journal archives and offers suggestions for improvement.

Different opinions exist about exactly what needs to be archived. Does the "look and feel" of each electronic journal need to be preserved? Can the archive be based solely on the articles themselves, or does the archive need to maintain the structure of the original journal issues? Does every publication really need to be archived for posterity, regardless of its quality? O'Donohue suggests that there may not be a single approach for determining what should be archived and in what format.[39] Potentially there might be multiple approaches with different long-term goals for retention.

The main entities that could take ownership of digital archives are libraries, publishers, third parties, or a combination of any of these. Different opinions have been offered as to who should take responsibility for long-term preservation. Libraries have always served as the repositories of information, and some argue that libraries should continue to serve in that capacity for the electronic format. Libraries are stable, long-term institutions that have always provided and maintained physical access and preserved the scholarly record. Others believe publishers should guarantee archival access as owners of the content. However, publishers may go out of business, merge with other groups, or be bought. Traditionally, publishers have had no historic responsibility for access once print journals were delivered. Some question whether commercial publishers, motivated by profits, may understand the need to guarantee a permanent scholarly record without charging exorbitant fees for the service. Third-party initiatives, such as bibliographic utilities, offer another option to address digital archival issues, but concerns have been raised over too much centralization and unclear funding and maintenance models. Collaborative efforts have also been suggested, combining local and national libraries, consortia, publishers, and others. Getting all groups to work toward the same goal, however, is seen as an additional challenge.

Questions of how best to archive electronic journals revolve primarily around business and technical considerations. Without any broad guidelines and consensus, individual approaches simply add complexities and costs. Effective preservation requires policy setting and planning from the outset when digital materials are created. Funding models are needed to ensure equitable costs and long-term sustainability. Collaborative, agreed-upon technical standards must be developed and broadly supported for hardware, software, and information architecture. The capacity for long-term compatibility with newer technologies must also be addressed.

At this time, various groups are experimenting with multiple digital archive initiatives. Some of the major entities of interest to health sciences libraries include the following:

- PubMed Central (PMC)—PMC <http://www.pubmedcentral.nih.gov/> is a free digital archive of biomedical and life sciences journals offered by the National Library of Medicine. Participation by publishers is voluntary, and publishers may delay release of their full-text content. Complete journal content is encouraged, and NLM is digitizing earlier print issues of many of PMC's journals.
- JSTOR (Journal Storage)—Founded in 1995, JSTOR <http://www.jstor.org/> is a not-for-profit organization whose goal is to create and maintain trusted archives of important scholarly journals. This subscription service includes journals from many disciplines with a one- to five-year embargo for most of the content.
- LOCKSS™ (Lots of Copies Keep Stuff Safe)—Initiated by Stanford University Libraries in 1999, LOCKSS <http://www.lockss.org/> is "open source software that provides librarians with an easy and inexpensive way to collect, store, preserve, and provide access to their own, local copy of authorized content they purchase." LOCKSS offers institutions the traditional custodial role for long-term preservation of a library's locally subscribed collection.

- CLOCKSS (Controlled LOCKSS)—CLOCKSS <http://www.lockss.org/clockss/Home> is a not-for-profit partnership among publishers and libraries begun in 2006 by Stanford University Libraries to develop a "distributed, validated, comprehensive archive" that would be triggered in the event of a catastrophic event or long-term disruption of publisher availability. It is also intended to provide access to orphaned or abandoned works for the scholarly community.
- Portico—Launched in 2005 and supported initially by the Andrew W. Mellon Foundation, Ithaka, the Library of Congress, and JSTOR, Portico <http://www.portico.org/> offers a permanent archive of electronic scholarly journals. In case of specific "trigger" events, Portico provides all libraries supporting the archive with campus-wide access to archived content.

At this time, digital archive support efforts are varied but growing. Major stakeholders are partnering to bring clarity to the issues and to develop collaborative approaches. The pace of progress on the development of archival technical standards has increased, and several community-based groups are now exploring issues and best practices. Experiments with funding models and pricing also continue to evolve with collaborative development and maintenance models, such as Portico's, with increasing broad-based support from publishers and libraries. Ultimately, there may be multiple digital archives to ensure the best possible long-term preservation and security of data. Despite the many unknowns, it appears that the major stakeholders are heading in the same direction, gradually reaching consensus that for digital archiving to be successful, it will need to be a shared responsibility.

CONCLUSION

Successful journal collection development efforts require varied approaches and skills from today's selectors. Librarians must be flexible while keeping an eye on the future. There is no clear road map for all decisions. The ability to deal with ambiguity is essential. In some cases, collection decisions will need to be made despite the lack of clear or desired information. Whether the issues involve open access, digital archives, or best value for cost, change is the common denominator. Change, however, is also an opportunity for improving services, and librarians must be advocates for what they believe is best for their patrons. It is critical for librarians to proactively stay abreast of evolving publishing and business environments, maintain open channels of communication and dialogue with all partners, and continue to broaden their knowledge base to include topics, such as licensing, that now impact journal selection. In spite of the volatile nature of the current environment, the tools, strategies, and information presented here can help librarians take calculated risks to continue to develop quality journal collections.

REFERENCES

1. Brahmi, F., and Kaneshiro, K. "The Online Journal of Current Clinical Trials (OJCCT): A Closer Look." *Medical Reference Services Quarterly* 12(Fall 1993): 29-43.

2. Walton, L.; Modschiedler, C.M.; Rodgers, P.M.; et al. *MLA DocKit #3, Collection Development and Management for Electronic, Audiovisual, and Print Resources in Health Sciences Libraries,* 2nd revised ed. Chicago: Medical Library Association, 2004.

3. Johnson, P. *Fundamentals of Collection Development and Management.* Chicago: American Library Association, 2004.

4. Eldredge, J. "Characteristics of Peer Reviewed Clinical Medicine Journals." *Medical Reference Services Quarterly* 18(Summer 1999): 13-26.

5. Weller, A.C. "Editorial Peer Review: Methodology and Data Collection." *Bulletin of the Medical Library Association* 78(July 1990): 258-68.

6. Richards, D.T., and Eakin, D. *Collection Development and Assessment in Health Sciences Libraries.* Current Practice in Health Sciences Librarianship, vol. 4. Lanham, MD: Scarecrow Press, 1997.

7. Garfield, E. "The History and Meaning of the Journal Impact Factor." *JAMA; Journal of the American Medical Association* 295(January 4, 2006): 90-3.

8. Garfield, E. "How Can Impact Factors Be Improved?" *BMJ; British Medical Journal* 313(August 17, 1996): 411-3.

9. Project COUNTER. Available: <http://www.projectcounter.org/index.html>. Accessed: December 2, 2006.

10. Standardized Usage Statistics Harvesting Initiative (SUSHI). Available: <http://www.niso.org/committees/SUSHI/SUSHI_comm.html>. Accessed: December 3, 2006.

11. Needleman, M.H. "The NISO Standardized Usage Statistics Harvesting Initiative (SUSHI)." *Serials Review* 32(September 2006): 216-7.

12. Chandler, A., and Jewell, T. "Standards—Libraries, Data Providers, and SUSHI: The Standardized Usage Statistics Harvesting Initiative." *Against the Grain* 18(April 2006): 82-3.

13. Medical Library Association, Collection Development Section. Available: <http://colldev.mlanet.org/resources/subjectlist.htm>. Accessed: December 10, 2006.

14. Medical Library Association, Dental Section. Available: <http://www.library.tmc.edu/mladental/reading.htm>. Accessed: February 13, 2007.

15. Medical Library Association, Cancer Librarians Section. Available: <http://www.selu.com/cancerlib/corelist.html>. Accessed: February 13, 2007.

16. "*Abridged Indexed Medicus (AIM)* Ceases Publication." *NLM Technical Bulletin* (September-October 1997). Available: <http://www.nlm.nih.gov/pubs/techbull/so97/so97_technote.html#aim>. Accessed: February 14, 2007.

17. "*Abridged Index Medicus* (*AIM* or 'Core Clinical') Journal Titles." Available: <http://www.nlm.nih.gov/bsd/aim.html>. Accessed: February 14, 2007.

18. Brandon/Hill *Selected Lists.* Available: <http://www.mssm.edu/library/brandon-hill/>. Accessed: December 10, 2006.

19. "Journals reviewed for the *ACP Journal Club.*" Available: <http://www.acpjc.org/shared/journals_reviewed.htm>. Accessed: December 10, 2006.

20. *2003 AACP Core Journals List* [Basic Resources for Pharmacy Education]. Available: <http://www.aacp.org/>. Accessed: December 10, 2006.

21. "InfoPOEMs Journals Reviewed." Available: <http://www.infopoems.com/product/methods_journals.cfm>. Accessed: January 8, 2007.

22. Shearer, B.S., and Nagy, S.P. "Developing an Academic Medical Library Core Journal Collection in the (Almost) Post-Print Era: The Florida State University College of Medicine Medical Library Experience." *Journal of the Medical Library Association* 91(July 2003): 292-302.

23. Curtis, D.; Scheschy, V.M; and Tarango, A.R. *Developing and Managing Electronic Journal Collections: A How-To-Do-It Manual for Librarians.* New York: Neal-Schuman Publishers, 2000.

24. "Fact Sheet: MEDLINE (U.S. National Library of Medicine, National Institutes of Health)." Available: <http://www.nlm.nih.gov/pubs/factsheets/medline.html>. Accessed: Feburary 14, 2007.

25. "Fact Sheet: Journal Selection for MEDLINE (U.S. National Library of Medicine, National Institutes of Health)." Available: <http://www.nlm.nih.gov/pubs/factsheets/jsel.html>. Accessed: December 10, 2006.

26. Eldredge, J.D. "Accuracy of Indexing Coverage Information As Reported by Serials Sources." *Bulletin of the Medical Library Association* 81(October 1993): 364-70.

27. Van Orsdel, L.C., and Born, K. "Journals in the Time of Google." *Library Journal* 131(April 15, 2006): 39-44.

28. EBSCO Information Services, Serials Prices 2002-2006 with Projections for 2007. Available: <http://www.ebsco.com/>. Accessed: December 10, 2006.

29. Collins, M. "Electronic Resource Management Systems: Understanding the Players and How to Make the Right Choice for Your Library." *Serials Review* 31(2005): 125–140.

30. U.S. Copyright Office. *Reproduction of Copyrighted Works by Educators and Librarians.* Washington, DC: Library of Congress, 1995, Web rev. June 1998. Available: <http://lcweb.loc.gov/copyright/circs>. Accessed: December 14, 2006.

31. Lehman, B.A. *The Conference on Fair Use: Final Report to the Commissioner on the Conclusion of the Conference on Fair Use.* Washington, DC: U.S. Patent and Trademark Office, September 1998. Available: <http://www.uspto.gov/web/offices/dcom/olia/confu/confurep.pdf>. Accessed: December 14, 2006.

32. Kronenfeld, M.R., and Gable, S.H. "Real Inflation of Journal Prices: Medical Journals, U.S. Journals, and Brandon List Journals." *Bulletin of the Medical Library Association* 71(October 1983): 375-9.

33. Hafner, A.W.; Podsadecki, T.J.; and Whitely, W.P. "Journal Pricing Issues: An Economic Perspective." *Bulletin of the Medical Library Association* 78(July 1990): 217-23.

34. Schlimgen, J.B., and Kronenfeld, M.R. "Update on Inflation of Journal Prices: Brandon/Hill List Journals and the Scientific, Technical, and Medical Publishing Market." *Journal of the Medical Library Association* 92(July 2004): 307-14.

35. Hugo, J., and Newell, L. "New Horizons in Adult Education: The First Five Years (1987-1991)." *The Public-Access Computer Systems Review* 2, no. 1 (1991): 77-90. Available: <http://epress.lib.uh.edu/pr/v2/n1/hugo.2n1>. Accessed: December 12, 2006.

36. "PMC Frequently Asked Questions (FAQs)." Available: <http://www.pubmedcentral.nih.gov/about/FAQ .html#q16>. Accessed: February 28, 2007.

37. Tenopir, C.; King, D.W.; and Bush, A. "Medical Faculty's Use of Print and Electronic Journals: Changes Over Time and in Comparison with Scientists." *Journal of the Medical Library Association* 92 (April 2004): 233-41.

38. DeGroote, S.L., and Dorsch, J.L. "Online Journals: Impact on Print Journal Usage." *Bulletin of the Medical Library Association* 89(October 2001): 372-8.

39. O'Donohue, K. "The Accessing and Archiving of Electronic Journals: Challenges and Implications Within the Library World." *The Serials Librarian* 49(2005): 35-87.

Chapter 4

Monographic and Digital Resource Collection Development

Esther Carrigan
Mori Lou Higa
Rajia Tobia

SUMMARY. This chapter presents an overview of collection development issues and processes for all nonjournal print and digital information resources. It provides general concepts, often clarified by real world examples, and offers practical suggestions and tools for accomplishing the work of collection development. The first section provides a broader context and framework for collection development challenges and issues within health sciences libraries. Section two presents selection tools and policies for print and multimedia resources. The third section focuses on the selection, evaluation, and the varying nature of fee-based digital resources. The topics of preservation and collection weeding are explored in the fourth section, and section five concludes with an overview of challenges that will impact collection development.

INTRODUCTION

It is a widely accepted notion that journals are the heart of a health sciences library collection, with all other resources playing a more secondary role. In the most recent era of primarily print collections, double-digit journal cost inflation threatened collection budgets for all other types of information resources in many health sciences libraries. As libraries expand their digital collections, there are even greater pressures on collection budgets from both print and electronic journals, as well as other digital resources that carry recurring costs. Electronic full-text journals are enthusiastically preferred by users over their print counterparts, but there is still a significant print component to health sciences journal collections.[1] Electronic books are beginning to gain wider acceptance, but the reality remains that print and digital monographs are largely complementary. Information resources and their associated costs can be compared to an ever-enlarging pie. New product types and aggregations of different types of resources are being produced and marketed at an accelerated pace. Most health sciences libraries are not enjoying a level of collection budget growth that allows them to keep pace with the ever-expanding information resource pie. Publishing industry and vendor consolidation continues, with the net result being fewer

Authors' note: The Texas Trio (Esther, Rajia, and Mori Lou) successfully joined together to develop and write this chapter. We'd like to thank Sandy Wood for this tremendous opportunity to share Texas words of wisdom with y'all and the surprisingly gratifying collaborative experience. We would also like to acknowledge the patience and support of our library colleagues while the Texas Trio contributed to the permanent annals of library knowledge.

choices for content providers, less price competition, and pockets of information resource monopolies.[2] There are few easy choices in this marketplace. A complex and rapidly changing world of information resources is the context and rationale for both collection development chapters—to help build the skills and provide the tools to make librarians the best possible stewards of information resource dollars.

OVERVIEW AND RELATIONSHIPS

Decision-Making

It is difficult to discuss collection development without at least mentioning the opportunities for bias in all aspects of information resource management. Personal and institutional biases can influence what librarians select and reject for purchase, as well as what they choose to preserve. Documented collection policies and clearly articulated collection development guiding principles are some of the best balances for bias. Solicitation of broad input from a variety of key user groups, library staff, and external colleagues can also assure a more balanced approach to collection decisions. Judicious use of data and objective criteria as the basis for collection decisions also protects against bias.

Relationship to Acquisitions

Acquisitions activities and collection development functions are closely related, regardless of the type of library. Richards and Eakin describe the relationship in health sciences libraries as "intertwined," involving responsibilities that are sometimes combined into a single position.[3] The widespread capability for online ordering through publishers and vendors can make the separation of the two functions seem very artificial; those who review and select library materials online can also easily place the order. Licensing of electronic resources—which includes a complex array of activities, such as identifying the possible resource for licensing, planning for trials and user feedback, and negotiating and signing the contract—weaves collection development and acquisitions activities together into a seamless fabric.[4] Regardless of library size and numbers of staff involved, collection development and acquisitions staff must communicate and work well together since they support symbiotic functions.

Staffing and Workflows

Collection development activities in all types of libraries follow some variation on one of two basic staffing patterns: centralized or decentralized. In the centralized model, one librarian manages all collection development responsibilities; in the decentralized model, collection development responsibilities are shared among several librarians. Each approach has strengths and weaknesses.[3] Library size is a key factor in the choice of approach; other factors include organizational history, organizational culture, and the need for change. Because the library's collection impacts many other library functions and services, collection development processes can serve as a powerful tool in leading or facilitating organizational change.

The actual selection work of collection development can be done at the individual resource title level or on a broader subject level. Selection done at the resource title level usually occurs when a high level of selectivity for collection additions is required or when one is attempting to build a specialized collection in a particular area. An **approval plan,** discussed at greater length in the second section of this chapter, is an example of selecting materials on a broader subject basis, rather than choosing each individual title. Use of an approval plan can be an effective way to extend the staffing complement by outsourcing a portion of the process to a materials vendor.

Skill Sets for Collection Development

What skill sets would equip a librarian to successfully accomplish collection development? The standard fare of specialized subject knowledge, analytical skills, knowledge of the publishing industry and technology, and critical judgment form the basic skill set. Other essentials include communication skills, flexibility, ability to embrace change and tolerate ambiguity, negotiation skills, commitment to continual learning and exploration, a willingness to take risks, and a sense of humor.

Budgeting

Regardless of the type or size of library, "budgeting is an integral part of collection development."[3] Most collection development decisions are made within a budgetary context. Approaches to budgeting and budget specifics vary across libraries depending on the size and complexity of the collection budget as well as the financial requirements of the library's parent institution.[5]

Several levels of decisions are involved in developing the collection budget. One of the first decisions to be made is exactly what will be included in the collection budget. The actual collection materials and information resources form the core of the budget, but there are additional choices about whether the collection budget will include more tangential areas, such as binding, interlibrary loan and document delivery fees, or collection security expenses. Once the overall parameters for the collection budget are set, the decision-making shifts to how the collection funds will be allocated. They may be allocated on the basis of subjects, academic departments, or material types. The allocation approach is influenced by the collection officer's or administrator's preferences for tracking collection expenditures and the method that best supports collection development plans. Details of allocation will vary across libraries, depending on the particular environment and the goals of the budgetary process.

In essence, a budget is a plan for how to spend limited resources which will impact more than the immediate collection. A collection budget plan should support and help accomplish the library's strategic plan and be consonant with the mission and priorities of the parent institution. For a broader-based discussion of library budgets, see Chapter 13, "Management in Academic Health Sciences Libraries," and Chapter 14, "Management of and Issues Specific to Hospital Libraries."

Analysis

Collection development activities offer many opportunities to develop and employ a thoughtful, analytical approach. The possibilities cover all aspects of the collection and its use. The analytical focus can be quantitative (numbers, size, growth) or qualitative (benchmarking, user surveys).[5] Qualitative analytical efforts can explore particular sections of the collection to determine relative age or condition and also to benchmark subject areas to another library's collection or an authoritative list. A balanced approach to collection analysis is recommended, integrating both collection-focused data and user-focused data or comments.[3]

Needs Assessment (Market Research) and Marketing

Successful collection development cannot be accomplished in a vacuum. In order for a collection of information resources to meet the needs of the user, there must be an active, two-way communication pathway between a library and its users. Sections two and three of this chapter provide numerous examples of the integration of user feedback into collection development processes. Beyond basic needs assessment, ongoing regular communication can make it possible for the collection developer to address user problem reports, encourage resource suggestions, and promote the library's resources. For more general information see Chapter 9, "Marketing, Public Relations, and Communication."

MONOGRAPH SELECTION AND COLLECTION DEVELOPMENT POLICIES

Although collection development policies and selection guidelines for monographic materials are similar to the collection development policies and selection criteria outlined for journals in Chapter 3, "Journal Collection Development: Challenges, Issues, and Strategies," librarians often use different criteria to build monograph and nonjournal collections. In general, print monographs, and in some cases electronic books, require a one-time purchase, while journal subscriptions are a continuing commitment that must be renewed annually, often with escalating subscription costs. Because the decision to purchase a book for the collection is a one-time decision, librarians may deliberate less and make quicker decisions when purchasing a book. However, it is still important for librarians to have a coherent collection development policy that guides book selection and ensures that acquired books fill a need within the institution and community served by the library.

Book Selection

Selection responsibilities for books differ with the type and size of the library. As discussed earlier in this chapter, selection responsibilities can be assigned to one librarian or to several librarians depending on the size and needs of the library. Collection development librarians often have primary responsibility for book selection, with feedback from other librarians. Some libraries have a head of reference or other reference staff who select materials to be housed within the reference or reserve collections. In both small and large libraries, an advisory group such as a library committee may provide feedback or general direction for book selection. Some health sciences libraries have librarian liaison programs in which a librarian is matched with a department, and the librarian liaison or a departmental representative provides input on book, journal, or electronic resources required by the department for research or teaching needs.[6]

Most librarians with a book collection of any size choose to work with a commercial book vendor to select and order books for their collections. Working through a book vendor simplifies and standardizes the order, receipt, invoice, and payment process. In addition, most book vendors will discount the list price of a book, with the discount percentage varying according to purchase volume or other factors such as governmental purchase contracts. Several book vendors specialize in health sciences and other scientific materials, and these vendors are a good resource for keeping up with the latest books being published in the field.

Resources for Book Selection

A number of resources can be used alone or in combination to assist the health sciences librarian with selection of books.

Approval Plans

Many health sciences librarians use approval plans as time-saving selection tools to acquire books. Approval plans allow librarians to identify a profile based on subjects or titles that they wish to receive from a vendor as books are published. Richards and Eakin describe an approval plan itself as a selection tool.[3] The approval plan profile details subject areas, publishers, and types of publications to include or exclude from the plan. For example, a library for a health sciences campus with a dental school will include dental titles within its profile, while a hospital library may choose to receive new editions for a small number of prominent dental textbooks or may completely exclude dentistry in the library profile. The profile should detail types of books the library wants to receive upon publication, such as new textbooks, health science reference books, lab manuals, and core titles. The profile should also identify types of books to exclude, for example, proceedings, examination review books, or books such as programmed instruction designed for individual use.

Books received on approval are normally reviewed by one or more librarians and are either accepted for addition to the collection or sent back to the vendor. Approval plans may need to be adjusted at least annually to reflect any changes in book acquisitions due to budget increases or decreases or hospital or campus shifts in focus.

Brandon/Hill List

From 1965 to 2003 the *Selected List of Books and Journals for Small Medical Libraries,* referred to as the *Brandon/Hill List* and discussed in greater detail in Chapter 3, defined a core collection of medical books and journals for small libraries.[7, 8] Despite discontinuation of the list, book vendors continue to identify "Brandon/Hill" books as new editions of the books are published. Eventually, the *Brandon/Hill List* of core titles will become dated since newly published books are not being added to the core title list. For the time being, however, librarians continue to use the "Brandon/Hill" designation as an important selection tool.

Doody's Core Titles

Doody's Enterprises, Inc., provides literature updates in the health sciences field, including *Doody's Core Titles.*[9] *Doody's Core Titles* was developed in 2004 to partially fill the void left by the discontinuation of the *Brandon/Hill List.* Although sponsored by a commercial company, core titles are identified and recommended by content specialists associated with the Doody's Book Review Service and library selectors.[10] *Doody's Core Titles* can be purchased for a nominal price from the company in either a basic or premium version. The premium version includes book reviews from the Doody's Book Review Service.

Other Core Lists

Over the years, various organizations and librarians have compiled lists of books recommended for a number of disciplines. Many of the lists are either no longer published or dated; however, the lists can be useful starting points for librarians seeking to update older editions of core texts with newer editions. The Collection Development Section of the Medical Library Association (MLA) maintains a Web site that documents many of the core lists that have been published over the years.[11]

Book Vendors

Book vendors, particularly those that specialize in the health sciences, can be useful sources of information for book selection. Book vendors normally provide services useful for collection development, such as these:

- weekly lists of newly published books in their inventory;
- catalogs of books in particular subject areas (consumer health, for example);
- foreign language titles;
- Brandon/Hill titles;
- approval plans;
- special sales or discounts;
- summaries of a library's book purchases and average costs; and
- customer service representatives who can assist librarians with collection development issues.

The Collection Development Section of MLA provides a list of library vendors through its Web site.[12]

Book Reviews

A number of prominent medical journals provide book reviews that can be useful for selection of titles. *JAMA* and *New England Journal of Medicine* are examples of weekly journals that many health sciences librarians use as sources for book reviews. Because there is usually a delay between the time a book is published and when it may be reviewed in a journal or magazine, book reviews can best be used as an adjunct to other sources for timely book selection.

Consumer Health

For consumer health information, *Library Journal* and *Publishers Weekly* provide book reviews for recently published health-related titles. The *Consumer Health Information Source Book* by Alan M. Rees, now in its seventh edition, has been used extensively over the years for building consumer health collections.[13] Barclay and Halsted's *Consumer Health Reference Service Handbook* also provides an extensive list of recommended consumer health books.[14]

Other Sources for Book Selection

Although not an unbiased source of information, publisher's mailings can provide information about new publications. Fliers and catalogs from university presses, societies, and other organizations may often be the only source to inform the librarian of publications produced by these small publishers. Publisher Web sites, as well as courtesy visits from vendors and publisher representatives, can provide useful information for keeping up with book publishing.

Collection Development Policies

A collection development policy is a written guide to the desired collection practices of a library. A collection development policy can range from a simple statement to a complex document, depending on the size and needs of a library. A small hospital library may develop a one- or two-page document that outlines categories of strength within the hospital and how the library will support those strengths through its acquisition of books, journals, and electronic resources. An academic health sciences library serving an institution with research, teaching, patient care, and outreach missions will likely require a more detailed policy due to the many needs of its diverse clientele. Many accrediting organizations require the library to have a written collection development policy and will ask for a copy of the policy as part of the accreditation documentation. Because of the rapidly changing information resource environment, a collection development policy should be a vibrant document, reviewed on an annual basis for its continued relevance and updated accordingly. Chapter 3 discusses collection development policies for journals in detail, and many of the same principles apply to both journals and books. The following sections address criteria to include in the collection development policy for print books and multimedia resources. Depending on the needs of the library, all or some points can be included.

Description of Institutional Environment

Most collection development policies briefly describe the institutional mission and environment to help guide selection decisions. A hospital may wish to identify particular areas of strength, such as pediatrics or cardiovascular medicine. Academic health sciences libraries should describe academic programs served, any research strengths of the university, and branch campus locations, if applicable. Some libraries include background and historical information about the library at the time the policy is written: for example, the number of books and journals that are owned and when the library was founded.

Selection Responsibilities

The policy should address who makes selection decisions. In a one-person library, selection responsibility may seem obvious, but even in a one-person library, there might be a committee that has responsibility for advising the librarian or another individual who must approve purchases. In a larger setting, the responsibility for selecting books might be divided among librarians with varying expertise, or an acquisitions or collection development librarian may make book selections. If a director or other superior must approve selections once they are made, this should be documented in the policy.

Budget

Every library has finite resources. Although budgets usually increase or decrease on an annual basis, the collection development policy should address the collection budget in general terms. What percentage of the library's collection budget will be expended on books? If a percentage is not documented, expenditures for journals and electronic resources can quickly devour collection funds. If possible, the policy should address what course of action to take during times of financial constraint. Will book purchasing be reduced or curtailed altogether? On the brighter side, the policy might also delineate areas for growth should a windfall of money present itself.

Advisory Groups

In some settings, advisory groups might be involved in recommending or approving book purchases. Library committees, curriculum committees, or other advisory groups are important to document in the collection development policy because these committees establish the relationship between librarians and their constituencies. Advisory groups are more likely to be involved with giving general direction to librarians for a collection development policy rather than recommending specific purchases. For example, rather than asking the librarian to purchase a particular book on bioinformatics, the committee may advise that bioinformatics is a growth area for the institution and, as a result, the book collection should be expanded in this discipline to support the increased need.

User Recommendations

The policy should document how user recommendations for book purchases will be handled. Journals represent a long-term commitment for libraries; however, a book is a one-time purchase and represents a smaller financial commitment over time. Many librarians choose to purchase virtually all books requested by their users, as long as the budget is robust, while the selection of journals requires a more rigorous review. Will all book requests be honored, or will there be a review of the requests? Will requestors be required to document the need for the book purchase, such as the book's use as required reading in a course or background reading for a new research area?

Subject Scope

The detail used to describe subject scope among collection development policies varies widely among health sciences libraries. Some collection development policies describe the subjects to be collected by outlining a profile according to the **National Library of Medicine** classification or some other classification system. Other policies may outline subject scope with broader strokes, such as nursing, allied health, medicine, public health, pharmacy, dentistry, and other broad subject categories. Some policies identify the level of collecting, for example, undergraduate, graduate, and research levels or basic, advanced, and research levels. The second revised edition of the *MLA DocKit #3, Collection Development and Management for Electronic, Audiovisual, and Print Resources in Health Sciences Libraries* provides a few excellent examples of collection development policies that show the detail used in defining the subject scope of various collections.[15]

Language and/or Country of Publication

For most health sciences libraries in the United States, English will be the predominate language for most book purchases. The collection development policy should state whether books in other languages or published outside the native country will be collected. For example, a hospital library serving a large Hispanic community may document in its collection development policy that consumer health materials will be purchased in both English and Spanish. For an academic health sciences library in the United States, the policy should document whether books published in Europe or other regions will be purchased as well as whether or not foreign language publications will be added to the collection. Likewise, if the policy is to collect only in the native language, such as English, this should be stated in the policy.

Retention of Older Materials

The collection development policy is particularly useful for identifying how older materials, superseded editions, or infrequently used materials will be handled. **Weeding** the collection will be discussed later in this chapter, but some aspects of routine weeding should be addressed in the collection development policy:

- When a new edition of a book is purchased, will all older editions be retained, or will they be withdrawn?
- In a smaller library with a primarily clinical focus, does the library maintain a cut-off date for the collection? For example, will only those books published within the last twenty years be retained?
- If a book has not circulated within the last ten years, will it be automatically withdrawn?

- If the library keeps older materials in storage, what is the trigger year for moving a book into storage?

Preservation

Preservation of library materials will be discussed in more detail later in this chapter, but preservation plans should be mentioned in the collection development policy. For some libraries, the preservation plan may be extensive enough to warrant a separate policy devoted entirely to preservation issues. For a library whose collection has a primarily current clinical focus, a preservation plan for older or damaged materials may not be as critical.

Textbooks

Some libraries choose to include a statement in their collection development policy about the responsibility of students to acquire textbooks for course work and study. Many libraries purchase textbooks and include them in the circulating collection or in the reserve collection. If textbooks will be purchased, a statement to this effect might be included in the policy, along with any particulars, such as working with a campus bookstore to identify textbooks or reviewing course syllabi for required and recommended texts.

Exam Study and Review Books

Health sciences libraries with student or postgraduate users may need to document whether or not they will purchase student study materials for exams and board reviews, such as the **USMLE (United States Medical Licensure Examination), NCLEX-RN (National Council Licensure Examination—Registered Nurse),** and specialty boards. Because these types of study materials are generally designed for individual use and often include sections to be completed by the student, many libraries do not purchase them. On the other hand, librarians may use these materials as a way to make the library more relevant to their student population. Some institutions may provide special funding for student review materials, such as funding through a dean's office or a student fee. This type of special funding should be documented in the policy.

Multiple Copies

The collection development policy should detail whether multiple copies of books will be purchased and in what circumstances. For example, if an instructor requests multiple copies of a book for reserve use, will the library purchase the multiple copies, or will purchase of multiple copies be designated a departmental responsibility? In times of financial constraint, many libraries by policy do not collect multiple copies of books.

Standing Orders

Jones and Wilkerson define a category of publication called "nonperiodical serials" that blurs the lines between a monographic publication and a serial, stating that there is little agreement as to what constitutes a nonperiodical serial.[16] Nonperiodical serials are generally published irregularly and are invoiced and paid as published rather than in advance of publication. A library may arrange with a vendor or publisher to receive new volumes as they are published, thus assuring that all volumes will be received in a timely manner. Librarians often refer to these publications as "**standing orders**" while publishers tend to identify them as "continuations." The *Physician's Desk Reference (PDR)* is an example of a title that many health sciences librarians keep on standing order with a book vendor. This title is published on an annual basis, and many librarians seek to have the newest editions added to their reference collections through prearranged standing orders.

The collection development policy should state whether a standing order plan will be maintained with a vendor or publisher. It is usually not necessary to list all titles to be placed on standing order because this information may change frequently. Instead, the collection development policy should state in general terms whether standing orders will be used as a method for acquiring new series volumes and new editions of books published on a continuous basis. The librarian will need to work with one or more vendors and publishers to initiate standing orders, defining whether each new volume will be acquired, or, in the case of new editions, whether each new edition will be acquired or an alternative frequency defined, such as every other edition.

Books with Accompanying Nonprint Media

Publishers are increasingly producing books with accompanying compact discs, DVDs, or Web sites. Because management of accompanying media can be problematic, the policy should state how accompanying media will be handled upon receipt. Libraries handle DVDs and compact discs in a number of ways. Some libraries leave the discs in the book while others choose to shelve the discs in a separate location, such as the reserve collection or within a separate disc collection. Still other libraries simply choose not to retain compact discs and DVDs that accompany books, under the assumption that they will eventually be lost, stolen, or damaged.

Books with accompanying Web sites are becoming more common, and the collection development policy should address how these sites will be handled. A publisher's instructions for access to its Web site must be carefully reviewed in order to determine whether the Web site is designed for individual use or whether institutional use is allowed. In some cases, use of the Web site on an institutional basis will require execution of an institution-wide license.

Nonprint Materials—DVDs, CDs, Audiovisuals

Most health sciences libraries will require some nonprint materials within their collections to support teaching and learning. Nonprint materials can include DVDs, CDs, slides, videos, audiocassettes, models, and formats yet to be developed. The collection development policy should detail how nonprint materials will be selected, subject needs within the nonprint collection, and format and equipment considerations. Some libraries may require departments to share in the purchase costs of costly nonprint materials, and this should be documented in the policy.

Gifts

Libraries often have a separate policy regarding in-kind donations of books and other materials. At some institutions, gifts of any kind, including books and journals, must be initially fielded through an office external to the library, such as a campus or hospital development office. The collection development policy should document whether the library accepts donations of books, journals, and other materials and how these donations will be handled, since acceptance or rejection of gifts can have implications for the parent institution. Some libraries choose not to accept gifts because of the amount of staff time required to process the material. If gifts are accepted, then the policy should document whether there are limitations, such as the age of materials the library will accept, subjects, condition of the material, and whether gifts are only accepted from faculty or other identified groups. Responsibility for acknowledging the gift and any appraisal or tax considerations should also be documented.

Historical Materials

Some libraries will have special collection areas for historical or rare materials, while others will not have the facilities to house these types of materials. If a historical collection is in place or planned, the collection development policy should describe the types of materials that will be housed in this collection. Will books published prior to a certain date or of a certain age be moved to the historical collection or permanently retained in the regular collection? Will the special collections area house an archival collection of university documents, local documents, or other historical documents? If the library will not retain historical materials, possibilities for disposition of the materials should be documented. Will the materials be transferred to another library or archive or sold to a rare or out-of-print book dealer? More information about historical materials can be found in Chapter 17, "Health Sciences Librarianship in Rare Book and Special Collections."

Institutional and Local Authors

Some libraries treat publications by authors from the institution or the local area in special ways. Books published by institutional or local authors or for which they have been contributors might be housed in a special collections area. Publications by institutional or local authors, whether these are journal articles, books, book chapters, or meeting presentations, might be included in a faculty/student publication bibliography compiled periodically by the library or included in an online institutional repository. If publications by institutional or local authors are to be handled in some special manner, this should be covered in the collection development policy, including the length of retention for these types of publications.

Government Documents

Government documents often contain important information for health sciences libraries, particularly in the field of public health. Librarians should monitor announcements of new government documents to determine titles to add to their collections. The Government Printing Office (GPO) Web site provides information about publications published by the U.S. government, and documents can be ordered through this site.[17] Bernan is a commercial company that also provides acquisition services for U.S. government publications and selected documents from international agencies and other governments.[18] Librarians have the option of establishing deposit accounts with either the GPO or Bernan for acquiring government documents. The collection development policy should discuss government documents and any varying acquisitions practices that may be in place for these types of documents, such as deposit accounts.

Specialized Books

Many librarians define specialized monographic materials in their collection development policies. Although specialized publications can take many forms, dissertations, technical reports, and proceedings are usually considered to be publications that have a specialized focus.

In the case of theses and dissertations, most health sciences libraries with graduate programs will have some responsibility for archiving these publications as part of the intellectual record of their institutions. Many graduate programs are eliminating print publication of dissertations and producing the dissertations only in digital form. Librarians should seek to define the library's role in collecting and archiving print and/or digital dissertations produced by their graduate students. Most health sciences libraries do not routinely collect dissertations published at other institutions, although the library may obtain dissertations through interlibrary loan or through other special arrangements.

Proceedings of meetings and technical reports often cover very specialized information, and as library collection budgets shrink, so does the ability to purchase specialized proceedings and technical reports. The collection development policy may detail whether the library will purchase proceedings and technical reports and in what subject areas.

Out-of-Print Books

On occasion, the library will be requested or will have need to purchase a book that has become out-of-print. A faculty member may need an out-of-print book for a course or for research purposes, or the library may need to replace a book that has been lost or damaged. It is useful for the collection development policy to document sources that library staff can use to acquire out-of-print books.

Ephemera

Ephemera are generally defined as printed materials with a short intended lifetime.[19] Examples include invitations, pamphlets, posters, tickets, photographs, and other materials considered to be of limited usefulness beyond a certain point in time. Depending on the source of the ephemera, libraries may choose to retain some ephemera while discarding other types. For example, ephemera published by the parent institution of a library or photographs of historical interest might be considered for archival retention, while ephemera printed by an outside organization might be discarded after its usefulness has passed. To avoid confusion about what to do when a piece of ephemera is acquired by the library, the collection development policy should identify disposition of these items.

Consumer Health

Many health sciences libraries maintain a consumer health collection, and Chapter 18, "Consumer Health Information," discusses consumer health services in detail. In hospital libraries, a consumer health collection may be used by patients or by patient education personnel. In academic health sciences libraries, a consumer health collection may be maintained for community users or for students who need to use the materials for class projects or for background reading. Some health sciences libraries may choose not to collect consumer health because this type of material does not fit their mission or for budgetary reasons. The collection development policy should document whether or not consumer health titles will be purchased; subject focus, if relevant, such as women's or children's health; literacy levels; and language considerations.

Leisure or Popular Reading

Some health sciences libraries choose to have small collections of leisure reading books and magazines for rest and relaxation purposes for their users. These collections can also draw users, such as hospital or university support personnel who might be interested in popular reading materials but not professional books and journals. Some libraries acquire popular fiction and nonfiction books through rental plans, such as the McNaughton Plan from the Brodart Company.[20] This assures that titles are refreshed on a continual basis without expending much effort in selection and acquisition. Some libraries maintain a popular reading book exchange for their users as a service. If leisure reading materials will be provided for users, this should be documented in the collection development plan.

SELECTION AND EVALUATION OF DIGITAL RESOURCES

When evaluating digital resources for purchase, various criteria, strategies, and tools can help librarians assess the value and viability of potential products for particular communities. This section offers practical approaches to help librarians make informed decisions to both build and maintain collections that effectively support the needs of their users. By combining basic selection criteria such as content, usability, technical functionality, need, and cost with qualitative feedback, librarians can systematically assess a product's value and its likelihood of potential use. Understanding how products relate and compare to other digital resources can also help with both initial selection and ongoing evaluation activities.

In the context of this chapter, "digital resources" refer to searching tools, databases, combined or aggregated products, electronic books, and other information resources that require a fee to be paid in order to access. With the exception of **MEDLINE,** this section is not intended to address free information resources and Web sites. Many excellent resources, such as Louis A. Pitschmann's *Building Sustainable Collections of Free Third-Party Web Resources,* can be consulted for guidance on the selection, management, and manpower needed to build and maintain collections of free information resources.[21] Additionally, electronic journals will be addressed in this chapter only peripherally due to the aggregated nature of some products. For a detailed overview of journal selection and related issues, please consult Chapter 3, "Journal Collection Development."

Digital Resource Selection Criteria

Content

Content should be examined for currency, quality, uniqueness, permanence, and coverage (see Table 4.1). Answering specific content-related questions can help librarians judge the overall value of a product's content and gain an improved understanding of any issues that may raise concerns. Some issues may be more pertinent than others for particular libraries. For example, if a librarian chooses to rely solely on electronic editions of particular books, currency and archival rights will be critical. Those supplementing their print collections with electronic access may view these concerns differently. There is no one blueprint for every library and every situation. An understanding of each institution's environment and the library's collection policies must also be considered.

Usability

Usability is generally determined by the ease with which new users can operate a resource and how efficiently tasks can be handled once learned (see Table 4.2). Seamless integration is also making information seeking easier, and increasingly librarians and users desire and expect integration of products or "interoperability," which can also increase visibility of, and access to, other expensive resources.

Technical and Other Support Considerations

When considering technical functionality, it is important to consider both the librarian's expectations for vendor support and the library's own support capabilities (see Table 4.3).

TABLE 4.1. Content Considerations for Digital Resources

Characteristic	Questions to Consider
Currency	• How frequently is the content reviewed and updated? • Are critical updates (e.g., those with clinical impact) added immediately? • For book content, is the most current edition included? • If newer editions of books are included as part of a library's purchase, how quickly is access made available upon release? • If the resource contains journal content, are any embargoes (i.e., delayed access to the most current content) in place?
Authority	• Is content authored by or does it involve participation of those affiliated with institutions of higher education, scholarly associations or societies, established for-profit publishers, etc.? • Are methods in place to vet content, such as editorial review, peer review, publisher quality control standards, etc.? • Are clinical "evidence-based" products based upon expert opinions, case studies, randomized control trials, etc.? What is their level of evidence? • Are sources referenced? • How long has the content provider been in existence?
Accuracy	• Do the data (e.g., full text, citations, references, etc.) appear accurate? • Are there any gaps in coverage based on defined scope? • Do the data, textual guides, "about" information, etc., contain spelling or typographical errors?
Uniqueness	• What type of content is offered (e.g., databases, e-books, e-journals, continuing medical education, patient information, citation only, full text, aggregated content, etc.)? • Is the content unique or is it available through multiple sources? • Could the resource serve as a replacement for existing print content or another digital resource? • Does the resource provide some added value if not unique (e.g., a superior or specialized subject-based interface; additional access for heavily used items; easy-to-use portal; cheap alternative option)?
Perpetual access rights	• Is there a guarantee of archival rights to the content? • Are archival rights relevant and critical (e.g., abstracting and indexing databases may not offer such rights or be desired)? • What years will be covered? • Will the vendor continue to provide access through its existing or some other interface?
Scope/coverage	• What content is included or indexed? • Is comprehensive or selective coverage provided? • What years, editions, etc., are included? • Is the content's focus national or international? • Will a library's subscription automatically include additional backfiles currently in development? • Will additional, new content be included, or will it need to be purchased separately? • Does access to older editions disappear once newer editions become available?

TABLE 4.2. Usability Considerations for Digital Resources

Characteristic	Questions to Consider
Ease of use	• Does the resource offer an intuitive interface? • Can the information be easily browsed? • Are sources of support (e.g., online help, user aids, tutorials, technical assistance, etc.) provided? • Would training be required?
Navigation	• Is there a natural or logical flow to tasks, organization, and functionality? • Is one's location apparent at all times? • Can one easily find the home, forward, and back options?
Searching functionality	• Does the resource offer both basic and advanced searching capabilities? • How effective is the search retrieval? • Are multifile or cross-database searching capabilities offered?
Printing/saving/e-mail/ video capabilities	• Are these capabilities simple or complex? • Are these functions readily apparent?
Stability	• Is the platform stable? • Have past upgrades or enhancements resulted in downtime? • Is there a backup system such as a mirror site?
Response times	• Are there any delays in the resource's response time when initiating actions?
Integration capabilities	• Do multiple resources from the same vendor offer compatible interfaces or easy integration between resources? • Is integration with external resources [e.g., linking to licensed full text or integration with electronic health records (EHR) or electronic medical records (EMR)] possible or planned for the future? • Is the resource compatible with existing bibliographic citation management tools?

TABLE 4.3. Technical and Other Support Considerations for Digital Resources

Characteristic	Questions to Consider
Vendor support	• Are there clear support options for resolving technical problems in a timely manner (e.g., help desk phone numbers, e-mail support, FAQs, or interactive chat)? • Are mechanisms in place to proactively communicate information relating to product updates, upgrades, and problems? • Is free or fee-based training offered (e.g., in-person training, Webinars, tutorials, or demonstrations)? • Is product support offered for PCs, MACs, and different browser interfaces? • Are COUNTER-compliant usage statistics available or will they be? What is the frequency and format of the statistics? Are statistics offered for trial periods and for each institution when dealing with consortia purchases? • Is branding, or the library's ability to include its logo or name on a digital resource's interface, available?
Library support	• Is the library's current workstation environment compatible with the vendor's requirements (e.g., can the library's workstations support PDA downloading, graphics, e-mail options, video clips, plug-ins, etc.)? • Are there any potential conflicts with the library's or institution's security policies or state and federal rulings relating to access of electronic information by individuals with disabilities? • Is a user authentication system in place to control and monitor access? • Are there any special restrictions requiring a heightened level of technical compliance (e.g., some vendors may prohibit guest user access or restrict remote access)?

Need and Relevance

A library's collection development policy will define its audience or users, subjects to be collected, and desired formats. This policy should help assess the general relevance of the resource to the institution. An earlier section in this chapter, Monograph Selection and Collection Development Policies, and Chapter 3 should be consulted for additional information relating to collection policies.

Cost Considerations

All selection decisions must consider an item's cost and whether the benefits of the item warrant the cost. When examining the cost implications of a digital resource, the selector should understand how a resource has been priced (i.e., cost basis) and the value for cost. The cost basis for digital resource pricing generally depends upon an institution's size and type. Vendors often calculate an institution's size based upon the number of full-time staff, students, and faculty. However, depending on the intended audience for a product, vendors may request an institution's **full-time equivalent (FTE)** count for a specific user group, such as medical students only. The librarian should request the vendor's definition of FTEs since different vendors may interpret this in various ways and use separate FTE counts for different products. Vendors may also estimate an institution's size using other data, such as hospital inpatient admissions or outpatient visits. Finally, vendors will consider the type of institution, such as for-profit, university systems, individual universities, academic institutions that include medical schools or doctoral programs, and hospitals.

Various pricing models exist and continue to evolve, as Kristin H. Gerhard has documented.[22] This summation offers some of the most common pricing approaches. Price quotes are generally split between subscriptions with recurring costs or single, one-time purchases. Another variation involves both options for a single resource. For example, a purchase might involve an annual subscription cost for the most current years with a single, one-time purchase for a defined or rolling **backfile** purchase. As long as the library retains a current subscription, an additional year will "roll" or be added to the permanent backfile.

Pricing can also be affected by the number of users a library is willing to fund. An unrestricted site license provides the widest possible access with unlimited users and will also be the most expensive. Vendors may also offer a more cost-effective approach based on a defined number of simultaneous users or a restricted geographic locale. For products where limited use is anticipated or the cost is prohibitive, a restricted licensing approach may be a library's best option.

Librarians should also consider if joint or consortia purchases with other institutions may be possible. By approaching vendors from a consortia perspective, reduced fees and guaranteed price caps are frequently possible due to the increased buying power of multiple institutions. For additional information about the benefits and drawbacks of consortia purchases, readers should refer to Chapter 3.

When considering individual resource costs, librarians must assess such fees in the larger context of their library's budget. With the increasing reliance upon digital resources, there are also increased numbers of items with recurring costs. The librarian should consider whether a library is capable of currently funding the resource as well as the library's future ability to sustain funding. While only an estimate, ascertaining the vendor's annual inflation rate for the past few years is one strategy to help understand and plan for future years' costs.

Obtaining firm prices has become an art form, as any practicing collection development librarian can attest. Initial quotes are generally negotiable. Collection specialists should never make assumptions about how resources are priced and always ask for clarification when uncertain. Vendors may make inaccurate assumptions about a library's user groups or institutional environment, and discounts may be applicable for multiple product purchases or for being a member of certain groups. Professionalism, assertiveness, and good communication are critical skills for establishing good working relationships with vendors.[23]

Licensing Terms

Since an increasing number of digital resources involve contracts, licensing terms that define and restrict who can use the product, where it can be used, how it can be used, and for what period of time should be considered as part of the product's basic evaluation. For in-depth coverage of license considerations, consult Chapter 3 and other recent publications.[23, 24]

Assessment Strategies and Tools

In addition to selection criteria, a number of strategies and tools can help assess a resource's value and priority for a library. The following are some approaches that can supplement basic selection criteria. Environments vary, and some tools may be more relevant in some situations and not in others.

Trials/Usage Data

Vendors will usually offer trial access to a digital resource to provide an opportunity for hands-on testing before purchase. In general, thirty-day trials are fairly standard, although specific trial periods can vary or be extended upon request. Vendors may also be able to provide usage data for the trial period. If user input is desired, librarians should have a plan in place to promote the trial and gather feedback before the trial is activated.

Feedback Mechanisms

Obtaining feedback from a library's users in advance of purchase can be time well spent. Feedback can be solicited directly from users through various methods, such as one-on-one interactions, product demonstrations, Web-based surveys, or focus groups. The librarian should decide in advance whether the desired feedback will be collected through the use of a broad statement—"Tell us what you think"—or solicited through a series of structured questions, such as these:

- What did you like about the product?
- What didn't you like about the product?
- Would you use this resource if the library purchased?
- How satisfied were you with your results?

Library staff should also be encouraged to provide feedback since they can supply different insight regarding a product's value.

Colleagues

Colleagues who have already acquired particular resources can offer advice supported by their experiences. Most vendors will supply contact information for current library subscribers. Consortia groups can also offer opportunities for information sharing. Most librarians are quite willing to answer questions about their overall satisfaction with a product, a product's potential user base, product functionality, and vendor responsiveness.

Published Reviews and Other Information Sources

Various publications include pertinent reviews of digital resources in the health sciences field, while other sources can help librarians stay abreast of the constantly changing information industry with current news reports about products, services, and content providers. Some useful publications include the following:

- *The Charleston Advisor* <http://charlestonco.com/>
- *Information Today, ONLINE Magazine,* and *Searcher* <http://www.infotoday.com/>
- *Journal of Electronic Resources in Medical Libraries* <http://www.haworthpress.com/default.asp>
- *Journal of the Medical Library Association,* Electronic Resources Reviews section, <http://www.mlanet.org/publications/jmla/index.html>
- *Medical Reference Services Quarterly* <http://www.haworthpress.com/default.asp>

Discussion Lists

These lists allow librarians to draw upon the experiences of colleagues, exchange information and ideas, and monitor trends. Some useful lists, in addition to those listed in Chapter 3, include ACQNET (Acquisitions Librarians Electronic Network) <http://www.acqweb.org/acqnet.html> and COLLDV-L (Library Collection Development) <http://www.infomotions.com/serials/colldv-l/>.

Use of Selection Teams or Committees

Since digital resources require that the library assess a broader array of potential impacts and considerations than a single print item, many libraries draw upon the expertise of varied library staff when selecting new products.[25, 26] Selection teams with broad library representation (e.g., reference librarians, collection specialists, technical support, public services staff, educators, or Web site support) ensure that a product is reviewed from all possible angles to eliminate unwelcome surprises later on and to facilitate communication among various stakeholders.

Priorities

New digital resource options appear with increasing regularity, and alternative options for existing products may be offered. User needs evolve, budget situations change, and additional funding may be made available on short notice. All of these elements contribute to the need to establish a workable process to systematically capture new, relevant options and to establish priorities. Through the use of tools such as spreadsheets or databases, "wish lists," "under consideration groupings," or "desiderata" can be created to gather pertinent information, such as the name of the resource and brief description, pricing information if known, consortia interest, product restrictions if any, user or staff input, and a priority ranking.

Checklists

Checklists offer a systematic method to evaluate new digital products and to help ensure that librarians do not overlook any key considerations. Librarians may wish to customize checklists, which have been widely documented, for their particular environments or for particular types of resources.[4, 27-30] Such lists ensure that any unique considerations are addressed as part of a product's evaluation process.

Overlap or Added Value? General Categories of Digital Resources

Understanding digital resources' capabilities and content and how these may compare to other purchased resources is essential. In some situations, overlap with existing resources can be useful and justified. For example, tools such as PsychiatryOnline or Mosby's Nursing Consult offer specialized subject portals combining both journal and book content, which can save users time and effort.[31-33] Other resources containing overlapping content can offer added value by providing access to the most current content, additional access points for heavily used resources, or increased support for expanding user needs. Still other tools such as the Faculty of 1000 Medicine or Biology may offer value by providing newer approaches to established concepts such as current awareness.[34, 35]

Digital resources are increasingly blurring traditional lines and may be placed in multiple categories. Table 4.4 identifies some of the major categories that health sciences librarians will likely address, a brief description of the category, and a sampling of specific resources. While not intended to provide a comprehensive list of all available resources on the market or to address specialized selection considerations, the table provides a broad overview of the wide array of options and demonstrates the possibilities for duplication and overlap. Additional in-depth resources, such as the *Introduction to Reference Sources in the Health Sciences,* should be consulted when evaluating specific types of resources such as bibliographic databases.[36]

MEDLINE—Free versus Fee-Based Options

In today's budget-conscious environment, collection development librarians will want to give special consideration to MEDLINE (Medical Literature Analysis and Retrieval System Online) due to its availability as both a free resource and a fee-based option. MEDLINE, the premier health sciences bibliographic database from the U.S. National Library of Medicine, includes journal citations and abstracts covering medicine, nursing, dentistry, veterinary medicine, the health care system, and the preclinical sciences. Coverage is generally from 1950 to the present, and citations are included for more than 5,000 international biomedical journals.[37]

Since 1997, MEDLINE access has been offered at no cost through PubMed, a database that was developed by the National Center for Biotechnology Information (NCBI) at the National Library of Medicine as part of the Entrez retrieval system.[38] When using PubMed, searchers can limit their retrieval to MEDLINE citations only or broaden their searches to include additional PubMed information, such as

- selected life sciences journals not included in MEDLINE;
- in-process citations for articles prior to inclusion in MEDLINE;
- citations preceding a journal's selection for MEDLINE indexing; and
- OLDMEDLINE citations not yet updated for MEDLINE status.[39]

In addition to PubMed, the National Library of Medicine leases its MEDLINE journal citation data at no charge to third parties who develop separate search software and interfaces to the data.[40] These interfaces are offered at no cost through providers such as Infotrieve and Medscape with free registration or involve separate databases fees through third parties such as Ovid.[41-44]

While cost is certainly one consideration, the decision to choose a free or fee-based MEDLINE interface will involve a number of other factors, such as budget, user and staff preferences and needs, ease of access, and search capabilities and interface. Countless comparisons of features and functionality exist, but ultimately it will be an individual library's decision whether the added value from a fee-based MEDLINE version is justified for its particular needs.[45-50]

TABLE 4.4 Categories of Digital Resources

Resource Category	Examples
TYPE: Databases. Abstracts and indexes; full text. DESCRIPTION: Searchable interface to bibliographic citations. May contain or provide links to full-text content.	BIOSIS Previews, *Chemical Abstracts,* CINAHL, Current Contents, EMBASE, MEDLINE, PsycINFO, Science Direct, Scopus
TYPE: Databases. Aggregated collections; aggregators. DESCRIPTION: Searchable mix of formats and content such as electronic books, electronic journals, databases, patient education, drug information, continuing education, etc. Content may be offered by a single content provider or a content aggregator hosting content from multiple providers.	AccessMedicine, MD Consult, PsychiatryOnline, ScienceDirect, STAT!Ref, Wiley InterScience Aggregators: CSA, EBSCO*host,* Ovid
TYPE: Databases. Citation indexes. DESCRIPTION: Interface for article retrieval with citation tracking and cited reference searching.	Google Scholar (free), *Science Citation Index,* Scopus, *Social Sciences Citation Index,* Web of Science
TYPE: Databases. Clinical decision or support; evidence based medicine. DESCRIPTION: Synthesized information to assist with clinical decisions, some at the point of care. Expert or evidence based, with varying levels of evidence. May support electronic medical or health records integration.	ACP PIER, Clinical Evidence, Cochrane Database of Systematic Reviews, Database of Abstracts of Reviews of Effectiveness (DARE), DXplain, DynaMed, eMedicine, Evidence Matters, FIRSTConsult, InfoRetriever, UpToDate
TYPE: Databases. Current awareness. DESCRIPTION: Keeps users informed about new published information. Can be configured for selected topics. Includes journal tables of contents or highlights/evaluations of recommended articles.	Current Contents Connect, Faculty of 1000 Biology, Faculty of 1000 Medicine
TYPE: Databases. Hybrids; "pseudo"-databases. DESCRIPTION: Searchable collections of full-text information created by publishers or vendors. Content is generally governed by availability, not formal journal selection policies such as MEDLINE's <http://www.nlm.nih.gov/pubs/factsheets/jsel.html.>	Academic Search Premier, ScienceDirect
TYPE: Databases. Images; 3D anatomy. DESCRIPTION: Image resources and tools to locate images, tables, figures, graphs, and illustrations.	Anatomy.tv, CSA Illustra, images.MD, Primal Pictures, SMART Imagebase
TYPE: Databases. Research support tools. DESCRIPTION: Assists with research process (research/writing/publishing) via citation management, journal performance indicators, institutional expertise, and grant funding opportunities.	Community of Scholars, Community of Science, EndNote, *Journal Citation Reports,* Reference Manager
TYPE: Databases. Specialty focus. DESCRIPTION: Information that supports specific disciplines or focus areas. May contain factual information, citations, full text, or other specialized content.	AccessSurgery, BioMedProtocols.com, Clinical Pharmacology, EXAM MASTER OnLine, MICROMEDEX, Natural Medicines Comprehensive Database, Natural Standard, Mosby's Nursing Skills or Consult
TYPE: Electronic books. DESCRIPTION: Platform offering access to electronic books from a single content provider or multiple publishers.	AccessMedicine, BioMedProtocols.com, Ebrary, MDConsult, Mosby's Nursing Consult, netLibrary, Books@Ovid, PsycBooks, R2 Library, STAT!Ref
TYPE: Electronic journals. DESCRIPTION: Full-text digital access to current and archival journals supplied by publishers, aggregators, other hosts.	EBSCO*host,* HighWire, JSTOR, Journals@Ovid, PsycArticles, ScienceDirect

A Day in the Life of a Collection Development Librarian

Name: Mori Lou Higa, MLS
Position: Manager, Collection Development, University of Texas Southwestern Medical Center Library

Job description: The Collection Development Manager leads, manages, and plans for all aspects of the library's collection development activities, including preparation and monitoring of a $2 million plus collection budget; selection, renewal, evaluation, and deselection of electronic and print resources; and negotiation, execution, and maintenance of license agreements. She works collaboratively with consortia, vendors, clients, and staff in support of her responsibilities and participates in various internal teams and library initiatives. Additionally, she manages the library's collection development department, which includes three full-time employees.

Sample Day

8:00 a.m.
- Respond to campus contract's office request for information and other inquiries.
- Request feedback from the library's educational staff about client needs relating to PDA (personal digital assistant) access (in response to a consortia inquiry).
- Research information related to specific faculty journal recommendations.
- Prepare for a morning meeting with vendor and afternoon interview with library school student.

9:00 a.m.
- Respond to faculty requests and vendor renewal notices.
- Process invoices for payment and update collection budget.
- Contact vendor to establish a trial for a potential new resource.

10:00 a.m.
- Attend vendor meeting.

11:00 a.m.
- Seek out and assess vendor usage statistics for items due for renewal.
- Begin preparation to lead next week's library project management seminar.
- Follow up with vendor on the status of a new license.
- Read and respond to more phone and e-mail requests.

Noon (Lunch)

1:00 p.m.
- Respond to library school student's phone interview questions relating to the economics of library information.
- Address library staff inquiry about loss of access for a licensed electronic product.
- Receive new license and begin review cycle.

2:30 p.m.
- Attend library managers' meeting.

4:00 p.m.
- Finalize staff member's annual performance appraisal.
- Resolve accounting problem relating to renewal payment.
- Try to catch up on e-mail and phone calls for the tenth time today.

Summary statement: Today's collection development librarians thrive on constantly learning and expanding their current responsibilities and vision for their clients' future information needs. Successful collection development librarians will be skilled at multitasking and time management, have high levels of energy, enjoy communicating, see the humor in everyday challenges, and take pride in quietly making a difference in the lives of today's students, physicians, researchers, other health care professionals, and patients.

Evaluation of Digital Resources

After resources have been acquired, ongoing evaluation is essential to ensure that a resource continues to provide good value for the library and adequately addresses the needs of its users. Rarely is evaluation based on a single factor, and a combination of different qualitative and quantitative approaches, such as those listed here, are usually combined as part of an assessment effort. With any evaluation project, librarians should determine their goals in advance of any information-gathering efforts. Gathering information can be time-consuming and, as Vicki L. Gregory points out, may not result in any useful data unless one is clear about the intent of a library's evaluation efforts.[27]

Usage Trends

Monitoring usage is one of the best methods to determine the value of a particular resource. An international initiative, COUNTER (Counting Online Usage of NeTworked Electronic Resources), was formed in 2002 to address the need for a consistent measurement approach to usage data.[51] For more information on COUNTER, refer to Chapter 3 and the COUNTER Codes of Practice relating to journals, databases, books, and reference works.[52, 53]

When considering usage data, data for multiple years are generally required for effective decisions. Since it often takes time for users to become aware and familiar with new resources, making a judgment call based on a single year's worth of data is not advisable. Trend data or multiple years' data are a more accurate reflection of real usage and can demonstrate either increases or reductions in use.

Content Analysis

As mentioned earlier, content analysis can be used to judge not only if a product is worthy of initial selection, but also, when combined with other data, if a product is worthy of retention. The overlap or uniqueness of a product's content should be evaluated on an ongoing basis. For example, when Elsevier's Scopus was introduced, some speculated whether Scopus might serve as an alternative to Thomson Scientific's Web of Science.[54-56] While several later comparisons suggest that the products are complementary rather than duplicative, librarians must remain knowledgeable of potential opportunities for content overlap as new products are introduced and continue to develop.[57-60]

As the market for digital resources is continually growing and evolving, librarians must monitor the information market to determine if their current resources are the best options among competing products. Examining the uniqueness of a product is another way to determine content value. For example, in the not too distant past, most libraries were looking to add one of the newer **clinical decision tools** to expand their available resources. With the increasing number of products in this area, libraries are now actively comparing and evaluating such resources.[28, 29] Two or more clinical decision tools may be warranted if each offers some unique value.

Budget, Cost-Benefit Analysis

Librarians must consider digital resources in the context of the library's overall budget situation. Since an increasing number of resources are now tied to recurring annual costs, it is essential that librarians review resource costs with each renewal. The cost-benefit evaluation for the library could easily change with increased inflation rates or changes in consortia participation.

Cost per use is one common approach to help clarify a resource's value. Determining a product's cost per use can be obtained by dividing the annual cost by the number of uses for the year:

annual subscription cost / annual uses = cost per use. This formula, when applied across multiple resources, can provide a broad overview of the value per resource in comparison with other resources or with print counterparts.

Budget shortfalls may also force libraries to quickly evaluate their digital collections. In such situations, all digital resources will need to be scrutinized and priorities or rankings established. When the University of Maryland at College Park faced a shortfall, they evaluated all electronic resource subscriptions using a quantitative criteria-based approach.[61] This allowed the librarians to provide systematic justification for their cancellation decisions.

Feedback

Soliciting feedback from library users can help to determine if a particular resource is continuing to provide value. If a library is contemplating the cancellation of a resource, communicating that possibility and asking for feedback can help to either justify or argue against such a decision.

User input can be challenging to obtain, as has been documented in the literature.[62] Faculty and other professionals are often busy and may be biased toward particular subjects or disciplines. On the other hand, they can supply subject expertise that may not be available through any other option. Student opinions may also vary widely from faculty, and they may lack the in-depth knowledge of particular subjects. Increased remote use has also made it more difficult to determine who is using particular resources and how well their needs are being addressed.

Various methods, such as surveys, focus groups, and usability studies, can be used to gather user feedback.[62, 63] User surveys can be delivered in person, by phone, electronically by e-mail, or via Web sites. Written questionnaires can be mailed or delivered inside the library. Regardless of which mechanisms are used to gather feedback, asking the right questions to get the desired feedback can be challenging and should not be pursued without thorough planning and consideration.[5]

PRESERVATION

Preservation of library collections is a fairly straightforward concept that can be defined in a number of different ways, depending on one's perspective. It can refer to a whole range of activities intended to preserve or maintain the physical information package for future use. It can also refer to actions taken toward the more fundamental purpose of maintaining or ensuring continued intellectual access to the information content carried by the container, regardless of the particular format. Examples of efforts to preserve the physical information package are binding and collection security; examples of efforts to ensure continued intellectual access include digitization and requiring archival access guarantees in licensing electronic resources.

The relative scope and intensity of preservation efforts will vary across health sciences libraries depending on the type and size of the library. For example, a small hospital library may determine that the level of use and retention plans for the collection do not merit preservation efforts. The larger academic health sciences library or those libraries with a specialized collection will have a more intense and varied preservation plan. These activities could include a strong preference for cloth binding in book purchases, an active repair and conservation program, the use of collection security measures for each individual collection item, and digitization or other format transfer for physically deteriorating collection items.

Preservation, like most aspects of collection management, should be tied to the collection development policy. If the collection development policy is detailed enough to contain individual subject policy statements, those subject policy statements could also indicate the long-term plans for retention of the collection and provide logical guidance for preservation decisions within subject areas. In essence, a decision to preserve a collection item is a second selection decision and can also be guided by the selection criteria specified in the collection development policy.[3]

Preservation policies in most health sciences libraries have been impacted in general by the efforts of the National Library of Medicine (NLM) to preserve the biomedical literature. NLM has outlined a preservation program that can serve as a comprehensive model.[64-65] This national plan provides a framework and larger context for local preservation decisions. Preservation of the biomedical literature is no small undertaking, and individual library decisions can strongly impact the cumulative result. For this reason, libraries should follow a process for preservation plan development that includes gathering and sharing of information with other institutions, including NLM.[66]

Binding

Binding is the most common preservation activity. Most librarians associate binding with the combination of individual journal issues into a hardbound volume, but the binding of monographic items can be an important piece of a comprehensive collection building policy.

From a preservation perspective, the purpose of binding is simply to prolong or extend the circulating life of an information package. The Library Binding Institute Web site is an excellent online source of information concerning binding, standards for the binding process, and lists of certified library binders.[67] Collection budgets can become strained by several factors outside the control of the library, such as materials inflation. In times of limited budgets, the expense of binding can be viewed as a cost savings target to help lessen budgetary stress, with the elimination or reduction of book binding as the most obvious cost savings candidate. Elimination or reduction of binding can be a short-term cost savings tactic, but any long-term decisions should be carefully reconciled with the library's preservation plan.

Repair and Conservation

Libraries of all types have some degree of a repair and conservation program as part of their standard operating procedures, even though they may not consciously consider it part of a preservation plan. All health sciences libraries must deal with the physical environment in which their collections exist. Those physical conditions can either prolong or shorten the life of the information packages. Collections are affected by several factors:

- General housekeeping standards (Is the library kept clean? Are materials regularly dusted?)
- Library regulations concerning food and drink on the premises
- Physical environmental factors (air temperature, humidity, direct sunlight)
- Staff training (Do staff know how to handle collection materials? Are staff trained how to shelve items, including how tightly to pack shelves?)[5]

In the best of all worlds, librarians are able to establish standards for the physical environment that will prolong the life of their library collections. Decisions concerning the extent and approach taken to provide basic collection repair and conservation should be based on the collection development policy and its implications for long-term retention plans for specific parts of the collection.

Most simple repairs and collection cleaning can be accomplished with products sold by standard library supply companies. If the item to be repaired is heavily used or has long-term importance to the collection, it is wise to let a professional binder handle the work. Most library binders can provide reasonable rebinding services as well as a full range of conservation treatments; all activities will then be done following Library Binding Institute standards.[67]

Collection Security

Collection security covers a wide range of activities that focus on keeping the collection safe. All types of libraries must deal with this in one way or another. There are some basic measures to ensure collection security that are common among most libraries:

- Maintain an accurate listing of the materials contained in the collection.
- Identify clearly all collection materials with library ownership stamps or labels.
- Place theft detection devices within each collection item so that an alarm sounds if material is removed from the library without first being properly checked out.
- Use controlled access shelving for collection items that are likely theft targets due to their content or price.
- Install security cameras in the library.

All collection security measures carry a cost. Some of those costs are financial, but some are less quantifiable and may involve user perceptions about ease of use or access restrictions. The costs and potential impact of collection security measures should be considered. A reasonable approach is recommended, where security measures are balanced with actual or potential collection loss, and collection access is balanced with collection security.

All of the environmental factors mentioned also impact the general security of the collection. In addition to the everyday variety of environmental factors that impact the health and security of the collection, the extremes of environmental forces can have drastic and far-reaching effects on the collection. Natural disasters, fires, and water breaks are all examples of potential collection destroyers. Libraries have varying levels of formal preparations for meeting these extreme situations, depending on their size and parent institution. Some have developed extensive preservation plans with detailed instructions for how to cope with specific disasters and emergencies; others have much simpler documents. At a bare minimum, every library should have simple procedures outlining the immediate response, plus a listing of key personnel to contact who will take responsibility for the library and the collection in a particular emergency situation.[5, 68] The recent disasters of Hurricanes Katrina and Rita reveal some interesting ideas and new perspectives relative to preservation. In view of the widespread destruction, many libraries focused on how to maintain access to information and services, rather than simply finding a way to salvage or restore the physical collection.[69] The widespread destruction seen in this particular natural disaster encourages librarians to consider not only preserving the physical package, but the information content.[70, 71]

Preservation of Content

Up to this point the focus of this preservation discussion has been the physical item, or information package. Another focus for preservation can be the information content itself, without regard for the packaging. Preservation microfilming has long been one of the most common techniques used to preserve information content. The newest technique to preserve content is digitization, making an electronic or digital copy of the intellectual content. The most likely monographic candidates for digitization would be content no longer protected by copyright and locally created or locally published content when the copyright holder can grant permission for digitization. As with basic preservation planning, all health sciences libraries should gather and share information with colleague institutions in creating a digitization preservation plan. The Google Book Search Library Project, with its goal to create a huge virtual library by digitizing the content of several major libraries and making it searchable, will test the feasibility of large-scale cooperative projects and the limitations imposed by current copyright laws.[72]

Weeding

Weeding, deselection, or deaccessioning is the practice of removing and disposing of books, journals, or other materials from the library's collection due to age, condition, space, online availability, or other factors. Most libraries, unless they are large research libraries, will need to practice some type of judicious weeding of their collections. Hospital libraries will need to weed to keep their materials current and because of space limitations. Academic health sciences libraries will need to weed to make room on the shelves for new materials and increasingly to repurpose space for study, computer access, and classrooms. In some cases, weeding may take the form of moving dated material to designated storage space; in other cases, weeding means that the material will be permanently removed from the collection.

Many librarians establish continuous weeding practices. For example, only the most recent two editions of a core textbook will be retained in the collection, or books published more than twenty years ago will be automatically withdrawn. In addition to continuous weeding, many librarians conduct comprehensive weeding projects to examine particular subject areas, shelf locations, or the entire collection for materials to weed.

Before a comprehensive weeding project can begin, librarians must consult with the institutional legal or inventory office to determine the requirements for disposing of material purchased with institutional funds. In some cases, weeded material must be offered to other institutions, such as other components of a university system or other hospitals within a network. The institution may have specific guidelines for how material can be disposed of, such as recycling or "giveaways" to hospital or campus faculty, staff, and students. Despite valid reasons for weeding, some librarians may be reluctant to weed due to possible repercussions from administration, faculty, or the community when large numbers of books are discarded.[73]

Weeding Library Collections by Slote provides a comprehensive review of weeding methods for libraries and is a good starting point for any librarian preparing to embark on a weeding project.[74] Criteria for weeding library material can include age, condition, duplication, superseded edition, dated information or presentation, subject matter not in scope for the collection, shelf crowding, and lack of use evidenced by circulation or in-house use data. To avoid unnecessary weeding in libraries with older material, particular attention should be paid to books that may have historical value.

Procedures for identifying material to be weeded and ultimately withdrawn will vary with each library. Common elements to define when developing criteria for a weeding project include, but are not limited to, the following:

- Subject or shelf areas that might need immediate attention due to overcrowding
- Time factors, such as any imposed deadlines for completion of the project
- Personnel who will be involved in identifying materials to weed and withdrawing these materials
- Disposition procedures for withdrawn materials
- Involvement of faculty or other experts who might be called upon to determine retention of important materials
- Replacement of dated material with more current publications
- Repair or replacement of damaged volumes
- Public relations or marketing for the weeding project

Criteria and procedures for weeding should be documented in writing so that they can be applied consistently by the library personnel who will be involved in the project.

CONCLUSION

The focus of this chapter has been to present a practical view of collection development processes within a broader library, institutional, and information industry context. The examples and suggestions offered are anchored in those traditional skills and approaches that are still valid, valued, and needed. They are presented through a real world lens of collection development as a work in progress, continually evolving and changing. Beyond the current collection development challenges presented in this chapter are several larger issues that will impact collection development in the future. These issues are both external to the library environment and internal to library operations and organizations.

External factors include these:

- Explorations of new models for scholarly communication that employ digital technologies and networking for teaching, research, and learning
- Open access campaigns to increase the free availability of quality literature and research reports
- Refinement of copyright and intellectual property rights in the digital environment
- The future of both book and journal "packaging" since digital publication may radically impact the need for the traditional book and journal publication structure
- E-commerce impacts on user expectations for information system interfaces and the impact of "disruptive" technologies
- Competition from freely available sources of both reliable and unreliable health information, such as Google, Wikipedia, and other Web-based resources
- Generational differences in expectations for access to information resources, particularly from the "wired generation" whose expectations have been nurtured by the Internet from the cradle
- Trends in publisher marketing directly to users, such as pay-per-view article access, information product development that bypasses the library as intermediary, and direct marketing to health care professionals by publishers and vendors

Internal factors include these:

- The need for change in a library's organizational structure to accommodate a drastically changed information environment
- The need to abandon traditional tasks such as journal check-in and binding and repurpose staff positions to more directly benefit user needs
- New approaches to marketing the library's role in delivering information
- The increased importance of determining user needs and capturing and analyzing data to support library decision-making
- The need to partner with other campus or hospital departments to deliver information to the bedside through mechanisms such as the electronic medical record
- The need to balance the strain on library budgets with an ever-increasing array of information resources

By fine-tuning traditional practices with new approaches and ideas in response to the myriad of external and internal factors impacting library collections, collection development specialists can continue to successfully nurture and grow relevant, valued collections.

REFERENCES

1. Crawford, W. "Beware What You Wish For: Online Journal Quandaries." *American Libraries* 33(November 2002): 65.

2. Mahon, B. "Study Addresses Europe's Scientific Publications System." *Information Today* 23(May 2006): 50.

3. Richards, D.T., and Eakin, D. *Collection Development and Assessment in Health Sciences Libraries.* Current Practice in Health Sciences Librarianship, vol. 4. Lanham, MD: Scarecrow Press, 1997.

4. Lee, S.D. *Electronic Collection Development: A Practical Guide.* New York: Neal-Schumann, 2002.

5. Johnson, P. *Fundamentals of Collection Development and Management.* Chicago, IL: American Library Association, 2004.

6. Tennant, M.R.; Cataldo, T.T.; Sherwill-Navarro, P.; and Jesano, R. "Evaluation of a Liaison Librarian Program: Client and Liaison Perspectives." *Journal of the Medical Library Association* 94(October 2006): 402-9.

7. Hill, D.R., and Stickell, H.N. A History of the Brandon-Hill Selected Lists. Available: <http://www.mssm.edu/library/brandon-hill/history.shtml>. Accessed: February 2, 2007.

8. Hill, D.R., and Stickell, H.N. "Brandon/Hill Selected List of Print Books and Journals for the Small Medical Library." *Bulletin of the Medical Library Association* 89(April 2001): 131-53.

9. Doody's Enterprises, Inc. Available: <http://www.doodyenterprises.com/>. Accessed: February 2, 2007.

10. Shedlock, J., and Walton L.J. "Developing a Virtual Community for Health Sciences Library Book Selection: Doody's Core Titles." *Journal of the Medical Library Association* 94(January 2006): 61-6.

11. Medical Library Association. Collection Development Section. Subject-Based Resource List. Available: <http://colldev.mlanet.org/resources/subjectlist.htm>. Accessed: February 2, 2007.

12. Medical Library Association. Collection Development Section. Vendor-Based Resource List. Available: <http://colldev.mlanet.org/resources/vendorlist.htm#books>. Accessed: February 2, 2007.

13. Rees, A.M. *Consumer Health Information Source Book.* 7th ed. Westport, CT: Greenwood Press, 2003.

14. Barclay, D.A, and Halsted, D.D. *Consumer Health Reference Service Handbook.* New York: Neal-Schumann Publishers, Inc., 2001.

15. Walton, L.; Modschiedler, C.M.; Rodgers, P.M.; et al. *MLA DocKit #3, Collection Development and Management for Electronic, Audiovisual, and Print Resources in Health Sciences Libraries,* 2nd revised ed. Chicago, IL: Medical Library Association, 2004.

16. Jones, D.H., and Wilkerson J.C. "Serials Acquisitions." In *Acquisitions in Health Sciences Libraries.* Edited by A. Bunting. Current Practice in Health Sciences Librarianship, vol. 5, 109-10. Lanham, MD: Scarecrow Press, 1996.

17. GPO (Government Printing Office). Keeping America Informed. Available: <http://www.gpo.gov/>. Accessed: February 9, 2007.

18. Bernan. Essential Government Publications. Available: <http://www.bernan.com/>. Accessed: February 9, 2007.

19. *The Encyclopedia of Ephemera: A Guide to the Fragmentary Documents of Everyday Life for the Collector, Curator, and Historian* by Maurice Rickards et al. London: The British Library; New York: Routledge, 2000.

20. McNaughton Popular Reading. Available: <http://www.books.brodart.com/products/mcnaughton.htm>. Accessed: February 8, 2007.

21. Pitschmann, L.A. *Building Sustainable Collections of Free Third-Party Web Resources.* Washington, DC: Council on Library and Information Resources, 2001. Available: <http://www.projectcounter.org/index.html>. Accessed: February 15, 2007.

22. Gerhard, K.H. "Pricing Models for Electronic Journals and Other Electronic Academic Materials: The State of the Art." *Journal of Library Administration* 42, no. 3/4 (2005): 1-25.

23. Anderson, R. *Buying and Contracting for Resources and Services; A How-To-Do-It Manual for Librarians.* New York: Neal-Schuman, 2004.

24. "Licensing in Libraries: Practical and Ethical Aspects." *Journal of Library Administration* 42, no. 3/4 (2005). *[Note: Complete issue with multiple authors.]*

25. Lord, J., and Ragon, B. "Working Together to Develop Electronic Collections." *Computers in Libraries* 21, no. 5 (May 2001): 41-4.

26. McGinnis, S., and Kemp, J.H. "The Electronic Resources Group: Using the Cross-Functional Team Approach to the Challenge of Acquiring Electronic Resources." *Library Acquisitions: Practice and Theory* 22, no. 3 (1998): 295-301.

27. Gregory, V.L. *Selecting and Managing Electronic Resources: A How-To-Do-It Manual.* New York: Neal-Schuman Publishers, Inc., 2000.

28. Trumble, J.M.; Anderson, M.J.; Caldwell, M.; et al. "A Systematic Evaluation of Evidence Based Medicine Tools for Point-of-Care." Paper presented at the South Central Chapter of the Medical Library Association (SCC/MLA) Conference, October 2006. Available: <http://ils.mdacc.tmc.edu/papers.html>. Accessed: February 24, 2007.

29. Schulte, S. "Ten Tips for Evaluating EBM Tools." *iHealthBeat.* (December 1, 2005). Available: <http://www.ihealthbeat.org/index.cfm?action=dspItem&itemID=117293&changedID=117272>. Accessed: February 24, 2007.

30. Stewart, D.C. "Electronic Textbook Vendors: An Evaluation." *Journal of Electronic Resources in Medical Libraries* 1, no. 3 (2004): 1-11.

31. PsychiatryOnline. Available: <http://www.psychiatryonline.com/>. Accessed: February 19, 2007.

32. Mosby's Nursing Consult. Available: <http://www.nursingconsult.com/offers/standard.html>. Accessed: February 19, 2007.

33. Blanck, J.F. "Review of Mosby's Nursing Consult." *Journal of the Medical Library Association* 94, no. 3 (July 2006): 356-7. Available: <http://www.pubmedcentral.nih.gov/articlerender.fcgi?artid=1525315>. Accessed: February 24, 2007.

34. Faculty of 1000 Biology. Available: <http://www.f1000biology.com/home/>. Accessed: February 19, 2007.

35. Faculty of 1000 Medicine. Available: <http://www.f1000medicine.com/home/.> Accessed: February 19, 2007.

36. Perry, J.; Howse, D.K.; and Schlimgen, J. "Indexing, Abstracting, and Digital Database Resources." In *Introduction to Reference Sources in the Health Sciences.* 4th ed., edited by J. Boorkman, J.T. Huber, and F.W. Roper, 53-98. New York: Neal-Schuman Publishers, 2004.

37. National Library of Medicine. "Fact Sheet: MEDLINE." Available: <http://www.nlm.nih.gov/pubs/factsheets/medline.html>. Accessed: February 4, 2007.

38. "PubMed Celebrates Its 10th Anniversary." *NLM Technical Bulletin*, no. 352 (September-October 2006). Available: <http://www.nlm.nih.gov/pubs/techbull/so06/so06_pm_10.html>. Accessed: February 4, 2007.

39. National Library of Medicine. *Fact Sheet: What's the Difference Between MEDLINE and PubMed?* Available: <http://www.nlm.nih.gov/pubs/factsheets/dif_med_pub.html>. Accessed: February 4, 2007.

40. National Library of Medicine. "Leasing Data from the National Library of Medicine." Available: <http://www.nlm.nih.gov/databases/leased.html>. Accessed: February 4, 2007.

41. Infotrieve. Available: <http://www4.infotrieve.com/default.asp>. Accessed: February 24, 2007.

42. Medscape. Available: <http://www.medscape.com/home>. Accessed: February 24, 2007.

43. Ovid MEDLINE. Available: <http://www.ovid.com/site/index.jsp>. Accessed: February 25, 2007.

44. Katcher, B.S. *MEDLINE: A Guide to Effective Searching in PubMed and Other Interfaces.* 2nd ed. San Francisco, CA: Ashbury Press, 2006.

45. DeGroote, S.L. "PubMed, Internet Grateful Med, and Ovid: A Comparison of Three MEDLINE Internet Interfaces." *Medical Reference Services Quarterly* 19, no. 4 (Winter 2000): 1-13.

46. Henner, T.A. "Free MEDLINE and Implications for Library Operations." *Medical Reference Services Quarterly* 19, no. 3 (Fall 2000): 71-9.

47. Parker, S. "MEDLINE on Ovid, SilverPlatter, FirstSearch and PubMed." *The Charleston Advisor* 1, no. 3 (January 2000): 5-10. Available: <http://www.charlestonco.com/comp.cfm?id=3>. Accessed: February 24, 2007.

48. Shultz, M., and De Groote, S.L. "MEDLINE SDI Services: How Do They Compare?" *Journal of the Medical Library Association* 91, no. 4 (October 2003): 460-7. Available: <http://www.pubmedcentral.nih.gov/articlerender.fcgi?artid=209512>. Accessed: February 24, 2007.

49. Drexel University Libraries. "MEDLINE: OVID and PUBMED, a Comparison." Available: <http://www.library.drexel.edu/resources/tutorials/medlinecomparison.html>. Accessed: February 23, 2007.

50. Thomas Jefferson University. "A Comparison of MD Consult, PubMed and Ovid Web." Available: <http://jeffline.jefferson.edu/SML/helpaids/handouts/comparison_chart.pdf >. Accessed: February 23, 2007.

51. COUNTER. Available: <http://www.projectcounter.org/about.html>. Accessed: February 18, 2007.

52. *Release 2 of the COUNTER Code of Practice for Journals and Databases.* April 2005. Available: <http://www.projectcounter.org/code_practice.html>. Accessed: February 25, 2007.

53. *Release 1 of the COUNTER Code of Practice for Books and Reference Works.* March 2006. Available: <http://www.projectcounter.org/code_practice.html>. Accessed: February 25, 2007.

54. Scopus. Available: <http://www.scopus.com/>. Accessed: February 24, 2007.

55. Web of Science. Available: <http://scientific.thomson.com/products/wos/>. Accessed: February 24, 2007.

56. Deis, L.F., and Goodman, D. "Web of Science (2004 version) and Scopus." *The Charleston Advisor* 6, no. 3 (January 2005). Available: <http://www.charlestonco.com/comp.cfm?id=43>. Accessed: February 24, 2007.

57. Deis, L.F., and Goodman, D. "Update on Scopus." *The Charleston Advisor* 7, no. 3 (January 2006). Available: <http://www.charlestonco.com/comp.cfm?id=55>. Accessed: February 24, 2007.

58. Goodman, D., and Deis, L. "Update on Scopus and Web of Science." *The Charleston Advisor* 8, no. 3 (January 2007). Available: <http://www.charlestonco.com/comp.cfm?id=59>. Accessed: February 24, 2007.

59. Burnham, J.F. "Scopus Database: A Review." *Biomedical Digital Libraries* 3, no. 8 (March 2006): 1. Available: <http://www.bio-diglib.com/content/3/1/1>. Accessed: February 23, 2007.

60. Bakkalbasi, N.; Bauer, K.; Glover, J.; and Wang, L. "Three Options for Citation Tracking: Google Scholar, Scopus and Web of Science." *Biomedical Digital Libraries* 3(29 June 2006): 7. Available: <http://www.bio-diglib.com/content/3/1/7>. Accessed: February 23, 2007.

61. Foudy, G., and McManus, A. "Using a Decision Grid Process to Build Consensus in Electronic Resources Cancellation Decisions." *The Journal of Academic Librarianship* 31, no. 6 (November 2005): 533-8.

62. Blake, J.C., and Schleper, S.P. "From Data to Decisions: Using Surveys and Statistics to Make Collection Management Decisions." *Library Collections, Acquisitions, & Technical Services* 28(2004): 460-4.

63. Kupferberg, N. "Evaluation of Five Full-Text Drug Databases by Pharmacy Students, Faculty, and Librarians: Do the Groups Agree?" *Journal of the Medical Library Association* 92, no. 1 (January 2004): 66-71. Available: <http://www.pubmedcentral.nih.gov/articlerender.fcgi?artid=314104>. Accessed: February 24, 2007.

64. National Library of Medicine. *Fact Sheet: Preservation Program.* Available: <http://www.nlm.nih.gov/pubs/factsheets/preservation.html>. Accessed: February 15, 2007.

65. National Library of Medicine. *National Preservation Plan for the Biomedical Literature.* Bethesda, MD: National Library of Medicine, 1988.

66. Byrnes, M.M., ed. "Symposium: Preservation of the Biomedical Literature." *Bulletin of the Medical Library Association* 77(July 1989): 256-98.

67. Library Binding Institute. "For the Love of Books." Available: <http://www.hardcoverbinders.org/home.htm>. Accessed: February 15, 2007.

68. Halsted, D.D.; Jasper, R.P.; and Little, F.M. *Disaster Planning: A How-To-Do-It Manual for Librarians with Planning Templates on CD-ROM.* New York: Neal-Schuman, 2005.

69. Texas State Library and Archives Commission. "Hurricane Relief and Recovery Resources." Available: <http://www.tsl.state.tx.us/ref/abouttx/katrita.html>. Accessed: February 26, 2007.

70. State Library of Louisiana. "Katrina and Rita." Available: <http://www.state.lib.la.us/la_dyn_templ.cfm?doc_id=580>. Accessed: February 26, 2007.

71. Association of American University Presses. "Library and Book Relief Programs for the Gulf Coast." Available: <http://aaupnet.org/news/katrina.html>. Accessed: February 26, 2007.

72. Google. "Google Book Search Library Project: An Enhanced Card Catalog of the World's Books." Available: <http://books.google.com/googlprint/library.html>. Accessed: February 26, 2007.

73. Tobia, RC. "Comprehensive Weeding of an Academic Health Sciences Collection: The Briscoe Library Experience." *Journal of the Medical Library Association* 90, no. 1 (January, 2002): 94-8.

74. Slote, S.J. *Weeding Library Collections.* 4th ed. Englewood, CO: Libraries Unlimited, Inc., 1997.

Chapter 5

Organizing Resources for Information Access

Maggie Wineburgh-Freed

SUMMARY. This chapter discusses the development and current practices in health sciences cataloging and classification, and includes a description of some of the new methods of organizing information resources in health sciences libraries. It includes information about current standards in cataloging, sharing catalog records, MeSH and NLM classification, and the MARC record. Software used in organizing information for libraries is also discussed, both the more traditional integrated library system and new systems for organizing digital information. An appendix with a list of resources is included.

INTRODUCTION

This chapter will present an overview of information organization in health sciences libraries. It will begin with a very brief historical look at how libraries began to organize information through library cataloging and classification and continue with an overview of the development and details of current methods and systems for organizing information. It will provide some specific information on current cataloging practices and also will include a discussion of how libraries organize some special types of materials common to health sciences libraries, and how they have integrated and continue to integrate new material formats into their organizational systems. Finally, it will examine the way in which the explosion of electronic resources has moved librarians to consider other methods of information discovery and access, and how some people think libraries will organize information in the future.

BRIEF HISTORY OF INFORMATION ORGANIZATION BY LIBRARIES

Libraries developed through the centuries first as mere collections of recorded works, from clay tablets, papyrus scrolls or books, to hand-lettered volumes, then printed books. These libraries began to develop descriptive lists of what was contained within them with varying amounts of information, and little consistency. One of the earliest documented Western European sets of rules for organization of a catalog was developed by Anthony Panizzi for the British Museum and published in 1841.[1] In the United States, Charles Ammi Cutter published *Rules for a Printed Dictionary Catalog* in 1876, where he described the objectives of the catalog, including enabling the user to find known items, or all items on a given topic or by a given author.[2]

The American Library Association (ALA), the Library Association (Great Britain), and the Library of Congress (LC) worked together in various degrees during the twentieth century to further develop standardization of description and organization that would fulfill Cutter's objec-

Introduction to Health Sciences Librarianship
© 2008 by The Haworth Press, Taylor & Francis Group. All rights reserved.
doi:10.1300/6041_05

tives. The rules that were hammered out by the end of this period were published in 1967 as the *Anglo-American Cataloging Rules (AACR).*[3]

OVERVIEW: CURRENT METHODS

Current Rules and Standards for Organizing Information in Libraries

The *Anglo-American Cataloging Rules,* Second Edition, 2002 Revision, with 2003, 2004, and 2005 updates (*AACR2R*),[4] is the current iteration in use in the United States and much of the English-speaking world. It is the authority for describing materials and providing **access points** to them that is used by both LC and the **National Library of Medicine (NLM)** in constructing **bibliographic records.** The Joint Steering Committee for Revision of AACR (JSC), the organization charged with maintaining and revising the rules, includes representatives from the United States, the United Kingdom, Canada, and Australia. This committee is working on a revision of the standards titled *RDA: Resource Description and Access,* due to be published in 2009.

Rules for description provide for consistency among libraries in describing works in all formats: printed books and serials, video recordings, sound recordings, electronic resources, and even what are called "realia," objects which can be naturally occurring or man-made, such as anatomical models and microscope slides. The rules are meant to be flexible enough to cover additional formats as they come into use. Rules for description and for selecting and constructing access points, such as personal and corporate names, make it possible to identify the particular item in hand and distinguish it from other similar items. The standards and the consistency they engender allow libraries to share records.

These rules for description of materials and for constructing authoritative name headings are complemented by the standards for classification and subject assignment, by which information can be organized and identified by topic. These are more varied, with a number of schemes in current use. LC classification and NLM classification use a combination of letters and numbers in their systems and are in widest use among academic and other health sciences libraries, while the Dewey Decimal System, a numerical system, is more commonly used in public libraries. The NLM classification is currently updated annually and is available online.[5]

Medical subject headings (MeSH) and LC subject headings (LCSH) are the two authoritative schemes in current use by health sciences libraries for describing material by subject. Both of these systems produce lists of approved **descriptors** from which catalogers select the most appropriate terms to describe the material by topic. Using controlled subject vocabularies such as these is meant to assist library users in retrieving all materials on a subject, no matter how they are described by the author or originator. With the ubiquitous use of Google and other search engines on the Web, library users have become accustomed to using keyword searches. When keywords include controlled vocabulary terms, they can provide more comprehensive retrieval on a particular topic.

Other controlled vocabulary lists may be used in specialized libraries. For example, the CINAHL® (*Cumulative Index to Nursing and Allied Health Literature*) database has its own subject heading list, which is modeled after MeSH but includes more specific headings for nursing and allied health topics. Another example, ERIC (Education Resources Information Center), a database of education literature from the U.S. Department of Education, maintains a thesaurus of descriptors with detailed and specific education-related terms. Thomson Scientific, publisher of *International Pharmaceutical Abstracts,* has developed the *IPA Thesaurus,* with specific terms for pharmacy and pharmacology topics.

Sharing Catalog Records

Sharing catalog records began with the LC catalog card distribution system in 1902, eventually discontinued in March 1997. As computer usage became widespread in the early 1960s, staff at LC designed a data format for the exchange of bibliographic information, the MARC (MAchine Readable Cataloging) format. McCallum[6] provides a thorough examination of the development and importance of this complex data format. The MARC format enabled LC to share catalog records and eventually led to the development of the Online Computer Library Center (OCLC), the Research Libraries Information Network (RLIN), and other bibliographic utilities, including commercial firms, such as Auto-Graphics' AGent MARCit™, all of which supply catalog records via the Internet to libraries of all sizes and types.

Book cataloging information is also shared via LC's Cataloging-In-Publication (CIP) program. Through this program, publishers submit a book or relevant portions of it at the proof stage, and catalogers at LC prepare a bibliographic record for it. They return this information to the publisher, who prints the record on the copyright page. This information is thus made available to any library (or individual) purchasing the book. NLM has participated in the CIP program, and now in its replacement, the Electronic CIP (ECIP) program.[7] In this way, many books arrive in health sciences libraries with records that already include NLM classification and MeSH.

Integrated Library Systems (ILS) and Other Resource Organization Products

Over the past twenty years, a large number of integrated library systems, which encompass cataloging, circulation, acquisitions, serials, and online public access catalogs (OPACs), have come and gone, developing, merging, and splitting. Marshall Breeding's Library Technology Guides[8] is an excellent resource for information about integrated library systems. This Web site lists forty-one companies in the United States alone which supply automation systems to libraries of all sizes. The systems most widely used by academic libraries include: Endeavor Information Systems' Voyager, Ex Libris' Aleph, Innovative Interfaces' Millennium, and SirsiDynix's Unicorn and Horizon (being merged into a new product called Symphony). Some systems that cater to special libraries, including hospital libraries, are EOS International's EOS.Web, CyberTools for Libraries, Inmagic's Inmagic Genie, Softlink's Liberty3, and SydneyPLUS.

Many academic health sciences libraries share OPACs with their parent institutions, requiring that only one subject heading system be chosen for use; that subject heading systems be mixed in the subject index, as in the Yale University Library catalog and others; or that separate indexes for LC subjects and MeSH be used, as is done at the Indiana University Libraries, Boston University, and others. At some institutions, the university library and health sciences library use completely different ILSs, such as the situation at Stanford University, where the main library uses SirsiDynix's Unicorn, while the Lane Medical Library uses Endeavor's Voyager, or at the University of Arizona, where the university library uses Innovative Interfaces' Millennium, while the Arizona Health Sciences Library uses SirsiDynix's Unicorn.

Methods for managing electronic resources, primarily electronic journals, have been developing as well, with a number of companies creating electronic resource management systems (ERMS). These are sometimes linked through the integrated library system or offer bibliographic records that can be imported into the online catalog, but they may also provide separate listings on the library's Web pages. They may include only title listings or may also include subject listings, which may or may not use controlled vocabularies such as MeSH or LCSH. Some ILS suppliers include an ERMS as an optional module with their systems, or one can be purchased separately.

In addition to the more traditional catalog and its supporting modules, many libraries are digitizing and organizing for retrieval a variety of materials that in the past would not have been included in the library catalog. They may be research papers written by faculty or students, reports, institutional archival documents, historical photographs, pathology or anatomy slides, or other information. These digital objects may be included in the online catalog or may be mounted separately on the library or institutional Web pages. There are many enterprise content management systems that are available to help organize and make these materials accessible, including these:

- OCLC's CONTENTdm Digital Collection Management Software <http://www.oclc.org/contentdm/>
- ETD-db software developed at Virginia Tech <http://scholar.lib.vt.edu/ETD-db/>
- Open Text <http://www.opentext.com/>
- FileNet <http://www.filenet.com/>
- Madison Digital Image Database (MDID) <http://mdid.org/mdidwiki/index.php?title=Main_Page>
- AGent Digital Collections <http://www4.auto-graphics.com/products/agentdigitalcollections/agentdigitalcollections.htm>
- EMC Corporation's Documentum <http://software.emc.com/products/product_family/documentum_family.htm>

These are a few of the many systems that libraries currently use to facilitate content digitization projects. These products use **metadata**[9] of various kinds to organize material for discovery. Some of the standard metadata schemas in current use include: Dublin Core, Resource Description Framework (RDF), Encoded Archival Description (EAD), Metadata Encoding and Transmission Standard (METS), and Metadata Object Description Schema (MODS).

Copy Cataloging and Health Sciences Libraries

"The Program for Cooperative Cataloging (PCC) is an international cooperative effort aimed at expanding access to library collections by providing useful, timely, and cost-effective cataloging that meets mutually accepted standards of libraries around the world."[10] Two important components of the PCC are the Monographic Bibliographic Record Component (BIBCO) and the Cooperative Online Serials (CONSER) programs. Participants in these two programs, including catalogers at LC and NLM, contribute authoritative records to OCLC and thus provide a basis for the copy cataloging of both monographic and serial materials that is conducted by smaller libraries without the resources to do extensive cataloging. Copy cataloging is the process of using or adapting a bibliographic record obtained from another source, instead of creating an original record, and allows for more efficient processing of materials.

Thanks to these cooperative programs, it is unnecessary for every small health sciences library to have staff devoted entirely to cataloging, because a large percentage of books generally acquired by health sciences libraries will have **catalog copy** available. However, the librarian should have a basic knowledge of current cataloging standards and practices in order to review copy records and to facilitate processing of material for which catalog copy is not available.

As mentioned previously, books from major publishers generally include CIP information on the copyright page, providing basic descriptive and classification information. A smaller library may decide to enter this information manually into a database or ILS for each item. Another method of obtaining records is to download them from another library's online catalog, such as NLM's LocatorPlus. Alternatively, libraries may subscribe to a service that provides electronic MARC records for their purchases, which is available from many book vendors. Other libraries may subscribe to OCLC's Connexion service, or their more basic CatExpress service, for cataloging online.

However catalog records are obtained, the copy cataloger verifies that the correct record was selected and that there are no errors in the record. The call number is also verified and checked to ensure it doesn't conflict with items already in the collection. Often catalog records obtained from LC on peripheral subjects such as chemistry, veterinary sciences, or anthropology will lack MeSH and NLM classification, so the librarian must also be prepared to assign these. It is helpful to assign the subject headings first, then use the online "NLM classification"[5] to find the classification for that MeSH descriptor. The subjects can be identified by using the LC headings that are listed in the CIP information or in the copy catalog record, and searching the "MeSH browser"[11] to find the corresponding MeSH. If no corresponding descriptors are found, the material itself should be examined and subjects assigned from MeSH based on its content.

CURRENT CATALOGING PRACTICES

Descriptive Cataloging in Practice

The description of a book or other resource is based on information from the resource itself, using supplementary information if necessary. The chapters of *AACR2R* Part 1 govern the bibliographic description of various formats of materials. Each chapter prescribes the chief source of information to be used as the basis for transcribing the resource description. For example, books are governed by *AACR2R* Chapter 2, which lists the title page or its substitute as the chief source of information. For videorecordings the cataloger uses Chapter 7, and the title frames or attached cassette label are prescribed as the chief source of information. For Web sites (electronic resources that are considered "integrating resources"), the situation is more complex. The cataloger uses Chapter 9 in conjunction with other relevant chapters, depending on the nature of the site, and

> [f]or online integrating resources, the chief source of information is the resource itself (9.0B1). Prefer formally presented evidence such as title screens, home pages, etc., and encoded metadata. If the information varies in degree of fullness, select the source with the most complete information as the source of the title proper.[12]

A note is always included to state what was used as the chief source of information for online integrating resources (as well as for serials), to allow others using the record to verify that they are looking at the same resource. Serials cataloging differs from monographic cataloging in that the chief source of information is the first issue rather than the item that is in hand. The first issue may not be available, so the earliest available issue is used in its place, and a note added to that effect. When a serial title changes, a new record must be created, and the rules in *AACR2R* Chapter 12 are followed.

Table 5.1 lists the chapters of *AACR2R* and the formats they govern. Within each chapter, sections are arranged similarly, providing rules for each of the eight areas of description listed in Table 5.2.

Access points are selected according to *AACR2R* Chapter 21, and Chapters 22-24 provide guidelines for constructing the form of names and titles that are being used. A main entry is selected as instructed in Chapter 21 and, particularly for monographs, is generally used as the basis for a book number, or Cutter number, which is added to the LC or NLM classification to form the complete call number.

TABLE 5.1. *AACR2R* Chapters and the Formats They Govern

Chapter	Formats
2	Books, pamphlets, and printed sheets
3	Cartographic materials
4	Manuscripts (including manuscript collections)
5	Music
6	Sound recordings
7	Motion pictures and video recordings
8	Graphic materials
9	Electronic resources
10	Three-dimensional artifacts and realia
11	Microforms
12	Continuing resources
13	Analysis

TABLE 5.2. Areas of Description in *AACR2R*

Area	Content
X.1	Title and statement of responsibility
X.2	Edition
X.3	Material (or type of publication) specific details
X.4	Publication, distribution, etc.
X.5	Physical description
X.6	Series
X.7	Note
X.8	Standard number and terms of availability

Subject Assignment

If following NLM's practices, the cataloger uses MeSH, the controlled vocabulary for the health sciences, which is organized in a hierarchical structure. Table 5.3 shows the sixteen categories into which MeSH is divided.

The MeSH hierarchical structure (or tree structure) allows subjects to be assigned at various levels of specificity depending on the resource being described. For example, Figure 5.1 shows a portion of the hierarchy for nervous system diseases. If a resource is about viral encephalitis, for example, that specific heading is used. If it is about three of the specific diseases listed in that tree structure, all three are used. If it is about more than three specific diseases, the next broader heading is generally used instead of the individual headings. The broadest heading, Nervous System Diseases, would only be used for the most general works.

TABLE 5.3. MeSH Tree Structure Categories

Category	Designation
Anatomy	[A]
Organisms	[B]
Diseases	[C]
Chemicals and Drugs	[D]
Analytical, Diagnostic, and Therapeutic Techniques and Equipment	[E]
Psychiatry and Psychology	[F]
Biological Sciences	[G]
Natural Sciences	[H]
Anthropology, Education, Sociology, and Social Phenomena	[I]
Technology, Industry, Agriculture	[J]
Humanities	[K]
Information Science	[L]
Named Groups	[M]
Health Care	[N]
Publication Characteristics	[V]
Geographicals	[Z]

Nervous System Diseases [C10]
   Central Nervous System Diseases [C10.228]
     Central Nervous System Infections [C10.228.228]
       Brain Abscess [C10.228.228.090] +
       Central Nervous System Bacterial Infections [C10.228.228.180] +
       Central Nervous System Fungal Infections [C10.228.228.198] +
       Central Nervous System Parasitic Infections [C10.228.228.205] +
       Central Nervous System Viral Diseases [C10.228.228.210] +
       Empyema, Subdural [C10.228.228.227]
       Encephalitis [C10.228.228.245]
         Encephalitis, Viral [C10.228.228.245.340] +
         Meningoencephalitis [C10.228.228.245.550] +
         Leukoencephalitis, Acute Hemorrhagic [C10.228.228.245.670]
         Limbic Encephalitis [C10.228.228.245.700]

FIGURE 5.1. MeSH Tree Structure for Encephalitis

The introduction to the current edition of MeSH is posted online each year and explains NLM practices in detail.[13] An outline of the main features of MeSH and specific instructions about the use of MeSH for catalogers is also available:

> Catalogers use the most specific MeSH terms available to describe the subject content of an item. . . . A very general work may sometimes be described with a single MeSH term. Complex concepts are represented by pre-coordinated main headings when available. When an appropriate pre-coordinated term is not available in the MeSH vocabulary, the concept is represented by the coordination of two or more main headings, or by main heading and topical subheading combinations.[14]

A pre-coordinated term is a single subject heading that represents more than one concept. For example, Aortic Diseases is a pre-coordinated term that combines the concept of aorta with that of disease. Because there is no such combined term for pulmonary artery disease, the cataloger would use the separate headings Pulmonary Artery and Vascular Diseases. Topical subheadings, or **qualifiers,** may be added to provide more specificity to the subject description. For example, works about lung cancer are assigned the term Lung Neoplasms and may be further refined by using such subheadings as genetics, diagnosis, or surgery. Table 5.4 provides some examples of the various ways MeSH is used to express topical concepts.

By 2005, NLM's cataloging practices were changed to make them more consistent with NLM's indexing practices for the MEDLINE databases. With these changes, geographic and language qualifiers, which had previously been added to the subject heading following a topical qualifier, have been placed in separate fields or represented by fixed fields in the MARC record.[15] In addition, physical format terms such as videocassette, audiocassette, and CD-ROM are no longer added to the subject headings but are represented by the physical description area, or by coding in the MARC record.

Genre refers to the form of presentation of the work being described, such as congresses, encyclopedias, or handbooks. It may be indicated as in NLM's LocatorPlus catalog, or as it is in records distributed to OCLC. In LocatorPlus, genre is entered in a separate 655 **MARC tag,** rather than the 650 that is used for subjects. NLM adjusts records for distribution to attach the genre term to the subject headings. Figure 5.2 shows an example of this change.

Classification

Based on the subject content of the resource, a call number is usually assigned, which provides a method for shelving physical material and may be used with remote-access material to provide another means to identify it by topic. NLM classification, supplemented by LC classification, is most commonly used in health sciences libraries, with LC classification sometimes being used exclusively when a catalog is shared with a parent institution using that scheme, as

TABLE 5.4 Examples for Using MeSH

Category	Example
Single MeSH term	Surgery; Nursing
Pre-coordinated main headings	Nursing Research; Cardiovascular Physiology
Coordination of two or more main headings	For the topic diagnostic imaging in spinal cord trauma: Diagnostic Imaging AND Spinal Cord Injuries
Main heading and topical subheading (qualifier)	Cardiovascular Diseases—diagnosis; Diabetes Mellitus—therapy

Currently in LocatorPlus:

650 12 $a **Community Mental Health Services**

650 22 $a **Child** $9 n

655 _2 $a **Directory**

Currently on distributed records:

650 12 $a **Community Mental Health Services** $v **Directory**

650 22 $a **Child**

FIGURE 5.2. Example of Distributed Records from NLM with Genre Heading

described earlier. The NLM classification, outlined in Table 5.5, makes use of QS-QZ and W-WZ, sections left unused by LC in its classification schedules. In addition, health sciences libraries which use NLM classification do not use the LC schedules for Human Anatomy (QM), Microbiology (QR), and Medicine (R). Subjects outside the scope of the NLM classification are described using the LC classification.

Information about NLM's practices in classification is available on the Web. The basic rules for classification follow:

- The classification number assigned to a work is determined by the main focus or subject content of the work.
- A work dealing with several subjects that fall into different areas of the classification is classed by emphasis, or if emphasis is lacking, by the first subject treated in the work.
- A work on a particular disease is classified with the disease, which in turn is classified with the organ or region chiefly affected, regardless of special emphasis on form of therapy or diagnostic procedure used.[16]

The complete call number is formed from the classification number and a book number, or Cutter number, for which NLM uses the *Cutter-Sanborn Three-Figure Author Table*.[17] This is followed by the date of publication. For multivolume works issued together, the volume number follows the date, while for multivolume works issued over a span of years, the volume number usually follows the Cutter number, with the year as the final element. An example of a complete call number is provided in Figure 5.3.

The MARC Record

All of this information is entered in a MARC record in **fixed** and **variable fields** and **subfields.** MARC coding is a complex topic, and this introduction should be supplemented by the resources listed here and in Appendix 5.A. *Understanding MARC Bibliographic: Machine-Readable Cataloging* is a work originally published by the Follett Software Company, now published by LC, which gives an excellent description of the MARC bibliographic record.[18] It provides brief explanations and outlines the actual usage of MARC tags and is highly recommended for beginning catalogers. LC also makes the *MARC 21 LITE Bibliographic Format* available on the Web, and this will be helpful for the cataloger with questions about MARC usage.[19] MARC provides coding for all formats of materials, monographs, serials, video recordings, and others and adds new coding when needed. For example, coding for integrating resources was added to the MARC fixed fields to provide for Web sites, which are electronic resources that may be neither monographic nor serial in nature.

TABLE 5.5. Outline of the NLM Classification

Field	Section	Subjects
Preclinical sciences	QS	Human Anatomy
	QT	Physiology
	QU	Biochemistry
	QV	Pharmacology
	QW	Microbiology and Immunology
	QX	Parasitology
	QY	Clinical Pathology
	QZ	Pathology
Medicine and related subjects	W	Health Professions
	WA	Public Health
	WB	Practice of Medicine
	WC	Communicable Diseases
	WD	Disorders of Systemic, Metabolic or Environmental Origin, etc.
	WE	Musculoskeletal System
	WF	Respiratory System
	WG	Cardiovascular System
	WH	Hemic and Lymphatic Systems
	WI	Digestive System
	WJ	Urogenital System
	WK	Endocrine System
	WL	Nervous System
	WM	Psychiatry
	WN	Radiology; Diagnostic Imaging
	WO	Surgery
	WP	Gynecology
	WQ	Obstetrics
	WR	Dermatology
	WS	Pediatrics
	WT	Geriatrics; Chronic Disease
	WU	Dentistry; Oral Surgery
	WV	Otolaryngology
	WW	Ophthalmology
	WX	Hospitals and Other Health Facilities
	WY	Nursing
	WZ	History of Medicine

The cataloger can review how MARC is applied to NLM's cataloging record for a particular resource by selecting MARC display in LocatorPlus, the NLM online catalog. NLM's bibliographic records are also contributed to OCLC and are available from vendors who use those files.

Figure 5.4 shows several examples of MARC tags. The tag number is the first number in the line and identifies the type of information recorded there. The title and statement of responsibility are recorded in the 245 field, while the 260 field contains the publication and distribution information. **Indicators** are in the two positions following the tag number, and in the 245 both are used and the value is 0 (zero) for both. For the 245 field, indicators show that the title does not need an added entry (first indicator 0), and that the value in the title field is filed beginning with the first character (second indicator 0). The 260 field does not use indicators. Indicators and subfields are specific to the particular tag in which they are used. Subfields are demarcated by a double dagger (‡). In the 245 field, the data in ‡a represent the title proper, in ‡b represent other title information, and in ‡c represent the statement of responsibility. In the 260 field, the data in ‡a represent the place of publication or distribution, in ‡b represent the name of the publisher or distributor, and in ‡c represent the date of publication or copyright date.

Figure 5.5 is a MARC catalog record from OCLC. The LC classification appears in the 050 field, and the NLM classification appears in 060 fields. Descriptors, or subject headings, appear in the 650 fields, and the second indicator identifies its source. If the second indicator is a 0, it is from LCSH, and if the second indicator is a 2, it is from MeSH.

Figure 5.6 shows the MARC record for the same book, which was retrieved from NLM's LocatorPlus, where the LC information is not included, and Figure 5.7 shows the CIP record transcribed from the copyright page of the printed book.

Class number for: Cardiovascular Disease and Diabetes

WK   General class for endocrine system

840   Specific number for diabetes as a complication in other conditions

C267   Cutter number for the main entry (title)

2007   Publication year

FIGURE 5.3. NLM Call Number

Title and statement of responsibility area (245)

245 00 ‡a Cardiovascular disease and diabetes / ‡c editor, Luther T. Clark; associate editor, Samy I. McFarlane.

245 00 ‡a Schwartz's principles of surgery : ‡b self-assessment and board review / ‡c editor-in-chief, F. Charles Brunicardi ; associate editors, Mary L. Brandt . . . [et al.].

Publication, distribution, etc., area (260)

260 ‡a New York : ‡b McGraw-Hill, ‡c c2007.

260 ‡a New York : ‡b Thieme ; ‡a Rolling Meadows, Ill. : ‡b American Association of Neurosurgeons, ‡c c2007.

FIGURE 5.4. Examples of Two MARC Tags with Indicators and Subfields

010	‡a 2006046614
040	‡a DNLM/DLC ‡c DLC ‡d NLM ‡d BAKER ‡d UKM ‡d C#P ‡d YDX ‡d YDXCP
015	‡a GBA685346 ‡2 bnb
016 7	‡a 101281015 ‡2 DNLM
016 7	‡a 013572393 ‡2 Uk
019	‡a 72867929
020	‡a 0071436812 (alk. paper)
020	‡a 9780071436816 (alk. paper)
020	‡z 9780071436816 (alk. paper)
029 1	‡a NLM ‡b 101281015
029 1	‡a YDXCP ‡b 2476401
042	‡a pcc
050 00	‡a RC700.D5 ‡b C3722 2007
060 00	‡a 2007 B-282
060 10	‡a WK 840 ‡b C267 2007
082 00	‡a 616.1/071 ‡2 22
096	‡a ‡b
049	‡a CSZA
245 00	‡a Cardiovascular disease and diabetes / ‡c editor, Luther T. Clark ; associate editor, Samy I. McFarlane.
260	‡a New York : ‡b McGraw-Hill, ‡c c2007.
300	‡a xix, 635 p. : ‡b ill. ; ‡c 24 cm.
504	‡a Includes bibliographical references and index.
650 0	‡a Diabetic angiopathies.
650 0	‡a Cardiovascular system ‡x Diseases ‡x Etiology.
650 0	‡a Cardiovascular system ‡x Diseases ‡x Complications.
650 12	‡a Cardiovascular Diseases ‡x complications.
650 12	‡a Diabetes Complications ‡x therapy.
650 22	‡a Cardiovascular Diseases ‡x therapy.
650 22	‡a Diabetes Mellitus ‡x therapy.
700 1	‡a Clark, Luther T.
700 1	‡a McFarlane, Samy I.
856 41	‡3 Table of contents only ‡u
	http://www.loc.gov/catdir/enhancements/fy0661/2006046614-t.html
856 42	‡3 Contributor biographical information ‡u
	http://www.loc.gov/catdir/enhancements/fy0666/2006046614-b.html
856 42	‡3 Publisher description ‡u
	http://www.loc.gov/catdir/enhancements/fy0666/2006046614-d.html
938	‡a Baker & Taylor ‡b BKTY ‡c 75.00 ‡d .00 ‡i 0071436812 ‡n 0006888434 ‡s active
938	‡a YBP Library Services ‡b YANK ‡n 2476401

FIGURE 5.5. MARC Record from OCLC for the Title *Cardiovascular Disease and Diabetes. Source:* From the OCLC's WorldCat® database; used by permission of OCLC. WorldCat® is a registered trademark of OCLC Online Computer Library Center, Inc.

```
000 01180pam a22003854a 450
001 1281015
005 20070207134003.0
008 060705s2007 nyua b 001 0 eng
010 __ |a 2006046614
020 __ |a 9780071436816 (alk. paper)
020 __ |a 0071436812 (alk. paper)
035 __ |9 101281015
040 __ |a DNLM |c DNLM
041 09 |a eng
042 __ |a pcc
044 __ |9 United States
060 00 |a 2007 B-282
060 10 |a WK 840 |b C267 2007
245 00 |a Cardiovascular disease and diabetes/ |c editor, Luther T. Clark ; associate editor, Samy I. McFarlane.
260 __ |a New York: |b McGraw-Hill Medical, |c c2007.
300 __ |a xix, 635 p.: |b ill.
504 __ |a Includes bibliographical references and index.
650 12 |a Diabetes Complications |x therapy
650 12 |a Cardiovascular Diseases |x complications
650 22 |a Cardiovascular Diseases |x therapy
650 22 |a Diabetes Mellitus |x therapy
700 1_ |a Clark, Luther T.
700 1_ |a McFarlane, Samy I.
986 __ |a a020107
992 __ |p P1 |e E4 |a 20070201
993 __ |a AXE |b 20070206
994 __ |a CDN |b 20070206
995 __ |a AUTH |b 20060706 |c REV |d 20070207
996 __ |a rev. CIP |b 20070207
999 __ |a AUTH
```

FIGURE 5.6. MARC Record for *Cardiovascular Disease and Diabetes* from NLM's LocatorPlus Catalog, MARC View

Cardiovascular disease and diabetes / edited by Luther T. Clark; associate editor, Samy I. McFarlane.
   p. ; cm.
Includes bibliographical references and index.
ISBN 0-07-143681-2 (alk. paper)
1. Diabetic angiopathies. 2. Cardiovascular system—Diseases—Etiology. 3. Cardiovascular system—Diseases—Complications. I. Clark, Luther T. II. McFarlane, Samy I.
[DNLM: 1. Cardiovascular Diseases—complications. 2. Diabetes Complications—therapy. 3. Cardiovascular Diseases—therapy. 4. Diabetes Mellitus—therapy. WK 840 C267 2007]
RC700.D5C3722 2007
616.1'071—dc22

FIGURE 5.7. CIP Record Transcribed from Copyright Page of the Title *Cardiovascular Disease and Diabetes*. *Source:* Clark, L. T. *Cardiovascular Disease and Diabetes*. New York: McGraw-Hill Professional, 2007. Reproduced with permission of the McGraw-Hill Companies.

ORGANIZING SPECIFIC MATERIALS

Organizing Audiovisual Materials

Health sciences libraries' collections often include a variety of audiovisual materials, such as video recordings of surgical, nursing, or other procedures; sound recordings of lectures; anatomical models; or microscope slides. It is not always easy to find catalog copy for such materials, but copy for commercially produced audiovisuals can often be found. If original cataloging must be created, it should be cataloged using the rules for description from *AACR2R* Chapters 6, 7, 8, or 10.

As mentioned earlier, MeSH now provides only for the subject of material, not for its physical format, which is identified by information in the physical description area and through the MARC fixed field coding. Each OPAC is a little different, but the librarian should be sure that there is a way to identify this material in the OPAC. In smaller libraries a separate listing of audiovisual materials may serve the purpose of identifying and locating them.

Audiovisual materials are generally shelved separately from books, due to the requirement for using playback equipment for some of them, and their variety of sizes and shapes. Because of this it is useful to include them in the catalog to facilitate discovery.

Organizing Print Journals

When the library includes journals and other serials in the online catalog and assigns subject headings to them, they will be easily identified along with other materials on the same topic. Thus, better access is provided than if a title list alone is used.

Some libraries will arrange print journals by class numbers so that they will be interfiled with books in a subject arrangement, but most health sciences libraries follow an alphabetic title arrangement and shelve journals separately from books. NLM follows this practice and does not classify its serials by topic but places them in a single class, W1, Cuttered alphabetically by title. This does separate journals whose titles have changed from one section of the alphabet to another. For example, *Acta Medica Scandinavica* has the call number W1 AC8551, but it is continued by the title *Journal of Internal Medicine,* which has the call number W1 JO716N. However, journal citations are identified by the current journal title, rather than a previous title, and health sciences library users work extensively from bibliographic searches in databases such as MEDLINE, in which the results can easily be sorted alphabetically by journal title. Thus, searching through print journal stacks is made more convenient if the stacks are arranged alphabetically.

Organizing Electronic Resources

Because electronic resources are so important to library users, it is very important to make it as easy as possible to find and access them. Electronic journals, books, databases, and Web sites may be included in the OPAC but may be made available via the library's Web site, either in addition to or instead of being included in the catalog. The information used to create a Web list may be extracted by a search of the catalog, or it may be a simple database created in-house from the library's journal list and posted on the Web site. The list may also come from a homegrown or commercial ERMS, which includes links to individual abstracts, indexes, databases, and journal titles, as well as links to journals that are acquired as part of full-text databases. An electronic journal list may also be generated by a journal vendor from the library's list of subscriptions. Librarians have found many ways to present electronic resources to their users. Librarians at the Los Alamos National Laboratory described an early project to extract catalog records from their OPAC and provide them as a Web-based list.[20] Hospital librarians have also been creative in their management of electronic resources, creating simple databases to display titles on their Web sites. One example was the use of the EndNote bibliographic reference software to create and maintain an electronic journal list.[21, 22]

Including electronic resources in the catalog affords the opportunity to provide more detailed subject description than may be available in an ERMS or simple list, thus enhancing discovery. Many libraries contribute catalog records for electronic resources to OCLC, and libraries participating in the CONSER program provide authoritative records for serials (including electronic journals), so copy cataloging is available for many electronic titles. Catalog copy for Web sites is not as commonly available, but there are systems that have automated some of the cataloging process. For example, by entering the URL of a Web page or the path of a local electronic file, the OCLC system will create basic records for electronic resources by extracting metadata into a cataloging workform, which can then be edited as needed.[23]

The library Web site is often the first impression users have of the library and is an important tool in organization of resources for use, and particularly important for electronic resources. The Hardin Library at the University of Iowa maintains Medical/Health Sciences Libraries on the Web, a listing of links to U.S. medical school and other health sciences libraries.[24] A review of these sites demonstrates the wide range of designs used for grouping library resources. A few libraries have a minimalist approach, such as the University of Southern California's Norris Medical Library, which has very little text on the home page. Some include links to portals aimed at different constituencies among their users, such as Washington University's Bernard Becker Medical Library, which has tabs on the home page leading to pages with specific selections of resources for researchers, clinicians, students, instructors, administrators/staff, and alumni/members/visitors. Many library Web sites feature a list of "quick links" providing direct access to the most frequently used resources. It is important to think carefully about the usefulness of various Web site designs to assist users in finding the information they need.

GLIMPSES OF WHAT'S TO COME

Health sciences libraries are certainly affected by the environment in which they function. Technology is developing more and more rapidly, providing librarians with many new information-related tools. There are some interesting programs being developed in open source software, freely available and adaptable by users, which show great promise for more convenient searching. Additionally, ILS vendors are beginning to take advantage of technological advances to make catalogs more attractive to library users, and thus to facilitate access to libraries' print collections as well as electronic content that libraries have licensed.

The library catalog at North Carolina State University uses Endeca's Information Access Platform <http://endeca.com/technology/index.html> to allow a general search of the catalog to be refined by call number range, or by genre, topic, geographic area, or format. Antelman, Lynema, and Pace have provided a description of the development of this interesting catalog project, which offers a range of methods to hone in on the topic being searched.[25] In a similar manner, the Queens (New York) Public Library uses AquaBrowser software <http://www .tlcdelivers.com/aquabrowser/default.asp> to help refine the results of a broad search and also provides a graphical "web," which allows the user to follow links to related information. Innovative Interfaces is working on a product called Encore, "a complete search and discovery experience" <http://www.iii.com/encore/main_index2.html>, and Ex Libris is developing a system they are calling Primo <http://www.exlibrisgroup.com/primo.htm>, which facilitates the "discovery and delivery of print and digital information sources regardless of format and location." Both SerialsSolutions and Ex Libris use Vivisimo's Velocity Clustering Engine <http://

vivisimo.com/> in their federated search products. This product provides for the grouping of search results to allow refinement of search results. All of these products are meant to facilitate searching, which of course is based on the subject description and metadata information attached to records representing works or to the works themselves.

Open source programs are also being developed to offer alternatives to the traditional ILS. Two examples are LibraryFind <http://www.libraryfind.org/>, developed by the Oregon State University Libraries, and dbWiz (Database Selection Wizard) <http://dbwiz.lib.sfu.ca/dbwiz/>, a federated search tool developed by the Simon Fraser University Library as part of their larger suite of software called reSearcher. The Georgia Public Library Service is developing and maintaining an open source ILS called Evergreen <http://www.open-ils.org/>, which serves a consortium of public libraries in that state. And a blog called Open Source Software for Libraries <http://oss4lib.org/>, started at the Yale Medical Library, covers "free software and systems designed for libraries."

Library users have become accustomed to the ranking algorithms and relevance information that informs Google searching, which are only coming slowly to the world of library catalogs. For the most part, searches in the traditional ILS still generally rely on simple keyword or browse queries and sort by date, title, or author. Some have predicted the disappearance of the library catalog, while others, such as Karen Markey,[26] have looked at the changes and new technologies, such as those just described, as opportunities to make catalogs more useful and relevant in this age of electronic information. Because OPACs already contain a vast amount of information about print and audiovisual resources in addition to electronic resources, taking advantage of these new technologies for library catalogs will be a great service to library users.

APPENDIX 5.A. RESOURCE BIBLIOGRAPHY
FOR ORGANIZING INFORMATION

Basic Cataloging Tools

Cutter-Sanborn Three-Figure Author Table. Littleton, CO: Hargrave House, 1969. Available: <http://www.cuttertables.com/cutter3.html>. Accessed: March 2, 2007.

Furrie, B. *Understanding MARC Bibliographic: Machine-Readable Cataloging.* 7th ed. Washington, DC: Cataloging Distribution Service, Library of Congress, in collaboration with The Follett Software Company, 2003. Available: <http://www.loc.gov/marc/umb/>. Accessed: March 2, 2007.

LocatorPlus, the NLM catalog. Available: <http://locatorplus.gov/>. Accessed: March 2, 2007.

MeSH Browser. Available: <http://www.nlm.nih.gov/mesh/2007/MBrowser.html>. Accessed: March 2, 2007.

NLM Classification. Available: <http://wwwcf.nlm.nih.gov/class/index.html>. Accessed: March 2, 2007.

General Resources

Chan, L.M. *Cataloging and Classification: An Introduction.* 2nd ed. New York: McGraw-Hill Higher Education, 1994.

Coyle, K. Metadata: Data with a Purpose, a Brief Introduction to Metadata, Especially for Librarians. Available: <http://www.kcoyle.net/meta_purpose.html>. Accessed: February 8, 2007.

Eden, B. "Functional Requirements of Bibliographic Records." *Library Technology Reports* 42, no. 6 (November/December 2006): 1-49.

"A Brief History of AACR." Available: <http://www.collectionscanada.ca/jsc/history.html>. Accessed: October 2, 2007.

Intner, S.S.; Lazinger, S.S.; and Weihs, J. *Metadata and Its Impact on Libraries.* Littleton, CO: Libraries Unlimited, 2005.

Joint Steering Committee. Available: <http://www.collectionscanada.ca/jsc/>. Accessed: January 30, 2007.

Statement of International Cataloguing Principles. Draft approved by the IFLA Meeting of Experts on an International Cataloguing Code, 1st, Frankfurt, Germany, 2003, with agreed changes from the IME ICC2 meeting, Buenos Aires, Argentina, 2004, and the IME ICC3 meeting, Cairo, Egypt, 2005. Available: <http://www.loc.gov/loc/ifla/imeicc/pdf/statement-draft3_apr06cleancopy.pdf>.   Accessed: February 6, 2007.

Taylor, A.G. *Introduction to Cataloging and Classification.* 10th ed. Littleton, CO: Libraries Unlimited, 2006.

Taylor, A.G. *The Organization of Information.* 2nd ed. Littleton, CO: Libraries Unlimited, 2003.

Thompson, L. *Bibliographic Management of Information Resources in Health Sciences Libraries.* Current Practice in Health Sciences Librarianship, vol. 6. Lanham, MD: Medical Library Association and Scarecrow Press, 2001.

REFERENCES

1. Panizzi, Anthony. "Rules for the Compilation of the Catalogue." *Catalogue of Printed Books in the British Museum* (1841), vol. 1, pp. [v]-ix. Cited on the JSC Web site. Available: <http://www.collectionscanada.ca/jsc/history.html>. Accessed: February 2, 2007.

2. Cutter, C.A. *Rules for a Printed Dictionary Catalogue.* Washington, DC: Government Printing Office, 1876, p. 10. Cited by Tillett, B. "Cataloging for the Future," the 2004 Phineas L. Windsor Lecture at the University of Illinois Graduate School of Library and Information Science, October 13, 2004. Available: <http://puboff.lis.uiuc.edu/catalog/windsor/windsor_tillett.pdf>. Accessed: February 6, 2007.

3. *Anglo-American Cataloging Rules.* Issued in North American and British editions, 1967.

4. *Anglo-American Cataloging Rules.* 2nd ed., 2002 rev. Chicago: American Library Association, 2002, 2005 update.

5. National Library of Medicine. "NLM Classification 2006." Available: <http://wwwcf.nlm.nih.gov/class/>. Accessed: February 22, 2007.

6. McCallum, S.H. "MARC: Keystone for Library Automation." *2002 IEEE Annals of the History of Computing* 24, no. 2 (April-June 2002): 34-49.

7. "ECIP Program Expands to Include Clinical Medicine." *News from the Library of Congress* (November 6, 2000). Available: <http://www.loc.gov/today/pr/2000/00-170.html>. Accessed: February 20, 2007.

8. Library Technology Guides: Key Resources and Content Related to Library Automation. Available: <http://www.librarytechnology.org/>. Accessed: February 7, 2007.

9. Visual Resources Association. "Metadata." Available: <http://www.vraweb.org/metadata.html>. Accessed: January 31, 2007.

10. Library of Congress. "Program for Cooperative Cataloging." Available: <http://www.loc.gov/catdir/pcc/2001pcc.html>. Accessed: February 17, 2007.

11. National Library of Medicine. "Medical Subject Headings, MeSH Browser." Available: <http://www.nlm.nih.gov/mesh/MBrowser.html>. Accessed: February 25, 2007.

12. "Integrating Resources: A Cataloging Manual," Appendix A to the *BIBCO Participants' Manual* and Module 35 of the *CONSER Cataloging Manual,* 2005 rev. by the Task Group to Update Integrating Resources Documentation and Training Materials under the auspices of the PCC Standing Committee on Training. Available: <http://www.loc.gov/catdir/pcc/bibco/irman.pdf>. Accessed: February 12, 2007.

13. National Library of Medicine. "Features of the MeSH Vocabulary." Available: <http://www.nlm.nih.gov/mesh/intro_features2006.html>. Accessed: February 12, 2007.

14. National Library of Medicine. "Use of Medical Subject Headings for Cataloging—2006." Available: <http://www.nlm.nih.gov/mesh/catpractices2006.html>. Accessed: February 12, 2007.

15. National Library of Medicine. "Use of Medical Subject Headings for Cataloging—2005." Available: <http://www.nlm.nih.gov/mesh/catpractices2005.html>. Accessed: February 13, 2007.

16. NLM Classification 2006. "NLM Classification Practices." Available: <http://www.nlm.nih.gov/class/nlmclassprac.html>. Accessed: February 13, 2007.

17. *Cutter-Sanborn Three-Figure Author Table.* Littleton, CO: Hargrave House, 1969. Available: <http://www.cuttertables.com/cutter3.html>. Accessed: February 13, 2007.

18. Furrie, B. *Understanding MARC Bibliographic: Machine-Readable Cataloging.* 7th ed. Washington, DC: Cataloging Distribution Service, Library of Congress, in collaboration with The Follett Software Company, 2003. Available: <http://www.loc.gov/marc/umb/>. Accessed: February 11, 2007.

19. Library of Congress Network Development and MARC Standards Office. MARC 21 LITE Bibliographic Format. Annual. Available: <http://www.loc.gov/marc/bibliographic/lite>. Accessed: February 13, 2007.

20. Knudson, F.L.; Sprague, N.R.; Chafe, D.A.; et al. "Creating Electronic Journal Web Pages from OPAC Records." *Issues in Science and Technology Librarianship* (Summer 1997). Available: <http://www.library.ucsb.edu/istl/97-summer/article2.html>. Accessed: February 17, 2007.

21. Just, M.L. "Using EndNote to Maintain Electronic Journals Lists." *MLA News* no. 325 (April 2000): 12.

22. Just, M.L. "Using EndNote for Electronic Journal Management in a Hospital Library." Poster presented at the Medical Library Association Annual Meeting. Orlando, FL, May 28, 2001. *Special Supplement, MLA 2001 Abstracts,* p. 60.

23. Cataloging: Create Bibliographic Records [OCLC]. Available: <http://www.oclc.org/support/documentation/connexion/client/cataloging/createbib/>. Accessed: March 2, 2007.

24. University of Iowa. Hardin Medical Library. "Medical/Health Sciences Libraries on the Web." Available: <http://www.lib.uiowa.edu/hardin/hslibs.html>. Accessed: March 9, 2007.

25. Antelman, K.; Lynema, E.; and Pace, A.K. "Toward a Twenty-First Century Library Catalog." *Information Technology and Libraries* 25, no. 3 (September 2006): 128-39.

26. Markey, K. "The Online Library Catalog, Paradise Lost and Paradise Regained?" *D-Lib Magazine* 13, no. 1/2 (January/February 2007): 1-15.

SECTION III:
PUBLIC SERVICES

Chapter 6

Access Issues

Elizabeth R. Lorbeer
Cindy Scroggins

SUMMARY. This chapter examines the ways in which health sciences libraries make their information resources available and usable. Whether material is accessible in print format or electronically, in-house or via interlibrary loan, on-site or from a remote location, libraries face the challenge of providing their users with the information they need, when and where they want it. The chapter includes discussion of traditional and emerging trends in access services in general, with particular emphasis on the importance of information access within clinical and academic health care environments.

INTRODUCTION

As noted in nearly every chapter of this book, hospital and academic health sciences libraries share much in common with other types of libraries. This is true in the area of access services as well. All types of libraries are seeing a shift from their previous role of repository for print materials to that of gateway to the larger world of electronic information. All libraries are also experiencing greater demand for ease of access and timeliness of information delivery. In this sense, the health sciences library may serve as a model to other libraries, in that the accessibility and timely delivery of health-related information have always been of utmost concern to health sciences librarians.[1]

While health sciences librarians have always stressed timely access to information, the pool of people eligible for such access was, until relatively recently, quite limited. Historically, hospital libraries were available only to those associated with clinical care or research, and academic health sciences libraries were limited strictly to faculty and students. Access was considered a privilege, due in large part to the expensive nature of the resources and the fact that they were written specifically for those schooled in the sciences. Material was frequently not allowed to circulate and often kept in closed stacks. Patients or members of the general public in search of health-related information were generally limited to what they could glean from the family physician.

Today, health sciences libraries play a strong supportive role in all functions of clinical research, education, and patient care. Health sciences libraries provide information to health professionals, faculty and students, administrators, and the general public. The library of today provides quality information for all levels of educational background and language comprehension. Patients and their families generally have physical access to the entire library collection. Even during times when the physical library is closed, authorized users may access the library's electronic collection twenty-four hours a day.

Introduction to Health Sciences Librarianship

FUNDAMENTALS OF ACCESS

Simply put, access is about connecting users to the resources they need. This requires the health sciences librarian to take an active role in partnering with the community it serves to ensure that it is meeting the informational needs of its current clientele while being mindful of new partnerships with underserved populations. The more obstacles the library puts in the way of its users, the more likely users are to seek information elsewhere. Health sciences librarians need to continually ask, "Am I connecting my users to the information they need, without barriers? What impediments stand in the way of users coming either physically or virtually to the library?" Staff can test accessibility by surveying their clientele and designing interfaces that enable efficient opportunities to engage the collection.[2] User input should drive the customization of library services, operations, design, and delivery.

When discussing access issues, it is important to keep in mind that the goal is to get the user to the source of information as easily as possible. Today's health sciences library contains vastly more electronic resources than it was ever able to acquire in print in previous years. Much content is born and acquired digitally with no print counterpart, while some publications remain available exclusively in print format. Essentially, the modern health sciences library exists in a mixed-media realm where it is providing access to both physical and electronic content. Many library users want the library to remain as it has traditionally been known to them, as a physical destination to socialize, study, and browse. Others want nothing but virtual access and see little need for physical libraries to exist, beyond housing a qualified staff to acquire, maintain, and deliver information electronically. The primary concern of both groups is easy access to information *in the form that they want it.* Libraries face the challenge of meeting the expectations of both groups.

Ideally access is taken into consideration at every level and within every job in the library, toward the ultimate aim of making the library's collections accessible and usable to clientele. The following examples illustrate how various library departments are involved with issues of access:

- Catalogers mull over subject headings and classifications in consideration of whether the user will be able to find the material easily.
- Web services staff consider the overall design and functionality of the Web site in terms of how to best connect the user with electronic information.
- Shelvers carefully ensure that books and journals are returned to their proper locations so they may be readily found.
- An electronic services librarian enabling a link resolver[3] to provide the full text of an article from a citation database is facilitating greater ease of access.
- Reference librarians promote virtual reference service to expand access beyond the walls of the library.
- A collection development librarian develops a policy of purchasing books in electronic format when available as a means of increasing access.
- Administrators enter into consortial licensing arrangements to increase access and affordability of electronic information resources.

ACCESS SERVICES

Many health sciences libraries have access services departments that generally include the functions of circulation, reserves, and stacks maintenance (shelving). The position of head of access services or access services librarian has traditionally been held by a master's-prepared librarian. In many libraries, access services management has been transferred to capable and experienced paraprofessionals who work under the supervision of a librarian. Typical job duties of an access services librarian include supervision and scheduling of staff, often including student workers and volunteers; the establishment of guidelines for circulation and reserves; monitoring copyright compliance and fair use of library materials; customizing the circulation and reserve modules of the **integrated library system (ILS);** ensuring the security of personal information of borrowers; collecting and reporting circulation, gate count, and shelving statistics; monitoring overdue materials; and overseeing and documenting the collection of fines.

Many libraries are moving toward consolidation of services and staff under a single umbrella.[4, 5] These libraries utilize a centralized service desk to address users' changing service needs in a digital age. In such centralized service units, access services falls under the same umbrella as reference, electronic services, document delivery, and interlibrary loan. Under this model, each employee maintains expertise in his or her specified area, but everyone works as a team to address user needs. For example, staff traditionally working in access services might perform the photocopying, scanning, and mailing of interlibrary loan materials.

A skilled access services librarian should have the experience to plan for long-term growth of the physical collection while balancing the need to reallocate space for new services (see Chapter 15, "Library Space Planning," for further information on facilities planning). In addition, the access services librarian should work closely with supervisors in all areas of the library on coordinated service efforts, whether or not a centralized service unit exists. Perhaps the most important aspect of the access services librarian's role is to foster an environment of exceptional customer service.

PHYSICAL ACCESS

The role of the library as a physical destination is clearly changing. Most libraries are seeing declines in their number of annual visitors, as well as in the number of books circulated. In their published statistics for a composite library, the **Association of Academic Health Sciences Libraries (AAHSL)** indicates a gate count drop of 24.5 percent from fiscal year (FY) 2000 to FY 2006 (from 288,126 to 217,554), and a dramatic 78.2 percent drop in circulation during that same time period (from 240,749 to 66,189).[6, 7]

These declining numbers are important to consider when planning physical space needs, as well as spending and service priorities; however, the fact remains that, while libraries are not the physical destination they once were, many people still want or need physical access to the library. Although an ever-growing percentage of information is available in electronic format, much remains available only in print. While many people are enthusiastic about computer access to information, some have no computer available to them apart from those provided in the library, and still others have no desire to learn to use a computer—including some physicians. Health sciences libraries are, above all else, service units, and they must strive to accommodate both the physical and electronic access needs of their clientele.

Public Access

In the past ten to fifteen years, most hospital libraries have broadened their service population to include patients and their families.[8] Some hospitals and health care organizations have created separate consumer health libraries with the specific aim of providing information to patients and their families, as well as to the general public. Most publicly funded academic health sciences libraries have adopted a policy allowing members of the general public in-house access to the library's full print collection. Many academic health sciences libraries also negotiate licensing terms to allow the public on-site access to electronic resources. Further, health sciences libraries often collaborate with local, state, or regional networks to provide access to their resources, in some cases extending borrowing privileges to public library card holders.

Borrowing

Full borrowing privileges are generally granted only to patrons affiliated with or otherwise recognized by the institution. Many health sciences libraries extend borrowing privileges to adjunct and emeritus faculty, alumni, physicians with admitting privileges, visiting researchers, and volunteers. Further privileges may be extended to users affiliated with regional health networks in which the library's institution is a member. The loan period and the types of materials that circulate are determined by each library, though many tend to circulate material for fourteen days. Reference books and journals typically do not circulate outside the library. With the availability of more electronic resources, however, many health sciences libraries are broadening their policies to allow circulation of print materials that have traditionally been noncirculating.

Hours of Availability

To accommodate the study and work schedules of health care providers, residents and students, the hospital library may choose to operate twenty-four hours a day, with secured entry available to authorized personnel during periods when the library is not staffed. With the growing availability of electronic information, this practice is less common today than in years past, when physical access to the library was the only means of accessing information needed to address urgent patient care.

Academic health sciences libraries, on the other hand, generally operate on a set schedule of 90 to 120 hours per week,[7] often extending their hours during midterm and final exams. In response to student requests, many academic health sciences libraries are considering the possibility of operating twenty-four hours a day. The lack of operational funds and difficulty in securing the interior of the building have prevented widespread adoption of this practice.

Security

Library security is the responsibility of every staff member.[9] The library director is responsible for ensuring the overall safety of the library, but the day-to-day responsibility of protecting materials is generally left to the access services department. Many large academic health sciences libraries employ security guards. The library should work in conjunction with the institution's public safety department to ensure routine foot patrol. A clearly written security policy should be in place that addresses physical security of the library's equipment and collections as well as means for ensuring a safe environment for patrons and staff.

Preventing theft of library materials is an obvious concern. To reduce potential losses, items should be clearly branded with a property stamp. The library should employ an electronic security system that allows for the use of magnetic security strips in books and journals (the 3M Company's trademarked Tattle-Tape Security Strips are commonly used). If a patron fails to properly check out an item, the detection system sounds an alarm when the material is taken past a sensor, usually located near an exit door. Some libraries are moving to newer technologies, such as **radio frequency identification (RFID),** which allows the library to track and locate material using a cordless handheld device.[10] RFID tags can be programmed specifically to identify and track each item as it enters or leaves the library. Physical equipment, such as computers and printers, are secured by cable and property stamps. For libraries offering unstaffed access, programmable access control systems such as keypads or cards are generally used. To increase security, many libraries install panic buttons and alarm systems, along with video cameras to monitor the actions of users in areas where staff are not posted.[11]

Unfortunately, health sciences libraries can attract disruptive individuals. At times their behavior or actions can be harmful to the staff, other users, or the collection, and they must be quickly removed from the premises. The library should have a well-crafted document on how staff should deal with disruptive patrons. This document should conform to the institution's practices and be reviewed by legal counsel to make sure the library is not impeding on individual rights. Above all, staff should never be put in a situation of having to approach or physically remove a potentially violent person from the library. Best practices recommend that staff call their institution's public safety officer or local police department to have the person removed.[9]

Books

Academic health sciences and hospital libraries organize their book collections based on the **National Library of Medicine**'s **(NLM) Medical Subject Headings (MeSH).** Subject headings are divided by broad preclinical subjects (e.g., anatomy, physiology, biochemistry), then by clinical specialty. Physical works are cataloged and provided a corresponding call number according to NLM classification. This division allows all works on the same topic to be located together and is therefore well-suited to patrons who wish to browse the collection. Call numbers for the preclinical sciences are located in QS-QZ, medicine is W-WX, nursing is WY, and medical biography is WZ.

Consumer health libraries may choose to use the Dewey Decimal Classification (DDC) in arranging their collections. DDC is the most widely used classification system in the world, and most members of the public are familiar with the system. DDC is only recommended when the collection is designed to be a consumer health resource. Collection arrangement is discussed further in Chapter 5, "Organizing Resources for Information Access."

Journals

In a health sciences library, the journal collection is generally much larger than the book collection and most commonly arranged in alphabetical order by title. While some users of health sciences libraries browse print journals, most seek specific articles following a search of MEDLINE or other electronic database of health sciences literature. Journal holdings are generally included in the **online public access catalog (OPAC)** (discussed in more detail later in this chapter), and many libraries provide A-Z listings of journals available in both print and electronic formats. For users who need additional help in locating a journal, implementing manned information stations or direct-dial telephones throughout the library can be a worthwhile investment. Libraries are seeing a marked decrease in the use of their print journal collections, as more and more journals are becoming available in electronic format.

Media

In addition to books and journals, many health sciences libraries have large audiovisual (AV) collections. Academic and large hospital libraries often have an educational technology center where audiovisual materials can be viewed in private or small classrooms. Some allow the circulation of materials and equipment, though most only allow in-house use. As with the other physical collections in the library, newer technologies are changing the way traditional AV materials are accessed. For example, many continuing medical education (CME) courses now offer online accessibility through streaming video. Interactive 3D human anatomy Web sites, digital image databases, and streaming video allow students, faculty, and clinicians to connect to mixed-media formats from the classroom, hospital floor, or home.

Remote Storage Facilities

Lack of collection space remains an ongoing struggle for many libraries, especially those maintaining extensive journal backfiles or full historical book holdings. While it is very likely true that the availability of electronic books and journals will one day free up space in the library, many libraries are currently experiencing greater space demands than ever. Stack space is often compromised to allow for newer educational services demanded by users. Some libraries deal with the lack of space by utilizing remote storage facilities for lesser used material, such as older journals and texts. Depending on the design of the facility, the collection may be accessible to library users, but most often is restricted to staff retrieval of material as needed. To expedite service, a requested article or book chapter may be scanned and delivered electronically to the requestor's desktop.[12] Many storage facilities utilize high-density automated shelving.[13] Library materials are stored in bins and retrieved by robotic arm. Users request storage material through the library's Web site, thereby activating the automated retrieval system. If storage is located on-site, the item can be retrieved quickly by the robotic arm and delivered to the service point for pickup.

ELECTRONIC ACCESS

With the abundance of publicly accessible and subscription-based resources available through the Web, a "trip to the library" is now as simple as sitting down to a computer with Internet access. The library's Web site is an essential portal connecting users to a vast array of electronic biomedical resources. Providing access to the digital collection presents a unique set of issues quite different from those associated with physical access. While the library building generally allows universal access, remote access to most electronic resources must be limited to affiliated users. Electronic resources are more often licensed than purchased outright, and each publisher and vendor has its own set of terms and conditions for access beyond the walls of the library. Most publishers permit remote access only to a predefined user group, and some vendors prohibit remote access altogether. While many vendors argue that their license terms are "set in stone," such is generally not the case. After all, electronic information vendors are essentially selling a product, and they want the library's business. Libraries may—and should—negotiate remote access terms with vendors, and it is generally advisable to do so with the assistance of the institution's legal department. Chapter 3, "Journal Collection Development," and Chapter 4, "Monographic and Digital Resource Collection Development," address license negotiations more fully.

Before negotiating access terms with the publisher or vendor, the library must identify its user population. This sounds easy, but questions immediately arise. Does the library want to extend access to clinical faculty and residents of affiliated hospitals, or limit access to the home institution? Should the library seek remote access for all physicians with admitting rights, or only for attending physicians and residents? Should students on rotation be granted remote access rights? Each hospital and institution has unique affiliations within its own organization, and often a subgroup of users may need to be recognized in the license agreement. In general, publishers and vendors strictly prohibited remote access to alumni, the general public, patients, unaffiliated clinicians and nurses, and volunteers.

Another issue in licensing remote access is whether the vendor imposes limitations on where the material may be accessed. Some publishers restrict access to specific geographic locations, prohibiting, for instance, access to students and faculty located at an international branch of the institution. This poses a problem for those institutions that support fieldwork in other countries. The John Cox Associate's Licensing Model Web site <http://www.licensingmodels.com> offers a best practice definition of authorized users to which a majority of librarians and publishers agree to adhere. The best approach is to ask the publisher or vendor to add a specific user group or location if it is not specifically expressed.

User Authentication

Identifying the user population and negotiating terms for remote access mean very little without a means for securing access for that population. While some libraries' electronic resources may reside on local network servers, the vast majority of licensed resources reside on the Web. Anyone can type in a Web address and get to a site, so the vendor must have a way to identify who is authorized to access a licensed resource and who is not. A variety of tools and approaches are available to address these authentication needs, some of which are discussed in the following sections. Those seeking a more detailed discussion of authentication issues should read Blansit's "eTechnology" column in *Journal of Electronic Resources in Medical Libraries.*[14]

Username/Password

The simplest form of authentication is the use of a registered login name and password. This practice is not widely used in libraries, however. It is extremely inconvenient, requiring the library to maintain a list of usernames/passwords and communicate them with authorized users. Users are often unhappy about having to remember vendor-specific logins and passwords. And, finally, this method is insecure; authorized users can easily share a username/password with unauthorized users.

IP Authentication

IP (internet protocol) authentication is very commonly used as a means of granting access within the parameters of the institution. This method requires that the library register the IP ranges of the licensing institution with each vendor. This can become burdensome when a library manages hundreds or thousands of electronic resources, and it is especially difficult to manage in larger settings where IPs are added or changed on a frequent basis. But IP authentication is generally a good experience for the user, who may sit in his or her office on campus and click a link to a journal and be granted immediate access because the computer's **IP address** is recognized as legitimate. IP authentication only works on computers that are on the hospital or university network, however, and does not allow for access off-site without an additional authentication procedure, such as a **proxy server** or **virtual private network (VPN)**.

Proxy Server

A proxy server is a computer network service that allows clients to make indirect network connections to other network services.[15] The best way to describe how a proxy server works is through an example: A physician, who is included in the library's authorized user population, is at home but wants access to one of the library's electronic journals. The journal is authenticated by IP address, and, of course, the physician's home computer's IP address is not recognized by the vendor. So the physician logs onto the library's proxy server with his username and password. The proxy server has an address within the IP range of the institution, and the physician is now on an IP-authenticated computer *by proxy*. He goes to the library's Web site, clicks on the journal he wants, and he is granted access.

One popular and inexpensive proxy authentication program commonly used by libraries is EZproxy, a URL rewriting proxy server developed specifically for use by libraries.[16] For a full discussion of proxy servers, see the Proxy Server Tutorial at <http://compnetworking.about.com/cs/proxyservers/a/proxyservers.htm>.

Virtual Private Network

A VPN is a secured connection between two parties to communicate confidential information between each other.[17] VPNs differ from proxy servers in that they provide remote users with actual access to the university or hospital network. A VPN connection allows off-site users to authenticate to the library's electronic resources by reassigning the remote computer's network connection to appear as if it has originated from an on-site computer. Because they essentially open the institution's network to the outside world, VPNs must be tightly secured and often require cumbersome access procedures on the part of the remote user. VPNs are often associated with the **Health Insurance Portability and Accountability Act (HIPAA),** in which hospitals must comply with federal standards to provide secure transactions of electronic health care information between providers, health insurance plans, and employers.

Emerging Authentication Systems

While the systems outlined previously are the most commonly employed in U.S. libraries today, the field of authentication systems is growing. The Athens Access Management System,[18] developed for education and health institutions in the United Kingdom, was previewed in the United States at the 2006 annual meeting of the Medical Library Association.[14] Athens controls access to Web-based resources via a single, unified login, and it is currently being offered by Teton Data Systems <http://www.statref.com/ourproducts/athens/athens.htm>. Shibboleth is an open source software development that addresses the need to distinguish privileges among various user categories. The Shibboleth Project is housed at <http://shibboleth.internet2.edu/>.[14]

The authentication methods just listed are only a few of those available to libraries and their institutions. Additional information on authentication is available at <http://library.smc.edu/rpa.htm>.

SHADES OF GRAY: SERVICES STRADDLING
THE PHYSICAL AND ELECTRONIC DIVIDE

Many people view the role of libraries in a clear-cut manner. Some continue to think of them as they always have, as physical destinations for books and print journals. Others view them strictly as electronic gateways—they literally never set foot in the library, yet are regular users of the library's electronic resources. Some library services are in a greater state of transition than others. The online catalog, interlibrary loan/document delivery, and academic reserves straddle the physical and electronic library worlds, and they are discussed more fully in the following sections.

Online Public Access Catalog

OPAC is key in locating both print and electronic resources held in the library's collection. The term "online public access catalog" was coined in 1981.[19] From its inception to the present,

OPAC has served essentially as an electronic version of the card catalog, a finder's guide to the library's in-house collection. OPAC is generally part of a larger system, the ILS, which offers acquisitions, cataloging, circulation, and serials functions, in addition to the public catalog.

The explosion of electronic information resources in the late twentieth century left information seekers with the desire to broaden search capabilities beyond the walls of the library, to perform a single "federated" search across various databases and platforms.[20] Such federated search capabilities are now integrated into the traditional OPAC. A single search will retrieve results, not only of what is available within the library's own library collection, but from various search engines, databases, and other library catalogs. Since many health sciences resources are accessible on the Internet, and no library can catalog the entire Web, metasearch engines allow users to retrieve more content pertaining to their queries. The addition of a federated search feature allows users to retrieve merged results based on relevancy or other criteria from a collection of library databases and OPAC. A single search returns citations for books, journal articles, and Web sites across different platforms, all in a matter of seconds. Federated searching broadens the library collection beyond the confines of what is held physically, to that of what is held electronically as well as to resources freely available on the Web.

Interlibrary Loan and Document Delivery

In the spirit of cooperation, libraries have shared materials with one another for well over a century.[21] No single library contains all the content that their users may need, and libraries utilize **interlibrary loan (ILL)** services to supplement their book, journal, and media collections. The continued use of the term "interlibrary loan" is somewhat misleading. While books and microforms are loaned to requesting libraries, most ILL transactions involve the delivery of nonreturnable journal articles. Health sciences libraries approach the process of interlibrary loan differently than other types of libraries, in that journal articles may be needed for urgent patient care. Often, the library is asked to obtain an article in a matter of hours in response to a patient care emergency. Routine turnaround times are in days, not weeks, as in other types of libraries.

The library's ILL department is staffed by a librarian and/or paraprofessionals. To facilitate efficient document delivery service among members of the **National Network of Libraries of Medicine (NN/LM)**, NLM created **DOCLINE®.**[22] DOCLINE allows libraries to quickly communicate with one another for rapid transmission of needed documents, and it serves over 3,200 U.S., Canadian, and Mexican medical libraries at no cost. It is primarily used to fill requests for articles needed from clinical journals or evidence-based data files, such as the Cochrane Database of Systematic Reviews. The DOCLINE system is divided into eight Regional Medical Libraries (RMLs), with each geographic region having an NN/LM office that manages Resource Libraries and Primary Access Libraries in the network. The Resource Libraries are primarily academic health sciences libraries that have extensive holdings of health sciences journals and books. The Primary Access Libraries are mostly hospital libraries with smaller holdings of journal titles. DOCLINE is essentially a twenty-four-hour service, but most requests are filled during normal business hours. Turnaround time depends on when the request is placed and the relative availability of the article, but requests can generally be filled the same day in cases of urgent patient care. Articles are shipped by mail, facsimile, or, most often, via the Internet. The preferred method is to scan the article and transmit it electronically via a document transmission system such as **Ariel**[23] or Odyssey.[24] Scanned documents retain color images and higher resolution, whereas facsimiles transmit data in grayscale with images often appearing smudged. Once the scanned document is received, it can be printed or converted into a PDF and placed on a secure server, and the requestor is notified that the article is available.

In addition to ILL, many health sciences libraries offer an in-house document delivery (DD) service to affiliated users. Traditionally, this service involved library staff photocopying print materials on behalf of users. Today, DD has expanded to include scanning print materials for delivery as PDFs, as well as printing or e-mailing electronic documents from the digital collection. This service is especially useful for clinicians who might not have ready availability to the hospital's VPN, or clinicians who do not wish to determine availability of materials and prefer to pay for a library staff member's time to determine whether needed information can be supplied in-house or through interlibrary loan. Some libraries charge for DD service, while others offer it to affiliated users free of charge. DD is considered by many to be one of the most essential services of a health sciences library.

An offshoot of ILL and DD is **Loansome Doc®,** a service of NLM coordinated by RMLs. Loansome Doc is a simple and efficient method for ordering articles from a health sciences library through the PubMed interface. Participation in Loansome Doc requires an agreement with the providing health sciences library. The articles may be available as part of the supplying library's collection or acquired via DOCLINE. While most Loansome Doc libraries utilize the service for their primary clientele, many also allow unaffiliated users to register for Loansome Doc, delivering articles to them for a fee. More information on NLM, DOCLINE, and Loansome Doc can be found on NLM's Web site <http://www.nlm.nih.gov/>.

Course Reserves

Most academic libraries continue to place books and media items on course reserve at the request of faculty, but virtual learning environments are rapidly replacing the traditional course reserve section of the library. With the implementation of proprietary and open source **course management systems (CMSs),** required readings can easily be integrated into the e-learning environment. If material is available only in print format, faculty can request that library staff scan articles, book chapters, and exams for student use. The reserve materials are made available to registered students, who retrieve assigned readings by authenticating through the course management platform via username and password. Electronic reserves are managed in much the same way as print reserves, being removed from reserve at the end of the semester. Careful attention must be paid to ensure that the reserves comply with fair use guidelines of the U.S. Copyright Law,[25] and that their inclusion in a CMS does not violate terms of the library's licensing agreement with the publisher. The library should have a well-written electronic reserve policy explaining copyright, fair use, and faculty responsibility. An excellent example of a course reserve policy can be found at the Cornell University Library Web site <http://www.library .cornell.edu/services/reserveinformation.html>.

With the growth of student-centered learning and distributed education in the health sciences, librarians can contribute to class assignments by inserting suggested links to digitized content. A CMS allows the librarian to exert presence in the classroom and reach students who would not necessarily think to use the electronic resources of the library. A criticism of CMS is its failure to comply with industry standards for accessibility for persons with disabilities.[26] It is advisable before purchasing a CMS to inquire if it complies with Section 508 of the U.S. Rehabilitation Act of 1973 (Section 504 of this act is discussed in further detail under Access for Disabilities later in this chapter). A selected list of CMS services appears in Table 6.1.

WIRELESS NETWORK ACCESS

With the popularity of mobile computing devices for clinical care and education, offering wireless access to local area networks (LANs) is an attractive service. A wireless local area net-

TABLE 6.1. Popular CMS Services

Product	Type	Web Address
Blackboard, Inc.	Proprietary	<http://www.blackboard.com>
Moodle	Free, open source	<http://moodle.org>
Sakai Project	Free, open source	<http://www.sakaiproject.org>
Scholar360	Proprietary	<http://www.scholar360.com>
Vista, formerly WebCT	Proprietary, merged with Blackboard	<http://www.blackboard.com>

work (WLAN) allows the user flexibility to connect to the Internet from anywhere inside the library. WLAN technology is most commonly referred to as **WiFi,** which is a high-frequency radio wave. A mobile computing device equipped with a WLAN card can access the LAN if in range of the WLAN receiver. Wireless networks can be implemented in an entire building, part of a building, campus-wide, or city-wide.

There are several security risks associated with WiFi. WLAN equipment is generally sold with limited encryption tools, which makes the network vulnerable to unauthorized users. If clinicians are using the WLAN to pass patient information back and forth from a mobile device, it is possible for unauthorized persons to gain access to private patient information. Health sciences libraries, in particular, require additional security and encryption tools to combat hacking of information. Current best practices include an authentication database to verify each user accessing the network and a rotating encryption key. When authorized users request entry to the secure library network, they are required to enter a username and password to gain access to the WLAN. Secured WiFi lessens the chance that patient data are visible to unauthorized users; however, no wireless network is impenetrable. Wireless networks are more commonly available in academic health sciences libraries than hospital libraries. Many hospitals restrict wireless networks and rely on wired LANs or Ethernet.

ACCESS FOR THE DISABLED

The **Americans with Disabilities Act of 1990 (ADA)** and Section 504 of the Rehabilitation Act of 1973 require libraries to provide equitable access for persons with disabilities.[27] This includes access to the library's facilities, collections, equipment, and services. Though buildings have been remodeled and designed to accommodate for the disabled, most libraries still have some physical access limitations, such as high shelving, requiring that staff be available to assist persons with disabilities. The ADA pertains not only to physical accessibility, but electronic accessibility as well. A free online service called Bobby <http://webxact.watchfire.com> is available to test accessibility of the library's Web site.[28] It is advisable to consult the ADA compliance specialist at the hospital or institution before remodeling or purchasing assistive technologies. In addition, inviting the compliance specialist into the library to educate staff and review building accessibility will greatly enhance service to persons with special needs. Everyone who enters the library should be treated fairly and without prejudice. Overall, it is a social responsibility to make sure all users who enter the library have equal access to health care information, equipment, and space.

CONCLUSION

Health sciences libraries seek to provide ready access to a wide range of electronic and print materials, to a clientele ranging from researchers and physicians to community members with low literacy skills. Ensuring that clients are getting the information they need should be of central concern to every employee of the library. While the role of *how* information is accessed is in a state of flux, the principle underlying *why* such information is important remains constant: the timely delivery of reliable health-related information can improve, and sometimes save, lives.

REFERENCES

1. Weaver, C.G. "Electronic Document Delivery: Directing Interlibrary Loan Traffic Through Multiple Electronic Networks." *Bulletin of the American Library Association* 72(April 1984): 187-92.

2. Pizer, I.H., and Walker, W.D. "Physical Access to Resources." In *Handbook of Medical Library Practice*, edited by L. Darling, 15-64. Chicago, IL: Medical Library Association, 1982.

3. McDonald, J., and Van de Velde, E.F. "The Lure of Linking." *Library Journal* 129(April 1, 2004): 32-4.

4. Hersey, D.P. "The Future of Access Services: Should There Be One?" *Journal of Access Services* 2(2004): 1-6.

5. Allegri, F., and Bedard, M. "Lessons Learned from Single Service Point Implementations." *Medical Reference Services Quarterly* 25(Summer 2006): 31-47.

6. Shedlock, J., ed. *Annual Statistics of Medical School Libraries in the United States and Canada, 1999-2000.* 23rd ed. Seattle, WA: Association of Academic Health Sciences Library Directors, 2001.

7. Byrd, G. et al., eds. *Annual Statistics of Medical School Libraries in the United States and Canada, 2005-2006.* 29th ed. Seattle, WA: Association of Academic Health Sciences Libraries, 2007.

8. Deering, M.J. and Harris, J. "Consumer Health Information Demand and Delivery: Implications for Libraries." *Bulletin of the Medical Library Association* 84(April 1996): 209-16.

9. American Library Association. "Library Security Guidelines Document." (June 7, 2001). Available: <http://www.ala.org/ala/lama/lamapublications/librarysecurity.htm#securityduty>. Accessed: March 19, 2007.

10. Singh, J.; Brar, N.; and Fong, C. "The State of RFID Applications in Libraries." *Information Technology and Libraries* 25, no. 1 (March 2006): 24-32.

11. Gelernter, J. "Loss Prevention Strategies for the 21st Century Library." *Information Outlook* 9, no. 12 (December 2005): 12-4, 16, 18-22.

12. Deardoff, T.C., and Aamot, G. *Remote Shelving Services.* Washington, DC: Association of Research Libraries, 2006.

13. The University of Chicago Board of Trustees, Materials Prepared for May 11, 2005, *University of Chicago Library Additional Shelving.* Available: <http://www.lib.uchicago.edu/e/reg/addition/TrusteesMay11b.pdf>. Accessed: January 1, 2007.

14. Blansit, B.D. "Beyond Password Protection: Methods for Remote Patron Authentication." *Journal of Electronic Resources in Medical Libraries* 4(2007): 185-94.

15. Wikipedia. "Proxy Server." Available: <http://en.wikipedia.org/wiki/Proxy_server>. Accessed: March 30, 2007.

16. Useful Utilities, LLC. "EZproxy by Useful Utilities" Available: <http://www.usefulutilities.com>. Accessed: January 1, 2007.

17. Wikipedia. "Virtual Private Network." Available: <http://en.wikipedia.org/wiki/Vpn>. Accessed: March 30, 2007.

18. Eduserv Athens for Education. "Eduserv Athens Welcome." Available: <athensams.net>. Accessed: January 1, 2007.

19. Hildreth, C.R. Public-Access Computer Systems Forum, March 10, 1994. Available: <http://listserv.uh.edu/cgi-bin/wa?A2=ind9403b&L=pacs-1&T=0&P=3670>. Accessed: March 30, 2007.

20. Wikipedia. "Federated Search." Available: <http://en.wikiipedia.org/wiki/Federated_search>. Accessed: March 30, 2007.

21. Chudnov, D. "The History of Interlibrary Loan." Available: <http://old.onebiglibrary.net/mit/web.mit.edu/dchud/www/p2p-talk-slides/img0.html>. Accessed: March 30, 2007.

22. U.S. National Library of Medicine. "DOCLINE System." (November 30, 2006). Available: <http://www.nlm.nih.gov/docline>. Accessed: March 1, 2007.

23. Infotrieve. "Ariel." Available: <http://www4.infotrieve.com/products_services/ariel.asp>. Accessed: March 1, 2007.

24. Atlas Systems, Inc. "Odyssey." Available: <http://www.atlas-sys.com/products/odyssey/>. Accessed: April 2, 2007.

25. Copyright Law of the United States of America and Related Laws Contained in Title 17 of the United States Code, Limitations on Exclusive Rights: Fair Use, §107. Available: <http://www.copyright.gov/title17/92chap1.html#107>. Accessed: January 1, 2007.

26. University of Tasmania. "Accessibility—Is Vista Accessible?" (February 3, 2006). Available: <http://www.utas.edu.au/accessibility/webct/is_webct_accessible.html>. Accessed: January 1, 2007.

27. American Library Association. "Library Services for People with Disabilities Policy." (January 16, 2001). Available: <http://www.ala.org/ala/ascla/asclaissues/libraryservices.htm>. Accessed: January 1, 2007.

28. Center for Applied Special Technology. "Bobby World Wide." Available: <http://www.cast.org/pd/resources/masterref.html#Bob>. Accessed: January 1, 2007.

Chapter 7

Information Services in Health Sciences Libraries

Elizabeth H. Wood

SUMMARY. This chapter will discuss how librarians provide reference and information services in health sciences contexts. Current trends are described, followed by discussion of how technology has made drastic changes in the delivery of information services. Analysis of the needs of the various kinds of users served by health sciences libraries is followed by suggestions for how librarians can fill these needs. At the same time, librarians can promote and enhance the image of the library as a vital part of the overall information services of the institution, and of the librarians as experts at the forefront of the latest information technologies. Finally, ethical considerations for health sciences information services are discussed.

INTRODUCTION

Who needs and uses health sciences library information services? A surgeon needs a review of the latest opinions on bariatric surgery. A pharmacist needs the U.S. equivalent name for a drug prescribed in Europe. A nurse wants advice on pediatric terminal care. A physical therapist wants information on rehabilitation after a broken collarbone. A student is working on the biochemical explanation for the benefits (or not) of certain herbal teas. A rural physician urgently needs to update her skills in performing an appendectomy. A retired faculty member is writing a book on the arguments about using mitochondrial DNA for tracing population genetics. Intriguing? Whetting the appetite of the reference sleuth?

These users, and their requests, have changed little over the years. Most of these questions, or less modern variations thereof, could have been asked a decade or more ago. What has changed is the access to the information. Computers are now about as ubiquitous as telephones on office desks, in research labs, at nurses' stations, and in examination rooms. The health sciences institution and most of its departments now have a Web presence. Libraries' Web sites provide access to many of their information services, including the ability to ask reference questions, search databases, and read or download the full text of journals and e-books.

This chapter and the next, "Information Retrieval in the Health Sciences," do not, and cannot, pretend to be comprehensive treatises on all of the information resources, and services based on them, that are available in the health sciences. The latest edition of Boorkman, Huber, and Roper's excellent *Introduction to Reference Sources in the Health Sciences* gives an overview of the current situation.[1, 2] This book is a required text in reference courses and highly recommended for any new information services librarian.[3]

The provision of information services is crucial to the image of the library. As fewer users visit the physical library, librarians must go to them, to promote services, demonstrate the utility of the library Web site, and engender enthusiasm for using librarians' expertise. It is impossible

Introduction to Health Sciences Librarianship
© 2008 by The Haworth Press, Taylor & Francis Group. All rights reserved.
doi:10.1300/6041_07

to describe the "state of the art" in library information services because the picture changes almost daily. The important reality is that librarians must keep up with new technologies and transform their services to reflect the developments.[4]

Librarians are experts at finding, or "retrieving," information from resources. The role of the librarian, however, goes far beyond these mechanics. Health sciences librarians must know the mission and philosophy of their institutions. They must understand the corporate identity, the personnel, and the organizational structure. The specific examples of queries and users in this chapter are chosen to indicate the variety of information needs that health sciences librarians are likely to face. Chapter 1, "Overview of Health Sciences Libraries," provides an excellent overview of these users, their educational backgrounds, and their work environments. This chapter discusses how their diverse information needs can be met. The reference librarian of the past, who was usually found behind a reference desk, has now expanded into information services, which involves provision of electronic access to databases, e-books, full-text journals, and meta-analyses of the literature. Many of the new information resources provide "user-friendly" interfaces, so that users can help themselves as they would have regularly browsed the journal shelves or the book stacks. As in the past, users also have the choice of asking for **mediated searching** where librarians do the searching and present users with the results they need.

INFORMATION IN THE HIGH-TECH ENVIRONMENT

All providers of information services have to keep up with new knowledge, developments in technology, and the world around them. Whether librarians already have training or experience in the sciences or as health professionals, have worked as paraprofessionals, or have taken classes in medical terminology or other health disciplines, continual professional development is essential. Not only are there breakthroughs in medicine and the latest health-related arguments in government and business, but librarians must have personal awareness of the world of technology. What is **RSS (really simple syndication)**? What are blogs and mashups? Do you use podcasting? As irritating as the daily onslaught of mail and e-mail from vendors and publishers may be, every librarian must know what is being developed, what updates are available, and how library users are also being bombarded with the same information. The librarian should not be the last to discover that library users have already subscribed to alerting services for their **PDAs (personal data assistants)** or are arranging to share their personal online passwords and subscriptions.

Professional organizations, national and local, are an essential part of this growth and development. Professional networking and support are important components of employment and advancement among health sciences librarians. While continuing education for health sciences librarians is not the focus here, it must be mentioned as a vital element in timely and up-to-date delivery of information services.

Information services librarians continue to answer factual reference questions, write guides and instructions, and give tours, but their roles have increased in the areas of teaching classes in searching databases and performing mediated searches. These databases are no longer only bibliographic but now provide links to the full text of journals.

The ubiquity of the Internet, with resources such as Google and Yahoo!, means that library users are now accustomed to finding information for themselves, at their own desktops, where in the past they would have visited the library in person. Ironically, the apparent ease of use but lack of quality control in many Internet resources means that the librarian or "informationist" is in fact needed more than ever.[5] The concept of the librarian being involved in **filtering information**—not just running the search, but actually making decisions as to what information the clinician or researcher needed—created a potential new role, that of the "informationist."[6, 7] In the clinical arena, the rising awareness of "**evidence-based medicine (EBM)**" (the expression has been a **MeSH** [Medical Subject Heading] since 1997) has further developed the definition of the informationist.[8, 9] Part of librarians' advocacy role for the library is in proving the value of the information services they provide and making sure users are aware of what is available.[10]

TYPES OF HEALTH SCIENCES INFORMATION NEEDS

Users in health sciences libraries can be divided by the areas in which they serve in the institution: patient care, education, and research. It must be noted that these are functions, and that individuals may have more than one role; for example, many clinicians also teach, and teachers are commonly involved in research.[11]

Academic health sciences libraries and hospital libraries serve their parent institution by providing information services to support a tri-fold mission of patient care, research, and education and, in many cases, a fourth mission of community service. In an academic health sciences center, there is also a distinction between clinical faculty (MD or DO, for example) and basic science faculty (PhD).

Chapter 1 describes users who fall in the various roles of patient care, education, and research. Information-seeking behavior varies greatly among the members and the needs of these groups.[12, 13] Librarians who serve different clientele have to be attuned to the different ways in which their patrons will approach the library and expect to be served.[14-16]

Patient Care

It should not be a surprise to librarians that many health care professionals rely on one another as a first resource when taking care of patients.[17] They also use the Internet, not necessarily for searching databases such as **MEDLINE** or CINAHL (*Cumulative Index to Nursing and Allied Health Literature*), but for many other electronic resources, especially to keep themselves up-to-date.[18, 19] Knowing this, librarians can strive to be part of these conversations, as one practitioner may recommend to a colleague that he or she contact the library. Once the practitioner has visited or contacted the library, these requests are often high on the librarian's list of priorities. Patient care requests can come from physicians, nurses, allied health personnel, or other clinical practitioners. As determined by a reference interview (discussed later), a subject request from a physician, versus the same subject request from a nurse, might result in different retrieval.[20, 21] On occasion, information services librarians may be required to locate information for a clinical emergency. Patient care requests of an emergency nature often must be handled immediately, or within minutes or hours, and must be prioritized above others.

The subject matter defines the question in the "patient care" category. However, these queries may not be emergencies. A question about the effectiveness or potential outcome of a therapy, a procedure, or a drug may not come from an urgent patient care case, but because the user is preparing a lecture or writing an article or book chapter.[19] The information needed is very different in each case. As described in a later section, The Reference Interview, the librarian needs to inquire further as to the purpose of the question:

- Is a patient about to undergo a procedure or be given a drug?
- Does the lecturer need to verify facts before presenting them to students?
- Does the author need the latest update for his or her bibliography?

The librarian may know several ways to answer the question but must ascertain from the user the type of information he or she needs:

- Several articles (or better yet reviews or meta-analyses, or material from an evidence-based database) discussing the pros and cons of the issue
- An overview of the topic with a comprehensive bibliography
- The very latest research on the topic

In any of these cases, the user may want the full text of articles.

Research

Researchers can be among the heaviest users of library services, and the resources they need are also the most expensive (subscriptions in the basic sciences are generally multiple times more costly than clinical titles). Scientists working in laboratories, competing for **National Institutes of Health (NIH)** or other grant funds, will need access to the most current literature and may use updating services to keep track of their competitors' publications. Researchers or post-doctoral students who are writing up their results for publication in a scholarly journal, or doctoral students preparing dissertations, may need exhaustive searches of the literature.[22, 23]

Librarians' investigations in support of research may be ongoing. As the research progresses, the scientist may need to modify and expand the search request.[24, 25] Part of the excitement of the librarian's job is to be part of the team, consulting with students assisting the scientist, and even sharing the "glory" with an acknowledgement in the resulting publications.

Education

Information services librarians have a major role in the education of the many types of students and interns who come to the institution. Residents, medical and nursing students, students in allied health sciences, graduate students in the basic sciences—all have special needs, starting with assignments from classes and moving on to their own research for clinical presentations, term papers, or dissertations. Librarians often engage in one-on-one instructional sessions teaching students how to develop search strategies and guiding them to appropriate resources.

Depending on their previous experience, students may not expect the librarians to be particularly helpful. Orientations provide opportunities to give students the more prosaic information about how to use the information services on campus, and also to let students know that librarians are there to help and welcome their questions.

Information services librarians may assist students in finding the answers to assignments. Librarians may meet with the faculty to ask how the teacher expects the assignment to be done. Good relationships with faculty can be profitable for their students. Faculty members know what students need, and librarians can hone their reference skills in those areas. If the students understand the librarians' time constraints from the beginning, they will be more likely to outline what they are going to need in advance. On the other hand, librarians must understand students' time constraints and respond as best they can.[26]

LIBRARIAN-USER INTERACTION

This section on librarian-user interaction will discuss ways in which information requests are received by the librarian, including the differences between real-time and offline requests. This will be followed by a section that describes and defines virtual reference. Then, the reference interview will be described in the context of virtual reference, and, finally, the idea of the single service desk and information triaging will be discussed.

Receiving the Information Request

In all libraries, not just health sciences libraries, the process of receiving an information request from the library user is likely to undergo even more radical change in the immediate future as Web 2.0 technologies are adopted by both librarians and their users.[27, 28] In the health sciences, the nature of both the users and their information needs has also played an important role in user-librarian interactions. The immediate needs of patient care, resulting in time-sensitive clinical information requests—needed sometimes in hours, not days—have always driven the health care setting. Besides institution-wide networks, other new technologies, such as PDAs, have facilitated the delivery of information.

Real-Time Requests

Synchronous, or real-time, interactions, either face-to-face, via telephone, or "live" chat online, are the most efficient and effective ways for library staff to answer questions about holdings, renewals, locations, directions, and straightforward cases of citation verification. Real-time conversations also allow information services librarians to determine more precisely what users really need. Virtual reference, discussed and defined later in this chapter, encompasses services such as "Ask a Librarian," which can either be real-time chat (with posted hours of librarians' availability) or a link on a Web site to leave questions to be answered at a later time.[29] See Figure 7.1 for an example of a Web site with virtual reference links.

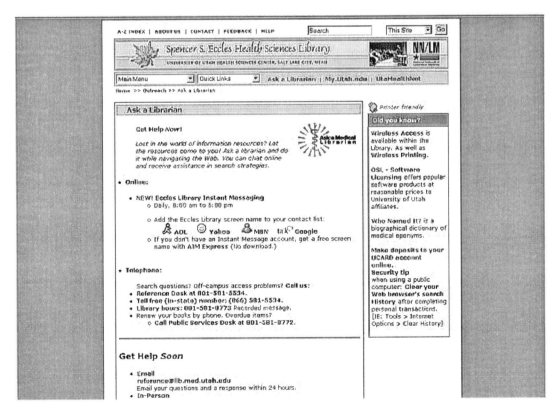

FIGURE 7.1. University of Utah Virtual Reference Web Page <http://library.med.utah.edu/or/asklibrarian.php>. Used with permission.

Users who do come to the library, or invite the information services librarian to their office or lab, need the librarian's full attention, patience, and a friendly approach. The librarian must be totally frank about his or her understanding of the question and the purpose of its answer. Does the surgeon need to know about bariatric surgery because it keeps coming up at meetings and he or she feels inadequately informed on the subject? Or does the surgeon have a patient requesting the procedure? Or is a patient who has had the procedure asking the surgeon about reversing the surgery? Some of these aspects of the question may be personally sensitive to the surgeon, who finds it easier to discuss the request verbally, in a private place. If the request requires a mediated search, some users appreciate being able to "look over the shoulder" of the librarian to see the terms being used, spot references that are exactly right, and make suggestions about further terms the librarian has not considered. This personal rapport builds a collaborative atmosphere that perhaps helps ensure that the user will come back, and also that he or she will tell colleagues about this excellent cooperative relationship with the library.

Live telephone calls and online "chat" are substitutes for face-to-face interactions, though somewhat less effective, especially for the first contact. It is important that an information services librarian be available most of the time to take the call or handle the chat session.

Offline Reference

Asynchronous, or offline, communication gives librarians time to reflect, to perform triage, to investigate, and to make test runs into the literature before getting back to the user. Both real-time and offline methods of initial contact may result in ongoing conversations before the librarian has fully clarified the request. How the librarian retrieves the information from complex online resources is described further in Chapter 8.

As discussed earlier, reality is that few users have time to darken the door, and life, including professional life, is lived through the computer monitor. As little as fifteen years ago, librarians wondered about their future roles in the new world of technology,[30, 31] but these concerns have proved to be unfounded as the availability of full-text content became common. Now, librarians' skills are needed both to provide access through links from databases or the library Web site, and as users require an unprecedented amount of help (as end users or through mediated searches) in reaching the various routes to full text.

A further consideration in offline communication is that the user who sends e-mail, or leaves voicemail, may not expect an immediate reply. In fact, the library user may not *want* an immediate reply because he or she is too busy at the time and would prefer to come back later from clinic or lecture hall to read the response when he or she has time.

Many users, especially in the clinical arena, have no interest, or time, for developing their own expertise in searching the literature. Some may have been requesting mediated MEDLINE searches for many years, and despite the availability of **PubMed** and user-friendly vendors' Web-based offerings, they may prefer and want to continue to have the librarian perform searches and do reference work. They still appreciate the new technology, such as being able to fill out a search request form online, or sending messages and requests offline, when they have time. They may also use their staff to assist in the interaction.

As mentioned earlier, offline transactions give the librarian time to download, print, or just review the requests, sort them, and decide which are more urgent and which are going to take considerable more time and effort to find the answer; this allows the reference librarian to triage and generally organize the workday. Thus, the librarian also has the advantage of responding as time permits. If these offline reference interviews require repeat communications to clarify the request or show the user what has been found so far, this is done as everyone has time.[32]

VIRTUAL REFERENCE

Librarians should anticipate that **virtual reference** will play an increasingly important role in the future of information services in health sciences libraries.[33] As the reader might have noted, virtual reference appeared in the discussion of real-time and offline requests, as it plays a role in both. The MARS Digital Reference Guidelines Ad Hoc Committee of RUSA (the Reference and User Services Association) defines virtual reference as follows:

> Virtual reference is reference service initiated electronically, often in real-time, where patrons employ computers or other Internet technology to communicate with reference staff without being physically present. Communication channels used frequently in virtual reference include chat, videoconferencing, Voice over IP, co-browsing, e-mail, and instant messaging.
> While online sources are often utilized in provision of virtual reference, use of electronic sources in seeking answers is not of itself virtual reference.
> Virtual reference queries are sometimes followed-up with telephone, fax, in-person, and regular mail interactions even though these modes of communication are not considered virtual.[34, 35]

The RUSA Guidelines go on to specify how to prepare for and organize the service, how to address the needs of individual clientele, and issues of privacy.[35]

In a recent study, Cleveland and Philbrick found that "over 90 percent of academic health sciences libraries offer virtual reference services with Web forms being the most common form of delivery."[36] Their definition of virtual reference includes all real-time and offline types of electronic communication. Their discussion provides overviews of the terminologies and types of virtual reference services; products available, both for a fee or for free; issues in delivering virtual reference services; and also reviews of the literature. Issues—both positive and negative—related to the initiation of virtual reference in health sciences libraries are detailed in numerous papers. In a two-part article in *Medical Reference Services Quarterly* (*MRSQ*) in 2003, Dee explores features of chat reference[37] and also discusses trends in medical school libraries.[38] Additional reports by Parker and Johnson,[39] McGraw, Heiland, and Harris,[40] Jerant and Firestein,[41] and MacDonald[42] detail planning, implementation, and usage of virtual reference. A case study of virtual reference published in the *Journal of the Medical Library Association* (*JMLA*) in early 2005 found virtual reference to be "a costly and problematic way to handle a low number of reference questions at the present time."[43] Follow-up articles by Dee in 2005 continue to document trends and barriers to virtual reference in health sciences libraries.[44, 45]

Readers looking for more information about implementing virtual reference services will find many articles by searching the librarianship literature in databases such as Library Literature or Library and Information Services Abstracts (LISA). Several new books are also recommended.[46-48]

As the new technologies become more pervasive, and the new generation of users, the so-called **Millennials,** become the "norm" rather than the minority of users, virtual reference will be an expected service that all health sciences libraries will need to offer. With this has come the need to adapt the reference interview for use in the electronic world.

THE REFERENCE INTERVIEW

The reference interview that is so vital a part of information services can be described in four stages: the receipt of the request; the triage process as the librarian organizes the requests and how they should be addressed; the location of the best possible information to answer the question; and the delivery of the requested information as the librarian ensures that the user's needs have been met. Numerous texts and articles document the complete process of the reference interview.[49-51] The following partial definition of the reference interview is from ODLIS (*Online Dictionary for Library and Information Science*):[52] "The interpersonal communication that occurs between a reference librarian and a library user to determine the person's specific information needs, which may turn out to be different than the reference question as initially posed." The emphasis in this chapter is on how the librarian interacts with individual users in the process of the reference interview.

Users may not know how to express their needs, or not realize that what they are saying is not conveying their real needs to the librarian. The ideal solution is the face-to-face reference interview, where the information services librarian can assess body language and tone of voice or help the user by demonstrating a quick preliminary search. These encounters are increasingly being replaced by e-mail, filling out forms (in print or online), or the "Ask a Librarian" links on library Web sites. Telephone and response to voicemail can provide a more personal contact. Whatever the method, the librarian must keep asking questions until he or she is confident in understanding what the user really wants.[53, 54]

The importance of understanding a user's information needs cannot be overstated. Experience is needed for effective reference service. This is due to the very personal and unique nature of every request. Real requests are rarely as straightforward as the examples used in a reference class, especially in health sciences libraries. It is essential that the librarian understand what the needs are beneath the question. For example, "Do you have this book?" may mean that the user assumes the answer to a particular question is likely to be found in this book. If the reference librarian is able to elicit the "real" question from the patron, he or she may know better sources for the answer. There are many subtle clues as to the ultimate nature of the information need.

Because of the time constraints on some health sciences library users, they may send someone else (a proxy[55]) to the library with their request. For example, a clinician may send a resident, medical student, or secretary, or a researcher may send a graduate student or lab tech. The delivery of a request via a proxy may present a barrier to a good interactive interview because the proxy may imperfectly understand the request, misspell important words, or not have understood the scope of the request.

Research questions are more inclined to include specialized scientific language. Rather than look up words in dictionaries or thesauri *after* contact with the user, the librarian should ask on the spot for further explanation; scientists are usually only too happy to explain their special projects. Once more, when the librarian may find a possible "hit" or two, sending these hits to the user with a query, such as, "Is this the kind of thing you had in mind?," will help clarify the information need. This will encourage the scientist to further explain the request, assisting the librarian in finding exactly what is needed. If enough information was not obtained, the librarian would recontact the user to request more information.

This ease of access may greatly enlarge the workload of the single librarian. Academic medical centers have reassigned job responsibilities and redesigned public areas (more than once in the past couple of decades) to remove the card catalog, provide computer terminals, and revise how both walk-in and online users express their needs and receive assistance. If the reference desk itself disappears, the "reference interview" is transformed, as in the following discussion.

SINGLE-SERVICE DESKS AND TRIAGING REQUESTS

One development in response to the decreased need for the physical reference desk has been to combine reference and more general information services into one desk; the next step is to put the reference librarians "on call" or readily available in adjacent offices.[56] This enables librarians to multitask by taking care of virtual reference but also to be available for in-person interviews. Where librarians in large libraries may have spent assigned hours daily at the reference desk, they can now deal with online requests and searches and spend less time at the desk. These changes do not mean that long-time users will not still insist that only "their" reference librarian can really help them. There are still users who enjoy the "refuge" of the library building, and library staff may be more welcoming and helpful than personnel in other areas of the institution with which they have contact.

SELECTED INFORMATION SERVICES

Certain information services are provided by most health sciences libraries, while other services may be so highly specialized that they are available at only a few of the larger academic health sciences libraries. This section describes some of the most frequently provided information services.

Informational and Factual Questions

All health sciences libraries will provide some sort of basic reference service, where the librarian will answer factual questions or direct library users to appropriate sources, in print or electronic, where users can locate the answer themselves. Responding to informational questions, and in the process determining whether the requestor in fact needs the answer to a more complicated question, is the most basic of information services provided by all libraries, not just health sciences libraries.

Mediated Search Services

Most health sciences libraries also offer mediated search services utilizing databases such as MEDLINE or CINAHL, via a variety of search interfaces. Database searching is the topic of Chapter 8, "Information Retrieval in the Health Sciences," so the reader is referred to that chapter for more detailed information.

User Education (Information Literacy)

All information services providers are, necessarily, involved in teaching information literacy to library users. This occurs through formal instruction, but also during informal, one-on-one encounters through what is often termed "the teachable moment." As reference librarians direct users to appropriate information sources, they simultaneously teach the patron where he or she might find answers to similar questions in the future. A full discussion of the librarian's education role is available in Chapter 10, "Information Literacy Education in Health Sciences Libraries."

Information Update Services

In the past, librarians went to elaborate lengths to provide "selective dissemination of information" (SDI) or table-of-contents services (sometimes called **TACOs**). Publications such as *Current Contents,* at first in print and later as online databases, alerted users to what was in the latest journals. More recently, both bibliographic database vendors and journal publishers provide alerting services, often in advance of print publication. Newer technologies, such as RSS feeds, facilitate alerting users and librarians about new products and services. Results are usu-

A Day in the Life of a Reference Librarian

Name: Marie FitzSimmons, MS
Position: Reference Librarian, Penn State College of Medicine, Hershey Medical Center, George T. Harrell Library

Job description: Reference Librarian and Webmaster. This position provides front-line reference and research assistance to faculty, staff, the general public, and medical, graduate, and nursing students; performs mediated literature searches in specialized databases; and provides point-of-use and bibliographic instruction. Responsibilities include Web site development and maintenance, participation in the Library Management Team, campus liaison to University Libraries Marketing Team, liaison to campus Information Technology Department, and coordinator of library public relations.

Sample Day

7:00 a.m.—10:00 a.m. Reference Desk Duty
- Reboot eighteen public access computers (launches a program that deletes all previous user profiles).
- Answer phone calls, directional and reference questions.
- Monitor e-mail and "comments" submitted to reference account from library Web site; this activity frequently consists of deleting spam.
- Log patron from the public onto computer and initiate a MedlinePlus search.
- Guide employee on Password Reset Workstation.
- Look up impact factors for journals in which a faculty member has published.
- Work with Information Technology staff to establish network connections for a new color printer for patrons.
- Help patron download and print full-text article.
- Fix printer jam.
- Schedule and complete paperwork to proctor an exam for a nursing student.
- Respond to resident calling to report a journal Web site that requires a username and password. After questioning, it is revealed the patron is trying to access full text beyond the date range of our subscription. Direct patron to Interlibrary Loan form on Web site.

10:00 a.m.—Noon. In Office
- Work with Education Librarian to create a flyer advertising technology fair.
- Edit the EZ Proxy Server configuration file for journal additions.
- Collaborate with in-house graphic artist to create a poster for technology fair.
- Add database links to Library Web page.

1:00 p.m.—4:00 p.m. Reference Desk Duty
- Answer phone calls, directional and reference questions.
- Monitor and respond to professional e-mail.
- Configure student's laptop computer for wireless secure network.
- Guide another employee on Password Reset Workstation.
- Recover search for patron who closed database.
- Demonstrate how to find IP address for staff member.
- Collaborate with a library school student/intern working on a collection development project.
- Attempt to find medical specialist for phone patron interested in glyconutrient supplements; made referral to a physician in the nutrition department.
- Update library pamphlet to reflect increase in printing charges.
- Called Information Technology to repair a computer.

ally sent to the requestor's e-mail. Many library users find these services for themselves; other users can be pointed to them.

Because of the importance that early access to current research and clinical studies plays in a health sciences setting, helping library users to set up an alerting service can be one of the most important functions provided by the reference department. One example of an alerting service is *My NCBI* (National Center for Biotechnology Information), offered through PubMed, where individuals can set up their own user profile. Information services librarians can help users to set up search strategies in appropriate databases. Often the opportunity to suggest an updating service arises following a mediated database search. The user may point out some examples of articles that he or she considers to be "right on target," and the information services librarian can use those to help determine a search strategy. In many cases, the requestor will want the librarian to actually input the search terms and initiate the alerting service with the vendor rather than investing his or her own time to handle the "mechanical" aspects of the alerting service.

Librarians must themselves keep current with issues (both positive and negative) affecting the institution so they can provide helpful, proactive services. For example, a department or program may have been granted monies for a new research enterprise and the library might monitor the literature or media coverage to locate appropriate information. Some libraries now use blogs and Web feeds for this purpose.[57] Grantees will be aware of the library's efforts and collaborate on suggesting appropriate journals or databases. Ideally, of course, some of the grant money will assist with these acquisitions.

Clinical Librarians

Early leaders in medical librarianship would often be physicians, and the relationship continues, as hospitals still include librarians in clinical practice. Health sciences librarians who have changed careers from medicine, nursing, physical and occupational therapy, emergency medicine technology, or other health professions are ideally suited for assisting with clinicians' requests. Some librarians participate in clinical rounds and collect topics to be researched as they learn of the patients' and physicians' needs. **LATCH (literature attached to chart)**[58, 59] has now been largely replaced by integrated research results in **clinical information systems** (CISs)—a major upgrade from paper charts. These integrated patient records usually require physicians to do their own computerized order entry and can have evidence-based literature and other useful material attached. Librarians may sit on committees that investigate and select these large-scale systems and may have input into the final decisions.[60, 61] Clinical librarians are discussed further in Chapter 14, "Management of and Issues Specific to Hospital Libraries," and CISs are described in Chapter 12, "Health Informatics."

Departmental Liaisons

Health sciences libraries are more frequently advertising for positions labeled as departmental liaisons or are listing departmental liaison responsibilities as part of the duties for an information services librarian position. Departmental liaison librarians are assigned to work specifically with one or more departments, serving their information needs, which may range from the provision of mediated searches, to collection development in the department's subject area, to performing informationist-level functions for department faculty. Often, liaison librarians will have particular subject expertise, or prior work experience, or interest in particular areas. For example, librarians who have been nurses or whose undergraduate work included microbiology may be assigned to provide reference services to a school of nursing or a group of bench scientists. Even without special knowledge, librarians can offer their personal services to a department by asking for a brief slot on the agenda of a departmental meeting where they can drop off promotional material and introduce the faculty, staff, or students to the services that the library can offer them. Liaison programs usually ensure that librarians leave the confines of the library and actively promote services in the department's own clinics or offices.

Institutional Publications

Several years ago, MEDLINE began including the first author's address or institutional affiliation. *Science Citation Index,* and its siblings in the Web of Science, gives addresses of all authors (discussed more fully in the next chapter). This makes it possible to create bibliographies of the institution's publications. These references can be stored in an electronic filing system, where they can be a useful resource for "data mining" or analysis, or they can be used to create an actual database of publications by institutional authors. Many health sciences libraries have become involved in creating such a database or publications list.

More recently, many institutions are creating **institutional repositories (IRs),** placing full-text (often PDF) copies of authors' publications on the institution's Web site. The existence of IRs has been fueled by the open access movement and an author's right to retain control of his or her own publications. Health sciences librarians are vocal supporters of the open access movement and many have become actively involved in their institution's IR.

Printed institutional publications may be displayed on regularly updated shelving in the library or advertised as lists that users may download. Now that **impact factors** from the *Journal Citation Reports* (once more, described in the next chapter) have become so popular for prestige and ranking of publications, information services librarians may be asked to assess the rankings of the institutions' publications, though some researchers question their validity as tools to this end.[62]

Other Services

It is not possible to detail all of the possible functions of an information services librarian. Some additional duties might include serving as the department's Webmaster, troubleshooting the library's computer learning center, assisting in grant-writing, teaching medical terminology, or providing translation services.

It is the responsibility of all health sciences librarians to investigate the needs that are pertinent to the institution. Departments such as administration, human resources, or information technology may send out regular questionnaires; the responses may provide suggestions to the library. Surveys and focus groups conducted by the health sciences library also elicit ideas for further services unique to the institution.[63, 64]

INFORMATION SERVICE ETHICS

Librarians in all types of libraries have standards relating to the provision of services, and to protecting the privacy of users. The American Library Association (ALA) has its own code; the following is from the ALA's "Position Statement":

> The members of the American Library Association, recognizing the right to privacy of library users, believe that records held in libraries which connect specific individuals with specific resources, programs or services, are confidential and not to be used for purposes other than routine record keeping: i.e., to maintain access to resources, to assure that resources are available to users who need them, to arrange facilities, to provide resources for

the comfort and safety of patrons, or to accomplish the purposes of the program or service. The library community recognizes that children and youth have the same rights to privacy as adults.[65]

Health sciences librarians should become familiar with the official Medical Library Association (MLA) Code of Ethics for Health Sciences Librarianship. The code is divided into six sections related to health sciences librarians and their users. The discussion here is from the perspective of an information services librarian and follows the outline of the code.

Goals and Principles

Information services require not only knowledge and expertise but also respect for the profession, the users, and society. That respect is expressed in the ethical use of that knowledge and expertise.

Code of Ethics for Health Sciences Librarianship

GOALS AND PRINCIPLES FOR ETHICAL CONDUCT
The health sciences librarian believes that knowledge is the sine qua non of informed decisions in health care, education, and research and the health sciences librarian serves society, clients, and the institution, by working to ensure that informed decisions can be made.

SOCIETY
The health sciences librarian promotes access to health information for all and creates and maintains conditions of freedom of inquiry, thought, and expression that facilitate informed health care decisions.

CLIENTS
The health sciences librarian works without prejudice to meet the client's information needs.
The health sciences librarian respects the privacy of clients and protects the confidentiality of the client relationship.
The health sciences librarian ensures that the best available information is provided to the client.

INSTITUTION
The health sciences librarian provides leadership and expertise in the design, development, and ethical management of knowledge-based information systems that meet the information needs and obligations of the institution.

PROFESSION
The health sciences librarian advances and upholds the philosophy and ideals of the profession.
The health sciences librarian advocates and advances the knowledge and standards of the profession.
The health sciences librarian conducts all professional relationships with courtesy and respect.
The health sciences librarian maintains high standards of professional integrity.

SELF
The health sciences librarian assumes personal responsibility for developing and maintaining professional excellence.

Society

The health sciences are particularly fraught with ethical and moral dilemmas as they deal with life-and-death decisions, the most intimate details of patients' lives, and, in the United States, with insurance and governmental decisions about universal coverage. Health issues appear in regular columns of newspapers and magazines as the population struggles with abortion rights, the "morning-after" pill, gay couples' rights to information about each other's health care, availability of affordable drugs, profits in the drug development industry—just to name a few current topics. This means that beyond the universal concerns of every reference librarian for accuracy, thoroughness, appropriateness, professionalism, privacy and confidentiality, and awareness of cultural diversity, librarians in the health sciences have to keep up with these many other issues.

Users

Professional service is the connection between the users' needs, or expressed desires, for information and the best possible sources for that information. The ethical librarian is responsible for carefully discovering and understanding those needs, identifying the best source of information to match them, and completing the transaction by ensuring that there is a successful and satisfying delivery of that information to the user or population. Often users can find "an answer" for many information requests by themselves. The librarian must ensure the delivery of "the answer" that best satisfies the users' needs. Examples in this chapter have demonstrated some of the particular difficulties the health sciences librarian may face.

Institution

Hospitals and academic medical centers each may have patient and professional libraries that can be visited by patients or their families. If the institution has separate libraries for these user populations, the libraries need to cooperate, have access to one another's collections and policies, and understand how to deal with users in severe emotional distress, or even exhibiting anger and frustration.

Larger institutions may have multiple libraries, and visitors may find that their access to some of them is restricted. For example, Stanford has more than two dozen libraries, with varied access policies for noninstitutional users.[66]

Profession

The health sciences librarian must keep up with new technology, updated policies from other libraries, and all the issues that arise from changes in the book publishing and database production industries. Continuing education and attendance at professional meetings are essential to stay current. If the librarian's employer does not provide travel money for attending meetings, many organizations have useful Web sites, newsletters and other publications, and opportunities for online discussion. MLA <http://www.mlanet.org> has sections on various topics and chapters throughout the United States and parts of Canada (Canada has its own Canadian Health Libraries Association/Association des bibliothèques de la santé du Canada <http://www.chla-absc.ca/>). Regions and states often have their own organizations. Health sciences librarians new to a city or area can find out about local library groups by contacting librarians at a nearby academic medical center or hospital.

Self

Health sciences librarians must be careful not to bias information that they provide with personal opinions. For example, they may provide access to "best doctors" books, explain what "board certification" means, or indicate the board's Web site, but they cannot make a personal recommendation.[67] A complicating factor may occur when the librarian has, or has had, a particular personal diagnosis or therapy. There may be a fine line between personal conversations with library staff and users and sharing advice. It is a judgment call to decide whether the conversation is strictly personal—from one sufferer to another—or borders on whether the librarian is acting in a professional role.

Other Ethical Considerations

The health sciences librarian cannot reveal that a patient in the institution has a particular condition or reveal to one user what another has requested. One practitioner may ask about another's request for information relating to the same patient's condition. This is not unique to the health sciences since ALA has taken firm stands on refusing to release library records.[68] The more recent **HIPAA (Health Insurance Portability and Accountability Act)** regulations provide more detailed information about government regulations on privacy.[69]

If a health care provider refers a patient to the hospital or academic health sciences library, or if the patient is also himself or herself a health care provider, the same rules apply. In the case of the general public, the librarian may not "interpret" the technical language but must refer the user back to the provider. With such questions as "Is my child's cancer always fatal? I want something authoritative!" from a frustrated parent who has exhausted the resources readily available online, the information services librarian can only assist in finding further information, not in translating it into simpler language. Librarians who are not trained to help consumers could develop a good relationship with an easily accessible consumer health library for referral.

A type of "triage" is needed for the librarian to prioritize requests and provide the most efficient service to users. This may call for simple judgment: the surgeon who is operating this afternoon may have a more urgent need than the researcher who does not expect to receive the interlibrary loan until next week. However, if the need for triage comes up frequently, or becomes an issue among users, the librarian may need to post a policy on prioritization of requests. An example of another type of emergency is the immediate need for information that might occur when the press is about to interview an administrator. However, the student who has postponed working on an assignment until the last minute may have to be made aware of the reference librarian's limitations in providing immediate service.

All librarians are necessarily trained in copyright law and intellectual property issues, and this is no different in the health sciences. Increasingly in recent years, part of "virtual" information services has been the ability to provide scanned copies, such as PDF files, of full-text material from books, journals, and online resources. The librarian has no control over whether and how clinicians and researchers share these among themselves. Disclaimers may be attached to documents, and policies clearly stated.

Library policies on providing information services beyond the institution, even where the library is tax-funded, will be coordinated with the overall institutional policies on service provision.

CONCLUSION

This chapter has attempted to enhance awareness of the myriad ways that librarians can provide information services. Literature from past years at the beginning of the Web explosion suggested that the physical library was in danger of being replaced by the Web and purely electronic resources. As the complexity of the resources has developed, information services librarians' roles have in fact expanded. The next chapter explores in detail how these changes have affected information retrieval and describes many of the new resources.

The message here is that information services librarians know they can help in areas their users have not realized. They must advertise and promote their services to users and potential users and offer the assistance that will enable their institution to grow and succeed.

For some users, the perception of "the library" may still be the inviting, calm place to peruse the latest received journal, look up older journal articles that are not available online, or check out a book for reading elsewhere. For many, if not most users, this is not the image they need or expect. Apart from the availability of what used to be only in print, but now is offered in electronic formats, the *services* provided by librarians are a vital part of what the library provides. While the physical library is either easily visible or appears on institutional maps or directional signs, the *services* may not be so obvious. It is essential for the development and success of the institution that all of its personnel, whether involved in direct patient care, research, or education, be aware that their highly trained and helpful librarians can assist them. Librarians may have to go to clinics, offices, and labs to ensure that their information services are known and utilized to their fullest extent.

REFERENCES

1. Boorkman, J.A.; Huber, J.T.; and Roper, F.W. *Introduction to Reference Sources in the Health Sciences.* 4th ed. New York: Neal-Schuman, 2004.

2. Connor, E. *"Introduction to Reference Sources in the Health Sciences:* An Interview with Jo Anne Boorkman; Jeffrey T. Huber; and Fred W. Roper." *Medical Reference Services Quarterly* 24(Fall 2005): 1-15.

3. Homan, J.M. "Review of *Introduction to Reference Sources in the Health Sciences.*" *Journal of the Medical Library Association* 93, no. 1 (January 2005): 135. Available: <http://www.pubmedcentral.nih.gov/articlerender .fcgi?artid=545138>. Accessed: March 20, 2007.

4. Absher, L.U.; Bowman, M.S.; Jackson, R.M.; and Schroeder, R. "Rethinking Reference: Shaken Foundations, Predictions, and What Really Happened Between 1988 and 2005." *ACRL Twelfth National Conference, April 2005, Minneapolis.* Available: <http://www.ala.org/ala/acrl/acrlevents/absher-etal05.pdf>. Accessed: February 20, 2007.

5. Slader, R.M.; Pinnock, C.; and Phillips, P.A. "The Informationist: A Prospective Uncontrolled Study." *International Journal for Quality in Health Care* 16, no. 6 (2004): 509-515.

6. Davidoff, F., and Florance, V. "The Informationist: A New Health Profession?" *Annals of Internal Medicine* 132(June 2000): 996-8.

7. Shearer, B.S.; Seymour, A.; and Capitani, C. "Bringing the Best of Medical Librarianship to the Patient Team." *Journal of the Medical Library Association* 90, no. 1 (January 2002): 22-31.

8. Giuse, N.B.; Koonce, T.Y.; Jerome, R.N.; Cahall, M.; Sathe, N.A.; and Williams, A. "Evolution of a Mature Clinical Informationist Model." *Journal of the American Medical Informatics Association* 12, no. 3 (May/June 2005): 249-55.

9. Banks, M.A. "Defining the Informationist: A Case Study from the Frederick L. Ehrman Medical Library." *Journal of the Medical Library Association* 94, no. 1 (January 2006): 5-7.

10. Florance, V.; Giuse, N.B.; and Ketchell, D.S. "Information in Context: Integrating Information Specialists into Practice Settings." *Journal of the Medical Library Association* 90, no. 1 (January 2002): 49-58.

11. Jerome, R.N.; Giuse, N.B.; Gish, K.W.; Sathe, N.A.; and Dietrich, M.S. "Information Needs of Clinical Teams: Analysis of Questions Received by the Clinical Informatics Consult Service." *Bulletin of the Medical Library Association* 89, no. 2 (April 2001): 177-84.

12. Gonnerman, K. "The Health Sciences Library and Professional Librarians: Important Resources for Busy ED Nurses and Nurse Managers." *Journal of Emergency Nursing* 29(April 2003): 183-6.

13. Haigh, V. "Clinical Effectiveness and Allied Health Professionals: An Information Needs Assessment." *Health Information & Libraries Journal* 23(March 2006): 41-50.

14. Wessel, C.B.; Tannery, N.H.; and Epstein, B.A. "Information-Seeking Behavior and Use of Information Resources by Clinical Research Coordinators." *Journal of the Medical Library Association* 94, no. 1 (January 2006): 48-54.

15. Dawes, M., and Sampson, U. "Knowledge Management in Clinical Practice: A Systematic Review of Information Seeking Behavior in Physicians." *International Journal of Medical Informatics* 71(August 2003): 9-15.

16. Dee, C., and Stanley, E.E. "Information-Seeking Behavior of Nursing Students and Clinical Nurses: Implications for Health Sciences Librarians." *Journal of the Medical Library Association* 93, no. 2 (April 2005): 213-22.

17. Coumou, H.C.H.; Zorgverzekeringen, A.G.I; and Meijman, F.J. "How Do Primary Care Physicians Seek Answers to Clinical Questions? A Literature Review." *Journal of the Medical Library Association* 94, no. 1 (January 2006): 55-9.

18. Bennett, N.L.; Casebeer, L.L.; Kristofco, R.E.; and Strasser, S.M. "Physicians' Internet Information-Seeking Behaviors." *Journal of Continuing Education in the Health Professions* 24(Winter 2004): 31-8.

19. Casebeer, L.; Bennett, N.; Kristofco, R.; Carillo, A.; and Centor, R. "Physician Internet Medical Information Seeking and On-Line Continuing Education Use Patterns." *Journal of Continuing Education in the Health Profession* 22(Winter 2002): 33-42.

20. Booth, A. "What Research Studies Do Practitioners Actually Find Useful?" *Health Information & Libraries Journal* 21(September 2004): 197-200.

21. Green, M.L.; Ciampi, M.A.; and Ellis, P.J. "Residents' Medical Information Needs in Clinic: Are They Being Met?" *American Journal of Medicine* 109(August 15, 2000): 218-23.

22. Doyle, J.D., and Harvey, S.A. "Teaching the Publishing Process to Researchers and Other Potential Authors in a Hospital System." *Journal of Hospital Librarianship* 5, no. 1 (2005): 63-70.

23. Harris, M.R. "The Librarian's Roles in the Systematic Review Process: A Case Study." *Journal of the Medical Library Association* 93, no. 1 (January 2005): 81-7.

24. Perry, G.J., and Kronenfeld, M.R. "Evidence-Based Practice: A New Paradigm Brings New Opportunities for Health Sciences Librarians." *Medical Reference Services Quarterly* 24, no. 1 (Winter 2005): 1-16.

25. Tennant, M.R.; Tobin Cataldo, T.; Sherwill-Navarro, P.; and Jesano R. "Evaluation of a Liaison Librarian Program: Client and Liaison Perspectives." *Journal of the Medical Library Association* 94, no. 4 (October 2006): 402-9.

26. Cogdill, K.W., and Moore, M.E. "First-Year Medical Students' Information Needs and Resource Selection: Responses to a Clinical Scenario." *Bulletin of the Medical Library Association* 85, no. 1 (January 1997): 51-4.

27. Connor E. "Medical Librarian 2.0." *Medical Reference Services Quarterly* 26(Suppl. 1, 2007): 5-23.

28. Web 2.0 Summit. Available: <http://www.web2con.com/>. Accessed: April 16, 2007.

29. Tenopir, C. "Rethinking Virtual Reference." *Library Journal* (November 1, 2004): 34.

30. Malinconico, S.M. "Information's Brave New World: Could Displace Librarians—or Magnify Their Importance." *Library Journal* 117(May 1, 1992): 36-40.

31. Fialkoff, F. "Retail Reference: Are We Downgrading Reference Just As Questions Get Harder?" *Library Journal* 131(March 2006): 8.

32. Taher, M. "The Reference Interview Through Asynchronous E-mail and Synchronous Interactive Reference: Does It Save the Time of the Interviewee?" *Internet Reference Services Quarterly* 7, no. 3 (2002): 23-34.

33. Ronan, J. "The Reference Interview Online." *Reference & User Services Quarterly* 43, no. 1 (Fall 2003): 43-7.

34. American Library Association. "Guidelines for Implementing and Maintaining Virtual Reference Services." (2006). Available: <http://www.ala.org/ala/rusa/rusaprotools/referenceguide/virtrefguidelines.htm>. Accessed: April 17, 2007.

35. MARS Digital Reference Guidelines Ad Hoc Committee. Reference and User Services Association. "Guidelines for Implementing and Maintaining Virtual Reference Services." *Reference & User Services Quarterly* 44, no. 1 (Fall 2004): 9-13.

36. Cleveland, A.D., and Philbrick, J.L. "Virtual Reference Services for the Academic Health Sciences Librarian 2.0." *Medical Reference Services Quarterly* 26(Suppl. 1, 2007): 25-49.

37. Dee, C.R. "Chat Reference Service in Medical Libraries: Part 1—An Introduction." *Medical Reference Services Quarterly* 22, no. 2 (Summer 2003): 1-13.

38. Dee, C.R. "Chat Reference Service in Medical Libraries: Part 2—Trends in Medical School Libraries." *Medical Reference Services Quarterly* 22, no. 2 (Summer 2003): 15-28.

39. Parker, S.K., and Johnson, E.D. "The Region 4 Collaborative Virtual Reference Project." *Medical Reference Services Quarterly* 22, no. 2 (Summer 2003): 29-39.

40. McGraw, K.A.; Heiland, J.; and Harris, J.C. "Promotion and Evaluation of a Virtual Live Reference Service." *Medical Reference Services Quarterly* 22, no. 2 (Summer 2003): 41-56.

41. Jerant, L.L., and Firestein, K. "Not Virtual, but a Real, Live, Online, Interactive Reference Service." *Medical Reference Services Quarterly* 22, no. 2 (Summer 2003): 57-68.

42. MacDonald, M.H. "Planning, Implementing, and Using a Virtual Reference Service." *Medical Reference Services Quarterly* 22, no. 2 (Summer 2003): 69-75.

43. Bobal, A.M. "One Library's Experience with Live, Virtual Reference." *Journal of the Medical Library Association* 93, no. 1 (January 2005): 123-5.

44. Dee, C.R., and Newhouse, J.D. "Digital Chat Reference in Health Science Libraries: Challenges in Initiating a New Service." *Medical Reference Services Quarterly* 24, no. 3 (Fall 2005): 17-27.

45. Dee, C.R. "Digital Reference Service: Trends in Academic Health Science Libraries." *Medical Reference Services Quarterly* 24, no. 1 (Spring 2005): 19-27.

46. Kovacs, D.K. *The Virtual Reference Handbook: Interview and Information Delivery Techniques for the Chat and E-mail Environment.* New York: Neal-Schuman, 2007.

47. Lankes, R.D.; Abels, E.; White, M.; and Naque, S.N. *The Virtual Reference Desk: Creating a Reference Future.* New York: Neal-Schuman, 2006.

48. Lipow, A.G. *The Virtual Reference Librarian's Handbook.* New York: Neal-Schuman, 2003.

49. Werts, C.E. "Just Ask. The Best Way to Get Your Clients the Right Information Is to Find Out Exactly What They Want." *Information Outlook* 10(April 2006): 33-5.

50. Alexander, K. "Getting to 'the Real Question.'" *Journal of Hospital Librarianship* 6, no. 3 (2006): 121-5.

51. Doherty, J.J. "Reference Interview or Reference Dialogue?" *Internet Reference Services Quarterly* 11, no. 3 (2006): 97-109.

52. ODLIS—Online Dictionary for Library and Information Science. "Reference Interview." Available: <http://lu.com/odlis/odlis_r.cfm>. Accessed: April 15, 2007.

53. Quint, B.E. "The Return of the Reference Interview." *Information Today* 19(February 2002): 8, 10, 14.

54. Kluegel, K. "The Reference Interview Through Time and Space." *Reference & User Services Quarterly* 43, no. 1 (Fall 2003): 37-43.

55. Gross, M. "The Imposed Query." *RQ* 35, no. 2 (1995): 236-43.

56. Personal communication with numerous librarians at health sciences libraries of various types.

57. McKiernan, G. "This Just In: Web Feeds for Enhanced Library Services." *Knowledge Quest* 3(January-February 2005): 38-41.

58. Brenner, L. "A Report on LATCH (Literature Attached to Charts)." *Medical Records News* 47(August 1976).

59. Hargrave, S. "LATCH—It Works!" *Hospital Libraries* 1(September 1, 1976): 4-5.

60. Finegan BA. "Access Denied; Care Impaired: the Benefits of Having Online Medical Information Available at the Point-of-Care." *Anesthesia & Analgesia* 99(November 2004): 1450-2.

61. Calabretta N., and Cavanaugh SK. "Education for Inpatients: Working with Nurses Through the Clinical Information System." *Medical Reference Services Quarterly* 23, no. 2 (2004): 73-9.

62. Baker R., and Jackson D. "Using Journal Impact Factors to Correct for the Publication Bias of Medical Studies." *Biometrics* 62 (September 2006): 785-92.

63. Higa-Moore, M.; Bunnett, B.; Mayo, H.B.; and Olney, C.A. "Use of Focus Groups in a Library's Strategic Planning Process." *Journal of the Medical Library Association* 90, no. 1 (January 2002): 86-92.

64. Glitz, B.; Hamasu, C.; and Sandstrom, H. "The Focus Group: A Tool for Programme Planning, Assessment and Decision-Making—An American View." *Health Information and Libraries Journal* 18(March 2001): 30-7.

65. Code of Ethics of the American Library Association. Available: <http://www.ala.org/ala/oif/statementspols/codeofethics/codeethics.htm>. Accessed: March 24, 2006.

66. Stanford University Access Policies. Available: <http://library.stanford.edu/how_to/borrow_get_access/non_stanford_users/access.html>. Accessed: March 23, 2007.

67. Connolly, J.J. "America's Top Doctors." New York: Castle Connolly Medical Limited, 2006.

68. American Library Association Position Statements. Available: <http://www.ala.org/ala/aasl/aaslproftools/positionstatements/aaslpositionstatementconfidentiality.htm>. Accessed: March 15, 2007.

69. HIPAA. "General Overview of Standards for Privacy of Individually Identifiable Health Information." Available: <http://www.hhs.gov/ocr/hipaa/guidelines/overview.pdf>. Accessed: March 15, 2007.

Chapter 8

Information Retrieval in the Health Sciences

Elizabeth H. Wood

SUMMARY. Information retrieval is the process by which librarians find the answers or data that the user has requested. Sources formerly published only in print are now increasingly available online. The chapter begins with definitions of primary, secondary, and tertiary literature. One of the most important tasks for librarians, and a major part of the provision of information services, is searching the indexing and abstracting "bibliographic" databases. Descriptions of the major bibliographic and full-text databases in the health sciences include their histories as printed indexes. The enhanced features of the online versions are explained and demonstrated with examples. Even though many of these online resources are designed for end users, busy health professionals and students may prefer to request "mediated" searches, performed by a librarian. This chapter explains how various types of users and requests are satisfied with information retrieval techniques.

INTRODUCTION

Defining "information retrieval" is a moving target in this world of stunning technological developments. As the Web and the availability of full-text documents, linked to bibliographic databases and library Web sites, increasingly dominate our lives, the distinctions between the types of information sources become blurred. Users' factual reference questions can often be answered through standard tools, such as dictionaries, directories, encyclopedias, and textbooks—and even through Google. The more difficult and time-consuming requests require searching bibliographic databases and, often, providing the full text of the journal articles. An understanding of the authority and quality of information sources, based on descriptions of their history and development, helps the information services librarian to choose the best resources. Whether the ultimate answer to a user's request is a fact, a bibliography, full-text articles, or monographs, the librarian new to the health sciences needs guideposts through the complex world of biomedical information and how to search it.

A particularly outstanding example of the utility of online databases is how they can provide rapid access to the answer to questions like, "Um, there was an article in *JAMA* (or was it *Annals*?), a couple of weeks ago (or last month?), about a new appendectomy technique. Guy was from Johns Hopkins—or was it Northwestern? Name's John Something." Before online databases, locating such an article could be impossible. The librarian would run (literally, because the user needed it for a staff meeting in half an hour) to the stacks and thumb through the latest issues of *JAMA* or the *Annals of Internal Medicine*. No luck. *Index Medicus* would not have the citation for this reference for weeks or months; and before the Internet was widely available, there was no Web site for the suggested universities, no e-mail to contact the authors, and no way to "Google" for "appendectomy." The librarian could go back to the user and ask where he or

Introduction to Health Sciences Librarianship
© 2008 by The Haworth Press, Taylor & Francis Group. All rights reserved.
doi:10.1300/6041_08

she had heard about the article, hoping to take the "rumor" back to a more reliable source. Today, there is a much better chance that the article can be unearthed.

Barbara Quint, editor of *Searcher* magazine, and prolific teacher and lecturer, suggested to incredulous students at the University of Southern California's library school that a library information service could be provided with nothing but a computer terminal. This was in 1980, before the Internet as it is known today, let alone the Web. Her frank, witty, controversial (if not outrageous) discussions of online searching provide food for thought, for fans and those who will become fans.[1] One of many classic quotes from "bq" is the following:

> A library is a building, and, as such, is accompanied by static verbs such as "stands," "is located," or "contains," etc. A librarian is a person for whom action verbs are appropriate, such as "coordinates," "designs," or "eliminates," etc. One illustration: libraries do not cooperate, librarians do.[2]

TYPES OF LITERATURE IN THE HEALTH SCIENCES

The definitions described here vary in other disciplines. For example, in many of the humanities, "primary" sources refer only to autobiographies, letters, manuscripts, original works of art, and the like. There are numerous, mostly academic, Web sites that describe the distinctions in different ways.[3, 4] Searching "primary secondary tertiary" on the Internet provides many variations. Some classifications place reviews (journal articles that review the literature on a topic, rather than original research) and textbooks in the "secondary" category. Some only include guides to the literature in the "tertiary" category. In the context of information retrieval in the health sciences, the following definitions are provided to explain why database searching is still one of the most important skills that health sciences librarians must master.

Primary Literature

The primary literature consists of the published case and research reports in health sciences journals. For purposes here, review articles and meta-analyses published in journals are included, as are editorials and letters. Over the past several years, more journals are available online through direct subscriptions to individual or bundles of journals, through aggregators, and via the **open access** movement.[5] Links to full text are provided in numerous places: attached to bibliographic databases, attached to library online catalog entries, or in separate lists on library Web sites, called something like "Current Journals" or "Health Sciences e-journals." Journal articles and other journal content, either in a bibliography or provided in full text, are among the most-requested information resources in the health sciences.

Secondary Literature

Secondary literature in this discussion includes all the indexing and abstracting sources that are used to retrieve the primary literature. For the past forty-plus years, these sources, once originally published only in print, have become the **bibliographic databases** that are crucial to information retrieval. Printed indexes provided access by author and subject. *Science Citation Index* also provided its unique citation listings, and *Chemical Abstracts* had additional search capabilities. When these sources became available online, many other parts of the records were searchable: abstracts; links to full text; words in titles and abstracts; publication types; and authors' addresses; and the ability to "limit" retrieval by language, type of research subject (species, age, gender), and date of publication. Publishers and vendors, and libraries, are adding links to full-text articles from the references in bibliographic databases, but these primary sources added to secondary sources do not change their role in information retrieval.

The most important and widely used indexing and abstracting resources in the health sciences have been selected for discussion and explanation in this chapter. Searching in these secondary sources leads to the primary literature. The databases, their subject coverage, special features, and techniques for searching them will be covered later.

Tertiary Literature

Tertiary literature sources include textbooks and reference tools such as dictionaries, directories, and drug resources. These sources are increasingly available online and often referred to as "e-books." They are considered "tertiary" here because they are derived from the primary literature, or from a compilation of data from other sources, often providing copious references, which were located using secondary sources.

Users who come to the library in person can often be referred to these resources on the shelf; however, with the availability of more e-books, it is more likely that the information services librarian will guide users, either in person or remotely, to the online version of the sources. Publishers go to great lengths to make them user-friendly, but users who rely on their librarians to find information for them may not have the time to find the e-books, search them, and download or print what they need; or they may simply prefer not to take the time. Clinicians who also teach and publish are often under particular time constraints. Librarians can assess their urgency by asking when the information is needed, and taking this into account in the triage process. As discussed in the previous chapter, "Information Services in the Health Sciences Libraries," users may not know where to look, making the knowledgeable information services librarian indispensable.

A category of resources that blurs lines among these definitions are **systematic reviews,** and the evidence-based practice sites and the monographs in Web-based products such as DynaMed, InfoPOEMs, MDConsult, and UpToDate. These are discussed in more detail in the section Full-Text Databases, which appears later in this chapter.

DATABASES IN THE HEALTH SCIENCES

This section covers the major databases available in health sciences libraries; only a carefully selected group of files is discussed as space precludes a more comprehensive approach. An excellent source for a more complete listing of databases is found in Boorkman, Huber, and Roper's *Introduction to Reference Sources in the Health Sciences.*[6]

Printed indexes, usually searchable by subject and author, preceded the online bibliographic databases used in the health sciences. *Index Medicus,* for example, the ancestor of **MEDLINE,** began in 1879. Larger libraries will have entire sets of the older printed indexes, which are useful for historical research. Librarians worry whether patrons who only use online databases for their background research and do not search back farther in time using the printed indexes are truly finding everything relevant to their topic; a comprehensive approach to locating vital information could prove crucial. MEDLINE, for example, now goes back to 1950, but in 2001 it only went back to 1965 (with a few earlier records), and a Johns Hopkins researcher failed to investigate a drug back in time, resulting in the death of a volunteer subject.[7, 8]

Technological developments, in particular the Web, have greatly complicated library services and forced librarians to make many decisions regarding how both librarians and users find information. The ability to electronically search many other parts of the database record has greatly expanded searching capabilities, enabling librarians to find and verify citations when only fragments are known, or some of the details are suspected to be incorrect. As competition among database vendors grows, the additional enhancements that experienced librarians enjoy can add layers of complexity for users, who may therefore choose **mediated searching,** just as they did before the retrieval systems were user-friendly.

One decision that information services librarians must make involves the selection of search interfaces. For example, many libraries choose the **National Library of Medicine (NLM)**'s own **PubMed** interface to search MEDLINE, perhaps because it is free of charge. If a library subscribes to more than a few databases, it is easier for both librarians and users to have a single interface where possible. Vendors such as Dialog <http://www.dialog.com>, EBSCO*host* <http://www.ebscohost.com>, and Ovid <http://www.ovid.com> provide a common interface to MEDLINE, CINAHL (*Cumulative Index to Nursing and Allied Health Literature*), PsycINFO, and evidence-based resources, along with other biosciences databases, such as BIOSIS, and drug resources. These indexes and many of their features will be discussed later in this chapter.

Bibliographic databases, the offspring of printed indexes, are not the only kind of database used in health sciences research. Full-text and factual resources are available from NLM and commercial vendors, aimed at consumers as well as health professionals. To facilitate access, many health sciences libraries provide lists of resources on the library's Web site. An example of an access page to electronic resources is shown in Figure 8.1.

Considerable space is given here to MEDLINE, one of the oldest (counting *Index Medicus* back to 1879) and most widely respected and used health sciences databases in the world, especially since its availability free of charge since 1997 via PubMed. Although originally intended for physicians, its subject coverage has expanded over the years. After the MEDLINE discussion, selected major databases are listed by subject, followed by a discussion of special features such as citation indexing and full text.

MEDLINE

MEDLINE, produced by the U.S. National Library of Medicine, currently indexes more than 5,000 journals and contains more than 15 million citations to journal articles in the life sciences from 1950 to the present.[9] As described in the front matter of the first volume of *Index Medicus* in 1879, its scope is international and its purpose has always been to enable practitioners around the world to share their knowledge and expertise. It is designed to be used primarily by health care providers and biomedical researchers and covers only articles published in a carefully selected group of biomedical journals. It does not cover meeting abstracts, books, Web sites, or other kinds of publications. It does index editorials, letters, comments, and corrections.

History and Training

Librarians have searched MEDLINE through increasingly sophisticated techniques since it first appeared in the mid-1960s. The Internet and Web greatly facilitated searching in the 1990s, and both commercial vendors and institutions created interfaces and subsets of the MEDLINE database, all part of the history of MEDLINE, as new features were introduced and access became streamlined.

Training for librarians in what was then called MEDLARS began as a four-month course on indexing and searching at NLM in Bethesda, Maryland. Librarians remember pulling **MeSH** (Medical Subject Headings; discussed in detail in the next section) punch-cards out of a rotating bin and mailing them to NLM to be run against the database. Results came back weeks later. With the advent of MEDLINE (MEDLARS Online), the training developed into a three-week-long course at NLM, and eventually a three-day course taught at Regional Medical Libraries

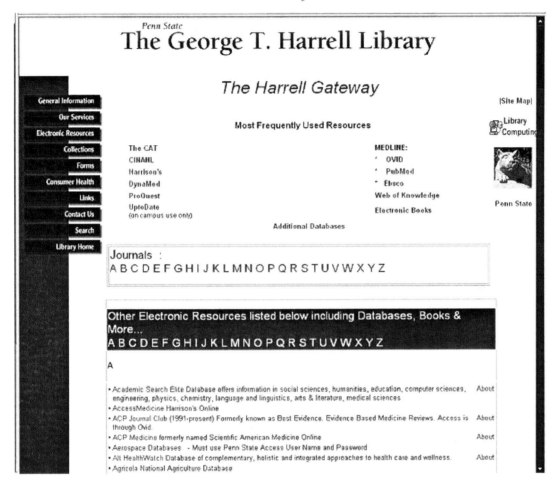

FIGURE 8.1. George T. Harrell Library Electronic Resources Page (Harrell Gateway). *Source:* This image is courtesy of Penn State George T. Harrell Library <http://www.hmc.psu.edu/library> at Penn State College of Medicine <http://www.psu.edu/college/>.

around the country (now called **NN/LM,** the National Network of Libraries of Medicine <http://nnlm.gov/>). MEDLINE was fee-based (libraries varied widely in whether, and how much, they charged users) in the years before PubMed and was definitely designed for information professionals, who learned somewhat arcane commands and were taught how the database was put together and how the search engine worked. The long training periods, and time taken to mail punch-cards and receive results, obviously did not help urgent patient care needs, but it was a big improvement over perusing printed journals as they were received, or waiting for *Index Medicus* to arrive weeks later.

Searching progressed from mailing punch-cards to NLM for MEDLARS searches, to an experiment called AIM-TWX, which used TWX (teletype) machines to search *Abridged Index Medicus (AIM),* a subset of 100 core clinical journals, to online access via telephone connections through dial-up modems, to text-based interfaces from commercial vendors, and eventually to Web access.[10] By the early 1990s, CD-ROM was the "hot" topic in database searching.[11, 12] With the arrival of the Web in the mid-1990s and with widespread access to the Internet, the earlier technologies have faded into history.

In the early 1980s, NLM produced a "simple" interface on a floppy disk designed to make searching easy for physicians; this was wittily titled Grateful Med (after a rock group at the time, the Grateful Dead). Its very simplicity limited its searching power. This evolved into Internet Grateful Med, which was eventually retired. A similarly "punny" interlibrary loan program for individual physicians, **Loansome Doc®**, continues to operate. The **National Center for Biotechnology Information** (NCBI) then produced a user-friendly interface to MEDLINE called PubMed; there are clues to its NCBI origins in its URL <http://www.ncbi.nlm.nih.gov/entrez .fcgi?db=PubMed>. NLM announced the availability of this free interface in 1997. Initially it was announced by then-Vice President Al Gore. He said at a conference that MEDLINE would now be available free to all U.S. citizens. Somehow he did not mention that the whole world actually had access. For those interested in this gradual development, there are articles that describe the history of MEDLINE at various points in time.[13-15]

Before PubMed, NLM licensed MEDLINE data to institutions that wanted to provide their own versions. Examples: PaperChase appeared quietly on a computer at Beth Israel Hospital, Boston, in 1981 and was an immediate hit.[16] Georgetown University produced miniMEDLINE, which led to discussion of how to create subsets of the database.[17]

There are now online tutorials designed for librarians and end users. Continuing education courses on searching are available from the **Medical Library Association (MLA),** from NLM, and from most database vendors. The "NLM Gateway" <http://www.nlm.nih.gov/pubs/fact sheets/gateway.html> provides access to, and information about, many searching sources.

Vendors

Since the days of dial-up modems, commercial vendors have offered their own interfaces to MEDLINE along with their other databases, and they continue to do so. Among the earliest were BRS (later acquired by Ovid), and Dialog, now owned by Thomson Corporation but still called Dialog. These and many journal publishers frequently change their offerings, buy and sell one another, change policies, and "improve" search features.

Fields

The MEDLINE "unit record" (or simply "record") consists of many **fields.** The searcher can limit the search by concepts such as language, existence of an abstract, whether the subjects were human or animal, age group, and more. PubMed and the various commercial interfaces allow searching with MeSH, and also words from titles and abstracts, authors, journal titles, and years. The address of the first author is provided, as it appears in the journal. Since there is no required structure for this field, searchers must consider alternate ways of discovering, for example, whether "USC" means University of Southern California or South Carolina. For citation verification, many interfaces allow the searcher to specify page numbers, or volume and issue numbers. Figure 8.2 shows a "complete" MEDLINE record.

Apart from MeSH (discussed in more detail in the following section), most of the fields in a MEDLINE record are derived directly from the journal article itself and are provided to NLM directly from the publisher. For instance, there are fields for the journal title, the article title, the authors' names, the year, the volume, the issue number, and the complete abstract if one was published in the journal. NLM does not write its own abstracts. There are fields for the country in which the journal is published, and the international standard serial number for the journal. Some of these fields have a "fixed" format (e.g., authors' names, journal titles) while others, notably the abstract and first author's address, depend on how the journal lists this information.

It should be noted here that NLM also provides "In Processing and Other Non-Indexed Citations," which have not yet been assigned MeSH but are the very latest references available from

Unique Identifier	17333990
Record Owner	NLM
Authors	Jain P, Nihill P, Sobkowski J, Agustin MZ.
Authors Full Name	Jain, Poonam. Nihill, Patricia. Sobkowski, Jason. Agustin, Ma Zenia.
Institution	Department of Growth, Development, and Structure, Southern Illinois University School of Dental Medicine, Alton, USA.
Title	Commercial soft drinks: pH and in vitro dissolution of enamel.
Source	Gen Dentistry. 55(2):150-4; quiz 155, 167-8, 2007 Mar-Apr.
Abbreviated Source	Gen Dent. 55(2):150-4; quiz 155, 167-8, 2007 Mar-Apr.
NLM Journal Name	General dentistry
Publishing Model	Journal available in: Print Citation processed from: Print
NLM Journal Code	fl0, 7610466
Journal Subset	D
Local Messages	Journal not owned by PSUHMC Library ; use Interlibrary Loan.
Country of Publication	United States
MeSH Subject Headings	Carbonated Beverages / cl [Classification] *Carbonated Beverages / to [Toxicity] Cola *Dental Enamel / de [Drug Effects] Dental Enamel Solubility Humans Hydrogen-Ion Concentration Sweetening Agents Tea *Tooth Erosion / ci [Chemically Induced]
Abstract	Most soft drinks are acidic in nature and exposure to these drinks may result in enamel erosion. This study sought to measure the pH of 20 commercial brands of soft drinks, the dissolution of enamel resulting from immersion in these drinks, and the influence of pH on enamel loss. Comparison of the erosive potential of cola versus non-cola drinks as well as regular sugared and diet versions of the same brands was undertaken. The pH was measured immediately after opening the soft drink can. Enamel slices obtained from freshly extracted teeth were immersed in the soft drinks and weighed at baseline and after 6, 24, and 48 hours of immersion. Non-cola drinks had significantly higher pH values than cola drinks but showed higher mean percent weight loss. By contrast, sugared versions of the cola and non-cola drinks showed significantly lower pH values and higher mean percent weight loss than their diet counterparts. The pH value of the soft drink did not have a significant influence on the mean percent weight loss (r = -0.28). Prolonged exposure to soft drinks can lead to significant enamel loss. Non-cola drinks are more erosive than cola drinks. Sugared versions of cola and non-cola drinks proved to be more erosive than their diet counterparts. The erosive potential of the soft drinks was not related to their pH value.
CAS Registry/EC Number/Name of Substance	0 (Sweetening Agents).
ISSN Print	0363-6771
Publication Type	In Vitro. Journal Article.
Language	English
Date of Publication	2007 Mar-Apr
Entry Date	20070320
Update Date	20070321

FIGURE 8.2. MEDLINE Record

the publishers. Without MeSH, searchers must create "hedges" of possible **textwords.** For example, authors may have used *myocardial, heart, cardiac,* or *cardiovascular* in articles about similar conditions, so all of these words may need to be searched. Each article is "tagged" with an "entry date," which is the field that is used to identify the actual date the article was entered into the database versus its publication date. The entry date for the citations allows NLM itself and the vendors/search interfaces that provide access to MEDLINE to offer "alerting" services where a librarian or library user can set up and store a strategy that searches MEDLINE for the latest records on a regular basis, usually sending the retrieval to the requestor's e-mail. Alerting services are described in Chapter 7.

In addition to these fields, the MEDLINE record includes a number of value-added, controlled vocabulary fields added by NLM indexers. For instance, there is a field for the CA (*Chemical Abstracts*) registry number and the registry name of particular drugs and chemicals mentioned in the article. Enzyme Commission (EC) numbers may also be included. There is also a "publication type" field, which identifies the article as a review article, case study, clinical trial, or any of a number of other carefully defined phrases allowed for this field.

The registry number, registry name, and publication type fields are particularly useful because of their controlled vocabulary—words and phrases which have one and only one meaning in their context. Controlled vocabulary allows the user to search for an article about a particular chemical compound or a particular kind of study without having to rely on either being mentioned in the title or abstract of the article.

The international scope of MEDLINE means that many languages are included. The English translation of the title is enclosed in square brackets, followed by the name of the language. In languages using the Latin alphabet, the complete reference gives the original title. The journal name will be transliterated as necessary.[18]

MeSH

One of the strengths of MEDLINE is its use of a hierarchical list of "Medical Subject Headings," or MeSH.[19] MeSH are organized into "trees" from broader to more narrow concepts, for example, Cardiovascular Diseases > Heart Diseases > Heart Valve Diseases > Aortic Valve Insufficiency. Unlike many Web-generated search engines, human indexers actually examine each article and assign the most specific applicable MeSH. The main points of the article are assigned "major" MeSH, and lesser points "minor" (some vendors call major headings "Focus"). MeSH also uses subheadings, such as diagnosis, therapy, or epidemiology, which further describe or subdivide the assigned MeSH.

The importance of MeSH becomes evident when constructing a search strategy in MEDLINE. The assignment of specific subject headings gives MEDLINE the added dimension of structured subject searching to complement the use of textwords. The differences between using subject headings and textwords, and the concepts of searching using "explode" and "focus," and how these capabilities affect retrieval is demonstrated later in the chapter, in the section "Explode."

Full Text

The growing trend toward open access publishing means that PubMed is able to offer the full text of an increasing number of journals in a linked database called **PubMed Central.**[20] PubMed also provides a feature called LinkOut, which allows libraries to identify their electronic journal holdings so that authorized library users can link directly from PubMed to publishers' sites to obtain full-text articles.[21] Commercial database vendors may themselves be publishers, or have made arrangements with publishers, to offer access to full-text journals linked to the MEDLINE records. Libraries may notify PubMed Central and database vendors that they subscribe to certain full-text journals, and these links are added so that MEDLINE search results lead librarians and users directly to those journals. This section has only discussed how the full text of journal articles to which the library subscribes may be obtained or linked to through a bibliographic database such as MEDLINE or CINAHL. There are other types of full-text databases which are discussed in the section Full-Text Databases.

MEDLINE and PubMed

It is important to differentiate between MEDLINE—the database—and PubMed—the free interface provided by NCBI/NLM. Even librarians sometimes conflate the two terms. MEDLINE was searched through librarian-friendly and end-user interfaces long before NCBI created PubMed. Commercial vendors followed suit with their own user-friendly interfaces. Since its introduction in 1997, PubMed has continued to develop new search features along with the other vendors. An alerting service, links to full text, links to individual library holdings, easier access to MeSH trees, the ability to verify a single citation (called "Single Citation Matcher"), and instructions for command-line, field-specific searching are among the many capabilities that have all greatly enhanced this interface.

Since MEDLINE is now free to the world, many nonmedical libraries include a PubMed link in their database offerings, even though the articles are often technical and full of medical and scientific terminology. In recent years, NLM has created MedlinePlus, which is designed for consumers. NLM has greatly increased its outreach to consumers in the past several years.[22, 23]

OTHER MAJOR DATABASES IN THE HEALTH SCIENCES

Given the scope and size of this chapter, it is not possible to discuss the entire range of databases that health sciences libraries might provide. Libraries in other disciplines or contexts (optometry, podiatry, veterinary medicine, business and corporate settings) may have highly specialized needs. This section briefly describes some of the bibliographic, full-text, monographic, and evidence-based resources most commonly found in health sciences libraries.

Health sciences librarians probably search MEDLINE more than any other database, but it is certainly not the only one available. Indeed, other databases may be more appropriate or should be searched instead of, or as well as, MEDLINE. NLM itself produces many more databases than MEDLINE. Dozens of resources, bibliographic, full text, and directories, are available from NLM and cover topics such as AIDS, drug information, toxicology, the history of medicine, chemical data, hazardous substances, genetics, research projects, information for specific ethnic groups, material in Spanish, and beautiful images of historic books. Readers are encouraged to visit the NLM site <http://www.nlm.nih.gov/databases/> to view the complete list of NLM databases.

The following highly selective group of health sciences databases, primarily produced by commercial vendors, is organized by subject specialty or special features, such as citation indexing. The title of the printed original is listed in parentheses after each database discussed in this section.

Nursing and Allied Health

CINAHL (*Cumulative Index to Nursing and Allied Health Literature*) <http://www.cinahl .com/prodsvcs/cinahldb.htm> indexes not only journals in those disciplines (and library science), but also books, pamphlets, audiovisuals, software, dissertations, and research instruments. It includes the full text of state nursing association journals, legal cases, standards of practice, government documents, and other publications. CINAHL's subject headings were originally based on MeSH and have a similar hierarchical structure.[24]

CINAHL provides the bibliography of references, where publishers have given permission, in a field called "Citations." This is useful for looking up related articles. They are not used for relating articles to those that later cite them, as described later in the section Citation Indexing.

ProQuest also publishes a nursing index <http://proquest.com/products_pq/descriptions/pq_nursingahs.shtml> with direct links to full-text nursing journal articles. Additional nursing journals were added to *Science Citation Index* in 2006.

International Coverage

EMBASE (printed *Excerpta Medica*) <http://info.embase.com/embase_com/about/index.shtml>, produced by the publisher Elsevier, contains more than 18 million citations to biomedical and pharmacological journal literature from 1974 to the present and emphasizes international research. It has its own extensive subject heading system. Most studies comparing EMBASE with MEDLINE have discussed specific subjects or areas of research.[25, 26] Conclusions are that the two are complementary (except for EMBASE's inclusion of international and pharmaceutical literature), and libraries that can afford EMBASE will enjoy the additional coverage.

Psychology and Social Sciences

PsycINFO (*Psychological Abstracts*) is important for psychological and social aspects of medicine; in addition to journal articles, books, and book chapters, it includes dissertations. PsycINFO's references include the authors' full names. PsycINFO does write its own abstracts, with authorship provided. Another index, *Social Sciences Citation Index,* is part of the Web of Science family discussed later under Citation Indexing.

Pharmacology and Drug Names

Micromedex (owned by Thomson) is found in hospitals and schools of pharmacy. Specific subsections, such as consumer information, or complementary and alternative medicine, can be purchased separately. *Physicians Desk Reference (PDR*—it now has offspring in specialty areas) used to be provided free of charge to doctors' offices. It contains the package inserts that are included with prescriptions, but also photographs of drugs and other useful information. PDR Electronic Library is also available through Thomson <http://www.thomsonhc.com/hes/librarian>. The FDA Web site <http://www.fda.gov> has both professional- and consumer-level information.

Selected Other Health-Related Databases

Other databases that may contain relevant material include AGRICOLA (from the National Agricultural Library), BIOSIS (*Biological Abstracts*), CA SEARCH (*Chemical Abstracts*), or **TOXNET** (Toxicology Data Network from NLM). Academic libraries or those affiliated with larger university libraries are more likely to have access to BIOSIS and/or CA SEARCH. Dialog, now owned by Thomson Scientific, allows per-minute searches of CA SEARCH. Academic health sciences libraries may have access to CA SEARCH through their parent university via SciFinder Scholar <http://www.cas.org/products/sfacad/index.html>, which is based on "seats" (number of simultaneous users).

Citation Indexing

Eugene Garfield and the Institute for Scientific Information (ISI) devised another enhancement to bibliographic database construction, called **citation indexing.** This produced a series of printed indexes, now available online in Thomson's Web of Science. The two indexes most often subscribed to in health sciences libraries are *Science Citation Index* and *Social Science Citation Index* along with *Journal Citation Reports.* In citation indexing, the references at the end of articles are analyzed to show how often they were cited (i.e., quoted) over the years since publication. Searchers can trace a topic back in time and identify the seminal articles at its origin. Each reference shows how often the article has been cited.

It must be noted that this is not an inexpensive database and is only available from the producers. Libraries may reduce their cost by subscribing to a more recent range of years, although this obviously limits how far back in time citations can be traced. A "Cited Reference Search," however, partly solves the year-range problem when only recent years are subscribed to by the library. When a Cited Reference Search is conducted, the searcher looks for specific articles or authors, and the results show how often the articles were cited. Articles within the range to which the library has subscribed have "live" links back to the cited articles; those beyond the range are also displayed, but without the links.

The accompanying database, *Journal Citation Reports (JCR),* provides an analysis of citation patterns that results in a ranking of journals, called **impact factors,** according to how often that journal has been cited overall (see Figure 8.3). *JCR* does not analyze citations of individual articles or authors. Mathematical formulas take into account how many articles the journal has published. The impact factors are recalculated annually. If this database is new to an institution, or new researchers are hired that have not seen it before, librarians must be prepared to explain what the impact factors do and do *not* indicate. It is usually the summer of the following year before the previous year's rankings have been calculated. Requests like, "I would like to know my rankings for the past ten years . . ." require that the librarian explain that a journal's ranking may have little or nothing to do with articles this author may have written. The best the researcher can be told is that there may be a certain prestige in having published in journals that have consistently high impact factors.

Like all of the databases discussed in this chapter, the journal title coverage of each database affects search retrieval. Impact factors only apply to the journals indexed in Web of Science. For example, the impact factor for *JAMA* for 2006 was 23.175, which made it third in a list of 103 titles in the category "Medicine, General & Internal." It means that the number of times articles published in *JAMA* in 2006, taking into account the total number of articles in each publication, ranked this high. Newer journal titles obviously will take a few years to gain a ranking, as authors must first become aware of the new journal, evaluate the quality of the articles, and decide to cite articles from the new journal.

Current Contents is an alerting service, also published by ISI in print and later online. It was particularly useful when journals were only available in print. *Current Contents* shows articles that are about to published. Many journals and publishers now provide their own alerting services for those users who are particularly interested in specific journals. MEDLINE and CINAHL also have a similar capability, but their journal coverage is not the same as Web of Science. No additional subscription is needed for these alerting services.

Searchers who are new to using the Thomson citation indexes need to know that the "keyword" field in these records is based on the authors' own suggestions and the occurrence of words in the references of the articles. These keywords do not have the authority of the human-assigned MeSH used for MEDLINE. Indeed, they can be misleading; for example, if enough of the references discuss that a particular biomarker is *not* an indicator of breast cancer, just the occurrences of "breast cancer" will cause it to be added to the keywords.

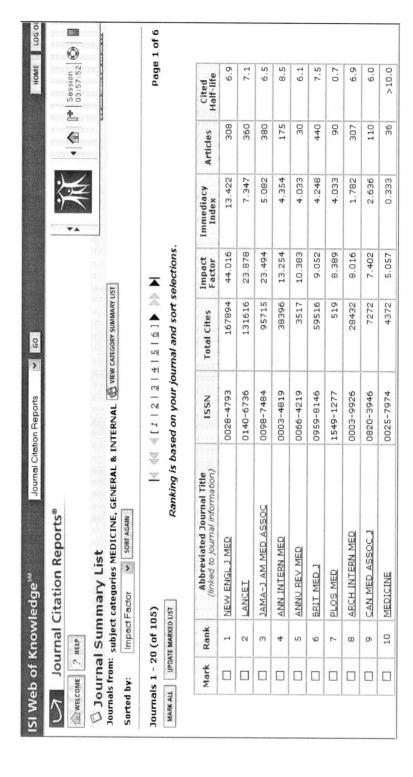

FIGURE 8.3. Impact Factor for *JAMA* in *JCR*. *Source:* Data from the 2005 Science Edition of the *Journal Citation Reports*™ from Thomson Scientific.

FULL-TEXT DATABASES

Evidence-Based Databases

The "randomised [*sic*] clinical trial" was largely the invention of Archie Cochrane, the British (hence the original spelling) researcher whose name lives on in the "Cochrane Collaboration."[27] Meta-analysis of several studies provides the "**evidence-based medicine**" (or nursing, or dentistry, or practice, or librarianship). Journals such as *ACP Journal Club, BMJ Clinical Evidence,* and *Evidence-Based Nursing* are devoted to evidence. MEDLINE and CINAHL are good sources for investigating this topic. The MeSH "Evidence-Based Medicine" appeared in 1997. CINAHL added the subject heading "Nursing Practice, Evidence-Based" in 2000. By the time the database adds a subject heading, the indexers have already noticed enough articles on the topic to recommend its addition. Earlier articles must be located in the databases via textwords, to supplement the subject headings.

Other vendors have produced full-text databases based on, or claiming to be based on, evidence. DoctorEvidence <http://www.doctorevidence.com/>, DynaMed <http://www.ebscohost.com/dynamed/>, InfoPOEMs <http://www.infopoems.com/>, MDConsult <http://home.mdconsult.com>, and UpToDate <http://www.uptodate.com/>—all claim to be based either on evidence or on systematic searches of major journals. Their monographs are not necessarily designed for the specialist and may be interesting for health sciences librarians and their users. The whole topic of "evidence" is discussed in detail in Chapter 11, "Evidence-Based Practice."

Other Full-Text Providers and Web Searching

Numerous professional organizations and government departments have Web sites with useful monographs; the FDA (U.S. Food and Drug Administration) <http://www.fda.gov> is a good example. Some, such as Medem <http://www.medem.com>, which derives much information from medical societies and organizations, are fee-based.

Mention must be made in this discussion of the way many (millions) of people look for medical topics and advice through Google. Google Scholar <http://scholar.google.com/> is more like a bibliographic database that combs the literature to provide links to scholarly journal articles and other relevant material. It may be added to the other databases being searched to answer a question. Elsevier's Scopus <http://scopus.com> and EBSCO's Academic Search Premier <http://www.epnet.com/thistopic.php?marketID=1&topicID=1> (login required) provide similar services, and this trend is spreading; Yahoo!, Ask Jeeves, Microsoft's own search system, and numerous other Web crawlers and popular interfaces are moving into the more scholarly arena. Health sciences students are particularly fond of searching for their library assignments using crawlers, even after the librarian has patiently demonstrated MEDLINE and other structured databases. Unfortunately, these systems are so vast that they often *do* lead to useful sites, especially disease-specific professional organizations, academic lecture notes, and even published articles. They also lead to spurious sites and downright commercial advertising. Students who have grown up with Web crawlers and have become experts in searching them, may find the answer to a particular question in the assignment, but when the time comes to do a comprehensive search for patient care or research, they must know how to search the professional literature in full.

PROVIDING SEARCH SERVICES

Mediated Searching

As discussed in the previous chapter, working with a user's information request must be refined to the point that the librarian understands exactly what is needed. Whether face-to-face or via e-mail or other messaging systems, this initial conversation is never more important than when providing search services. If the librarian does not quite understand the scientific terminology, or needs more detail on the patient case, he or she must ask further questions. The librarian may have considerable work to do before beginning the search. The requestor may be using terminology (drug names are a classic case) that must be searched as keywords to reveal the subject headings. The librarian may need to create a "hedge" of synonyms and related terms to ensure comprehensive retrieval. If the subject matter warrants it, nursing questions may need CINAHL; psychological, social, and emotional topics may need PsycINFO or *Social Science Citation Index;* biochemistry and microbiology may need *Science Citation Index.* If the vendor allows for simultaneous searching of multiple databases, perhaps with the ability to remove duplicates, this may indicate whether the search should use more than one database. A caveat: removing duplicates (sometimes called "de-duping") will indeed remove identical records, but some that actually refer to the same article may have fields that look sufficiently different that the de-duping may not find them all.

The initial search may retrieve nothing, or thousands of references. If the librarian is not having much success, or needs to further clarify the request, the user must be contacted again. If the request was urgent, the user must be contacted immediately, to discuss further avenues for searching. Whether urgent or not, the user could be invited to the library to watch the search and make suggestions, or, if the user prefers, the librarian could go to the office, clinic, or lab with printouts, or use the requestor's workstation to demonstrate the search. If the request came to the librarian through an intermediary such as an administrative/clinic assistant or secretary, the librarian may endeavor to reach the original requester for clarification.[28] More detail on the actual process of conducting a mediated search appears later in this chapter.

End Users

Database producers (including NLM) promote and market their user-friendly interfaces to individuals. Just as there are users who never have any intention of doing their own searching, there are others who enjoy the thrill of the hunt. This is the audience that attends both on-site vendor demonstrations and library classes. The literature abounds with discussion of the pros and cons of end-user searching. These analyses have dwindled over the years as user-friendly interfaces have proliferated and improved, and computers have appeared on every desk.[29]

Vendors are usually very willing to provide on-site training, with printed handouts, when libraries buy a new interface or database, or when information services librarians feel they and their users need an update. Some vendors will provide prerecorded demonstrations; some will provide training via **"webinars,"** online interactive training sessions. Users should be invited to attend sessions in the library or be notified of the availability of online sessions. Those who participate (in person or virtually) will be users who regularly do their own searching; others may be interested in a better understanding of the features of the interface and/or the databases, so they know what the librarians can do for them. Flyers, institution-wide e-mail, or other methods of advertisement are also good for enhancing the image of the library as a place that is state-of-the-art and providing the very latest information-seeking methods.

THE MEDIATED SEARCH PROCESS

Receiving the Request

There are innumerable ways to advertise and receive mediated search requests Examples of ways to receive a request include the following:

- Asking users who come to the library, especially those who ask for help at the information desk, or are sitting at computer terminals, if they are aware of this service
- Including this service in every library tour, demonstration, or class
- Flyers and posters with the library URL, e-mail, or phone number
- "Ask a Librarian" on the Web site, offering virtual reference, or inviting e-mail or telephone calls
- Printed search request forms at the information/service desk, or the library Web site, to be filled out and sent back online
- Conversations in the hallway, after a meeting, or even in the cafeteria that lead to users' discussing their information needs

Triage

As discussed in Chapter 7, all information requests may need to be ranked by urgency, prioritizing patient care requests, or by length of time the answer may take, so that easier questions can be answered speedily, giving time for reflection on the more difficult ones. Larger libraries may have literature searching assigned to one or two librarians who specialize in this. Triage can be problematic in searching: urgent requests obviously come first, but after that a seemingly simple topic may turn out to be hard to find and require more research than was anticipated. At the time a search request is received, asking when the results are needed helps to prioritize requests. If the user is kept apprised of the librarian's progress when a search does take a long time, he or she will appreciate that a thorough job is being done.

Conducting the Search

The librarian is now ready to conduct the search. It must be noted that all of the techniques described here are not provided by all vendors, and methods for applying them differ greatly. Librarians, and users who prefer to run their own searches, need to become familiar with the particular techniques used by each system.[30, 31] Published guides to online searching can be helpful,[32, 33] but librarians must be aware that the picture changes constantly.

There is an old saying of which experienced searchers are well aware: "You get what you ask for." When searching a database, the information services librarian must familiarize himself or herself with its structure, the specific search techniques that are applicable to that database, and how Boolean operators are used in different interfaces, and he or she needs to be able to adjust and modify the search depending on results. Understanding why a search retrieved nonrelevant results is important to ultimately obtaining valid, relevant retrieval.

Preliminary work has already been done:

- The librarian has already conducted one or more extensive interviews with the user, in person or via telephone, e-mail, or chat, to clarify exactly what is needed, for what purpose, and when it is needed. This is the "reference interview."
- Trial searches have determined which databases should be searched.

- Trial searches have also shown which subject headings, keywords, or textwords (or combinations thereof) should be used.

Many of the features of the most important health sciences databases have been mentioned. Beyond these, there are several other features that the new searcher needs to be aware of and investigate in each database.

Natural Language Processing

Not everyone thinks that a **controlled thesaurus** such as MeSH is the best way to search a database. Students of the science of information retrieval will have discussed "natural language processing" or NLP.[33] NLP may use techniques such as "weighting" to evaluate how occurrences of words, or proximity of words and phrases, are likely to indicate relevance, eliminating the possibility of error or bias by human indexers assigning subject headings. These techniques work well for "mining" huge databases such as patient records or large blocks of text. Experienced searchers may indeed add textwords (usually considered to be words in the title and abstract) into a search strategy with Boolean "OR" for more comprehensive retrieval.

Boolean Logic

A mathematician named George Boole devised an algebraic use of "operators," called "Boolean logic," to combine concepts. It is usually explained with overlapping circles, as shown in the more complete set of examples from Colorado State University (see Figure 8.4).[34] In a real search statement the terms would be qualified with which field they come from, for example, subject, author, animal species, textwords. The Boolean operators and basic logical combinations include the following:

- AND means that all words, subjects, or concepts must be present. For example, "asthma AND cat" or "Smith J AND Brown C" or "asthma AND Smith J AND Chicago."
- OR means that either word may be present; it will retrieve comprehensively from both terms separately: "cat OR dog."
- Boolean operators are searched in specific order. OR precedes AND, so the OR terms would be dealt with first, then added to the AND terms: "asthma AND (cat OR dog)." This nesting assures that both "cat" or "dog" are found first, then that set is combined with "asthma."
- NOT eliminates the specified words: "allergies NOT (cat OR dog)."

Truncation

Truncation is used to find variants of words and names. The truncation symbol is different among vendors (PubMed = *, Dialog = ?, Ovid = $, Web of Science = *). Truncation is mostly used at the end of words, but some interfaces allow truncation at the beginning or in the middle of words; this is useful for those British spellings that include Greek diphthongs: orthop(a)edic, an(a)esthesia; also wom?n for singular or plural. These insertions are sometimes referred to as "wildcards." They can be used with abstracts, textwords, and authors. Wildcards usually cannot be used for subject headings and other controlled vocabulary, which must usually be spelled exactly and completely.

Venn Diagrams

Venn diagrams are a useful way to visualize Boolean logic.

AND looks like this:

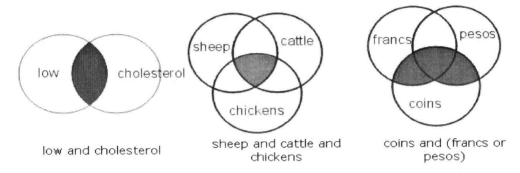

| low and cholesterol | sheep and cattle and chickens | coins and (francs or pesos) |

Scenarios:

> I need articles about low cholesterol.
> He needs information about running a farm with sheep, cattle, and chickens.
> She need francs and pesos in coins.

OR looks like this:

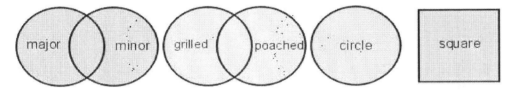

FIGURE 8.4. Boolean Operators. *Source:* From <http://lib.colostate.edu/hotto/others/venn/html> by Naomi Lederer, Reference Librarian, Associate Professor, Morgan Library, Colorado State University. Used with permission from the author.

Institutional Affiliations

Science Citation Index (SCI) provides affiliations for all authors. There are two things to understand: unlike most databases, *SCI* does not use the address or affiliation exactly as listed in the journal. *SCI* has standard abbreviations, e.g., UNIV for University. This can be very useful: City of Hope National Medical Center is a cancer hospital in California. The search *AD = city and hope* produces the correct place but also *Hope* Circle, in Salt Lake *City*. The searcher notices that CITY HOPE is the *SCI* abbreviation that retrieves only the correct address. A second consideration: an article may have nine authors and five addresses. The addresses are in the same order as the authors, but apart from the first and last authors, it is not possible to determine which authors belong to the same address.

"Explode"

In hierarchical subject headings, as used in MEDLINE and CINAHL, the "explode" command will add all the headings indented, i.e., more specific, in the "trees" under the chosen heading. Indexers are instructed to assign the most specific heading. Searching only with the more general heading without "exploding" the term may omit huge numbers of articles that were assigned more specific headings. EDUCATION (as a subject heading) in CINAHL, for example, retrieved 1,075 references in late March 2007. Making this the "major" heading or the "focus" of the article reduces this to 543. These articles are about education *in general*. Under EDUCATION in the "trees" are 52 more specific headings. Many have more postings than the overall heading (for example, CURRICULUM has 6,784). Exploding EDUCATION results in 233,338 citations, or "hits." Adding "major" or "focus" to this yields 111,933. Using EDUCATION as a textword (it must appear in title or abstract) gives only 61,754. Clearly, the searcher must understand how the assignment of subject headings works! In summary:

- EDUCATION (subject heading) 1,075
- EDUCATION (*major* or *focus*) 543
- Explode EDUCATION 233,338
- Explode EDUCATION (*major* or *focus*) 111,933
- EDUCATION as textword 61,754

Readers are encouraged to consult other sources for a more detailed explanation of this advanced searching concept.[35, 36]

Limits

Depending on the database and the interface, "limits" are handled differently. Basic limits (English, Human, Abstract, Publication Year, Full Text, Local Holdings) may be offered on the top page of the search interface, with the lines of search strategy. Further limits may be offered in drop-down lists: Language (other than English), Gender, Age, Publication Type, Animals. Adding a limit to a subject search is the equivalent of "ANDing" another term, thus reducing the size of the retrieval.

Display, Sort, Print, E-Mail, Download

There is great variation among databases and vendors in the way retrieval can be output. Displays can be altered to include abstracts and subject headings/keywords, or the "full" record with the unique identifier (in MEDLINE) codes for journals, journal subsets, dates the article was entered and revised, and (in *Science Citation Index*) the number of times articles have been cited.

Retrieval can be sorted in a variety of ways. For example, sorting by journal title facilitates finding the printed journals on the shelf or searching the full text in the journal's database; sorting by authors' names gives the user a good idea of who is doing the most work in the field of interest; or sorting by date of publication, from most recent to oldest, may be the most important element for other users. Sorting can usually be done before printing or e-mailing results.

Print options usually include the ability to choose which fields to print and whether they will appear with vendor information and field tags. They can also be "formatted for print," creating a list that looks more like a regular bibliography.

Some vendors provide the ability to send retrieval via e-mail in most of the formats that have just been described. References can be in the body of the message or attached as formatted files.

When using a less familiar interface, or if the information services librarian performing a mediated search is unsure of the formatting, it is a good idea to send the e-mail to himself or herself first, as a test.

Personal Filing Systems

Another way to control formatting and output is to download records into a personal filing system. In recent years, Thomson Corporation has acquired most of the major personal filing software programs, specifically EndNote, Reference Manager, and ProCite. They are so similar in this context that only EndNote will be mentioned further. Databases in the Web of Science, and other vendors, provide easy access to these programs. EndNote requires that the searcher choose from a long list of databases and interfaces used for the retrieval, for correct formatting by EndNote. Programs such as EndNote offer various formats for creating subset files, for printing or formatting according to the requirements of a journal, since one of the main purposes of these programs is to lay out bibliographies in manuscripts. Some library users may request that the information services librarian send the search retrieval to them as EndNote "libraries," as the files are called.

EVALUATING AND DELIVERING THE RESULTS OF THE SEARCH

The librarian needs to examine the search results, to determine which are the best matches for the request, and to eliminate "false drops." The latter are records that match what the searcher asked for, but not what the requestor wanted, e.g., AIDS, the disease, or "aids" meaning assistive devices. The librarian may know from experience with a particular user whether he or she would prefer a few "high quality" (right on target) references/articles, or a broader approach. The next big question is whether the user wants a bibliography or some full-text articles. Once more, the librarian has either asked the user in advance or knows the user's preferences.

The searcher is now ready to send the final result to the user. This may not, however, always be the *final* result. If the librarian is comfortable that the retrieval really is just what was requested, it can be sent by the user's preferred method: internal mail, U.S. mail, FAX, PDF attached to e-mail, or as a direct e-mail to the requestor from the database vendor. If the librarian has any qualms, he or she should also send the user a message, asking if this is acceptable, or if the user can pick out the best articles and send the list back to the librarian, which will give him or her clues on how to refine the search.

In either case, the information services librarian should keep records of the searches. These could be Word files, or stored in EndNote. The records should be retrievable or searchable by the user's name, the subject, and the final search strategy. This enables the librarian to see whether a user has requested searches in the past, and what he or she seems to be researching. A library with a large volume of search requests may find that this subject, or a similar one, has been searched before, so the search strategy will assist in a future search on the same topic. If a user requests a repeat search on the same topic, the librarian might suggest that the user set up an alerting service to receive search results on a regular basis.

CONCLUSION

Retrieval of information is a major service provided by health sciences libraries. Subscriptions to as many databases as possible from the same vendor gives a common interface, facilitating searching by both librarians and end users. There will still be resources that have their own interfaces and special methods for logging in. This means that while librarians will endeavor to become fluent in the use of all vendor products to which the library subscribes, many users will opt for mediated searches rather than learn all of the search interfaces.

Typing words into Google or Yahoo! is becoming increasingly popular. Searchers will probably retrieve only a small percentage of what they really want. It is important that this be explained at every possible opportunity. The authority and quality behind the construction of the health sciences databases and resources described in this chapter must be fully understood and appreciated by librarians, and continually promoted and explained to the users that health sciences librarians serve. This is essential for the health of all.

This rather prosaic discussion of retrieving biomedical information for library users may not sound exciting. It *is*! It may not be as profitable as gold mining or as thrilling as a bungee jump, but finding *the* article that assists in diagnosis or modifying the surgical procedure, identifies better ways to give the patient comfort and peace of mind, or aids the faculty member investigating stem cells—these bring *Eureka!* moments, gratitude and appreciation, and the indescribable, inexpressible satisfaction of a job well done.

REFERENCES

1. Quint, B. "'No Guts, No Glory': Information Professionals March into the 22nd Century." Luminary Lectures @ Your Library (lecture to Library of Congress; phone conference). Available: <http://www.loc.gov/rr/program/lectures/quint.html>. Accessed: March 31, 2007.

2. Quint, B. Quote from Searcher, January 1996. In *The Quintessential Searcher; The Wit & Wisdom of Barbara Quint,* edited by M. Block. Nedford, NJ: Information Today, Inc., 2001. Available: <http://books.infotoday.com/books/QuintSearcher.shtml>. Accessed: March 31, 2007.

3. Cooper, J.C. "Organization of the Biomedical Literature." Available: <http://people.musc.edu/~cooperjc/organizationoflit.htm>. Accessed: March 30, 2007.

4. Berard, G.L. "Session One—Lecture Notes." Carnegie Mellon University. Available: <http://www.andrew.cmu.edu/user/lberard/Ses1Notes.html>. Accessed: March 30, 2007.

5. Wood, E.H. "Open Access Publishing: Implications for Libraries." *Journal of Electronic Resources in Medical Libraries* 2, no. 2 (2005): 1-12.

6. Boorkman, J.A.; Huber, J.T.; and Roper, F.W. *Introduction to Reference Sources in the Health Sciences.* 4th ed. New York: Neal-Schuman, 2004.

7. Alliance for Human Research Protection. "OHRP Suspends Johns Hopkins Research License for Fed Funded Research." Available: <http://www.ahrp.org/infomail/0701/19.php>. Accessed: April 12, 2007.

8. Perkins, E. "Johns Hopkins' Tragedy: Could Librarians Have Prevented a Death?" *Information Today.* Available: <http://newsbreaks.infotoday.com/nbreader.asp?ArticleID=17534>. Accessed: April 12, 2007.

9. National Library of Medicine. "Fact Sheet MEDLINE®." Available: <http://www.nlm.nih.gov/pubs/factsheets/medline.html>. Accessed: March 12, 2007.

10. National Library of Medicine. "History of MeSH." Available: <http://www.nlm.nih.gov/mesh/intro_hist2006.html>. Accessed: April 2, 2007.

11. Wood, E.H., and Chiang, D. "Introduction and Overview." In *CD-ROM Implementation and Networking in Health Sciences Libraries,* edited by M.S. Wood, 31-44. Binghamton, NY: The Haworth Press, Inc., 1993.

12. Wood, E.H., and Kittle, P. "CD-ROM: The Past and the Future." In *CD-ROM Implementation and Networking in Health Sciences Libraries,* edited by M.S. Wood, 45-55. Binghamton, NY: The Haworth Press, Inc., 1993.

13. Williams, J.F. II. "MEDLINE Training and the Transition to Online." *NLM Technical Bulletin* 209, Spec Issue (September 1986): 13.

14. van Bemmel, J.H. "Knowledge for Medicine and Health Care—Laudation at the Occasion of the Honorary Doctorate Bestowed to Donald A.B. Lindberg by UMIT, University for Health Sciences, Medical Informatics and Technology in Innsbruck, Tyrol, Austria." *Methods of Information in Medicine* 44, no. 4 (2005): 596-600.

15. Wood, E.H. "MEDLINE: The Options for Health Professionals." *Journal of the American Medical Informatics Association* 1(September/October 1994): 372-80.

16. Horowitz, G.L., and Bleich, H.L. "PaperChase: A Computer Program to Search the Medical Literature." *New England Journal of Medicine* 305(October 15, 1981): 924-30.

17. Laynor, B.; Calabretta, N.; and Ross, R. "Building a miniMEDLINE Database: Which Journals to Choose? *Bulletin of the Medical Library Association* 76, no. 2 (April 1988): 146-50.

18. Wood, E.H. "SEARCH TIP: Translating with MEDLINE." *Online* 15(November 1991): 48.

19. The Basics of Medical Subject Headings. Available: <http://www.nlm.nih.gov/bsd/disted/mesh/index.html>. Accessed: March 15, 2007.

20. PubMed Central. Available: <http://www.pubmedcentral.nih.gov>. Accessed: March 23, 2007.

21. Schott, M.J. "PubMed Enhancements: Fulfilling the Promise of a Great Product." *Medical Reference Services Quarterly* 23, no.4 (Winter 2004): 1-11.

22. National Library of Medicine. "MEDLINEplus Website Launched. New Database Is Geared to Consumers' Health Information Needs." *NLM Newsline* 53, no. 3 & 4 (July-December 1998). Available: <http://www.nlm.nih.gov/archive/20040423/pubs/nlmnews/juldec98.html#MEDLINEplus>. Accessed: April 1, 2007.

23. Stephenson, J. "National Library of Medicine to Help Consumers Use Online Health Data." *JAMA* 283(April 5, 2000): 1675-6.

24. CINAHL. "The CINAHL® Database." Available: <http://www.cinahl.com/prodsvcs/cinahldb.htm>. Accessed: March 16, 2007.

25. Wong, S.S.; Wilczynski, N.L.; and Haynes, R.B. "Comparison of Top-Performing Search Strategies for Detecting Clinically Sound Treatment Studies and Systematic Reviews in MEDLINE and EMBASE." *Journal of the Medical Library Association* 94, no. 4 (October 2006): 451-5.

26. Wilkins, T.; Gillies, R.A.; and Davies, K. "EMBASE Versus MEDLINE for Family Medicine Searches: Can MEDLINE Searches Find the Forest or a Tree?" *Canadian Family Physician* 51(June 2005: 845.

27. Cochrane Collaboration. "The Name Behind the Cochrane Collaboration." Available: <http://www.cochrane.org/docs/archieco.htm>. Accessed: March 20, 2007.

28. Wu, M., and Liu, Y. "Intermediary's Information Seeking, Inquiring Minds, and Elicitation Styles." *Journal of the American Society for Information Science and Technology* 54(October 2003): 1117-33.

29. Arnott Smith, C. "An Evolution of Experts: MEDLINE in the Library School." *Journal of the Medical Library Association* 93, no. 1 (January 2005): 53-60.

30. Katcher, B.S. *Medline: A Guide to Effective Searching in PubMed and Other Interfaces.* 2nd ed. San Francisco: Ashbury Press, 2006.

31. Stave, C.D. *Field Guide to Medline: Making Searching Simple.* Philadelphia: Lippincott Williams & Wilkins, 2003.

32. Bell, S.S. *Librarian's Guide to Online Searching.* Westport, CT: Libraries Unlimited, 2006.

33. Hersh, W.R. *Information Retrieval: A Health and Biomedical Perspective.* 2nd ed. New York: Springer, 2003.

34. Colorado State University Libraries. "Venn Diagrams." Available: <http://lib.colostate.edu/howto/others/venn.html>. Accessed: March 25, 2007.

35. National Library of Medicine. "PubMed Tutorial." Available: <http://www.nlm.nih.gov/bsd/pubmed_tutorial/m1001.html>. Accessed: March 12, 2007.

36. CINAHL. "CINAHL Search Tools." Available: <http://www.cinahl.com/prodsvcs/prodsvcs.htm>. Accessed: March 16, 2007.

Chapter 9

Marketing, Public Relations, and Communication

Patricia C. Higginbottom
Lisa A. Ennis

SUMMARY. Marketing library resources and services in the digital age is essential in every library. This chapter will explain the need for marketing and public relations and will distinguish how these activities are different in health sciences libraries. This chapter explores and compares the many ways for librarians and libraries to connect with users. This discussion also includes an overall approach to developing marketing plans and securing funding for public relations activities.

INTRODUCTION

Libraries are more than just collections of books and other materials. Libraries are dynamic forces in their communities with the power to improve lives. Modern marketing demands that librarians look beyond their traditional roles ("outside the book") to find new ways to connect with people and further their success.[1]

Libraries exist to serve their users. Libraries and librarians connect people with sources of information and entertainment in order to enrich their lives. In today's electronic environment, librarians must promote and market both library resources and themselves to the people they intend to serve. This chapter describes marketing and **public relations** in health sciences libraries both in the academic and clinical settings. Marketing concepts are not difficult to understand, and most marketing techniques are easy to implement. For some librarians, the very notion of marketing is difficult to accept. Why should something so obviously good as libraries have to be promoted? Sometimes librarians are their own worst enemies, because they refuse to promote themselves and libraries as fundamental parts of their communities. However, it is because libraries and librarians are such an integral part of the American tapestry that marketing them can be so easy and fun. People cannot use or support what they do not know about, understand, or value. In marketing librarians and libraries, users must be made to realize that they need and want these services and resources, thereby generating extra value. So, it is up to librarians to awaken that need and want within their potential users.

Marketing Basics

Marketing is about building relationships with the people who use one's goods or services. According to Kotler and Armstrong, in the tenth edition of their *Principles of Marketing*, the aim of marketing activities is "to build and manage profitable customer relationships."[2] In *Marketing/Planning Library and Information Services*, Weingand describes marketing as "an exchange relationship: a process providing mutual benefit to both parties in the transaction."[3] A term closely related to marketing is public relations or PR. At its most basic, PR is "the art and technique of relating to the public."[4] Weingand goes on to say that the communication aspects of public relations consist of publicity and personal contact.[3]

There are many informative introductory books that describe the basics of marketing and the marketing mix, as portrayed in Table 9.1. Good overviews are found in the aforementioned *Principles of Marketing* text, or in *Marketing: An Introduction* by the same authors.[5] Additional recommended books are found in the selected readings in Appendix 9.A. Librarians should note, though, that general marketing works are often targeted to for-profit businesses, not libraries. Therefore, the strategies and information in general marketing textbooks are not always applicable to the activities, goals, and missions of libraries. As a result, consulting sources that relate marketing to the social sector is necessary. A helpful introduction to library marketing is Ash and Wood's chapter in *Administration and Management in Health Sciences Libraries*.[6] Owens's "Marketing in Library and Information Science: A Selected Review of the Literature" serves as a good review of the library literature related to promotions and marketing.[7]

Effective marketing is not rocket science. As Wisniewski and Fichter explain in their article, "Electronic Resources Won't Sell Themselves: Marketing Tips," there are basically six elements needed to effectively market anything: a defined market, something to promote, a targeted audience, a venue, an appropriate message, and a way to evaluate the effort and outcomes.[8] By outlining these six elements ahead of time, librarians can create an efficient and effective marketing strategy. Wisniewski and Fichter go on to explain:

> Our users' attention is a finite resource. If we fill it with white noise, where nine out of 10 announcements aren't relevant, then users will simply tune us out. The unfortunately rather ubiquitous "database of the month" or "resource of the month" is a perfect example of this.[8]

Promoting a specific resource or service to a targeted audience at a crucial time is the most effective way to market anything.

Branding

Another important part of marketing is the concept of "branding." When most people think of branding, they think of a snazzy logo or a catchy jingle, but branding is much more than just a simple image or tune. Branding is about creating an identity in the users' minds and hearts. As Shaffer states, branding is internal and "lies at the heart of those intangible attributes that define a product, service, or entity."[9] Branding is anything and everything that gives libraries and librarians a unique identity and fosters a connection between the users and that identity. Branding is a set of elements like a logo, name, slogan, services, Web presence, events, colors, mascot, or

TABLE 9.1. Marketing Mix

Focus	Characteristics
Product	Resources and services offered
Price	Includes more then the amount paid for the service; can include costs saved
Place	Can include both physical and virtual spaces
Promotion	All the ways you communicate with users

theme. To understand the power of branding, all one needs to consider are everyday images such as "golden arches" and a "swoosh," or slogans like "Just Do It" and "A Few Good Men." Most college athletic departments, for instance, understand branding very well. In essence, branding means positioning the library and its librarians so that when users think of them they feel good and maybe even smile.

MARKETING IN LIBRARIES

With the vast proliferation of electronic resources today, a number of popularly held beliefs seem to signal the downfall and irrelevance of physical libraries in today's virtual world.[10] Librarians have traditionally gone about their work in a quiet behind-the-scenes sort of way. In the past, when people used library resources, they immediately recognized the connection between their need for information and the physical existence of the library. Today, however, many people think that libraries are extraneous and outdated. People also believe that libraries are no longer necessary because everything appears to be on the Internet. They fail to realize that very little full-text, high-quality information is freely available on the Internet, and, further, they do not see the role librarians play in licensing, creating, organizing, and providing access to reliable resources. To combat this shortsighted perspective, librarians have turned to marketing, public relations, and advertising to get their message across to users. Library marketing is about finding out what users need and filling that need as well as getting people to want what libraries have. While most of the literature on marketing comes from the corporate world, health sciences librarians can take the best from business and meld it to the special environment of their library and their institution, remembering that businesses and libraries often have very different goals and missions and measure success differently.

In their efforts to remain relevant to users, librarians must market both their libraries, including the collections and physical spaces, and their services. Because potential library customers cannot use services they do not know exist, libraries have always had to come up with different ways to inform their target populations about events, materials, activities, and services. Librarians must market themselves and their libraries for a number of reasons: first, to create a user demand for the library's resources and services, so that the library can in turn advocate for the money to maintain those resources and services; and, second, to promote new programs and services that will enrich users' lives. The key to marketing, however, is much more than just advertising already existing services. Marketing entails actively learning what users want and need, and finding dynamic ways to provide those things as well as creative ways to let users know about them.

HOW MARKETING HAS CHANGED

Even though modes of communication have multiplied and advanced in recent years, fifteen or twenty years ago it was actually easier to find out what users wanted and to get that information to them, because to use the library, they had to visit the building. Librarians had ample opportunities to connect with users; as people came in to check out books or read print journals, they would see strategically posted flyers and announcement boards, and library employees were able to place brochures in the books that had just been checked out. In short, librarians were able to talk face-to-face with their users.

Today, however, people physically visit libraries less often and instead use the library's resources and services virtually. For health sciences libraries, this change means that people who once came into the library to photocopy a journal article now access it online and print it out in their offices or homes. They no longer see the various notices by the copy machine alerting users to new resources or events. They do not drop by the reference desk to request a search and talk a bit because now they generally do their own searching online, and many times, if they do ask for help, they do so by phone, e-mail, or chat. People now use libraries from their homes and offices for convenience.

While librarians encourage users to access the library remotely, the unfortunate side effect is the loss of face-to-face contact with users. With people obtaining information in so many ways (newspapers, television, radio, magazines, the Internet, blogs, newsfeeds, mail, e-mail, phone, and more), librarians have to be skilled at marketing in order to get their message across and remain relevant and important in users' lives. The mission of libraries and librarians is to enrich people's lives and to serve as a public good; but to accomplish these goals, they must publicize what they do and how successful they are at doing it.

MARKETING IN HEALTH SCIENCES LIBRARIES

Marketing strategies and techniques have a variety of similarities no matter the type of library, whether public, academic, or health sciences. There are basic skills needed regardless of the type of library or services being marketed. There are, however, some aspects to marketing that are unique to health sciences libraries. As in any library, librarians need to tailor their messages to specific audiences. The clientele of a health sciences library is often very different from that of other types of libraries. The health professionals who use health sciences libraries generally have a very high level of education. They also tend to be very busy and are inundated with information. They will often have a higher level of skill or mastery in finding information—or at least think they do. When they need information, it often can be considered very urgent—literally life or death in a clinical situation. The users of health sciences libraries need to know what types of information they can get, how the various resources work, and how to get help at any time of the day or night; health sciences libraries never close and health sciences librarians never sleep, as there are doctors and other health care professionals on the job all the time. In addition, like many other libraries, health sciences libraries frequently serve the general public, so staff must be able to relate to this group as well.

METHODS FOR PROMOTING LIBRARIES

Once a librarian has gained a basic understanding of the terminology and concepts involved with marketing and promoting a library, the next step is to consider the various methods and approaches to promotion of the library. The next few sections of this chapter will describe categories of materials and services that can be used to market libraries. While examples are provided for each area, more information can be found in the additional readings in Appendix 9.A.

PRINT/PHYSICAL MATERIALS

Handouts

No matter how fast the world changes to keep up with the digital medium, there will always be a need for printed materials to hand out to users. Items like flyers, newsletters, handouts, and, predictably, bookmarks are very effective ways of marketing the library. Figure 9.1 illustrates an example of a cover page of a library newsletter. While newsletters can be published quite inex-

Volume 16, Number 8

August 2006

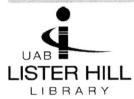

UAB
LISTER HILL
L I B R A R Y

UAB Lister Hill Library

Lister Hill Letter

Lister Hill Library of the Health Sciences

The UAB Lister Hill Library of the Health Sciences (LHL), established in 1945, is the largest biomedical library in Alabama and one of the leading such libraries in the South.

The Library offers a variety of services and information through its website—see web address below. Access to electronic resources is available across campus and remotely to authorized users. The library catalog is available from the web site and can be searched to find print, electronic, and media holdings.

The Library provides a variety of reference and educational services plus extensive educational opportunities. These include one-on-one instruction at point of need or through scheduled workshops on using library resources or searching for information. To contact the library for assistance, see http://www.uab.edu/lister/qpask/.

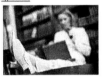

Lister Hill Home: http://www.uab.edu/lister/

Visiting the Library: Everyone is Welcome

Our library is open 94.5 hours per week and open to everyone at UAB. Members of the public are also welcome to come into the library. In addition to books, journals, historical manuscripts and artifacts, and audio-video materials, the library provides access to online materials. There are over 60 computers with Microsoft Office, Internet access and other tools. Some of these computers require a Blazer ID and password to use, others are open to anyone. Printing is available from all stations, though you must buy a card to pay for copies.

Wireless access to the UAB network is available throughout the building to authorized users. Specialized equipment available includes:
-Station with tools for the disabled
-Scanner
-TV/VCR
There are a variety of service points throughout the library where you can find help. If you have a question, ask any staff member.

Library Hours

Monday–Thursday
7:00 am–11:00 pm

Friday
7:00 am–7:00 pm

Saturday
9:30 am–6:00 pm

Sunday
12:00 pm–10:00 pm

Some service hours may vary.

Look for holiday hours on the library website.

FIGURE 9.1. Lister Hill Library's Newsletter, First Page

pensively utilizing in-house talent and printing with existing library equipment, the cost savings can sometimes be apparent in the overall lower quality of the materials. Unless the library or parent institution has staff members with graphic design skills, it may be best to contract with a professional to design the materials. The library can also commission a graphic designer to develop a bookmark or newsletter template that can then be adjusted for different situations and used to tie or brand materials together. Similarly, producing materials on library printers can work if high-quality paper is used, but going with a professional printing service may increase the overall impact of the materials. It is also worthwhile to determine if the library's parent organization includes a print shop or has signed a contract with a local printing business; these arrangements can generally help to decrease costs. On the other hand, if a good color printer and nice paper are used, the library has the ability to print on demand and update the materials as often as necessary. Often a mix of in-house and professional printing is ideal. It is important to keep in mind that the quality of the presentation of promotional materials goes hand-in-hand with branding the library as a source of quality information.

In addition to ensuring that all promotional materials look as professional as possible, it is also important to make sure that printed materials are accurate and kept up-to-date. Providing materials that contain inaccurate information is often much worse than using items with poor quality or those that are badly designed. Also, the library will want to make certain that the information presented is consistent and that it matches the information provided on the library Web site and in policy manuals.

In the initial stages of developing and designing promotional materials, it is important to follow any policies, practices, and images that the library's parent institution has concerning the use and creation of printed materials. In many cases, organizations such as universities and hospitals have style guides that dictate what can and cannot be printed. For example, if the library has a logo or graphic element, it should be used on all materials. However, one must also determine whether the parent organization's logo should be used on library materials as well. In addition, staff will need to decide what common features should be on all handouts. Should handouts include the author, date, file name, or URL if posted on the Web? What else should be included? Again, the key is to be consistent across all materials no matter what library department, staff member, or print service has developed them. Logos and graphics used consistently equate with branding, which equates with the library's identity.

Once materials and handouts are created, staff should then consider when and how to use them. A bookmark with contact information, for example, may be appropriate for all library patrons. Items like bookmarks can be located throughout the library and given to users when they check out materials or stop by the reference desk. Other handouts may apply only to particular populations. Materials geared for students, for example, are not necessarily appropriate for physicians. Information about certain events might also go to a specific target audience. Promotional materials such as flyers and posters should be posted outside of the library where target users would be likely to view them. For an academic health sciences library, this may mean putting materials in the hospital, clinic, and academic departments. Certainly anytime library staff members go to events outside the library, they should take handouts and flyers with them for distribution.

Promotional Items

Give-away items are great promotional tools for a library. Magnets with library information, for example, are typically welcomed by users. Today a number of companies make these kinds of items, and a library does not need to spend much money to purchase them. Pens and pencils are also popular marketing items that are usually inexpensive. For special events, spending money for water bottles, T-shirts, tote bags, or other items may be worthwhile. As with print materials, the library logo should be placed on all giveaway items. If the same vendor is used for multiple items, it may be cost-effective for the library's logo to be designed for use in a variety of formats (see Lister Hill's logo in Figure 9.2). The fee is generally inexpensive and is a one-time charge. Contact information should be included on all promotional items.

IN-PERSON EVENTS

The very best part of marketing in the library world is that the marketing campaign can be big or small, as needed or wanted. An in-person event can consist of a tour for one person, a class for fifty, a lecture series for 100, or a reception for as many people as the library will hold or has space for outside (see Figure 9.3). Further, in-person events can also entail librarians getting out of the library building and going to the users. Volunteering to speak at events on library topics or other research interests, for example, or volunteering to help at library stakeholder events, such as health fairs and student organizations, is also part of marketing the library and its services.

Motivating busy health care professionals and students to come into the library is often a daunting task; they just do not have time. There are, however, some really clever ways to lure potential library users into the building. The most traditional method is to offer classes. The technique for making classes successful is to target a specific group that has a known need; however, the class should always be advertised to everyone. For instance, creating a basic class on teaching nursing students how to use CINAHL (*Cumulative Index of Nursing and Allied Health Literature*) is very relevant. Once the dates and times for the class are set, the class should not only be announced to the nursing school but be directed to other audiences as well. Posting a flyer in the clinical nurses' and doctors' lounges may also increase participation. Just because the class is targeted at one group does not mean that there are not others who would also find the class helpful. Further, when the classes are announced, a note should also inform potential attendees that they can also call and schedule another time for instruction. Libraries need to make it as convenient as possible for people to use their resources and services. This is especially important for librarians who serve practicing clinicians whose schedules change often and usually without notice.

Depending on the library's size, allowing outside groups to use library space can also be an easy way to get people into the building. It is also a free marketing opportunity! Much of marketing is exploiting opportunity, so if a group of physicians wants to hold a meeting in the library conference room, it presents the perfect opportunity to place flyers about library services offered to physicians on the conference room table, along with a library pen and pad if available. A "Let Us Help You Search PubMed Faster!" flyer may attract the attention of one of the meeting

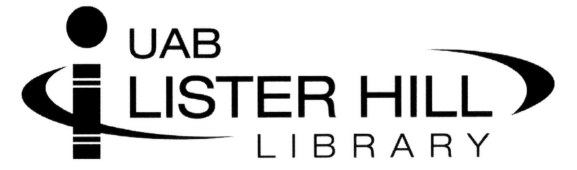

FIGURE 9.2. Lister Hill Library's Logo

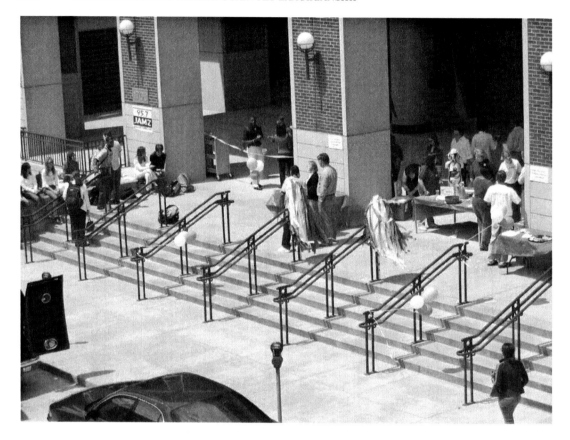

FIGURE 9.3. Lister Hill Library Moves Its Celebration Outside on a Plaza for National Medical Librarians Month

participants. Another clever approach is to create a display that is pertinent to the particular group. If a group of radiologists are using library space for a meeting, for instance, a display of radiology resources at the library entrance would be a sure attention grabber.

While hosting events in the library takes more time and money, it can be well worth the effort in terms of inserting the library into the community and creating an awareness of library services. Again, events can be as big or as small as needed. One of the most crucial aspects of event planning is timing. For instance, in a public library, holding a tax clinic in August most likely will not get the attention of users that the same clinic would if it were held in March. By the same token, scheduling a lecture during the week of finals is not likely to be well attended by students. However, advertising the health sciences library's study space as well as providing coffee and/or snacks to students during finals is likely to be very popular. For very little cost, showing that the library is sensitive to what is going on in the lives of its stakeholders can generate plenty of goodwill.

Recognizing important events and milestones of users and potential users can also be a good excuse to host an event. For instance, creating a display and inviting nurses to the library for impromptu visits is a wonderful way to mark National Nurses' Week. Further, National Breast Cancer Awareness Month could be used to highlight an oncology department, and National Heart Month is a good opportunity to let the cardiology department know the library has resources and services for them, too. Librarians should create information packets for those who visit and also send some to the school or hospital for those who could not make it to a scheduled event.

Hosting large library events such as lecture series, book fairs, or conferences can be a daunting task, but the key is to get everything in writing, be organized, and make sure all the details are communicated to library staff. Spaces or rooms needed for the event should be reserved early, along with placing necessary food orders. If at all possible, the event space should be set up and ready to go the day before the event, and it's always wise to double-check on the food a few days before the event to be sure that everything is in order. Checking to make sure all the technology is in working order is also beneficial and can help prevent "event day" stress. Providing attendees with information packets on area restaurants, museums, and other attractions is also a good idea. Having a "plan B" is always prudent in the case of unexpected trouble like foul weather, a power outage, or faulty network connections.

Often, getting librarians out of the building is as difficult as getting other people into the building. The more the librarians are willing to go to the users, the more users will be willing to come to the library. Offering to visit users in their offices and classrooms is a great way to provide library services. Also, if the library wants and expects people to attend their events, then it is only fair that librarians should make a point to attend events within the community, school, clinic, or hospital. Even spending just ten minutes at a student or employee orientation can remind people that there is a library on campus or in the hospital, and that it is full of librarians who want to help. Volunteering to help out at other people's events is also a wonderful way to take the library to the users. This can be as easy as keeping an eye out for upcoming events and asking if any more volunteers are needed. Some libraries, like the Eskind Biomedical Library of Vanderbilt in Tennessee, have been so successful in marketing their research skills that they participate side-by-side with doctors as they go on rounds.[11]

In today's electronic environment, librarians should seize every opportunity to actually see and talk to a person face-to-face. For libraries, event planning is about relationship building and people—seeing people, meeting people, helping people—whether it is just one unit or an entire hospital or university. By taking advantage of other people's events and creating events and activities that focus on library user needs and interests, librarians can insert themselves into their users' everyday lives. In Figure 9.4, Lister Hill librarians take a popcorn machine into various schools for events.

Everyday encounters with library users, however, should not be overlooked. Every single contact between library staff members and library users is a chance to market and promote the library and hopefully create some healthy PR. By definition, public relations is the "ongoing interaction between the information agency and its current and potential target markets."[3] Thus, for every library staff member, marketing and promoting the library should be a way of everyday life. Chatting with people in hallways, at ball games, in the cafeteria, and the like are all opportunities to present the library in a favorable and friendly light. Even if the topic of conversation is the current weather, by being friendly and courteous, each employee has the opportunity to create goodwill so that when users think of the library the thoughts are pleasant.

THE VIRTUAL WORLD

Since today's library users primarily visit the library through virtual means, it makes sense to use the same virtual medium to market library resources. Just because a resource exists, however, does not mean that it is right for the job. As Wood states, librarians need to be able to tell the difference between trends, things that are "expected to continue in the same direction at about the same rate," and blips, "minor deflections from a trend."[12] The wired world offers librarians a

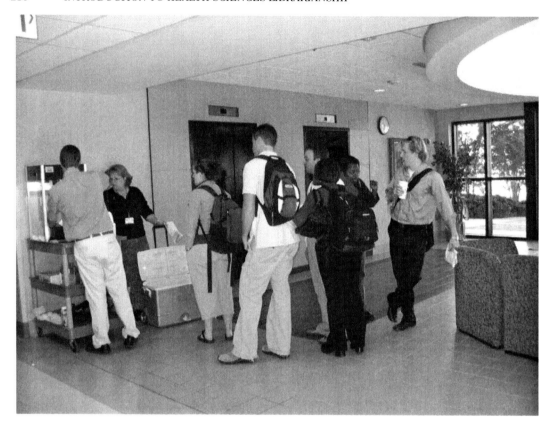

FIGURE 9.4. Jason Baker and Karen Giangrosso Take Lister Hill Library's Popcorn Machine to the School of Health Professions

whole host of cool and slick tools including **wikis, blogs, RSS (really simple syndication)** feeds, facebooks, podcasts, e-mail, e-surveys, chat, interactive tutorials, and more. But the caution here is to match the tool to the message and the message to the users. Librarians are uniquely situated to harness the power of the World Wide Web and Internet to reach more users in the ways that users want and expect. The key is to use and mold the technologies to find creative ways to do the things librarians do best. As Judith Seiss states in *The Visible Librarian,* librarians "need to position [themselves] in the minds of our customers as *the* experts in navigating and making the best use of the Internet."[13]

Every library should have a Web site, and hundreds of thousands of resources cover all aspects of good Web design. From a marketing point of view, however, there are a few things to keep in mind. It is important to remember that Web sites are about the content. The goal is to create a useful and informative Web site that users will visit again and again. All the bells and whistles are meaningless if the content is poor. Further, from a marketing standpoint, the library Web site and the services provided through it must be clearly branded as belonging to, or provided by, the library, as in the example Web page provided in Figure 9.5. The library marketer wants the user to know that, even though the user may be at home in a recliner, he or she is visiting and using the library and its resources. To accomplish this, each page on the site should include the library's logo or name and an easy way to navigate back to the main page. The Web site's navigation should be simple to use and intuitive. Contact information and hours should be easy to find, and the content and design should be current and free of typos or errors.

Lister Hill Library Programs & Promotions

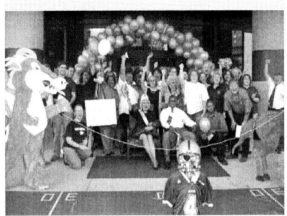

We'd like the whole UAB community to use library resources and librarian assistance to accomplish their goals. We want you to know what is available, how to get access to it and to ask for help when you need it.

To accomplish these goals, we have developed a liaison program, offer customized instruction, staff an Information Desk, offer online tips and help, and promote our services and resources through a variety of events.

Please let us know what we can do to meet your needs!

Past events:

National Library Week 2006

National Medical Librarians Month 2005

National Library Week 2005

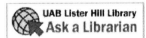

Add the "Ask a Librarian" Button to your UAB website! Here's how...

FIGURE 9.5. Lister Hill's Library Outreach and Promotions Web Site <http://www.uab.edu/lister/outreach/>

Today's users expect Web sites to be interactive and data driven. One of the simplest ways to do this is to include a form asking for user feedback. Forms, however, are becoming passé. The new generation of library users is more accustomed to social networking applications such as blogs and wikis. Luckily, libraries can test out both blogs and wikis for free. There are numerous free blog sites such as E-blogger <http://www.blogger.com>, while others like Typepad <http://www.typepad.com> charge a very small monthly fee. Wikis, such as PBwiki <http://pbwiki.com>, are other resources that librarians can try for free or for a small fee. The learning curve involved in using these technologies is minimal, and it does not take much time to become proficient at designing and posting messages. In fact, PBwiki claims to be "as easy to make as a peanut butter sandwich."[14] The same rules that apply to regular Web pages also apply to blogs and wikis. They both must be maintained and kept up-to-date and fresh. Further, if the library plans to allow users to make comments, a staff member must be designated to reply to them all.

Blogs, especially, are really useful for marketing. A number of libraries use blogs to communicate their library news, new book lists, new resources, and the like. Blogs can also be used to target specific user populations. For instance, in an academic library where librarians serve as liaisons to academic departments, blogs can be very useful tools for reaching those users. The liaison librarian should make sure that the posts are kept on topic and are relevant to the blog's scope. Examples of different types of library blogs can be found via a search engine like Google or Yahoo! by searching for "library blogs" or "medical library blogs."

Companions to blogs are RSS feeds, which are news aggregators that use XML to deliver new blog headlines directly to the user's desktop. Using RSS feeds allows users to sign up to receive notices when there is new content posted without having to check the library's Web site every day. No matter what tools the library chooses to use, they need to be publicized, kept current, and must be accurate.

With all of the new and wonderful tools available for librarians to use, e-mail still remains an important communication and marketing tool. The key to marketing with e-mail is to use it sparingly and make the messages brief and relevant to the particular users receiving the e-mail. With that said, e-mail is a fantastic way to let people know of a new blog, resource, or event. It's important, though, to place enough information in the subject line to let the recipient know who the message is from and something about the content, so it is not mistaken for spam.

COMMUNICATION

The ultimate goal of promoting and marketing the library is to increase the number of people who use the library's resources and services and to develop a better relationship with those users. So far, this chapter has discussed various ways to reach out and connect with users. Another fundamental aspect of marketing, however, is gathering user feedback. Anytime librarians come into contact with users, whether in the library, around the institution, or virtually, they have the opportunity to learn more about what users need and how the group (called a "market segment" in marketing terminology) utilizes the library and its services. Everyone associated with the library, from faculty, staff, and students to the library director, should stay alert to any opportunity to interact with library users and potential users. Staff should notice what the users say, how they say it, and what points they choose to emphasize. Ideally, the library will have a way to share and track this informal feedback, possibly through a blog or wiki, but more often it is shared informally in meetings and hallway chats.

While this information is valuable, it is important to go beyond this type of feedback, however, and routinely gather structured feedback from users. There are a number of ways to do this and many good resources are available for more information on each technique.

Focus Groups

Holding focus group sessions is a great way to gather user feedback. Much has been written about methods and uses of focus groups. Some of the best sources to use are included in Appendix 9.A.

While focus group sessions can be very formal and structured, they can also be more spontaneous and open. Either way, there is a lot of work involved in holding a focus group session. Steps include recruiting participants, scheduling sessions, finding or training someone to facilitate, planning what types of questions to ask, recording the session, and providing refreshments and a comfortable room. Keeping the participants on track without guiding their discussion is the key to having a successful focus group session. Focus group sessions can sometimes be costly, because refreshments or even a meal are typically provided for the people who participate. Many libraries also give participants some token of thanks as compensation for their time. Five to ten dollars per person is generally acceptable. After the session is complete, someone will also need to transcribe the recording of the session. Once transcribed, a report analyzing the results is usually generated.

When planning a focus group session, it is important to be clear on what information the library is seeking. Once the type of information is determined, then the specific questions must be developed. Before the focus group session is held, the librarian or facilitator should try out the questions with an uninvolved library staff member or friend to see if the questions elicit the desired responses.

Surveys

In addition to holding focus group sessions, a library can also use surveys to obtain user feedback. Library surveys have come a long way in the last five to ten years. Since the LibQUAL+ survey first became available in 2002, conducting institution-wide surveys has become a much easier task. LibQUAL+ is a "Web-based survey bundled with training that helps libraries assess and improve library services, change organizational culture, and market the library."[15] The LibQUAL+ survey is based on SERVQUAL, an online survey that measures the quality of service in libraries. Each LibQUAL+ question asks users to rank the minimum acceptable service level, the desired service level, and the level they feel their library currently meets. LibQUAL+ surveys provide results with a window or gap of perceived importance on a particular issue, including where the library falls within that range. Because the survey is commonly used and is often conducted in conjunction with other libraries, a particular library can also compare its results to those of peer institutions.

Also making the survey process easier is the advent of such Web tools as SurveyMonkey <http://www.surveymonkey.com/> and Zoomerang <http://info.zoomerang.com/>. These services are free (for a limited set of services) or available at low cost and are very easy to use. Not only is developing the survey straightforward and easy, but the results are collected and analyzed within the tool itself. Using a survey to gather information works well if there is an easy way to e-mail library users or potential users. This method is useful, for example, if the goal is to get people's opinions on specific issues, such as providing laptops for checkout or how late the library should stay open on weekends.

Web Usability Testing

In today's electronic world, library Web sites have become more and more important as they are often the library's front door to the community and the first place users encounter the library. Therefore, the need to ensure that the site is doing what it is supposed to do is of utmost importance. Using Web statistics and interactions with users can provide the library with information to refine and improve the library's site, but to really see how people are using the Web site, formal Web usability testing is needed. As with the other tools mentioned earlier, there is a lot of literature on this topic. Some of the best are listed in the additional readings in Appendix 9.A.

Usability testing is described as finding a typical user, developing a set of tasks to be completed using the library Web site, and asking the user to accomplish those tasks while being observed. Usually, the task is presented as a scenario that is read to the user. Then library staff members watch and take notes (or record the session) while the user navigates the library Web site, attempting to complete designated tasks. Librarians have a different depth and breadth of experience and do not think like typical users, so the only way to see how users find information on Web sites is to watch them do it. In some cases, users are monitored virtually, rather than in person. Uniformly, every librarian will be surprised at something the user says or does. Asking the user to think out loud as he or she works is very illuminating. The advantage of Web usability testing is that it highlights problems with Web pages that librarians may not see. On the other hand, a disadvantage is that Web usability testing does not provide clear instructions on how to remedy or correct the site.

Costs associated with usability testing are usually minimal—just a token thank-you gift to the user for his or her time. Once the test results are compiled, library staff will need to brainstorm ideas based on the initial testing and, ultimately, redo the test with another group. The report generated from usability testing should include the success rate of the participants and also some patterns in the way they used the Web site. The report should also include some observations, such as "people tend not to use the navigation bar at the top of the screen but instead use the back button on their Web browser."

User-Centered Design

User-centered design takes these feedback ideas a step further. This approach involves connecting with a group of users who will be available to provide feedback over a set period of time. This will help the library fix some problems, but librarians must remember that as the group's experience grows, these users become less and less like typical library users.

Friends Groups

Even beyond user-centered design are library friends groups. These groups are intended to support the library and can also provide feedback on resources and services. For state-supported institutions, friends groups can be political advocates for libraries. Friends groups should be used in an advisory role and should never have authority over the library's services.

Using the Feedback

One of the hardest things about user feedback is what to do with it once it is gathered. Each organization must first develop a culture of listening and responding to users and not assuming that the librarians know best. Responding to and utilizing feedback will be dependent on a variety of factors, including staffing and library budget.

FUNDING ISSUES

Throughout the chapter, there has been discussion of the costs associated with marketing and public relations activities. Costs of marketing and public relations programs can range from very little to quite expensive, depending on the types of activities the library wants to try and how many activities the library decides to undertake. To assure funding for those events, library administration must be convinced to commit to the concept that marketing and promoting the library is one of the institution's most important goals. This commitment can vary from developing a special position responsible for marketing, to designating some of the budget for marketing activities, to simply approving specific projects. It may be necessary to start small and work up to bigger things.

Initially, a marketing plan must be developed that can be used to lay out ideas for the year, detailing how much these activities and events will cost so that library administrators can see and understand the range of plans. There a number of ways to keep marketing costs low. For example, negotiating for the best possible price with an outside vendor is one way to lower costs. Some institutions may not be required to pay sales tax for certain items or may be eligible for educational discounts; librarians should know their tax status to take advantage of these tax or price breaks. Local businesses, vendors, or corporations that do business with the institution might be willing to donate prizes and/or sponsor events. Often, businesses are happy to donate food or money in return for some recognition at a library event. In such cases, follow-up thank-you letters, detailing how the business was promoted and how their donation was used, are essential. Before soliciting any donations, librarians must become knowledgeable about institutional policies for raising money or sponsorship for marketing activities. If institutional policy prohibits outside sponsorship, it may be possible for the library to use book sale money to fund different projects. It is very important to be clear on how money can be spent at individual institutions. Some accounts or funds may have restrictions on their use, so it important to know about such restrictions before any money is spent. Alternative funding, for example, the money collected in fines or late fees, might be used for marketing activities. It is important to be able to show how the money was used and what benefit the library and its users received from the expenditure. Even if a promotional event turns out not to be successful, it can still be money well spent if the library staff learn from the mistake and try again.

CONCLUSION

Library marketing requires flexibility and creativity. Libraries have a unique and special mission within their communities, and library marketing efforts should be as unique and special as the libraries and librarians themselves. Often, the hardest part of any marketing effort is just getting started, but once begun, library marketing becomes a natural part of working. The more marketing librarians do, the more opportunities evolve. Key to a successful marketing program is watching and listening to users, and then giving them what they both want and need in new and creative ways. Librarians should take the best lessons from the business world and mold them into marketing strategies that work for particular library environments and user populations. Health sciences librarians have specialized clientele, who have unique and sometimes individualized needs. Newer technologies will facilitate communication with these groups of users. It is important to remember that, no matter what is marketed, the library and librarians must follow through on promises made to users and must stay on top of current technologies and changes in user needs. Without follow-through, marketing is worthless.

APPENDIX 9.A. ADDITIONAL READINGS

Besant, L.X., and Sharp, D. "Libraries Need Relationship Marketing." *Information Outlook* 4, no. 3 (March 2000): 17-22.

Blake, B.R., and Stein, B.L. *Creating Newsletters, Brochures, and Pamphlets: A How-To-Do-It Manual.* New York: Neal-Schuman Publishers, 1992.

Caballero, C. "Strategic Planning As a Prerequisite to Strategic Marketing Action in Libraries and Information Agencies." *The Acquisitions Librarian* 14, no. 28 (2002): 33-59.

De Saez, E.E. *Marketing Concepts for Libraries and Information Services.* 2nd ed. London: Facet Publishing, 2002.

Dowd, N. "The M Word: A Blog Designed to Bring the Wonderful World of Marketing to Librarians." Available: <http://themword.blogspot.com>. Accessed: March 28, 2007.

Edsall, M.S. *Library Promotion Handbook.* Phoenix, AZ: Oryx Press, 1980.

Fern, E. *Advanced Focus Group Research.* Thousand Oaks, CA: Sage, 2001.

Fisher, P.H., and Pride, M.M. *Blueprint for Your Library Marketing Plan: A Guide to Help You Survive and Thrive.* Chicago: American Library Association, 2006.

Glitz, B. *Focus Groups for Libraries and Librarians.* New York: Forbes, 1998.

Gomez, M.J. "Marketing Models for Libraries: A Survey of Effective Muses from Far Afield." *Library Administration and Management* 15, no. 3 (2001): 169-71.

Hart, K. *Putting Marketing Ideas into Action.* London: Library Association Publishing, 1999.

Higa-Moore, M.L.; Bunnett, B.; Mayo, H.G.; and Olney, C.A. "Use of Focus Groups in a Library's Strategic Planning Process." *Journal of the Medical Library Association* 90, no. 1 (January 2002): 86-92.

Howe, N. *Millennials Rising: The Next Great Generation.* New York: Vintage Books, 2000.

Kyrillidou, M. "From Input and Output Measures to Quality and Outcome Measures; or, From the User in the Life of the Library to the Library in the Life of the User." *Journal of Academic Librarianship* 28, no. 1/2 (January/March 2002): 42-6.

Leerburger, B.A. *Promoting and Marketing the Library.* Rev. ed. Boston: Hall, 1989.

Lindsey, A.R. *Marketing and Public Relations Practices in College Libraries.* Chicago: Association of College and Research Libraries, 2004.

"Marketing Library Services: A 'How To' Marketing Tool Written Specifically for Librarians." Available: <http://www.infotoday.com/MLS>. Accessed: March 28, 2007.

Marshall, N.J. "Public Relations in Academic Libraries: A Descriptive Analysis." *Journal of Academic Librarianship* 27, no. 2 (March 2001): 116-21.

Owens, I., ed. *Strategic Marketing in Library and Information Science*. Binghamton, NY: The Haworth Press, 2002.

Rettig, J. "Beyond Cool." *Online* 20, no. 5 (September/October 1996): 52-61.

Rettig, J., and LaGuardia, C. "Beyond 'Beyond Cool': Reviewing Web Resources." *Online* 23, no. 5 (July/August 1999): 51-5.

Taylor, M.E. "It's Hard to Make New Friends: What to Think About in Creating a Friends of the Library Group." *Library Trends* 48, no. 3 (Winter 2000): 597-605.

Usherwood, B. *The Visible Library: Practical Public Relations for Public Librarians*. London: Library Association, 1981.

Vitale, J. *There's a Customer Born Every Minute: P.T. Barnum's Secrets to Business Success*. New York: AMACOM, 1998.

Walter, S. *Library Marketing That Works!* New York: Neal-Schuman Publishers, 2004.

Weingand, D.E. *Future-Driven Library Marketing*. Chicago: American Library Association, 1998.

Weingand, D.E. *Marketing for Libraries and Information Agencies*. Norwood, NJ: ABLEX Publishing, 1984.

Weldon, S. "Collaboration and Marketing Ensure Public and Medical Library Viability." *Library Trends* 53, no. 3 (Winter 2005): 411-21

Woodword, J.A. *Creating the Customer-Driven Library: Building on the Bookstore Model*. Chicago: American Library Association, 2005.

REFERENCES

1. Stover, J. "Library Marketing: Thinking Outside the Book." Available: <http://librarymarketing.blogspot.com/>. Accessed: March 28, 2007.

2. Kotler, P., and Armstrong, G. *Principles of Marketing*. Upper Saddle River, NJ: Pearson Education, 2004.

3. Weingand, D.E. *Marketing/Planning Library and Information Services*. 2nd ed. Englewood, CO: Libraries Unlimited, 1999.

4. Sherman, S. *ABC's of Library Promotion*. Metuchen, NJ: Scarecrow Press, 1980.

5. Armstrong, G., and Kotler, P. *Marketing: An Introduction*. Upper Saddle River, NJ: Prentice-Hall, 2003.

6. Ash, J.S., and Wood, E.H. "Marketing Library Services." In *Administration and Management in Health Sciences Libraries* (Current Practice in Health Sciences Librarianship, vol. 8), edited by R.B. Forsman, 75-100. Chicago: Medical Library Association, 2000.

7. Owens, I. "Marketing in Library Information Science: A Selected Review of the Literature." *The Acquisitions Librarian* 14, no. 28 (2002): 5-31.

8. Wisniewski, J., and Fichter, D. "Electronic Resources Won't Sell Themselves: Marketing Tips." *Online* 31, no. 1 (January/February 2007): 54-7.

9. Shaffer, R.I. "Using Branding to Make Your Mark(et): What Lessons Leaders Can Learn for Library and Information Science." *The Acquisitions Librarian* 14, no. 28 (2002): 81-91.

10. Cochrane, L.S. "If the Academic Library Ceased to Exist, Would We Have to Invent It?" *EDUCAUSE Review* 42, no. 1 (2007): 6-7.

11. Govern, P. "Eskind Librarians Make Move from the Stacks to the Bedside." *The Reporter* (April 16, 1999). Available: <http://wwwmc.vanderbilt.edu/reporter/index.html?ID=773>. Accessed: March 27, 2007.

12. Wood, E.J. *Strategic Marketing for Libraries: A Handbook*. Westport, CT: Greenwood Press, 1988: 21.

13. Siess, J.A. *The Visible Librarian: Asserting Your Value with Marketing and Advocacy*. Chicago: American Library Association, 2003: 72.

14. PBwiki. Available: <http://pbwiki.com>. Accessed: March 28, 2007.

15. LibQUAL+. Available: <http://www.libqual.org/About/Information/index.cfm>. Accessed: March 28, 2007.

Chapter 10

Information Literacy Education
in Health Sciences Libraries

Stewart M. Brower

SUMMARY. This chapter examines information literacy education activities as they apply to health sciences libraries. It includes general definitions of information literacy, as well as an examination of learning theories and pedagogies and their application to information literacy education. The chapter also includes discussion of information literacy programming and planning activities, and it outlines specific learning activities for classroom and online instruction. The chapter concludes on a brief discussion of assessment as applied to information literacy activities.

INTRODUCTION: WHAT IS INFORMATION LITERACY?

A term coined by Paul Zurkowski in 1974, **information literacy** is generally thought of as a minimally acceptable set of skills that enable one to locate, use, and synthesize information in a meaningful way.[1] The Association of College and Research Libraries (ACRL) defines information literacy as "the ability to locate, evaluate, and use information to become independent lifelong learners."[2] Both the term and the concept behind it have created a great deal of confusion and, at times, controversy.

While information literacy (IL) refers to the knowledge and skills of people—their overall facility with information—it has come to be associated primarily with user education programs developed by librarians. Library instruction itself is often described in terms such as information literacy training, information literacy programs, and information literacy instruction.

These terms have replaced older terminology such as "bibliographic instruction" or "user education," generally describing similar kinds of activities, although with some significant differences. Bibliographic instruction, in the traditional sense, taught skills related to specific resources and library functions: how to use a card catalog, how to use a bibliographic index, and how to file an interlibrary loan request, for example. Bibliographic instruction usually addressed educational needs specific to a situation, such as learning to use specific library resources to complete an essay. Modern information literacy instruction revolves around teaching lifelong information skills that can be adapted and used in many ways. IL is generally accepted as a broader concept than bibliographic instruction, reflecting the changing service values of librarians.

Librarians have not always been concerned with how well patrons could find or use information. Early librarians considered their roles to be almost exclusively related to the acquisition, organization, storage, and maintenance of books. It was not until the late 1800s that the concept of "reference service" became a legitimate part of library work, something to be codified and discussed among librarians as a matter of professional practice. In 1977, the ACRL created its

Introduction to Health Sciences Librarianship
doi:10.1300/6041_10

Bibliographic Instruction Section, one of the earliest formal recognitions of the role of librarians in user education.[3]

Health sciences librarians, particularly those in higher education, play a continuing role in user education. This chapter will examine this role in detail, including information literacy standards being adopted in medical libraries, learning theories and pedagogies that relate to IL, methods for developing IL programs, specific techniques in classroom and online instruction for medical librarians, and techniques for **assessment.** While it is hoped that this chapter will serve as a primer for medical librarians, it should be noted that information literacy and library user education are concepts with broader impact than just the health sciences information community, and that this chapter cannot cover the topic in any comprehensive way. Wherever possible, this chapter will focus on IL as it impacts the medical library, specifically.

INFORMATION LITERACY STANDARDS AND OBJECTIVES

Both professional library associations and nonlibrary organizations have recognized the need for information literacy training. Many of these groups have defined information literacy in terms familiar to their memberships, and these definitions are often accompanied by standards, recommendations, outcomes, or objectives. The most valuable of this kind of documentation includes measures of performance or skills ability, so a librarian can accurately assess the student after instruction.

Perhaps no definition of information literacy is more often quoted than that of ACRL, a branch of the American Library Association.[2] The standards outlined by ACRL, "Information Literacy Competency Standards in Higher Education," have been widely adopted, particularly in academic undergraduate and graduate school libraries:

> Standard One: The information literate student determines the nature and extent of the information needed.
> Standard Two: The information literate student accesses needed information effectively and efficiently.
> Standard Three: The information literate student evaluates information and its sources critically and incorporates selected information into his or her knowledge base and value system.
> Standard Four: The information literate student, individually or as a member of a group, uses information effectively to accomplish a specific purpose.
> Standard Five: The information literate student understands many of the economic, legal, and social issues surrounding the use of information and accesses and uses information ethically and legally.[2]

An exhaustive list of performance indicators and specified outcomes that should be met by students to be considered "information literate" accompanies these standards. While this document is remarkably detailed, it is also geared toward a general undergraduate population and does not necessarily specify any outcomes or measures for students of medicine, dentistry, nursing, pharmacy, or allied health disciplines. Oftentimes health sciences students have been exposed to some level of information literacy instruction during high school or undergraduate requisite courses but have not had classroom exposure to information literacy materials specific to health sciences disciplines.

Several accrediting agencies and professional associations in the health sciences have proposed their own standards and outcomes in information literacy education. In many cases, these discipline-specific standards may override any more general IL standards adopted by the college or university. They may also serve to supplement existing standards by addressing IL needs specific to that discipline, above and beyond those outlined by ACRL.

The Association of American Medical Colleges (AAMC) initiated the Medical School Objectives Project to outline skills and knowledge expected of all medical school graduates.[4] As part of this initiative, AAMC has designated "Medical Informatics and Population Health" as an educational objective, including specific outcomes related to lifelong learning and information literacy. These outcomes are detailed in Section II A of the project guidelines.

These outcomes, while specific, lack indicators for assessing performance or skill. This report also addresses several outcomes that the ACRL standards do not, including demonstrating skills in using specific resources such as MEDLINE and personal bibliographic database management, as well as critical thinking skills, "information skepticism," and protecting confidentiality of private information.

Medical educators and librarians alike have noted the Medical School Objectives Project Report II, *Contemporary Issues in Medicine: Medical Informatics and Population Health,* that was completed June 1998.[4] Many medical librarians have cited this report as foundational to their instructional initiatives. A commonly reported concern among instruction librarians is that it is difficult to involve teaching faculty and to spearhead changes to the curricula of the schools they

Section II A of Medical School Objectives Project

1. Demonstrate knowledge of the information resources and tools available to support life-long learning. Knowledge includes awareness of these resources, their content, and the information needs they can address. Relevant resources include MEDLINE and other relevant bibliographic databases, textbooks and reference sources, diagnostic expert systems, and medical Internet resources.
2. Retrieve information, demonstrating the ability to:
    a. Perform database searches using logical (Boolean) operators, in a manner that reflects understanding of medical language, terminology and the relationships among medical terms and concepts.
    b. Refine search strategies to improve relevance and completeness of retrieved items.
    c. Use a standard bibliographic application to download citations from a search and organize them into a personal database.
    d. Identify and acquire full-text electronic documents available from the World Wide Web or a local "virtual" library.
3. Filter, evaluate, and reconcile information, demonstrating the following:
    a. Knowledge of the factors that influence the accuracy and validity of information in general.
    b. The ability to discriminate between types of information sources in terms of their currency, format (for example a review vs. an original article), authority, relevance, and availability.
    c. The ability to weigh conflicting information from several sources and reconcile the differences.
    d. The ability to critically review a published research report.
    e. Knowledge of copyright and intellectual property issues, especially with regard to materials that are retrieved electronically.
4. Exhibit good "information habits." These reflect attitudes that support the effective use of information technology, and include:
    a. Using multiple information sources for problem solving.
    b. Maintaining a healthy skepticism about the quality and validity of all information. (This includes recognition that technology which provides new capabilities also has the potential to introduce new sources of error.)
    c. Making decisions based on evidence, when such is available, rather than opinion.
    d. An awareness of the many ways information becomes lost or corrupted and the need to take appropriate preventative action (for example, routinely employing backup procedures for personal and institutional data).
    e. Effectively using security procedures (for example, choosing "good" passwords, not sharing them, and changing them often).
    f. Protecting confidentiality of private information obtained from patients, colleagues, and others.

serve. With the AAMC report, medical librarians have been better able to directly address educational outcomes and bring reform to medical curricula, often with the full support of medical faculty and administrators.

The AAMC objectives are meant to address all medical school students equally. Other disciplines, such as nursing, have taken a different approach. The American Nurses Association (ANA) published *Scope and Standards of Nursing Informatics Practice* in 2001, outlining competency standards for "informatics nurse specialists," a specialty within nursing practice that integrates nursing with computer and information sciences.[5] While this book primarily addresses the needs of the specialist, there is a section on "Informatics Competencies" intended for all nurses. Information literacy skills are addressed, largely by citing the ACRL standards.

Specific informatics competencies for all nurses, outlined by the ANA, include

- identifying, collecting, and recording data relevant to the nursing care of patients;
- analyzing and interpreting patient and nursing information as part of the planning for the provision of nursing services;
- using informatics applications designed for the practice of nursing; and
- implementing public and institutional policies related to privacy, confidentiality, and security of information. These include patient care information, confidential employer information, and other information gained in the nurses' professional capacity.[5]

The ANA document, while addressing the nursing informatics specialty in some detail, lacks the authority found in the AAMC outcomes. While the scope of the AAMC outcomes clearly influences medical school curricula, the ANA document addresses only those nursing schools that have an informatics degree program. Because of this, many librarians who work with nursing schools might find it difficult to promote IL reform in the curriculum, even though many nurse educators do agree with the need for IL instruction.

Many pharmacy education programs recognize the need for strong IL instruction. The pharmacy profession deals in large part with the correct use of drug information, and IL education can better prepare pharmacists to do their jobs. The Accreditation Council for Pharmacy Education (ACPE) developed standards to which all accredited Doctor of Pharmacy (PharmD) programs must adhere, including *Standard 29—Library and Educational Resources,* which has the following subsection:

> Guideline 29.2
> The college or school should provide organized programs to teach faculty, preceptors, and students the effective and efficient use of the library and educational resources.[6]

One of the organizations that helps direct the ACPE is the American Association of Colleges of Pharmacy (AACP), which provides three of the ten members of the ACPE Board of Directors. This highly influential association represents faculty and student interests for over 100 U.S. schools of pharmacy and helps in the development of pharmacy curricula. The AACP has published an *Educational Outcomes* report, which includes the following as an anticipated PharmD outcome: "Retrieve, analyze, and interpret the professional, lay, and scientific literature to provide drug information to patients, their families, and other involved health care providers."[7]

Other agencies, such as the American Dental Association (ADA), allow for much more vague standards relating to information literacy. The ADA's accreditation standards for dental education programs only barely touch on IL in the curriculum:

Standard 6—Research Program

Research, the process of scientific inquiry involved in the development and dissemination of new knowledge, must be an integral component of the purpose/mission, goals and objectives of the dental school.[8]

Unfortunately, this reflects the current state of many such accreditation standards and documents as relates to information literacy. References to "process of scientific inquiry" and "development and dissemination of new knowledge" barely touch on the tenets of IL as outlined by the ACRL. Other agencies, such as the Council on Education for Public Health (CEPH) and the Council of State and Territorial Epidemiologists (CSTE), may only address IL as part of a specific informatics subdiscipline or as a professional competency to be expected following graduation, with no indication of the particulars of information literacy education as part of the process.[9]

On the whole, there exists a great deal of supporting documentation to assist librarians in developing IL programs and adapting these to specific health sciences disciplines. That does not mean, however, that these efforts are always welcome or without controversy.

CRITICISMS OF INFORMATION LITERACY

Many criticisms were leveled against both the concept and the term, "information literacy," especially in the early 1990s. Some librarians could not see a significant difference between information literacy and bibliographic instruction and held that the latter really subsumed the former, rather than the other way around. Other librarians believed the concept to be either too abstract to merit any significance or too insulting to their users to be of value.[10]

In 2005, Stanley Wilder published a letter in the *Chronicle of Higher Education* accusing librarians of making all manner of incorrect assumptions about library users and their need for training.[11] Fundamentally, his argument is that IL is all about teaching the user how to navigate difficult information systems, and that librarians should instead spend their time and energy creating new search interfaces and technologies to make it easier to use these systems.

There is much to consider in these arguments. Because of the negative connotations of "literacy," or more specifically "illiteracy," some reasonable alternatives have been suggested, including *information skills* and **information fluency.** The development of all of the aforementioned standards has helped greatly in not only codifying IL in specific health-related disciplines, but also demonstrating value to faculty and administrators.

Wilder's argument that librarians should build new systems instead of teaching old ones has merit but fails to address the current reality—a mixture of old and new information systems that have to be understood by library users. A suggested course of action is that librarians should try to develop better information systems, while also teaching information skills to library users, and adopt user feedback from these encounters to improve information system design.

Most important, librarians who engage in IL instruction should always be aware that some librarians and some faculty perceive information literacy, as philosophy and practice, very negatively. That said, many librarians and faculty fully embrace the concepts behind IL and welcome it into the classroom or curriculum.

Information Fluency—An Alternative Model

A new school of thought regarding library instruction has begun to emerge in recent years, one where information literacy is considered to be only a single piece of a larger puzzle. The Associated Colleges of the South (ACS) have developed another standard for instruction which they refer to as *information fluency.**

ACS outlines a fully integrated approach to learning information skills involving "traditional" library-oriented information skills training, computer literacy instruction from information technologists, and critical thinking skills taught by faculty within each discipline. Where these concepts meet becomes a new, more specialized set of skills, referred to as information fluency.

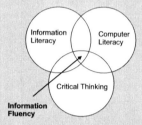

While the outcomes of the information fluency approach mimic, in many ways, the outcomes set forth by the ACRL, the responsibilities of instruction are more clearly defined. Furthermore, the integration of these skills suggests higher-order thinking skills as outcomes for all standards, as well as stronger lifelong learning skills that will adapt to new information technologies readily.

---

*<http://www.colleges.org/techcenter/if/>.

LEARNING THEORIES AND PEDAGOGIES

How do people learn? That question has plagued teachers since the earliest days of formalized education. While many learning theories have been proposed over the years, only a handful continue to have general acceptance today.[12, 13]

Learning Theories

One of the earliest theories, **behaviorism,** began with psychologist B. F. Skinner.[14] He proposed that all learning is "conditioned" in the learner, as a result of positive or negative reinforcement of learned behavior. Rewards for good behaviors (learning) might include praise, positive grades, or a better job upon graduation. Behaviorism began to be largely discounted in the 1950s, refuted as lacking the sophistication needed to explain more complex forms of learning and application of knowledge.

Cognitivism, on the other hand, states that all mental processes can be understood through the application of the scientific method.[15] While a reasonable enough case can be made for this view, the theory itself does not enhance our understanding of learning per se, except as a refutation of the behaviorist approach.

Another theory, **constructivism,** has proven to be much more effective in explaining the learning process and has gained acceptance among many educators.[16, 17] As a theory, it views all human learning as being "constructed," built upon by the perceptions and experiences of the learner. Constructivism suggests a role for the teacher that is more like that of a facilitator, providing framework and opportunity for a student to gain experience and knowledge. Constructivism has been very influential in the field of education and has guided much of the development of what is known as "modern education."

A radical new learning theory was proposed by George Siemens in 2004 that he has dubbed **connectivism.**[18] Siemens proposes that learning occurs as a part of the formation of networks, and that this learning can exist both within and outside of the human condition. One quote from Siemens's original article directly correlates to the goals of information literacy: "The pipe is more important than the content within the pipe. Our ability to learn what we need for tomorrow is more important than what we know today."[19]

Connectivism proposes that learning can be defined as the formation of networks and the ability to use them well. Siemens suggests that self-contained knowledge, in and of itself, is no longer the goal of education. Learning how to learn—the ability to find and use relevant information—is the primary goal. As a theory, connectivism has yet to gain credibility among educators, and it challenges more established theories like constructivism by shifting "learning" outside of the human experience. However, its central tenet of being able to correctly locate and use appropriate information correlates well with the principles of information literacy. Of all the learning theories, connectivism may have the most to offer the instruction librarian.

Pedagogies

All learning theories help define **pedagogies,** the practical applications of education and the science of teaching. If the learning theory addresses the philosophy of learning, then pedagogy deals with the practical application in the classroom. There are several formal pedagogies that have gained acceptance among educators.

Of the common pedagogies, **student-centered learning** is probably most closely identified with constructivism.[20] Student-centered learning emphasizes the student as an active participant who builds upon his or her own knowledge, rather than a receptive vessel into whom knowledge is fed by the teacher. Oftentimes, the latter approach is regarded as **teacher-centered learning,** although that is something of an oversimplification. Teacher-centered learning occurs whenever information or knowledge is transferred in a direct method from the instructor to the student, whether by lecture, course notes, or textbook.

A more specific form of student-centered learning is **problem-based learning (PBL),** which was developed by medical educators at McMaster University in the 1960s.[21] PBL involves students by asking them to work on challenging, open-ended problems, typically in small groups and with only minimal intervention by the instructor. One example of this in health education is the **case study method,** where a specific situation is codified into a "case," oftentimes as a medical patient or outbreak of a disease, and students are asked to develop solutions.[22] Many cases or problems may not have a specific solution and are designed instead to sharpen analytical skills and build knowledge.

Last, in his book *The Courage to Teach,* educator and philosopher Parker J. Palmer has suggested that there may be a very legitimate third pedagogy to consider:

> As the debate swings between the teacher-centered model with its concern for rigor and the student-centered model with its concern for active learning, some of us are torn between the poles. . . . Perhaps the classroom should be neither teacher-centered nor student-centered but subject-centered. Modeled on the community of truth, this is a classroom in which the teacher and students alike are focused on a great thing, a classroom in which the best features of teacher- and student-centered education are merged and transcended by putting not teacher, not student, but subject at the center of our attention. If we want a community of truth in the classroom, a community that keeps us honest, we must put a third thing, a great thing at the center of the pedagogical circle.[23]

Evidence-Based Physical Therapy—A Problem-Based Learning Example

To help a class of first-year physical therapy students better understand the principles of "evidence-based practice" (see Chapter 11), two health librarians at the University at Buffalo were asked to construct a problem-based learning experience for the students in fall 2004.

After a brief lecture on the research and publication cycle, the forty-three students were broken into smaller groups for an in-class exercise. Each group was given an abstract for a journal article describing a randomized controlled trial (RCT). Each group was then asked to answer a series of questions, identifying the number and type of participants in each experimental study, the clinical interventions and outcomes measured, and the research methods used. They were also asked whether they "trusted" the information in the article. A worksheet was distributed to facilitate this part of the exercise. After a reasonable amount of time, all the groups reported back to the entire class as to their conclusions.

Experimental studies, such as RCTs, can form the basis of much of the evidentiary literature used in health care practice. However, the vast amount of experimental research, and the varying quality of that research, has brought about the development of systematic reviews. By systematically reviewing the literature, results may be screened for their viability and value. Additionally, viable results from RCTs and other experimental trials may be incorporated into a meta-analysis, strengthening the scientific relevance of the results of individual studies by combining them into a larger statistical population.

This concept has been notoriously difficult to explain to students in the brief amount of time librarians had when teaching this course in the past. In this instance, however, students analyzed RCTs in their small groups and then the librarians showed them a systematic review that had incorporated those same RCTs as part of the review process. By demonstrating the RCTs and systematic reviews with meta-analysis in this context, the students' retention of these concepts increased considerably.

This concept of **subject-centered learning** is only just beginning to be discussed in the education literature in any significant detail.[24, 25] It suggests the basic tenet of putting the subject "in the middle," and using many different approaches to better understand and learn the subject. It also suggests that in a real community of learning, there will be times when the teacher is the student and vice versa, but that the greatest obligation of all parties is to the subject matter itself.

It would be a mistake to consider these pedagogies as being completely distinct and separate from one another. Real-world classroom techniques often blend pedagogies. For example, an instructor might use a lecture to develop a context for discussion, develop a fictitious case to illustrate a point, ask students to develop potential solutions on their own or in small groups, and then question the students about their findings. Many online courses use broadcast technologies like PowerPoint slides or audio lectures to transfer knowledge to students in ways that simulate more traditional teacher-centered instruction, but then use discussion boards and other forums to engage the student as an active learner. Pedagogy, in all of its forms, provides general educational methodologies but not necessarily the techniques. More examples of specific classroom techniques used in information literacy instruction will follow later in this chapter.

THE MILLENNIALS

Another factor to consider is the learning styles and preferences of the students themselves and how these influence IL instruction. The current generation of traditional college-age students have grown up with the Internet, cell phones, personal data assistants (PDAs), and other forms of information technology, and "Millennials" typically believe themselves to be intuitive and native users of electronic information. Much has been written about this generation, including several books, identifying them by several alternative titles, including "Net Gen," "Gen Y," and the "Entitlement Generation." *Millennials Rising* by Neil Howe and William Strauss is perhaps the best-known general work on this generation,[26] but the e-book *Educating the Net Gen-*

eration by Diana and James Oblinger reports on college students and their relationships with faculty, educational technologies, and libraries specifically.[27]

The Millennials, born between 1982 and 2001, have several identifiable traits that can impact their learning:

- Visual learners—They have significant visual-spatial skills and are adept visual learners.
- Inductive learners—Millennials are experiential learners who prefer to learn by doing or through discovery, instead of by reading or being lectured.
- Multitasking—They shift their attention from one task to the next fluidly and without much thought. They have been accused of lacking focus.
- Group learners—Most members of this generation are accustomed to small group activities and form social and political networks easily.
- Gamers—A significant portion of this generation are avid game-players and have developed unique "virtual" skills as well as significant problem-solving capabilities.
- Goals-oriented—Millennials are hopeful and believe in the future. They are willing to make sacrifices now in favor of their goals.[26, 27]

Instructional methods specific to the Millennial Generation will be addressed later in the chapter. However, two major points about these students should be considered carefully.

First, surveys have repeatedly pointed to the Millennials preferring to use general search engines such as Google instead of more specialized library databases and indexes. Seventy-three percent of college students indicated that they are more likely to use the Internet for research than the library.[28] This suggests that IL instruction cannot take place solely within the realm of traditional (or even nontraditional) library resources. For the Millennials, "information literacy" will need to address the state-of-the-art Internet as it is known today, as well as prepare them for changes in information that may come in the future.

Second, Millennials want to succeed in their careers and possess high standards of success. Recently, the Educational Testing Service, best known for the SAT college exams, developed a new exam called the Information and Communication Technology (ICT) Literacy Assessment. This exam tests the information literacy skills and knowledge of college applicants. Initial testing in Fall 2006 of 6,300 students indicated significant weaknesses in their abilities to judge the objectivity and authority of information found on the Internet.[29] Millennials can be made to understand that these skills are vital, not only to completing their education, but also to their future careers. If IL goals and outcomes are demonstrably linked to their future successes, Millennials can be motivated to learn.[30]

PLANNING AN INFORMATION LITERACY PROGRAM

Developing a sound information literacy program for health sciences schools requires careful planning. Information literacy program coordinators need to learn a great deal about their users, consider the points of view of many stakeholders, and try to design a program that meets the needs of the students and also satisfies the school's accrediting agencies, curriculum designers, teaching faculty, and deans. While IL planning can take many different forms depending on who is involved, some essential elements always play a role.

Information literacy planning usually begins with the end in mind. Goals-setting is the practice of knowing what outcomes are desired and planning with that in mind. Many of the IL outcomes have been documented already, including the ACRL guidelines, as well as those guidelines of various accrediting and professional agencies.

In the case of information literacy planning, goals-setting also means the ability to assess and document the progress of your IL program toward those goals. Assessment is discussed in greater detail near the end of the chapter.

IL programs do not exist in a void. They affect the daily activities of library staff, teaching faculty, students, and many others. These individuals are stakeholders in the IL planning process (see Figure 10.1). Consulting with stakeholders is vital in order to develop IL programs that can actually move forward. Stakeholders can be surveyed en masse for their opinions, or they can be selected individually to serve on task forces or planning committees. It may also be desirable for instruction librarians to serve on an existing curriculum committee as a stakeholder in that school. This arrangement can lead to IL planning as well.

Also important to the planning process is a thorough and objective look at library staffing and support. If the IL program is offered in addition to already existing library education services, staffing will be a significant consideration. Some IL planning initiatives try to balance this by eliminating less valued services, such as open-enrollment workshops, in favor of course- or curriculum-based IL programming. Other programs recognize the need for additional staffing and build it into the planning efforts.

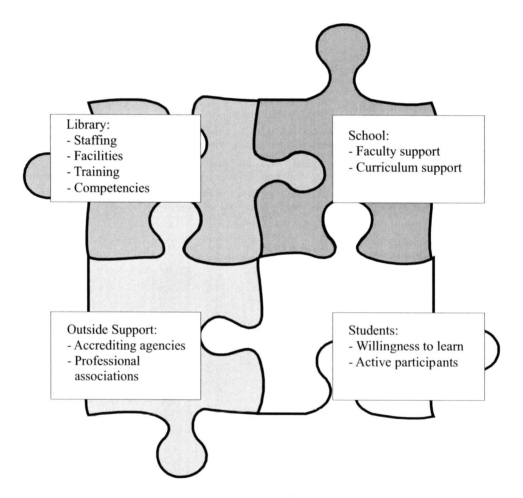

FIGURE 10.1. A Strong Information Literacy Program Relies on Many Different Factors

Library staffing has other considerations tied to it as well. Core competencies in education and classroom instruction, adequate funding for continuing education and professional development, and availability of appropriate classroom facilities all can have a significant impact on IL programming efforts. Core competencies and proficiencies have become a matter of some interest recently, and the Instruction Section of ACRL has developed standards for instruction librarians and program coordinators.[31]

INFORMATION LITERACY PROGRAM DESIGNS

After setting goals for the information literacy program, consulting and planning with stakeholders, and properly accounting for library resources and support, the coordinator then needs to design the program accordingly. There are many possible IL program designs, each with positive and negative aspects to consider.[32]

Many libraries offer open-enrollment workshops and seminars. Workshops are typically brief, require minimal preparation, and can be an outstanding tool for marketing and outreach. Workshops are highly flexible, allowing librarians to develop any educational content they choose without needing to meet the expectations of any particular group. They can be marketed to specific target audiences or can be widely promoted. If workshop content is already developed, then "workshop on demand" programs may be marketed to faculty and student groups on campus. Workshops can be timely, focusing on new library databases and resources or new Internet technologies, usually with minimal preparation.

The downside of workshops is their lack of impact overall. Only individuals with a particular interest in the workshop content will attend, and many librarians find it increasingly more difficult to justify the time and energy expended on developing new workshops due to low attendance, particularly among the students.

Perhaps the best-known form of library instruction is the so-called **one-shot.** Early adopters of bibliographic instruction (BI) in the 1970s relied on one-shot BI sessions as their primary opportunity to teach students how to use the library. One-shots are notoriously short, typically less than one hour, and almost always focus on a particular assignment that the students need to complete using library resources. Preparation time for a one-shot varies considerably, based on the nature of the assignment and the particular expertise of the librarian doing the teaching.

One-shots, like workshops, have gotten something of a bad reputation in recent years. Because one-shots are usually built around a single assignment, outcomes are very focused and do not always touch on all the tenets of IL. A student may learn how to search, but not to evaluate information, for example. One-shots may also be requested by faculty who have no specific library-related assignment, which can be frustrating for the students who may perceive such instruction as "filler."

One-shots are often confused with **course-based instruction,** sometimes called "course-integrated instruction," though there are some differences. While the one-shot consists of a single instructional opportunity by definition, course-based instruction can be spread out over two or more sessions within a single course. Course-based instruction typically implies a closer working relationship between the faculty and the librarian to develop content that meets course objectives, rather than a single assignment. For these reasons, course-based instruction can be a very valuable opportunity, allowing librarians to instruct to many or all of the facets of IL. Course-based instruction can even be used as an opportunity to satisfy ACRL standards, as well as the standards of other accrediting bodies.

Still, course-based instruction is not without its downside. If the class is not a required course in the major or discipline, not every student will benefit from the instruction. Also, should the course be reassigned to a new faculty member, as often happens in large academic departments, the librarian may not be asked to contribute each year.

Overall, the "gold standard" approach to IL instruction is **curriculum-integrated programming** (see Figure 10.2). A curriculum-integrated approach is defined as any programming that is consistently integrated into the requisite curriculum of the school. This type of IL program may exist within a single first-year course or may be spread out over several courses within the curriculum. While the methodology and practice of curriculum-integrated programming may vary, some elements are consistent:

- A curriculum-integrated IL program has *authority*. It should be recognized by the dean of the school or departmental chair and should have the general support of the school's faculty behind it. Likewise, such programming requires the full support of the library administration.
- A curriculum-integrated IL program meets *standards*. If there are information skill requirements in the discipline or department, or if standards have been addressed by their accrediting agency, those standards are being met by the IL programming.
- A curriculum-integrated IL program provides *uniformity,* in that all students enrolled in that program are exposed to the same material.
- A curriculum-integrated IL program is *customized,* so as to best meet the IL needs specific to that discipline or school.

While curriculum-integrated IL instruction can be very effective, it can also be exceptionally demanding to orchestrate well, and particularly hard on library instructors (see Figure 10.3). Librarians who have responsibility for these programs have reported high levels of stress and job burnout.[33] Other librarians have written about having remarkable teaching experiences with their students and immense job satisfaction, but it is clear that in either case the workload is considerable and demands on their time are high. Librarians involved with curriculum-integrated

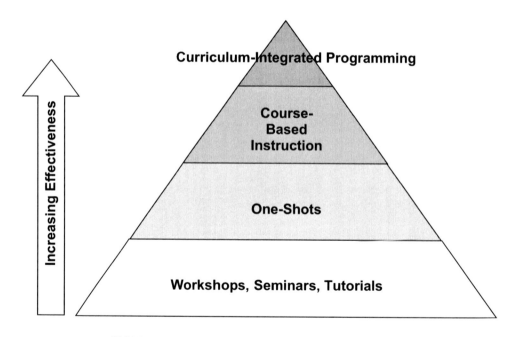

FIGURE 10.2. Increasing Effectiveness of IL Programs

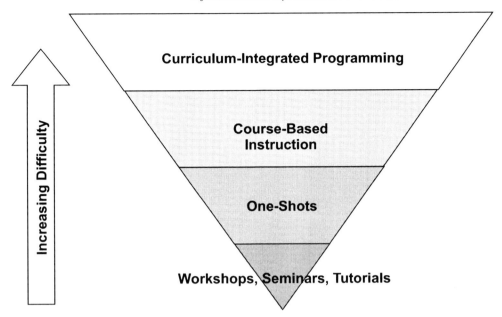

FIGURE 10.3. Increasing Difficulty of Developing IL Programs

programs spend a great deal of time preparing for class, developing course assignments, collaborating and meeting with faculty, conducting office hours and working with students, building online course guides, and conducting classroom and online instruction sessions. IL instruction activities and techniques will be described in depth in the following section.

Not all IL programs fit neatly into one of these categories. For example, some universities and colleges require a library skills assessment, such as an online workbook or test. Many libraries may blend programs as well. For example, a library might offer workshops throughout the year while also conducting curriculum-integrated instruction in the medical school each fall. Part of the IL planning process is determining which programmatic elements best fit the particular needs of the institution.

IL INSTRUCTION ACTIVITIES AND TECHNIQUES

The typical day of an instructional librarian is a busy one. The activities that make up the act of information literacy instruction require a variety of skills. This section will focus on what makes up instruction and will provide examples specific to health sciences libraries wherever possible.

Before Instruction Begins

For many instruction librarians, the first step in preparing for a class is drafting a **lesson plan.** Formalized lesson plans typically include such elements as a title for the lesson, projected time frame and lesson objectives, materials and facilities needed for the lesson, and an evaluative component to assure that the lesson was effectively learned by the students. This kind of lesson plan finds itself at odds, in some respects, with the more constructivist approach to education.

A Day in the Life of an Education Librarian

Name: Julia Shaw-Kokot, MSLS
Position: Education Services Coordinator, Health Sciences Library, University of North Carolina at Chapel Hill

Job description: This position leads the team that assumes primary responsibility for group instruction. Education programs are aimed at improving participants' understanding and skills in information problem solving, retrieval, and management. Education librarians work closely with faculty, staff, and administrators in health affairs schools, the library, the hospitals, and campus units to provide continuity of instruction from the classroom to other environments. Key responsibilities of this position include planning and evaluating, teaching, consulting, coordination of staff scheduling, training, and performance evaluation. This position also serves as the liaison to the School of Nursing.

Sample Day

8:30 a.m.–8:45 a.m.
- Do a walk around to see and talk with others about the day.

8:45 a.m.–9:15 a.m.
- Log onto the computer and check e-mail, check phone messages, etc.

9:15 a.m–10:00 a.m.
- Follow up on things that need to be done today.
- Prepare for meetings.

10:00 a.m.–12 noon
- Attend meetings, teach classes, hold one-on-one consultations, or respond to student assignments.

12 noon–1 p.m.
- Eat lunch and check e-mail or have lunch at a meeting.

1:00 p.m.–3:00 p.m.
- Attend meetings, teach classes, hold one-on-one consultations, or respond to student assignments.

3:00 p.m.–5:00 p.m.
- Prepare for upcoming classes.
- Work on presentations or professional work.
- Check e-mail, phone messages, etc.

5:00 p.m.–6:00 p.m. (2 days a week)
- Work at the services desk.

Summary statement: Some meetings/classes require a commute to another building or part of campus, often a fifteen-minute walk each way. This is an average day; some days are all one thing or another. For example, a day-long class or conference, multiple back-to-back meetings, or need to cover additional service or class hours. Never a dull moment!

This does not, however, invalidate the practice of writing up lesson plans. Lesson planning provides the opportunity for instruction librarians to get their thoughts out on paper, consider their goals for the lesson, and map out a method for teaching the class. The planning process itself often brings about new ideas for more effective instruction. A less formal lesson plan may include some of the following kinds of elements:

- Title/subject: What is the lesson supposed to cover, in general?
- General notes: How many students will there be? What is the time frame for preparation? For instruction? When and where does the class meet, or is this an online course? Will there be an assignment?
- Goals: What should the students know at the end of the lesson?
- Objectives: What should students be able to do at the end of the lesson?
- Materials: What resources will the session cover? What readings or other materials might the instruction librarian need?
- Examples: What examples might the instruction librarian use to illustrate various points?
- Activities: What activities will the instruction librarian guide the students through to improve their understanding of the material?
- Assessment: How will the instruction librarian evaluate the learning and the effectiveness of their instruction? Were goals/objectives met?

Instruction librarians may omit some of these or include other elements not listed here. Minimally, however, any IL lesson should have clearly defined objectives, educational activities to perform, and some form of assessment attached to it. Many examples of lesson plans can be found online.[34]

Instructional Proficiencies in the Classroom

When an instruction librarian outlines or plans a lesson, he or she does so with full knowledge of the format that instruction will take. In modern higher education, this typically will take one of two forms: classroom instruction or online instruction.

Classroom instruction is one of the oldest methods of education, but training in classroom instruction techniques seems to be reserved for K-12 teachers, primarily. Few college instructors receive any formal training in how to teach, and that includes librarians as well.

Teaching in front of a group of students can be mentally challenging, physically wearying, and a test of character as well. Simply put, teaching isn't for everyone. Many librarians may find that they are ill-prepared for classroom instruction, lacking some of the key instructional proficiencies and personal traits that expert instructors possess. Some of these skills can be taught; others can be learned through experience. It falls to the individual librarian to continue to improve his or her classroom skills, through experience and education, however he or she can. Some suggestions follow.

Presentation skills are an area of proficiency that can be addressed. The ACRL proficiencies statement specifies the use of voice, eye contact, and gestures to keep the class lively and engaged. Other presentation skills of value are timing, projection, patience, clarity, a sense of humor, and a "cool head" under pressure. For librarians lacking solid presentation skills, there are workshops and classes they can take. Toastmasters International and similar groups can also be beneficial to the inexperienced presenter.

Another helpful classroom instruction skill is proficiency with educational technologies. A successful instruction librarian should be proficient in the use of all manner of audiovisual equipment, be able to use software to create engaging multimedia presentations, and be capable of developing online course guides and tutorials to supplement the classroom experience. Many colleges and universities offer workshops in these technologies; some may have an educational technology department to give assistance to librarians and faculty.

Specific teaching methods can be used in IL instruction to help deliver a stronger educational message. One particularly well-established technique is demonstration and lecture. Using a Web-enabled workstation and a projector, the instruction librarian guides the students through the use of various resources. For example, by demonstrating a MEDLINE search and discussing the merits of the techniques used in the search, it is believed that the student will learn specific search techniques and be able to replicate them. Unfortunately, in a standard classroom setting where the students have no computers of their own, this method does not always capture the students' full attention, nor does it engage the students as active learners.

Lecture-based instruction can be aided with active learning techniques, however. Group learning exercises, in particular, can be effective with younger students. **Think-Pair-Share** was developed as a group learning technique that is particularly effective with large groups of students.[35] During a pause in a lecture, the instruction librarian will ask a question of the class, typically open-ended, though not always. The students are asked to think about the question briefly on their own, then to pair up with a neighbor or deskmate to discuss for a minute or two. The instruction librarian can then call on pairs to share their conclusions with the larger group. Think-Pair-Share adds structure to the discourse, allowing students to talk with each other about the topic, but without the discussion becoming uncontrollable.

Other IL-based group activities can benefit classroom instruction. Small group activities can include brief in-class projects or case studies. Students are typically grouped into tables of four to six students apiece, and a group leader is selected. Then the projects are distributed and clear instructions are provided on how to complete the work. For a group activity to be successful, it is important that it have very clear objectives or outcomes.

One IL-oriented example of a small group activity is "Understanding MEDLINE." In this example, each group is given a very short full-text article from a journal indexed in MEDLINE, typically no more than three pages long. Enough copies are provided that all students can read the article. Each group is also provided with a single, sealed envelope. They are then asked to list three keywords or phrases that would identify that article. Specifically, they might be asked, "What would you type into Google to find this article? Give me three examples and write them on the back of the envelope."

After the group has discussed their choices and written down their answers, the instruction librarian approaches each group in succession and asks the leader to open the envelope. Inside the envelopes are the full MEDLINE records for the articles, with major MeSH terms highlighted. The students are then asked to share with the class their keywords and the MeSH terms, and to discuss any variations between the two. This exercise helps students to understand the differences between MeSH searching and keyword searching, and gives an opening for a more extensive class discussion of the MEDLINE database and its features.

Other IL group activities can be similarly structured, perhaps looking at specific databases or the library's catalog as examples. The evidence-based physical therapy example provided earlier is another type of in-class group activity that requires no computer access to complete. Still, although IL instruction can benefit from the use of these techniques, classroom instruction without computers can be frustrating for students and instructors alike.

Using computer labs or e-classrooms and employing hands-on examples with the students have proven to be very effective IL instructional methods. Demonstration and lecture become more dynamic in the e-classroom, and many specialized tools can help make the session even more effective.

Many e-classrooms employ **classroom control software.** This software enables the instructor to "take over" student computers, to use as examples on the projector, or to provide immediate assistance even when the instructor is still at his or her own workstation. Classroom control software can be used to keep students on target with their work, by keeping them from indulging in chat or e-mail during the class. Most important, though, classroom control software allows the students to share their activities and examples with the rest of the class, enabling group learning techniques in an e-classroom setting. Classroom control software systems can take some effort to install, maintain, and use proficiently, however.

Another e-classroom tool is the wireless polling device, part of an **audience response system.** These handheld devices are usually very simple in design and allow an instructor to instantly poll larger classrooms in an unobtrusive way. For example, during an IL lecture, the librarian might ask, "What Boolean operator would be best for this search?" The students could then press a button on their polling devices to indicate their choice. The results are then transmitted to the instructor's workstation to share with the class, often in the form of a bar graph or chart. These devices are particularly useful in larger, hard-to-navigate classrooms, where the instructor is at a disadvantage in engaging the class in discussion. They can also be used to quickly assess the current knowledge of the students before instruction begins. (Audience response systems are discussed in detail in Chapter 16, "Special Services Provided by Health Sciences Libraries.")

Interactive whiteboards may also play a role in the modern e-classroom. Very commonly used in Europe, and being found in increasing numbers in K-12 classrooms throughout the United States, these electronic whiteboards provide a large projection screen that is linked to the instructor's workstation. Through pressure-sensitive touch points, the instructor can use the whiteboard to control the mouse, navigating Web pages or slide presentations without needing to be physically behind a podium or near his or her workstation at all. Some interactive whiteboards can also record any drawings or markings made on the screen, similar to how a Telestrator is used to illustrate plays during a football game. As many of today's college students are primarily visual learners, these illustrations may be fundamental in helping them to understand IL concepts and methods.

While e-classrooms and the computers and tools they provide can be helpful, it is ultimately the information literacy instruction itself that is key to the learning experience. Hands-on activities for the students can be used to enhance this instruction in many ways.

One simple method can be to have the students simply follow along with the examples used by the IL instructor, a sort of **"Mirror me"** approach. If the instructor is using a particular example to search MEDLINE, the students are encouraged to run the same search, closely following the exact keystrokes and clicks used by the instructor. This kind of mirroring can be effective early in an instructional session, when students may be unfamiliar with the basic navigation of a particular database or Web site. However, the technique loses its effectiveness quickly as students adapt. It can also cause a type of "separation anxiety" in some students who find themselves unable to keep up with the pace of the rest of the class.

Another method that combines hands-on exercises with a group learning approach is **round-robin searching.** The objectives of round-robins can be to compare and contrast different databases or demonstrate a variety of search methods and techniques. In this example, the instruction librarian breaks the class into groups. There should be enough groups so that each group will be able to search a different database. Each group is given a list of three to five specific searches to be run and instructed on a particular database to search, for example, MEDLINE, CINAHL (*Cumulative Index to Nursing and Allied Health Literature*), or Web of Science. They are also instructed to take notes on what searches worked well, what searches worked poorly, and why they think that was.

Example of Round-Robin Instructions

PHM 517. IN-CLASS SEARCH EXERCISE

Directions: Each group will search for answers to these questions in their assigned database:

- GROUP A—Ovid MEDLINE
- GROUP B—Ovid EMBASE
- GROUP C—Web of Science
- GROUP D—Health Reference Center
- GROUP E—Google Scholar

Not all searches will work equally well in all databases—that is to be expected. Give each search a good effort, but don't get hung up on questions you cannot answer. As you are searching for answers, write notes about which of these searches worked well and which did not, and whether that was because of the searching or the database itself. We'll compare results at the end of the session!

1. Locate articles that discuss pharmacies restricting access to over-the-counter pseudoephedrine in order to limit the illegal production of crystal meth. How many states have passed legislation on the matter? Are there any reported outcomes yet (e.g., less meth on the streets, fewer lab busts)?

2. Locate articles on the medical science behind the recent decision by Merck to pull Vioxx from the shelves. How long have we known about the possible risks of heart attack for users of Vioxx and other COX-2 inhibitors? (For Web of Science or Google Scholar searchers, what is the most-often cited article?)

3. Locate articles that discuss pharmacists refusing to distribute the "morning after" pill, otherwise known as emergency contraceptives. Are there any official remarks or statements from professional pharmacists associations? What is the AMA's position? Is this a U.S.-only problem or are there issues elsewhere?

After a few minutes of searching, the instructor tells the students to stop searching and then directs each group to search the next database in sequence. This process continues until all groups have searched all databases with all examples. Group leaders are then asked to share their notes with the class, indicating which searches did particularly well in which databases. This exercise will help cement the idea that not all databases are alike, and that some search methods work better than others. It can also open up a classroom-wide dialogue on these databases in general. It should be noted that this approach can make for a very busy and somewhat boisterous classroom and may not work well if the class is particularly large or if the exercise takes too much time to complete.

The classroom, whether electronic or classic, can be a chaotic environment. The ability of a good instruction librarian to instruct does not hinge on the order or chaos of the classroom, however, but on how well the students learn the material. Today's college student is accustomed to some degree of multitasking, and learning tends to come from many different places. Some learning occurs in the more disciplined and ordered environment of the classroom, and some in their dorm rooms or apartments in study sessions with their friends.

Proficiencies of Online Instruction

A great deal of learning in today's modern centers of higher education takes place online. On-line instruction can be as much a demand on the schedule of the instruction librarian as classroom instruction. Online instruction usually comes in two forms, **courseware** and tutorials.

Courseware (course management systems) is available now in almost every college and university in the United States. Commercial courseware products include ANGEL, Blackboard, and WebCT. Courseware is also available as noncommercial open source software, such as

Moodle. Some libraries are responsible for the administration of courseware, right alongside the catalog and other Web resources, but more often courseware is administrated by information technologies departments.

Instruction librarians can use courseware in the same way teaching faculty use it—to share learning materials such as slide presentations or class notes, to link to various library resources and Web pages of interest, to assign readings or other activities, and to post quizzes and tests for students to complete.

Many instructional librarians also develop online tutorials to help students learn. Tutorials are designed to give an individual student an educational experience by interacting with an online document, media, or software in a prescribed manner. Tutorials vary widely in terms of design and quality, but they do have one common factor—tutorials allow individual students to learn on their own time, outside of the classroom. Many IL instructors design tutorials to supplement the classroom instruction, to provide additional detail that may have been glossed over during instruction, or to provide a hands-on opportunity that the classroom setting could not physically support. Tutorials take many forms as well.

Interactive tutorials can be very complex. Following a model of computer-based education, the interactive tutorial typically requires that a student follow on-screen instructions to complete specific tasks or exercises. Construction of interactive tutorials can vary widely, from the relative simplicity of a series of HTML-scripted Web pages, to modules filled with complex animations and voiceover narration. Developing informative and effective tutorials can be a time- and labor-intensive process and typically requires significant experience with education technologies and instructional design.

A less complex form of tutorial is the **screencast.** Screencasts are essentially short movies of computer activity with a narrative voiceover, typically describing the actions on the screen. It is, in many respects, the online equivalent of demonstration and lecture in the classroom. Screencasts can be created with relative ease, using inexpensive or free software found online, and require minimal experience with educational technology. The instruction librarian simply scripts out what he or she wants to demonstrate, for example, how to run a basic MEDLINE search. The librarian then starts the screen capture software and runs the search while reading from the script. All of the onscreen activity is captured to a movie file, which can then be made available on the library Web site or through courseware for the students to access. While screencasts are easy to build, they lack interactivity. For this reason, many screencasts are partnered with online quizzes or other assignments to make certain that the methods demonstrated in the screencast are in fact learned by the students.

Instruction librarians have incorporated some newer Internet technologies into their online instruction as well, including **RSS (really simple syndication), blogs, wikis, podcasting,** and **vodcasting.** (Podcasting is also discussed in Chapter 16.) In application to IL objectives, RSS and blogs both lend themselves to the sequential and regular publishing of text-based IL learning materials and lessons. One example of this is the Case Studies in Health Sciences Librarianship blog as part of a Medical Library Association continuing education program.[36] Individual cases are examined through blog postings, and librarians participating in the tutorial engage one another through the comments feature of the blog.

Podcasting and vodcasting incorporate sequential learning with audio and video, respectively. The libraries at New York University publish a podcast series of audio tutorials, covering everything from the basics of finding an article to subject-specific tutorials for nursing students.[37] The University of Central Florida has developed a vodcast series to give students a virtual tour of the campus and to introduce them to the basics of online learning.[38]

Wikis, while not a form of tutorial per se, may offer some intriguing new ways to engage students in IL activities. PharmD students in a one-month clinical informatics rotation at the University at Buffalo may complete drug monographs in the wiki-based PubDrug.org for credit.[39]

Other wikis have been developed to support library workshops, including a course guide in evidence-based health care.[40]

For health sciences libraries that lack the resources needed to develop original tutorials, there are still options. Some libraries select and link to tutorials developed by other institutions. The **National Library of Medicine** and the library at the National Institutes of Health both offer extensive lists of tutorials on topics such as PubMed searching, finding drug information online, and using bibliographic software such as EndNote or Reference Manager.[41, 42]

INFORMATION LITERACY ASSESSMENT

An important element of effective information literacy programming, and one that is often misunderstood, is the concept of assessment. Integrating assessment protocols into an IL program can help the instruction librarian understand better what is being done right and what could be done better.[43] Assessment helps find ways to improve both individual instruction sessions, as well as whole curriculum-integrated programs. But the results of assessment can be difficult to understand, time- and labor-intensive to implement, and easily misinterpreted.

Assessment comes in two forms: summative and formative. **Summative assessment** comes at the end of instruction, often in the form of a grade on a paper or project, or a grade for the course, and it is used to tell whether the students learned what was expected of them.[44] Summative assessment may also include what is sometimes called "performance assessment," which assesses student learning through performance, often in the form of a portfolio or presentation. Summative assessment is sometimes called "assessment of learning," in that it is intended to address whether the student learned the material or not.

In contrast, **formative assessment** is "assessment *for* learning," and examines the educational process itself, the type and form of the instruction offered, the experiences of the students both in the classroom and online, to determine how learning occurred and whether the educational experience can be improved.[44] If summative assessment looks at what the student learned, formative assessment asks if the instructor learned how to be a better teacher.

Both forms of assessment play a role in higher education and may be used to quantify a student's progress in a program or a program's validity to the overall curriculum. In IL education, it is important to assess students for their ability to meet the objectives outlined by the program, often adopted from the ACRL or AAMC standards. Likewise, formative assessment of the IL instruction itself is crucial to finding ways for the librarians to improve as instructors, and to improve IL programming overall.

Assessment can be formal or informal. Informal assessment often takes place in the classroom, while instruction is taking place. To informally assess students, instruction librarians may observe activity in the class, conduct informal question-and-answer sessions with the students, or call upon students to participate in group activities or search examples. Informal assessment of the IL instruction itself might be done by inviting a colleague to the lecture for feedback, or briefly surveying students at the close of the lecture.

Formal assessment means that work will be done by the students for a grade. Developing strong IL assignments for students to complete, or the ability to assist teaching faculty in doing so, can be a key proficiency for the instructional librarian. An assignment that addresses key IL standards or objectives can be used as part of a comprehensive program assessment later on.

In undergraduate information literacy programs, the most common assignment is the essay. However, in health sciences disciplines, very few courses require students to write essays, and many instruction librarians may find themselves needing to develop other kinds of assignments. Health sciences require the clinical application of data and information from the literature, however, which opens up some opportunities to develop other kinds of assignments. A few examples:

- Executing a search in MEDLINE or another database: Given a topic to search, students can be evaluated on the techniques they use and whether or not they locate appropriate journal articles.
- Locating clinical information: Students can be given specific case studies to search in MEDLINE or other databases and locate appropriate clinical solutions.
- Evaluating clinical information: Students can also be required to assess or critically appraise information they have found in various ways, on a worksheet or through an activity like posting to an online bulletin board.
- Locating/evaluating statistical data: Particularly applicable to social medicine or public health disciplines, students can be required to use different resources to track down specific statistics or facts.
- Questionnaire or quiz: Through a series of multiple choice, matching, short essay, or other question formats, students will demonstrate general understanding of library and IL skills.

Examples of Questions from an IL Assignment

1. Using Ovid MEDLINE, search for all English language articles on the genetics of Bowen's disease. Print a copy of your search history and the first ten references.
2. When did "calcium channel blockers" become a Medical Subject Heading (MeSH)? "Calcium channel blockers" is used for what other terms?
3. In 1999 there was a review article published in the Netherlands about testing human hair for pharmaceuticals. The primary author was Gaillard. Please find the citation for this article. Be sure to include your search history.
4. When did "serotonin uptake inhibitors" become a Medical Subject Heading (MeSH)? List all the subjects for which "serotonin uptake inhibitors" is used. (HINT: Look at the Scope Note.) Also, print a copy of the MeSH tree structure for "serotonin uptake inhibitors," listing all the narrower drug terms beneath it. From examining the tree, when would it be appropriate to explode "serotonin uptake inhibitors"?
5. What is the appropriate EMBASE subject heading for "serotonin uptake inhibitors"? When did it become a subject heading? Does EMBASE allow you to use the MeSH term as well?
6. Using Ovid MEDLINE, search for all English language articles that specifically discuss using immunization programs to administer smallpox vaccinations in the United States.
7. Create a ten-item bibliography on a pharmacy-related topic of your choice. Write a single sentence (no more than twenty words) describing your specific information need. Outline an action plan for the database(s) you will search, and list the subject headings and keywords you intend to use to find your information. Execute your searches and e-mail your results.

Other Databases

Match the following searches to the most likely database (one match each; no searching necessary):

a. AARP Ageline	_____ environmental impact of asbestos exposure
b. Biological Abstracts	_____ nursing theorists
c. CANCERLIT	_____ patient information on chickenpox
d. CINAHL	_____ retirement and migration
e. Current Contents	_____ diagnosis of major depression
f. HAPI	_____ tests for job-related stress
g. Health Reference Center—Academic	_____ most cited articles by Dr. Francis M. Gengo
h. PsycINFO	_____ adenocarcinoma of the colon
i. TOXNET	_____ most recent articles on smallpox
j. Web of Science	_____ three different species of trapdoor spiders

Many of these assignments can be delivered either in print or online via courseware. Working with the teaching faculty to develop an in-course assignment is best, particularly if it creates a natural and purposeful reason for IL instruction, rather than an artificial construction to assess IL skills. Although essays are not always the norm, many health sciences courses still require major projects such as a class presentation or poster, which rely on many IL-related skills to complete. Learning how to develop strong IL student assignments can be a difficult process, but can be made easier through collaboration with experienced teaching faculty.

Developing a Library Assignment

Teaching faculty recognize, especially in this information-driven age, the necessity of getting their students thoroughly immersed in the library and its resources. The faculty of the health sciences schools are especially keen on giving their students library-specific assignments that require the use of MEDLINE, CINAHL, and other major bibliographic databases. When these assignments are done well, students often come away with a greater confidence and assurance in using library and Internet resources. Unfortunately, library assignments that are poorly designed or out-of-date often have the opposite effect, leaving students confused and frustrated and often unclear as to the purpose of the assignment.

When developing a library assignment, you may wish to consider the following:

* Names of resources should be specific and up-to-date. As an example, if you ask them to search MEDLINE, do you mean Ovid MEDLINE or PubMed from the National Library of Medicine? Do you want them to search all years of the database, or just the last five? Any assignment involving online systems and databases should have very detailed instructions and be checked for accuracy each semester.
* Be realistic about what the students will be able to find. Perform all searches yourself before assigning the work.
* If you will require all the students to find the same book or journal article, you should arrange for those items to be placed on reserve.
* Be sure that the reference librarians have a copy of your assignment, too, and that they are familiar with its contents and requirements.

Good library assignments are accurate and clearly understandable to both the students and the library staff who will assist them. These assignments should require critical thinking and analysis but also be flexible enough to provide students an opportunity to explore their own specific interests, or to modify their topics based on available resources.

Assessing whole information literacy programs requires combining many different elements in such a way that the assessor can objectively appraise the successes or failings of the program. For example, if an assessor can evaluate grades from the same assignment over successive semesters that the course has been taught, trends might be identified. He or she may then be able to identify variables that have affected those trends. Do the grades reflect a typical Bell curve? Did the grades go up in years that one type of instructional technique was used, but down in others? Has the assignment been given and graded consistently, or have there been changes? If the grades have always been high, and consistently remain high, is the assignment not challenging enough?

Informal elements will affect programmatic assessment as well. Do the students have favorable things to report about the IL instruction they receive? Do the teaching faculty likewise report good things? Has the librarian used active learning techniques, and does he or she try to learn ways to improve instruction? Has there been any peer assessment from other instruction librarians of this program?

In the end, a lot of assessment may reveal incremental ways to improve programs. After surveying students, reflecting on grades, and talking with instructors, an instruction librarian might find a way to slightly alter the class or the assignment that makes only a moderate improvement. All IL programming must be committed to a philosophy of continuous growth and improvement, however, to be of lasting value to the students and the institution.

THE FUTURE OF INFORMATION LITERACY

As Wilder has remarked, it is questionable what the future of IL instruction will hold in a world that moves toward smarter, faster, better information resources.[11] Certainly, as this chapter attests, the world of IL instruction is demanding and complex, and the work necessary to develop worthy information literacy programming is considerable. Many instruction librarians report burnout from the long hours and frustrating workload.

But the question of information literacy is bigger than just preparing better searchers and better information users. In the final analysis, IL is really about service to the users, meeting their needs in the here and now, and preparing them for whatever the future of information may hold. Information retrieval may become easier over time, but helping library users truly understand the nature of information, helping them become fully fluent participants in the marketplace of ideas, is a goal worthy of the effort.

REFERENCES

1. Zurkowski, P. *The Information Service Environment: Relationships and Priorities.* Washington, DC: National Commission on Libraries and Information Science, 1974.

2. American Library Association. *Information Literacy Competency Standards for Higher Education.* (January 25, 2007). Available: <http://www.ala.org/ala/acrl/acrlstandards/informationliteracycompetency.htm>. Accessed: March 7, 2007.

3. Dudley, M.; Laidlaw, S.; and Dudley, M. "Instruction Section: How It All Began." Available: <http://www.ala.org/ala/acrlbucket/is/welcome/howallbegan.htm>. Accessed: March 5, 2007.

4. "AAMC: MSOP: Medical School Objectives Project." Available: <http://www.aamc.org/meded/msop/start.htm>. Accessed: March 5, 2007.

5. *Scope and Standards of Nursing Informatics Practice.* Washington, DC: American Nurses Association, 2001.

6. Accreditation Council for Pharmacy Education. *Accreditation Standards and Guidelines.* [PDF File] (2007). Available: <http://www.acpe-accredit.org/pdf/ACPE_Revised_PharmD_Standards_Adopted_Jan152006.pdf>. Accessed: March 7, 2007.

7. American Association of Colleges of Pharmacy. *Educational Outcomes.* [PDF File] (2004). Available: <http://www.aacp.org/Docs/MainNavigation/Resources/6075_CAPE2004.pdf>. Accessed: March 5, 2007.

8. American Dental Association. "Standards for Dental Education Programs." (2007). Available: <http://www.ada.org/prof/ed/accred/standards/index.asp>. Accessed: March 5, 2007.

9. Council on Education for Public Health. "Schools of Public Health Criteria." (2007). Available: <http://www.ceph.org/i4a/pages/index.cfm?pageid=3352>. Accessed: March 7, 2007.

10. Snavely, L., and Cooper, N. "The Information Literacy Debate." *Journal of Academic Librarianship* 23, no. 1 (1997): 9-14.

11. Wilder, S. "Information Literacy Makes All the Wrong Assumptions." *The Chronicle Review* 51(2005): 18.

12. Wikipedia. "Learning Theory (education)." Available: <http://en.wikipedia.org/wiki/Learning_theory_%28education%29>. Accessed: March 5, 2007.

13. Gredler, M.E. *Learning and Instruction: Theory into Practice.* 4th ed. Upper Saddle River, NJ: Merrill, 2001.

14. Skinner, B.F. *About Behaviorism.* 1st ed. New York: Knopf [distributed by Random House], 1974.

15. Amsel, A. *Behaviorism, Neobehaviorism, and Cognitivism in Learning Theory: Historical and Contemporary Perspectives.* Hillsdale, NJ: L. Erlbaum Associates, 1989.

16. Piaget, J. *The Psychology of Intelligence.* [Translated from the French by Malcolm Piercy and D. E. Berlyne]. London: Routledge & Paul, 1967.

17. Wikipedia. "Constructivism (Learning Theory)." (2007). Available: <http://en.wikipedia.org/wiki/Constructivism_(learning_theory)>. Accessed: March 7, 2007.

18. Siemens, G. "Connectivism." (2007). Available: <http://www.connectivism.ca/>. Accessed: March 7, 2007.

19. Siemens, G. *Connectivism: A Learning Theory for the Digital Age.* (2004). Available: <http://www.elearn space.org/Articles/connectivism.htm>. Accessed: March 5, 2007.

20. Wikipedia. "Student-Centered Learning." (2007). Available: <http://en.wikipedia.org/wiki/Student-centered_learning>. Accessed: March 5, 2007.

21. Eldredge, J.D. "The Librarian As Tutor/Facilitator in a Problem-Based Learning (PBL) Curriculum." *Reference Services Review* 32, no. 1 (2004): 54-9.

22. Manuel, K. "Generic and Discipline-Specific Information Literacy Competencies: The Case of the Sciences." *Science & Technology Libraries* 24, no. 3-4 (2004): 279-308.

23. Palmer, P. *The Courage to Teach: Exploring the Inner Landscape of a Teacher's Life.* San Francisco: Jossey-Bass.

24. Showalter, E. *Teaching Literature.* Malden, MA: Blackwell, 2003.

25. Sternberg, R.J., and Grigorenko, E.L. "Are Cognitive Styles Still in Style?" *American Psychologist* 52, no. 7 (1997): 700-12.

26. Howe, N., and Strauss, W. *Millennials Rising: The Next Great Generation.* Cartoons by R.J. Matson. New York: Vintage Books. 2000.

27. Oblinger, D., and Oblinger, J.L. *Educating the Net Generation.* EDUCAUSE 2005. Available: <http://bibpurl.oclc.org/web/9463>. Accessed: March 5, 2007.

28. Oblinger, D. "Boomers, Gen-Xers, and Millennials: Understanding the 'New Students.'" *Educause Review* 38, no. 4 (2003): 37-47.

29. "College Students Fall Short in Demonstrating the ICT Literacy Skills Necessary for Success in College and the Workplace" (November 14, 2006). Available: <http://www.ets.org/portal/site/ets/menuitem.c988ba0e5dd572 bada20bc47c3921509/?vgnextoid=340051e5122ee010VgnVCM10000022f95190RCRD&vgnextchannel=d89d1 eed91059010VgnVCM10000022f95190RCRD>. Accessed: March 5, 2007.

30. Brower, S. "Millennials in Action: A Student-Guided Effort in Curriculum-Integration of Library Skills." *Medical Reference Services Quarterly* 23, no. 2 (Summer 2004): 81-88.

31. American Library Association. *Proficiencies for Instruction Librarians and Coordinators.* [PDF File] (2006). Available: <http://www.ala.org/ala/acrlbucket/is/newsacrl/proficiencies.pdf >. Accessed: March 5, 2007.

32. Rockman, I.F. *Integrating Information Literacy into the Higher Education Curriculum: Practical Models for Transformation.* San Francisco: Jossey-Bass, 2004.

33. Sheesley, D.F. "Burnout and the Academic Teaching Librarian: An Examination of the Problem and Suggested Solutions." *Journal of Academic Librarianship* 27, no. 6 (2001): 447-51.

34. Lorenzen, M. *Lesson Plans at LibraryInstruction.Com.* (2004). Available: <http://www.libraryinstruction.com/lessons.html>. Accessed: March 5, 2007.

35. Lyman, F. "Think-Pair-Share: An Expanding Teaching Technique." *MAACIE, Cooperative News* 1, no. 1 (1987): 1-2.

36. *JMLA Case Studies in Health Sciences Librarianship* (2007). Available: <http://jmlacasestudies.blog spot.com/>. Accessed: March 5, 2007.

37. New York University Bobst Library. *Research Tutorials.* (2007). Available: <http://library.nyu.edu/research/tutorials/>. Accessed: March 5, 2007.

38. University of Central Florida. *Video @ UCF.* (2007). Available: <http://video.ucf.edu/vodcast/index.cfm>. Accessed: March 5, 2007.

39. PubDrug. (2007). Available: <http://www.pubdrug.org>. Accessed: March 5, 2007.

40. University at Buffalo Health Sciences Library. "Evidence-Based Health Care: A Guide to the Resources." (2007). Available: <http://libweb.lib.buffalo.edu/dokuwiki/hslwiki/doku.php?id=ebhc_guide>. Accessed: March 5, 2007.

41. National Institutes of Health Library. "Resource Training." (2007). Available: <http://nihlibrary.nih.gov/ResourceTraining/default.htm?SelectedValue=Online>. Accessed: March 5, 2007.

42. National Library of Medicine. *PubMed Tutorial.* (2007). Available: <http://www.nlm.nih.gov/bsd/pubmed_tutorial/m1001.html>. Accessed: March 5, 2007.

43. American Library Association. *Assessment Bibliography.* (January 30, 2007). Available: <http://www.ala.org/ala/acrlbucket/infolit/bibliographies1/assessmentbibliography.htm>. Accessed: March 5, 2007.

44. Questionmark. "Glossary of Terms." Available: <http://www.questionmark.com/us/glossary.aspx>. Accessed: March 5, 2007.

Chapter 11

Evidence-Based Practice

Jonathan D. Eldredge

SUMMARY. Practitioners in many professions now employ evidence-based practice (EBP) to make informed decisions. EBP began as evidence-based medicine (EBM) to help physicians make sense of incomplete or contradictory information in order to diagnose and treat patients appropriately. EBM soon diffused as EBP to other professions including health sciences librarianship. EBP utilizes a sequential process of formulating questions, searching for evidence, critically appraising all relevant evidence, and then making decisions for implementation. This chapter describes the health sciences librarian's role in EBM and explains how librarians use their own version of EBP called evidence-based librarianship (EBL) to make their own informed decisions.

INTRODUCTION

How do you make decisions in your professional practice? How have you made important decisions in the past? Based on lessons learned from past experiences, how will you make important decisions in the future?

The term **evidence-based practice (EBP)** refers to a sequential process employed by professionals to reach informed decisions. EBP offers a process for reconciling the need to make sound decisions with the exponential growth of applied research-based knowledge. The EBP process involves formulating answerable questions, searching for relevant answers in the knowledge base, and then critically appraising any available evidence to make a decision.

EBP originated formally about fifteen years ago in medicine,[1] although its origins informally emerged long ago as professionals in many fields grappled with making informed decisions. Within a few years of the establishment of **evidence-based medicine (EBM)** as a social movement among clinical physicians, this innovation diffused first to several clinical specialties such as cardiology and pediatrics.[2] This diffusion soon spread to other health professions including

Author's note: First and foremost, the author wishes to thank Ann McKibbon of McMaster University. Ann has always been a mentor to me. She taught me the librarian's role in EBM during 1997 and encouraged me later to develop what was then the controversial concept of EBL. The following colleagues have provided valued guidance in my EBM activities at the University of New Mexico: Robert Rhyne, Craig Timm, Richard Hoffman, Thomas Becker, Angelo Tomedi, Martha McGrew, and Deana Richter. I appreciated the honest criticism and support of the following colleagues during those early years when EBL was controversial: Bob Wood, Eileen Stanley, Andrea Ball, Amelia Boutras, Andrew Booth, Anne Brice, Liz Bayley, Alison Bretting, Gary Byrd, Ellen Crumley, Denise Koufogiannakis, and Joanne Marshall. Since that time, other valued colleagues have included T. Scott Plutchak, Marie Ascher, Gillian Hallam, Helen Partridge, Kris Alpi, as well as my many colleagues in the MLA Research Section. Finally, I have appreciated all of the many participants in my MLA CE course on EBL, and my numerous students at the University of New Mexico, who have taught me so much.

Introduction to Health Sciences Librarianship
doi:10.1300/6041_11

public health, nursing, and health sciences librarianship. Finally, EBP diffused to professions outside of the health sciences that were as diverse as education, social work, and public policy analysis. A high-profile U.S. presidential candidate even recently discussed "evidence-based decision-making" in an interview.[3] A limited number of academic, public, school, and special librarians now are practicing EBP as well. Although EBP tends to be practiced most widely in developed, English-language nations, it has become an international social movement among most professions.

All forms of EBP appear to include a sequential process coupled to a system for critically appraising the acquired evidence in order to make a decision. Beyond these few commonalties, however, the various professions involved with EBP readily exhibit their differences. The types of questions formulated, the search strategies, and the ways that evidence will be appraised for relevancy and validity differ among professions. Clinical physicians are interested principally in answering diagnosis, prognosis (a predicted clinical outcome), and therapy questions to make decisions.[4] Nurses ask the same general questions as physicians, but they also ask questions on interpreting meaning in relation to patients.[5] Librarians are most interested in answering prediction, intervention, and exploration questions.[6] Public health practitioners are interested in answering questions pertaining to frequency (statistics), determinants of health, intervention, behavioral patterns with bearing on health in a population, and policy.[7]

This chapter focuses upon two aspects of EBP with particular significance to health sciences librarians: (1) the roles of health sciences librarians in EBM; and (2) **evidence-based librarianship (EBL).** Securing high-quality information plays a role in all forms of EBP. Librarians (and this discussion includes information scientists and informaticists) consequentially often play a role in this aspect of the EBP process. This chapter focuses on EBM because, as the grandparent of all other forms of evidence-based practices, EBM has been far more developed in both breadth and depth, so it suggests possible future directions for librarians involved with other forms of EBP; and because health sciences librarians have become so integral specifically to the current practice of EBM. The knowledge gained from the EBM discussions should be largely transferable to librarians' roles in other areas of EBP.

LIBRARIANS' ROLES IN EBM

What Is EBM?

Many physicians in clinical medicine cite the following definition of EBM:

> Evidence-Based Medicine is the conscientious, explicit, and judicious use of current best evidence in making decisions about the care of individual patients. The practice of evidence-based medicine means integrating individual clinical expertise with the best available external clinical evidence from systematic research.[8]

Definitions of EBM revolve around three key concepts:

1. The integration of the best current available evidence based on systematic research of the literature
2. Clinical experience as the basis for making judgments
3. Respect for the wishes and values of the individual patient

Experienced clinicians have the knowledge to recognize the relevance of any potential evidence to a pending decision. EBM then provides the skills to distinguish between poor, good, and the best available clinical evidence when making such a decision.

The EBM Process

The EBM process offers a sequential series of five steps to arrive at clinical decisions:

1. Convert an information need into a focused and answerable question.
2. Search for the best evidence to answer this specific question using the published literature, diagnostic tests, physical exam, or other reliable information sources.
3. Critically appraise the available evidence for its validity (closeness to the truth) and its relevance (clinical applicability to the individual patient) to make a decision.
4. Decide and apply the results of this appraisal to the individual patient.
5. Evaluate one's performance throughout the first four steps of this process.

Minor variations of this process exist,[9] but this description largely overlaps with other versions.

EBM represents the most significant and influential contemporary social movement in clinical medicine. The Medical Subject Heading (MeSH) term "Evidence-Based Medicine" first appeared during 1997 and was linked to 648 journal article references in the MEDLINE database via PubMed (hereafter simply referred to as PubMed) during that first year. These references were only to those articles on the subject of EBM itself, whereas an indeterminate number of more articles referenced in PubMed constituted the actual evidence that supported EBM during that year and during subsequent years. With each year since 1997, the numbers of references to articles on EBM in PubMed have steadily increased so that during the single year of 2005, the last full year available for analysis for this book chapter, there were 3,413 references published on EBM. From 1997 through late autumn of 2006, more than 22,500 publications had been indexed in PubMed on EBM. Another contemporary and parallel social movement in clinical medicine, "Disease Management," only represented a small fraction of the numbers of references compared to EBM for each year since its introduction as a MeSH term also in 1997. PubMed covered a total of about 4,850 references from 1997 to late 2006, with 514 references published on disease management during 2005, as a point of contrast with EBM.

The EBM Levels of Evidence

From its beginning as a social movement within clinical medicine, EBM has stressed the principle that all information is *not* equal.[10] Consequentially, some evidence is more important than other information. The extent to which a research report has relevance to a specific patient, and its research methodologies ensure validity, determines the value EBM attaches to that information. EBM utilizes the **Levels of Evidence,** a formal system of identifying bias in any given piece of evidence. The EBL section later in this chapter discusses bias in more detail. The systematic review, a methodology discussed momentarily, resides at the highest level of evidence because it synthesizes many studies. For individual studies marshaled to make a clinical therapeutic decision, the Levels of Evidence hierarchy places randomized controlled trials at the top for therapy questions, followed by cohort studies, case control studies, case series, and expert opinion in descending order of validity. The example in this chapter presents the Levels of Evidence for therapy, although comparable tables exist for other subjects, such as diagnosis.[11] This hierarchal Levels of Evidence principle seems disorienting, not only for some physicians, but also for librarians who are newcomers to EBM. The Levels of Evidence become particularly important to librarians in their support of EBM during the third critical appraisal step of the EBM process.

EBM Levels of Evidence for Therapy

Systematic Reviews (synthesizing multiple research studies)
Randomized Controlled Trials
Cohort Studies
Outcomes Research
Case Reports
Expert Opinion

Source: Adapted by Jonathan Eldredge from the Centre for Evidence Based Medicine, Oxford. A more detailed version of this can be accessed at: <http://www.cebm.net/levels_of_evidence.asp>.

Potential Roles for Librarians in EBM

Librarians' expertise has been tapped by participants in the EBM movement in a variety of both expected and, perhaps, unexpected ways since the very beginning of EBM. The more prominent roles of librarians in EBM include these:

- Searching for the best available evidence to support clinical decision-making
- Serving as a team member along with physicians, statisticians, and sometimes basic scientists in developing systematic reviews or meta-analyses to synthesize large amounts of original research data to make general recommendations for clinical care
- Producing and improving upon the information resources so essential for the existence of EBM, including, but not limited to, PubMed and commercial versions of MEDLINE, *BMJ Clinical Evidence,* DARE, the Cochrane Library, and the EBM journal titles *ACP Journal Club* and *Evidence Based Medicine*
- Training clinicians on how to conduct their own searches for needed evidence, or improving on these clinicians' existing searching and other information management skills
- Defining the relatively new **informationist** role in clinical medicine

These diverse roles offer options for librarians desiring to play key roles in EBM. Librarians have been conducting bibliographic database searches in support of clinical decision-making since the beginning of EBM. This service from librarians actually has existed since before the advent of bibliographic databases, although EBM now has redefined and elevated this role for librarians to an essential status. As the EBM approach becomes the dominant mode of providing medical services, the EBM process requires competent searches for the best available and highest-quality evidence for a given question. Previously, busy clinicians were far more likely to pass over what now are known as the search or critical appraisal steps in the EBM process. Instead, clinicians traditionally relied on intuition or limited past experiences when making clinical decisions.

Systematic Reviews

EBM practitioners recognize that **systematic reviews** are the highest form of evidence when making clinical decisions. Systematic reviews are scientifically conducted literature searches coupled to rigorous reviews and syntheses of all relevant evidence to answer focused clinical questions. Systematic reviews are distinctly different from **narrative reviews.** Narrative reviews are a familiar genre of literature review found in medicine, and they have existed for many years. Residents and medical students have relied heavily upon narrative reviews for advice on how to diagnose and treat, and generally to understand medical conditions. Narrative reviews are written by experts on the announced subject. Narrative reviews also have been demonstrated to offer biased, dated, and sometimes dangerous advice due to the lack of rigor in finding and appraising evidence in support of any recommendation.[12]

Systematic reviews overcome the common limitations of narrative reviews by beginning with the formulation of a focused and answerable clinical question, conducting a thorough and transparent search of the literature, and then a rigorous critical appraisal of all evidence found in the search. The clinicians, librarians, and statisticians on teams conducting systematic reviews are careful to document every step in this process so that a reader could replicate their study and achieve the same results. In this manner, a systematic review resembles any scientific protocol since a reader could replicate it on the basis of the described methodology, just like a thoroughly and clearly written methodological description of a laboratory experiment or a clinical trial. Librarians play several potential roles in systematic reviews.[13-19] First, librarians' daily expertise in helping others to formulate clearly defined questions in their roles as reference librarians or subject liaisons can be translated into helping the systematic review team to define the question to be answered by the completed systematic review. Second, librarians search for the evidence themselves, or they consult on searching for the evidence by identifying relevant databases and journals. Third, librarians provide guidance in selecting the highest-level evidence through use of filtering tools in bibliographic databases. Librarians sometimes advise on the creation of comprehensive bibliographies, some numbering in the thousands of citations, for all references considered while conducting a systematic review. Librarians often utilize tools such as EndNote or RefWorks in this bibliography-building aspect of systematic review creation.

Librarianship As Prerequisite of EBM?

At this juncture, it should be obvious that EBM has provided librarians with exciting opportunities to play essential collaborative roles in clinical medicine. Indeed, these opportunities have provided the added benefit of elevating their prominence within clinical medicine. Would EBM have ever emerged or, at the very least, attained its level of sophistication and influence without librarians? One might scoff at this suggestion until one considers that EBM probably would never have developed without the existence of sophisticated information resources such as PubMed that have been a necessary precondition for the emergence of EBM. The prehistory of EBM features the preliminary advances of James Lind, Ignez Semmelweiss, and Pierre Charles Alexandre Louis, who pioneered the cohort study design. This prehistory further includes members of the Medical Research Council in the United Kingdom who developed the first randomized controlled trial during the 1940s. Ernest Amory Codman, who studied outcomes of medical procedures, was another clinician who paved the way for EBM.[20]

Albert Allemann, Principal Assistant Librarian at what is now the **National Library of Medicine,** stands out as another pioneer who actually attempted to make EBM a reality during the 1920s. Allemann founded a short-lived journal during 1928 titled the *Medical Interpreter.* This journal summarized key findings in clinical journals, a move that anticipated the contemporary EBM format known as the structured abstract. In the foreword to the first volume of the *Medical Interpreter* Allemann wrote,

> Its purpose is to establish a system by which the most valuable and most practical attitudes will be selected from the great bulk of medical reports, international and national, and present them to the medical practitioner in a condensed form . . . and also will give daily Service by answering all medical questions that may help the physician at the bedside or in any of his [*sic*] special problems.[21]

Allemann's efforts to maintain this new resource ultimately were unsuccessful, but his successors in the medical library field built on the earlier work of John Shaw Billings, who created *Index Medicus,* to develop the MEDLINE database at the National Library of Medicine.[22] Not only did librarians create the information resources to make EBM possible, librarians continue to improve existing information resources in terms of speed and accuracy, and they are involved in the creation of new information resources that will further support EBM.

EBM Search Training

Most EBM physicians now regard librarians to be the experts on searching for the needed evidence. Yet, librarians have become trainers in the hope of making physicians in everyday clinical practice more capable and independent searchers. EBM informatics training begins for many future clinicians during medical school.[23] Recent evidence suggests that these efforts are most productive when students are experiencing the more clinically oriented phases of their medical school education.[24] Following graduation from medical school, physicians in pursuit of specialty training as house officers and residents also frequently experience EBM informatics training. Even after specialty board certification, practicing physicians benefit from additional EBM informatics training, oftentimes provided for continuing medical education credit at conferences. Librarians provide EBM informatics training in all of these educational venues.

At the University of New Mexico, students during their first year of medical school and residents and practitioners around the state have experienced "survival-level EBM informatics training." The **EBM Specific Search Method** assists busy physicians with finding about twenty to sixty high-quality references per EBM question in PubMed quickly and without an elaborate knowledge of search techniques. This Specific Search Method has been described elsewhere in greater detail[25] and will be utilized later in this chapter to illustrate how the reader actually might conduct his or her own EBM searches.

Informationist Role

During recent years, a new specialty generally known as the informationist has emerged in response to the need to bring the best evidence in the literature to the point of clinical care. This specialist has a solid understanding of the clinical environment, often backed by academic training, and a clear conceptual understanding of information linked to practical skills in its management. Informationists often report to a clinical director rather than to the library director.[26] Beyond these common elements, however, visionaries within the library profession have different ideas connected with this new specialty.[27-30] The Clinical Informatics Consult Service at Vanderbilt University Medical Center[31] has provided one model for this new specialty that includes the most common informationist elements.[32] Regardless of how this new role might eventually take form, a strong emphasis upon EBM will permeate this new specialty. In many ways this might become the most active among all possible roles for librarians involved in providing support as a team member implementing EBM.

EBM has proven to be an enduring, pervasive, and adaptable approach to decision-making in medicine. It clearly has thrived and become increasingly popular over the past fifteen years. Clinical physicians often refer to it as an overall approach for their practices or to their employing specific elements of the EBM process in aspects of their clinical practice. EBM also has proven to be adaptable. In the face of criticism early in its development, EBM advocates listened intently to critics and incorporated many of their suggestions as a means to improve EBM. As one example, early on, EBM tended to focus upon the health needs of broadly defined demographic profiles rather than the needs of the individual patient. By 2000, two key EBM publications reflected a change of focus to the individual patient.[4, 33] This adaptable stance of its proponents probably explains, in part, the breadth and depth of the profound influence of the EBM movement upon modern clinical medicine.

The Librarian's Role in EBM Searching

The librarian supports EBM in a variety of ways through multiple roles, as outlined earlier, but the librarian's principal role hinges on searching for the needed evidence. As already noted, EBM questions tend to cluster around three major types: therapy, diagnosis, or prognosis. Searching for the evidence for any of these questions takes years to master.

The EBM Specific Search Method

The EBM Specific Search Method might be one fairly easy way for the reader to try his or her hand at conducting actual EBM searches. The EBM Specific Search Method has been taught to medical students, residents, physicians, and other health care providers, such as physician assistants at the University of New Mexico, since 2002, and also to a variety of health care professionals in both rural and urban clinical settings around the state. By completion of these EBM informatics training sessions, nearly all participants report improved confidence and ability to conduct their own EBM searches. Figures 11.1 and 11.2 utilize the example of an EBM therapy search to answer the question "What diet therapies are most effective for treating people with diabetes?" Figure 11.1 focuses upon the initial search strategy in the detailed display section of the

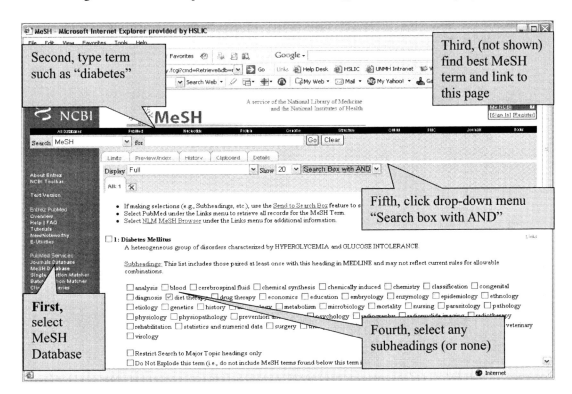

FIGURE 11.1. First Part of EBM Specific Search Method in PubMed. *Source:* Created by Jonathan Eldredge.

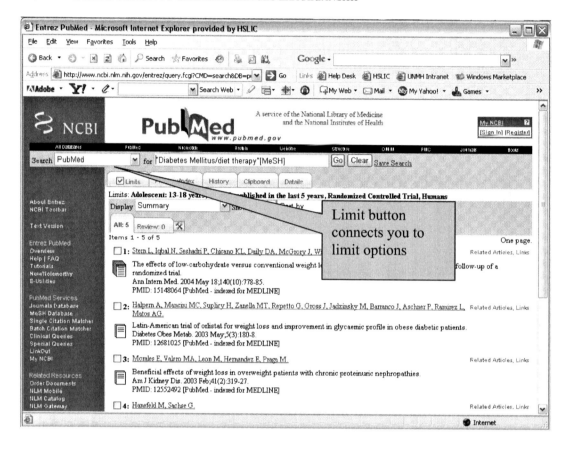

FIGURE 11.2. Second Part of EBM Specific Search Method in PubMed. *Source:* Created by Jonathan Eldredge.

MeSH Database in PubMed. Figure 11.2 focuses upon the limits applied to the results of this initial search strategy. The EBM Specific Search Method stands out as one of the simpler database searching techniques, so readers are advised to consult the more comprehensive coverage of database searching found in Chapter 8, "Information Retrieval in the Health Sciences," to obtain a broader perspective.

The EBM Specific Search Method in PubMed consists of the following easily remembered steps:

1. Define and refine your focused, answerable EBM question.
2. List the components for the question in descending order of importance from the most to least central concept.
3. Access PubMed at <http://www.nlm.nih.gov/>.
4. Access the MeSH Database in PubMed.
5. Enter the highest-ranked term.
6. Identify the MeSH term most relevant to your question based upon the definitions provided in the MeSH Database.
7. Click on the link under that MeSH term to access the detailed display; select the "Full" option under the "Display" menu.

8. Select only one relevant subheading, drop down the "Send to" menu, and select "Search box with AND" so you can review your search strategy.
9. Search PubMed.
10. Apply limits: human, English; possibly apply additional limits for publication type, subset, age, or date.

Examples of actual EBM questions using the major question types of diagnosis, prognosis, and therapy illustrate how the EBM Specific Search Method works in practice. Normally, the first resource to consult in these cases would be the Cochrane Library, but since the Cochrane Library requires little expertise to search and because it has a limited selection of systematic reviews that precisely match actual EBM questions posed, this chapter will demonstrate using PubMed instead. This chapter provides some possible search strategies for answering each sample question from the PubMed "History" mode.

EBM diagnosis searches. Here are some examples of EBM diagnosis questions collected from participants during training sessions:

- What are the most accurate indicators for diagnosing diabetes mellitus in adolescents?
- How effective is prenatal diagnosis for Down's syndrome during the third trimester?
- What is the sensitivity and specificity of different diagnostic tests for knee injuries?

Many diagnosis questions require simple, straightforward search strategies in PubMed. These questions involve identifying the appropriate MeSH term for the disease or condition in question (example: Diabetes Mellitus) and combining it with the subheading "Diagnosis" while in the MeSH Database within PubMed. Since so many articles cover diagnosis in passing, readers are urged to check the "Restrict Search to Major Topic headings only" box before searching PubMed to focus only on those articles concentrating on diagnosis. Limits on the references produced from this search might include English-language and human, but this search also might be limited by date of publication, age group, or the systematic reviews subset. The first question thus might be answered using the following search strategy in PubMed:

> "Diabetes Mellitus/diagnosis"[MAJR] Limits: Adolescent: 13-18 years, English, published in the last 3 years, Humans, Systematic Reviews

Some diagnosis questions require slightly more sophisticated approaches. The second question involves combining the three MeSH terms for prenatal diagnosis, Down syndrome, and the third trimester of pregnancy in PubMed, along with some limits to compose the following search strategy:

> "Down Syndrome"[MAJR] AND "Prenatal Diagnosis"[MAJR] AND "Pregnancy Trimester, Third"[MeSH] AND "Cohort Studies"[MeSH] Limits: English, Humans

Note that this search strategy also includes the fourth MeSH term "Cohort Studies." It will be recalled from earlier in this chapter that a cohort study is the highest level of evidence in the Levels of Evidence hierarchy for a single study for diagnosis questions. Thus, when a systematic review cannot be found by limiting the initial retrieval in this search, then the MeSH term "Cohort Studies" can be enlisted to focus the search results toward the highest level of evidence for a single study to answer a diagnosis question.

The third diagnosis question necessitates combining only two MeSH terms to answer, but then the searcher can seek out the highest level of evidence by limiting to systematic reviews:

"Knee Injuries/diagnosis"[MAJR] AND "Sensitivity and Specificity"[MeSH] Limits: English, Humans, Systematic Reviews

EBM prognosis searches. Most EBM prognosis questions are remarkably easy to answer via PubMed. The searcher simply needs to combine the disease or medical condition name with the MeSH term "Prognosis" to find an answer. Here are some actual EBM prognosis questions:

- What is the prognosis for using growth hormone to increase the height of Turner syndrome patients?
- What is the prognosis for an adolescent diagnosed with lymphocytic leukemia?

The first question involves combining the three MeSH terms "Turner Syndrome" and "Growth Hormone" and "Prognosis," and then limiting to systematic reviews:

"Turner Syndrome"[MeSH] AND "Growth Hormone"[MeSH] AND "Prognosis"[MeSH] Limits: English, Humans, Systematic Reviews

The second prognosis question combines the MeSH terms for prognosis and lymphocytic leukemia but adds the limit for the adolescent age group to the limits for English language and humans:

"Leukemia, Lymphocytic"[MAJR] AND "Prognosis"[MAJR] Limits: Adolescent: 13-18 years, English, Humans

EBM therapy searches. EBM therapy questions are the most common form of EBM question in clinical settings. Here are some examples of therapy questions to illustrate this approach:

- What diet therapies are most effective for phenylketonurias?
- What are the most effective drug therapies for adolescents with depressive disorder?

The majority of therapy questions require straightforward search strategies in the Specific Search Method approach. Like the previous diagnosis questions, the use of a medical condition or disease combined with the subheading "Therapy" using the Specific Search Method tends to retrieve a manageable number of relevant references. Search strategy effectiveness hinges on whether the broad, all-encompassing subheading "Therapy" for general and unspecified therapy or the possibility of multiple concurrent therapies really addresses the clinicians' exact EBM therapy question. Additionally, the subheading "Therapy" does not include certain therapeutic modalities, such as diet therapy, so it might produce a large number of unwanted references. Other narrower, more focused subheadings, such as "Diet Therapy" or "Drug Therapy" or possibly even "Radiotherapy," "Surgery," or "Rehabilitation," might be required instead.[34]

Consider the first EBM therapy question. This question initially might have been phrased in a less focused manner, such as, "What *therapies* are most effective for phenylketonurias?" The second question could have been similarly general rather than specific to drug therapy. The librarian or informaticist would need to determine if this more general question requires further refinement and focus, such as diet therapy or drug therapy, so that the clinical team obtains the truly needed information.

Focusing and refining of any EBP question takes an entire career to approach a satisfactory level of competency. All professionals struggle with formulating precisely the question really in need of an answer. This skill requires patience and persistence to develop. Even experienced practitioners fall into the common trap of thinking that they know what question they need answered—only to realize much further in the EBP process that they had an entirely different question. When librarians are involved with EBM therapy questions, this general observation takes on extra significance since one wants to balance the need to be open to different types of possible therapies, reconciled with what treatment options are really eligible for discussion by the clinical team.

Returning to the first EBM therapy question, the question genuinely had to be restricted in its focus on simply diet therapy due to a number of considerations revolving around the actual patient. The EBM Specific Search Method had to exclude merely "Therapy" as a subheading, and it even had to avoid identifying references to articles containing a brief mention of "diet therapy," so the search had to check the "Restrict Search to Major Topic headings only" box to focus on only references dealing with diet therapy as a major theme. As in most clinical situations, time was limited so only a short list of relevant references would be acceptable to the clinical team. The search strategy consisted of the following elements:

"Phenylketonurias/diet therapy"[MAJR] Limits: English, Humans, Systematic Reviews

The second EBM therapy question focuses on the varieties of drug therapies for depressive disorders in adolescents. The MeSH term "Depressive Disorders" combined with the subheading "Drug Therapy" as a restricted search produces an initial retrieval of references that need to be limited to English language, human species, and the age group adolescents. The large retrieval with these limits provides the opportunity to filter results to include publication types such as randomized controlled trials or meta-analyses, or perhaps the subset of systematic reviews to produce a highly satisfactory answer to this EBM therapy question:

"Depressive Disorder/drug therapy"[MAJR] Limits: Adolescent: 13-18 years, English, published in the last 3 years, Humans, Systematic Reviews

Some EBM practitioners, and the librarians who work with them, prefer to phrase EBM therapy questions in the PICO format. The components of a PICO question are P for *p*atient or *p*roblem or (sometimes) *p*opulation, I for *i*ntervention (i.e., the therapy), C for *c*omparison, and O for *o*utcomes. The PICO format can help clinicians and librarians focus their questions while incorporating all necessary elements. Interested readers should consult Strauss and her colleagues' book on EBM for a more detailed explanation of PICO and the other types of EBM questions not summarized in this introductory chapter.[35]

The best teacher for learning the EBM Specific Search Method involves repetitive practice coupled with increasing one's knowledge of medicine through education and gaining practical experience. The EBM Specific Search Method has continued to evolve through continuous experimentation. Interested readers are urged to practice using these examples, checking their work against the provided search strategies. Later, readers can graduate to begin assisting EBM teams as librarian consultants to expand their own searching skills. It should be noted that sometimes when teaching busy clinicians how to search PubMed, the instructor might opt to teach instead the less precise mode of Clinical Queries as a quick method for these clinicians to access needed references on therapy, diagnosis, or prognosis. This instruction should be coupled with an explanation of the Clinical Queries Filter Table[36] and supporting documentation accessible via PubMed's link to Clinical Queries.

Obstacles to Librarian Involvement in EBM

EBM has provided librarians with many opportunities to make meaningful contributions to improving patient care at either the educational phases of physicians' professional training or later when these physicians are in practice. As noted earlier, librarians have highly desirable skills and can play a variety of roles during the first three of the five steps in the EBM process.

Physicians who are newcomers to EBM sometimes resist or constrict librarian involvement in EBM activities for a variety of reasons stemming from their existing perceptions. First, physicians might be prejudiced against librarians because librarians are not physicians. Librarians are not alone in experiencing such prejudice. Even primary care provider physicians sometimes complain that they, too, have encountered elitist prejudice directed toward them from their specialist colleagues. Virtually every nonphysician health care professional actually has encountered this elitist prejudice, although, fortunately, this perception among physicians has begun to change. If a librarian encounters this negative attitude, he or she might consider proving himself or herself instead through performing well with other EBM physicians. Learning the culture and vocabulary of clinicians combined with providing good service can help overcome this elitism.

Second, physicians sometimes believe that librarians' contributions might be welcome during the question formulation and search steps, but that they have no place in the third critical appraisal step. Librarians might prove themselves to be helpful through limiting references to the publication types of randomized controlled trials or meta-analyses or through the subset for systematic reviews, as demonstrated in earlier examples. This skill is an important contribution, but a more enduring skill for engaging in a high-level dialogue with physicians would be for librarians to learn about the three highest levels of EBM evidence: systematic reviews for all types of EBM questions,[12] randomized controlled trials for single studies to answer intervention (therapy or prevention) questions,[37] and cohort studies for answering diagnosis or prognosis EBM questions.[38]

A third obstacle to librarian involvement in EBM might be termed the "little bit of knowledge can be a dangerous thing" syndrome. In this third obstacle, physicians delude themselves into believing that because they know how to type in terms without using the necessary tools, such as the MeSH database, and other features, such as subheadings, and then restricting searches to topic and limits that they, somehow, have mastered EBM searching. This third obstacle can be overcome by educating these physicians on what important references they missed and the many superfluous references they retrieved instead. By suggesting that physicians click on the "Details" tab in PubMed, librarians can begin to foster an appreciation of how PubMed has misinterpreted the physician's naïve search approach. If the librarian includes such warnings as part of his or her training sessions, most physicians are perceptive enough to heed the advice.

Becoming an EBM Librarian

EBM offers many opportunities for librarians who are willing to acquire new knowledge and skills to make meaningful contributions to improve patient care. These opportunities can range from helping physicians formulate questions, to providing searches or training on search strategies, to critical appraisal of the available evidence. The Medical Library Association (MLA) offers courses to equip health sciences librarians with the skills needed to perform various roles in EBM. Many health sciences centers and some hospitals offer courses for clinicians that might provide a more general background for the newcomer about EBM. This section has offered a glimpse on how librarians can make useful contributions, particularly if they overcome any inaccurate perceptions of their valued roles.

EVIDENCE-BASED LIBRARIANSHIP

What Is EBL?

Librarians, like other professionals, need to make important decisions on a regular basis. Bennett and Gibson have noted that making decisions also constitutes the defining characteristic of all managers and leaders.[39] EBL provides librarians with a sequential, structured process for making informed decisions.

Librarians probably have incorporated elements of EBL for as long as they have been entrusted by society to provide access to high-quality information resources.[40] During the twentieth century a number of early librarian pioneers of what later would become EBL developed the attitudes and research skills within librarianship that ensured its current acceptance. EBL represents a distinct break from the past, however, because it consciously uses a defined process coupled to the awareness that precautions must be taken to avoid making less than ideal decisions due to insufficient or conflicting evidence as well as human biases.

The term "evidence-based librarianship" and its initialism "EBL" first entered the professional vocabulary of health sciences librarians through a brief article published during 1997.[41] The MLA continuing education course on EBL was developed during 1998. Most of the early proponents of EBL were librarians involved in supporting the work of EBM physicians. These early proponents recognized the potential of adapting EBM principles to librarianship.[42] Since then, health sciences librarians have developed and revised some of the early principles of EBL. Health sciences librarians in Canada, the United Kingdom, and the United States additionally have facilitated the export of EBL to other types of librarians within their own nations as well as to librarians in other nations. International EBL conferences in the United Kingdom (2001), Canada (2003), Australia (2005), and the United States (2007) have tracked the unfolding diversification of EBL while underscoring the continued common features of EBL.[43-47] These conferences have brought together librarians from increasingly diverse libraries representing an ever-widening array of nations. These events reaffirm that the EBL process resides at the center of any definition of EBL, particularly the first three steps of that process. These international meetings also suggest that the diffusion process inevitably has required that EBL be adapted to different national contexts and different types of libraries. One now can find articles about EBL pertaining to academic, government, law, public, school, and special libraries.[48-60]

To avoid any confusion, particularly from the outset in this context of diffusion and diversification of EBL, this chapter will define EBL as follows:

> Evidence-based librarianship (EBL) provides a process for integrating the best available scientifically generated evidence into making important decisions. EBL seeks to combine the use of the best available research evidence with a pragmatic perspective developed from working experiences in librarianship. EBL actively supports increasing the proportion of more rigorous applied research studies so that these results can be made available for making informed decisions.

This definition implies inclusion of informaticists and information scientists in its use of the term "librarianship." In the United States, the term "evidence-based librarianship" and the initialism "EBL" enjoy great popularity among most librarians. Outside the United States, however, some librarians have begun to adopt the new term "evidence-based library and information practice" (EBLIP) for purposes of greater inclusiveness. In this chapter, however, the reader should equate the terms "EBL" and "EBLIP" in his or her mind.

Overview of the EBL Process

The EBL process consists of the following steps:

1. Formulating a clearly defined, relevant, and answerable question
2. Searching for an answer in both the published and unpublished literature, plus any other authoritative resources, such as high-quality data generated locally, for the best available evidence

3. Critically appraising the relevance and quality of the assembled evidence
4. Assessing the relative value of any expected benefits and costs, and then deciding upon an action plan
5. Evaluating the effectiveness of the action plan[61]

Most librarians seem to agree on the first three steps of the five-step EBL process. Consensus seems to fall away on steps four and five, perhaps due to the need to incorporate factors highly dependent upon particular library-type or national contexts. The years of experience required to form sound judgments as professionals probably also dominates steps four and five. Steps four and five overlap with skills sets normally associated with graduate training in public policy analysis, economics, educational administration, public administration, and management. Graduate library and information schools traditionally have not lent much focus to these skills sets. Insufficient research on why steps four and five reflect this diversity, however, prompts one to offer these speculations as to why so little consensus exists across different contexts.

Most librarians who practice EBL for making their important decisions do not conduct research projects themselves on a regular basis, although applied research studies provide the prerequisite information for making most sound decisions. Probably only 35 percent of the health sciences librarians in the United States during their careers would ever possess both the interest and workplace incentives to conduct applied research studies even on an occasional basis.[62] EBL therefore incorporates both practicing librarian "consumers" who utilize applied research results when making those decisions as well as the "producers" who generate the needed evidence for consumers to apply to making decisions.[61]

Obstacles to Making Sound Decisions

EBL provides a prescribed process for making informed decisions, while incorporating elements intended to reduce the likelihood of making poor decisions. EBL practitioners would be wise to review some of the obstacles identified by the social and behavioral sciences that are outlined in this section. Even when one practices EBL, the obstacles can threaten the efficacy of using the EBL process.

Every day professionals must find patterns in a vast volume of data, some of it incoherent, and make decisions. The physician must analyze a stream of patient information, discarding much irrelevant data, to find a series of seemingly unconnected findings to make an accurate diagnosis. Reference librarians and mediated database searchers decipher user questions and supplementary comments to search for needed information. The personnel aspect of the job responsibilities of any type of professional poses challenges in analyzing vast amounts of data about supervised employees in order to detect deficiencies in need of correction while recognizing the strengths that need to be channeled to serve organizational needs.

The term "**cognitive biases**" refers to a variety of common ways that the human mind fails to perceive a situation correctly or to think clearly about a decision. It is a universal by-product of mental processes intended to simplify complex, ambiguous, or large amounts of information. Even the most expert practitioners in a field can, *and do,* succumb to cognitive biases. Table 11.1 summarizes some of the more common cognitive biases thought to interfere with decision-making in libraries. Knowledge of these common forms of bias possibly can equip librarians to detect their presence in certain situations, and then to take action to avoid any unwanted effects in the decision-making process. Several forms of bias will be discussed later in this chapter in particular contexts within the five-step EBL process as a further guide to ensuring more sound decision-making. Beyond the immediate practical importance of protecting the integrity of the EBL process through knowledge of cognitive biases, this area of social psychology offers rich applied research opportunities for librarians wishing to better understand how these biases might interfere with decision-making within the profession.

TABLE 11.1 Common Forms of Cognitive Bias

Type	Definition
Anchoring	Relying on a single fact or a small number of facts disproportionate to all facts when making a decision.[1]
Attribution	Over-emphasizing the effect of someone else's personality in a situation while under-estimating the role and power of that person in this situation.[2]
Authority	Deferring to expert or other authority disproportionate to the extent of the expertise or the range of that authority.[3-6]
Confirmation	Reaching a conclusion prior to reviewing a situation and then focusing only upon those facts that confirm the prior conclusion.[2]
Déformation Professionnelle	Viewing a situation through the common perceptions of one's profession rather than by taking a broader perspective.[1]
Expectancy Effect	When a person with some authority or control such as a teacher manipulates the situation so that an expected outcome actually occurs (self-fulfilling prophecy).[7-10]
Groupthink	Believing in the autonomy of a group, stereotyping of those outside the group, self-censoring, censoring of dissenters, maintaining the illusion of unanimity, and enforcing a group "consensus" viewpoint.[11]
Halo or Horns Effect	Allowing another person's positive or negative characteristics to affect one's perception of this person in other unrelated contexts.[11]
Naïve Realism	Believing that one perceives the world accurately without considering that one's physiology and prior experiences have shaped one's unique perception of the world.[12-14]
Outcome Bias	Viewing an outcome retrospectively (hindsight) based on the specific outcome rather than by how events occurred leading up to this specific outcome.[2]
Perseverance of Belief	To persist in believing previously acquired information even after it has been discredited.[15-19]
Positive Outcome	Accentuating only the positive events or outcomes in a project rather than taking a more balanced view.[20]
Primacy Effects	Placing disproportionate importance upon information initially provided in a sequence of far more information rather than giving equal consideration to all information.[11]
Question Framing	Causing a decision to be directed by the way that it has been phrased and by the range of alternative considered or permitted outcomes.[2]
Recency Effects	Placing disproportionate importance upon information provided at the end of a sequence of far more information rather than giving equal consideration of all information.[2]
Selective Perception	Prior expectations cause one to filter how one perceives a situation despite the existence of facts that should contradict these prior expectations.[21-23]
Status Quo	Desiring to keep conditions relatively similar to one's present state and therefore predictable.[24]
Stereotype	Forming rigid perceptions based upon incomplete information about another individual or about a group.[25]
Storytelling	Granting more importance to a compelling anecdote rather than weighing all of the pertinent information when making a decision.[26-30]
Wishful Thinking	Assessing a situation incompletely according to a desired rather than a likely outcome.[31]
Worst-Case Scenario	Emphasizing or exaggerating those possible negative outcomes disproportionate to all possible outcomes.[32]

Source: Copyright 2007 Jonathan Eldredge. Reproduced by permission of the author.

1. "List of Cognitive Biases." *Wikipedia.* Available: <http://en.wikipedia.org>. Accessed: December 21, 2006.
2. Plous, S. *The Psychology of Judgment and Decision Making.* New York: McGraw-Hill, 1993.
3. Milgram, S. *Obedience to Authority: An Experimental View.* New York: Perennial Classics Editions, 2004, 1974.
4. Fearnside, W.W., and Holther, W.B. *Fallacy: The Counterfeit of Argument.* Englewood Cliffs, NJ: Prentice-Hall, 1959: 84-9.
5. Copi, I.M. *Introduction to Logic.* 7th ed. New York: Macmillan Publishing Company, 1986: 98-9.
6. Kilgore, W.J. *An Introductory Logic.* 2nd ed. New York: Holt, Rinehart and Winston, 1979: 22-4.

7. Rosenthal, R., and Lawson, R.A. "A Longitudinal Study of the Effects of Experimenter Bias in the Operant Learning of Laboratory Rats." *Journal of Psychiatric Research* 2, no. 2 (1964): 61-72.
8. Rosenthal, R., and Jacobson, L. *Pygmalion in the Classroom: Teacher Expectation and Pupils' Intellectual Development.* New York: Holt, Rinehart and Winston, 1968.
9. Rosenthal, R., and Rubin, D.B. "Interpersonal Expectancy Effects: The First 345 Studies." *Behavioral and Brain Sciences* 3(1978): 377-415.
10. Hock, R.R. *Forty Studies That Changed Psychology: Explorations into the History of Psychological Research.* 3rd ed. Upper Saddle River, NJ: Prentice-Hall, 1999: 92, 100.
11. Baron, J. *Thinking and Deciding.* Cambridge: Cambridge University Press, 1988: 259-61.
12. Ross, L., and Ward, A. "Psychological Barriers to Dispute Resolution." *Advances in Experimental Social Psychology* 27 (1995): 255-304.
13. Ross, L., and Ward, A. "Naïve Realism in Everyday Life: Implications for Social Conflict and Misunderstanding." *Values and Knowledge* (1996): 103-35.
14. Pronin, E.; Gilovich, T.; and Ross, L. "Objectivity in the Eye of the Beholder: Divergent Perceptions of Bias in Self versus Others." *Psychological Review* 111(2004): 781-99.
15. Gilovich, T. *How We Know What Isn't So: The Fallibility of Human Reason in Everyday Life.* New York: The Free Press, 1991: 86-7.
16. Levy, B., and Langer, E. "Aging Free from Negative Stereotypes: Successful Memory in China and Among the American Deaf." *Journal of Personality and Social Psychology* 66(1994): 989-97.
17. Anderson, C.A.; Lepper, M.R.; and Ross, L. "Perseverance of Social Theories: The Role of Explanation in the Persistence of Discredited Information." *Journal of Personality and Social Psychology* 39(December 1980): 1037-49.
18. Ross, L.; Lepper, M.R.; Strack, F.; and Steinmetz, J. "Social Explanation and Social Expectation: Effects of Real and Hypothetical Explanations on Subjective Likelihood." *Journal of Personality and Social Psychology* 35(1977): 817-29.
19. Wright, E.F.; Christie, S.D.; Johnson, R.W.; and Stoffer, E.S. "The Impact of Group Discussion on the Theory-Perseverance Bias." *Journal of Social Psychology* 136(1996): 85-98.
20. Yin, R.K. *Case Study Research: Design and Methods.* 2nd edition. Newbury Park, CA: Sage Publications, 1994.
21. Klapper, J.T. "Mass Communication: Effects: Selective Perception." In: *International Encyclopedia of the Social Sciences*, vol. 3, edited by D. L. Sills. New York: The Macmillan Company & The Free Press, 1968: 83.
22. "Selective Perception." *Wikipedia.* Available: <http://en.wikipedia.org>. Accessed: December 21. 2006.
23. Hastorf, A.H., and Cantril, H. "They Saw a Game: A Case Study." *Journal of Abnormal and Social Psychology* 49, no. 1 (January 1954): 129-34.
24. Samuelson, W., and Zeckhauser, R. "Status Quo Bias in Decision Making." *Journal of Risk and Uncertainty* 1(1988): 7-59.
25. Levy, B., and Langer, E. "Aging Free from Negative Stereotypes: Successful Memory in China and Among the American Deaf." *Journal of Personality and Social Psychology* 66(1994): 989-97.
26. Baumeister, R.F., and Newman, L.S. "The Primacy of Stories, the Primacy of Roles, and the Polarizing Effects of Interpretive Motives: Some Propositions About Narratives." *Advances in Social Cognition* 8(1995): 97-108.
27. Pennington, N., and Hastie, R. "Explaining the Evidence: Tests of the Story Model for Juror Decision Making." *Journal of Personality and Social Psychology* 62(1992): 189-206.
28. Baumeister, A.S., and Wotman, S.R. "Victim and Perpetrator Accounts of Interpersonal Conflict: Autobiographical Narratives About Anger." *Journal of Personality and Social Psychology* 59(1990): 994-1005.
29. McGregor, I., and Holmes, J.G. "How Storytelling Shapes Memory and Impressions of Relationship Events Over Time." *Journal of Personality and Social Psychology* 76(1999): 403-19.
30. McAdams, D.P. *Power, Intimacy, and the Life Story: Personological Inquiries into Identity.* Homewood, IL: The Dorsey Press, 1985.
31. Wohlstetter, R. *Pearl Harbor: Warning and Decision.* Palo Alto, CA: Stanford University Press, 1962: 397.
32. Merta, E. Interview by J. Eldredge, March 17, 2007.

The EBL Process

Step One: Formulate the Question

The EBL process begins with the raising of at least one question when faced with making an important decision. Members of the Arapaho Nation have noted, "If we wonder often, the gift of knowledge will come."[63] Librarians who frequently ask questions will be rewarded, not only by expanding their knowledge, but potentially by making better decisions. Identifying and articulating the question in step one of the EBL process can be a challenging experience, but clarifying the objective at the outset makes the four steps that follow much easier. This first step can be a disorienting phase, one that John Dewey described as a "troubled, perplexed, trying situation." This condition contains its own solution, moreover, when Dewey writes further that "a question well put is half answered."[64] Similarly, Cole has written that, "In science, feeling confused is essential to progress. An unwillingness to feel lost, in fact, can stop creativity dead in its tracks."[65] Because most people do not feel comfortable in this state of confusion or uncertainty, they tend to truncate this first step with the possible result of having to repeat the EBL process later when they realize, at a later step, that they needed to know the answer to a different question.

There are techniques to draw upon to make this first question-formulation step easier. Most important, it helps greatly to recall that the vast majority of EBL questions[66] fall into one of three question types, defined as follows:

1. *Prediction:* These questions seek to discover patterns that might be expected to occur under similar circumstances. Many collection usage studies and information literacy training pretest and posttest studies address these questions.
2. *Intervention:* These questions seek to determine the comparative efficacy of one course of action versus another course of action. For example, an instruction librarian might wonder if one method of instruction might be superior to another, when the two could be compared accurately and free of any bias.
3. *Exploration:* These questions often ask either overtly or indirectly "why" something either exists or does not exist. For example, why do some students use libraries? Or, conversely, why do some students not use libraries?

The examples of the three types of EBL questions provided in this chapter were collected from participants enrolled in the MLA's continuing education course on EBL. These three types of

---

Sample EBL Questions

Prediction

- Would a virtual tour of the library improve new users' skills in locating resources and services?
- What print reference books still need to be bought now that many reference questions can be answered with free Web resources?
- How will replacing print journal subscriptions with online subscriptions impact both the professional and clerical workloads?
- Does the teaching of searching skills to clinicians measurably improve the quality of their searches and the relevancy or recall of their retrieval? How long does this effect last?

Intervention

- What is the most effective method for teaching PubMed searching skills to third-year medical students during their clinical training?
- What approach will increase book circulation most among our users of a collection not weeded for twenty years: a drastic weeding of 40 percent of the collection OR a conservative weeding of about 15 percent that focuses on removing only items that have not circulated for ten years and editions now superseded?
- What teaching modality results in improved information literacy skills: the existing online-only training OR a proposed combined face-to-face and online training program?

Exploration

- How do our users prefer to learn about new developments in services and resources from our library?
- Why do some users visit our library building instead of just using our resources and services online?
- Why do some students rarely use the library resources and services despite a direct need to use these resources and services to ensure academic success?

EBL questions will be discussed in greater detail in the later section Step Three: Critical Appraisal.

Additional help with formulating productive EBL questions can be found in the following pragmatic suggestions:

1. Cultivate the habit of recognizing and recording questions as they occur to you.
2. Capture questions as soon as you recognize them, and before you forget them, if only recording them in the vaguest terms at that fleeting moment. Placing these questions in a single location, such as notebook, calendar, or computer file, aids retrieval later.
3. Refine your questions when you have a moment to reflect and focus your attention; if at all possible, ask colleagues to help you refine and clarify what you really need to know.
4. Reframe your questions; many questions really have other questions lurking behind the original questions.
5. Prioritize your questions: ask yourself how important these questions are to you, your institution, or the profession.
6. Courageously pursue all questions at the preliminary stage, no matter how vague, counterintuitive, or ridiculous. These muddled and awkward questions sometimes develop later into critically important questions.

Hundreds of health sciences librarians participating in the MLA's EBL continuing education course have demonstrated their newly learned skill in identifying and refining their EBL questions. Even the instructor for this course has formulated many questions during his career. Participants and instructor alike have agreed that this first step in the EBL process can be a humbling experience when seemingly straightforward questions initially can prove to be daunting challenges to articulate clearly in the long run. Thus, humility appears to be a helpful asset during step one, even for an experienced EBL-oriented librarian. Overall, though, this first step in the EBL process becomes much easier, faster, and likely to succeed with experience. Further guidance with the first question-formulation step can be found elsewhere in the professional literature.[67-70]

Step Two: Searching for the Evidence

Step one can impose a sense of humility due to the intellectual exercise of formulating a productive, focused EBL question. Step two also imposes humbling experiences regularly, but for the different reason that success in searching for the needed evidence in the published and unpublished library literature can be a daunting task. The two principal bibliographic databases in the field of librarianship are not as well organized and as consistently indexed as PubMed, so many health sciences librarians experience frustration when searching for the needed published evidence in their own professional knowledge base. These databases are both produced by commercial entities, so their lack of availability might present an added obstacle.

Library Literature, produced by the H. W. Wilson Company, indexes the contents of 600 journals, books, conference proceedings, and theses each year in librarianship, some of them published in languages other than in English. Because many of these indexed journals are published in North America, U.S. librarians tend to favor *Library Literature.* Librarians experience frustration while searching *Library Literature* due to the inconsistent coverage for key journals. During some years *Library Literature* provides full coverage for key journals, such as *Health Information and Libraries Journal, Journal of the Medical Library Association,* and *Medical Reference Services Quarterly.* On other years, this indexing coverage has been proven to be less complete.[71, 72]

The second bibliographic database serving the field is *Library and Information Sciences Abstracts (LISA)*. This database provides U.S. librarians with a largely unrecognized window to librarianship outside North America. *LISA* covers 440 journals from sixty-eight nations and in at least twenty languages. Carol Perryman and Dihui Lu, however, have discovered that *LISA* has indexing problems due to a lack of consistency and comprehensiveness of subject descriptor terms.[73]

Subject domains. Crumley and Koufogiannakis have noted that when searching the published literature, most EBL questions fall into six subject domains:

1. Reference
2. Education
3. Collections
4. Management
5. Information access and retrieval
6. Marketing/promotion

These investigators moreover have observed that three of the six subject domains—reference, collections, and information access and retrieval—are best searched via the library literature bibliographic databases. Three other subject domains—education, management, and marketing/promotion—are best searched through other databases serving the management or education fields.[74] Incidentally, Koufogiannakis and Crumley in a subsequent article, suggest that the marketing/promotion category might be subsumed under the broader heading of management.[75] Some useful references for answering education questions also can be answered with PubMed. In addition, PubMed indexes some key journals in the field of medical librarianship as well, and it can be accessed at no cost, in direct contrast to either *Library Literature* or *LISA*.

Alison Winning has built on Crumley and Koufogiannakis's work by detailing the mechanics of searching both within library literature databases and those databases outside the field.[76] Catherine Beverly has also developed practical strategies for searching for the evidence within the published and unpublished library literature to answer EBL questions.[77] These publications on EBL searching all point to the need to be creative, flexible, and resourceful when searching for the evidence.

Gray literature. When searching for the EBL evidence, one needs to include the gray literature, since many librarians work for institutions that apparently reward employees for presenting papers or posters at conferences by financing attendance at these conferences. Yet, many parent institutions do not offer similarly attractive incentives to publish the results from the same research. During recent years MLA has posted structured abstracts for posters and papers presented at annual meetings on the MLA Web site. Other sources of abstracts from this gray literature include the summer issue of the journal *Hypothesis,* some MLA chapter Web sites, the four international EBL conferences, and the biennial Research in the Workplace awards competition Web site in the United Kingdom.[78] The convention of using structured abstracts has improved the efficiency of librarians extracting the needed evidence from the gray literature as well as from the published literature.[79]

Psychological challenges in searching. Beyond the challenges just described, the second search step in the EBL process can offer psychological obstacles as well. Busy health sciences librarians many times will conduct their EBL searches in small blocks of time, as their schedules permit. This pattern might introduce two forms of cognitive bias into the EBL process. **Primacy effects** occur when evidence collected and reviewed early on during an incomplete juncture in the search phase begins to exert undue influence on the librarian making a decision on the pending EBL question. The librarian needs to maintain an open mind during these early periods in the search process until all of the evidence has been assembled and is ready for a comprehensive review in step three. **Recency effects,** the converse of primacy effects, occur when the most recently acquired evidence exerts greater influence over the bulk of previously acquired evidence.[80] Table 11.1 reviews these types of bias.

Step Three: Critical Appraisal

The critical appraisal step in the EBL process requires the skills associated with the formal rules of research evidence coupled with possession of keen critical thinking skills. The three types of EBL questions outlined in step one become important during step three, since these different types of questions rely upon different forms of evidence to answer them appropriately. Table 11.2 offers the EBL Levels of Evidence organized by each question type: prediction, intervention, or exploration. The Levels of Evidence are based upon the abilities of different research designs to manage various threats to validity, reliability, and the forms of bias already discussed previously in the EBL process section of this chapter.

TABLE 11.2. EBL Levels of Evidence

Prediction	Intervention	Exploration
Systematic review	Systematic review	Systematic review
Meta-analysis	Meta-analysis	Summing up*
Prospective cohort study	Randomized controlled trials	Comparative study†
Retrospective cohort study	Prospective cohort study	Qualitative studies‡
Survey	Retrospective cohort study	Survey
Case study	Survey	Case study
Expert opinion§	Case study	Expert opinion§
	Expert opinion§	

Source: Copyright 2002 Jonathan Eldredge. Reprinted with permission from the author. Originally published as part of Eldredge, Jon. "Evidence-Based Librarianship: Levels of Evidence." *Hypothesis: The Journal of the Research Section of MLA* 16, no. 3 (2002): 1-13. Available: <http://research.mlanet.org>. Accessed: November 14, 2006.

Note: This table assumes that neither any publication bias[1] nor what Rosenthal refers to as "File Drawer Problem"[2] has occurred when assembling relevant evidence.

1. Moscati, R., Jehle, D., Ellis, D., Fiorello, A., and Landi, M. "Positive-Outcome Bias: Comparison of Emergency Medicine and General Medicine Literatures." *Academic Emergency Medicine* 1(1994): 267-71.
2. Rosenthal, R. "The 'File Drawer Problem' and Tolerance for Null Results." *Psychological Bulletin* 86(1979): 638-41.

* Please see *Summing Up* by Richard J. Light and David B. Pillemer (Cambridge: Harvard University Press, 1984) for a comprehensive overview of creative ways to synthesize exploratory study data.
† A comparative study in the Exploration category involves two or more qualitative studies.
‡ Qualitative studies include but are not limited to focus groups, ethnographic studies, naturalistic observations, and historical analyses.
§ Expert opinion offered without rendering any supportive evidence.

The EBL Levels of Evidence. While no research design can eliminate all forms of these weaknesses, some research designs perform better than others due to their structural characteristics. Systematic reviews are designed to eliminate many forms of bias while retaining research methodology integrity. Table 11.2 indicates that the systematic review resides at the highest level of evidence for a prediction, an intervention, or an exploration EBL question. Systematic reviews are scientific literature reviews that epitomize the strengths of the EBL process. Systematic reviews in librarianship, similar to systematic reviews in clinical medicine, begin with focused and answerable questions that have high relevance to librarianship. Fully documented, comprehensive searches for the evidence follow. The creators of the systematic review should describe the search in sufficient detail so that readers can replicate the search to obtain the same results. Producers of systematic reviews critically appraise the evidence, employing precise rules for including and excluding evidence (many times, but not exclusively, contained in articles from peer-reviewed journals), perform any needed analyses, and then render their recommendations. Regrettably, health sciences librarianship has few systematic reviews to draw upon when making important decisions.[81]

Dropping down all the way to the bottom in each question type category column of the EBL Levels of Evidence in Table 11.2 one finds **expert opinion.** This low position might surprise newcomers to EBL since it might be assumed that expert opinion would hold a far higher position in the Levels of Evidence. First, this lowest level of the evidence hierarchy pertains only to expert opinion devoid of any supportive evidence. Yet, as Jonathan Baron has noted, "Because experts know the answer to most questions [within the area of their expertise], they usually do not have to consider alternatives or counterevidence."[80] Research findings on the inadequacy of expert opinion found in narrative reviews of the literature for clinical medicine formed a major original motivation for EBM clinicians to develop systematic reviews.[12]

The **case study** genre of research resides immediately above expert opinion at the second lowest rung on the Levels of Evidence for all three types of EBL questions, as depicted in Table 11.2. Case studies are a common form of research in all types of librarianship. Case studies are notorious for their susceptibility to many forms of bias, including most of the forms listed in Table 11.1. In contrast to this genre in other fields such as public policy analysis, case studies in librarianship additionally are prone to accentuating only positive outcomes while ignoring any negative events. This **positive outcome bias,** listed in Table 11.1, can be countered partially by including "lessons learned" to ensure the acknowledgment of some negative outcomes. Case studies might appear to be easily conducted forms of research because they seem to consist of constructing stories of how a project proceeded, but their proper execution, as detailed by Yin, requires a lot of rigorous effort.[82] Very few case studies in librarianship, however, even approach Yin's standards.

Case studies seem to be an appealing genre, not only for researchers, but also for practitioners critically appraising evidence in step three of the EBL process. Case studies pose problems for basing decisions due to their undue influence disproportionate to the quality of evidence produced from this type of research. For several decades behavioral scientists have documented how the human mind prefers processing information in narrative story form. In fact, the case study narrative story model otherwise can enhance teaching effectiveness in learning contexts.[83] **Storytelling** might be a comfortable mode of acquiring information, but it also leads to inaccurate perceptions of evidence as another form of cognitive bias listed in Table 11.1. The story model seems to be more memorable than other formats. This tendency of the human mind has serious implications when critically appraising evidence that includes case studies, since it gives a "good story" an advantage over more solid evidence presented instead through standard scientific reporting formats.[84-86] The story model also has wide appeal, possibly since humans construct self-generated life stories to form their essential self-identities.[87]

The three types of EBL questions rely on systematic reviews as their respective highest levels of evidence. The lowest levels of evidence for the three EBL question types consist of expert opinion at the lowest rungs in each hierarchy with case studies just above in the second lowest positions in each category. The highest levels of evidence for single research studies are unique across the three types of questions, however. Prediction questions rely upon **cohort studies,** intervention questions rely upon **randomized controlled trials,** and exploration questions rely upon **qualitative research studies.**

Prediction questions. Prediction questions probably are the most popular type of EBL question. Cohort studies answer the prediction type of EBL question at the highest level of evidence for a single research study. Cohort studies observe how a carefully defined population that shares a common experience or condition changes over time.[38] Cohorts might consist of all users of a book or journal collection, participants in a training class, a subset of users such as faculty members, or even a group of librarians such as library directors. Cohort studies are particularly helpful for detecting subtle changes in the cohort. Prospective cohort studies are slightly higher forms of evidence because they are designed prior to observed changes occurring in the cohort, whereas retrospective cohort studies recover data after the change has occurred to this population. Cohort studies are not the highest form of evidence for a single research study for answering intervention questions, but they are still commonly used to answer intervention questions. The biggest current obstacle to using cohort studies in EBL decision-making consists of identifying them in the librarianship knowledge base. While cohort studies are popular forms of research in librarianship, ranging from user education pretest and posttest studies to most collection resource usage studies, they rarely are identified as cohort studies by professional communications within librarianship. The goals of EBL would be greatly enhanced through the simple identification of all cohort studies by authors and editors.

Intervention questions. Intervention questions rely upon randomized controlled trials as the highest form of evidence for a single research study, as depicted in Table 11.2. Randomized controlled trials resemble prospective cohort studies in their protocols except that they enroll all members in a single population that then typically becomes randomized into a control group and an intervention (or "study") group.[37] The control group usually receives the normal treatment whereas the intervention group receives an experimental treatment. In this research design, a control group might participate in a regular library training course whereas the intervention group might participate in a new type of training class.

Exploration questions. Exploration questions rely upon qualitative research studies for the highest form of evidence from a single research study in the EBL Levels of Evidence depicted in Table 11.2. Qualitative studies vary from focus groups to participant observation. The specific form of qualitative study selected must match the EBL question appropriately. Exploration questions often answer EBL questions that might contain an explicit or subtle variation of the question of "why" some event or attitude has or has not occurred. Lisa Given provides an inventory of common qualitative research methods and has argued convincingly that they require rigor to conduct correctly.[88] Her perspective matches the experiences of others who have conducted their own qualitative research studies.

The Levels of Evidence must be supplemented in the third EBL step of critical appraisal with an evaluation of the quality of all relevant evidence. A systematic review might reside at the highest level of evidence of all three question type categories but be conducted so poorly that a lower level of evidence study trumps it on quality alone. Fortunately for newcomers to EBL, some useful guides help the novice navigate through a thorough critical appraisal of the available evidence when making an EBL decision. Andrew Booth and Anne Brice have developed a wonderful resource with their Critical Appraisal Checklist.[89] Booth and Brice developed this checklist while teaching critical appraisal skills throughout the United Kingdom, so it has been tested extensively with diverse audiences. Lindsay Glynn recently has built on this checklist and other resources in a more comprehensive manner.[90] While Glynn's Critical Appraisal Checklist holds great promise for EBL since it incorporates other validated checklists, it has not been tested widely itself.[91]

Step Four: Decision and Cost-Benefit Analysis

When engaging in EBL at the critical appraisal or decision-making steps, it seems most important to be aware of what biases might be exerting an influence while still keeping an open mind. While one must be deferent and respectful to legitimate authority, at the same time the pathological abuses caused by blind obedience to authority, as evidenced historically and experimentally,[92] require one to exercise independent judgment.

When a group of library professionals are debating the merits of a decision, some intuitively appealing yet fallacious forms of reasoning might become the basis for making a flawed decision. Newcomers to the profession who are unfamiliar with the types of fallacies that might emerge during such debates should consult a number of classic works on logic and fallacy. The **appeal to authority,** one of the forms of cognitive bias in Table 11.1, occurs when a recognized or admired authority figure becomes associated with a viewpoint outside the area of his or her expertise.[93-95] While this authority figure deserves respect within an area of expertise, this respect cannot be extrapolated to other domains.

Booth and Brice's Critical Appraisal Checklist

Is the study a close representation of the truth?

- Does the study address a clearly focused issue?
- Does the study position itself in the context of other studies?
- Is there a direct comparison that provides an additional frame of reference?
- Were those involved in collection of data also involved in delivering a service to the user group?
- Were the methods used in selecting users appropriate and clearly described?
- Was the planned sample of users representative of all users (actual and eligible) who might be included in the study?

Are the results credible and repeatable?

- What was the response rate and how representative was it of the population under study?
- Are the results complete and have they been analyzed in an easily interpretable way?
- Are any limitations in the methodology (that might have influenced results) identified and discussed?

Will the results help me in my own information practice?

- Can the results be applied to your local population?
- What are the implications of the study for your practice?
  —in terms of current deployment of services?
  —in terms of cost?
  —in terms of the expectations and attitudes of your users?
- What additional information do you need to obtain locally to assist you in responding to the findings of the study?

Source: Reproduced with permission from Booth, A., and Brice, A. "Appraising the Evidence." In: *Evidence-Based Practice for Information Professionals,* edited by A. Booth and A. Brice, 104-118. London: Facet Publishing, 2004.

Two additional obstacles to sound decision-making might predominate during the fourth step in the EBL process: **need for cognitive closure** and **groupthink.** The first, the need for cognitive closure (NCC), is not a psychopathological condition but actually a location on a personality continuum. This personality trait can manifest itself in different contexts, as either an advantage or disadvantage, depending upon the context. NCC can be highly advantageous in time-sensitive clinical situations when the traits of preferring order and structure, discomfort with ambiguity, desire for predictability, and decisiveness will ensure success. NCC can become an obstacle when this trait dominates in situations lacking the same kind of time sensitivity and the need for decision makers to consider more ambiguous issues.[96] Groupthink, a form of cognitive bias described in Table 11.1, represents a pathological hijacking of a group process that then causes poor decisions to occur.[80]

It can be worrisome that an EBL process can be conducted nearly flawlessly during steps one through three only to become warped beyond recognition during the fourth decision-making step. This derailment of the process probably will be disturbing to newcomers to the profession wanting to enact a sound EBL process. Not much has been written in a prescriptive manner about the fourth step in the EBL process, most likely because this step is immersed so thoroughly in particular contexts. Even within the same national contexts, libraries vary tremendously due to their broader parent institutions' missions. Specific libraries can have such vastly different organizational cultures, histories, and personalities that it is difficult to even generalize about, never mind prescribe, courses of action. Roughly parallel observations have been made about context and decision-making in medicine.[97] Newcomers to the profession need to pay close attention to their library institutional contexts when learning how to incorporate an EBL process. Newcomers also need to realize that cost-benefit analysis within a library includes a number of costs and benefits that are difficult to quantify or even assign literal monetary values; it takes time to understand how these calculations fit into any EBL process due to institutional contexts.

Step Five: Evaluate the Effectiveness of the Action Plan

Booth has outlined three levels of evaluation: practitioner, institution, and profession.[98] The North American context for all three of these levels differs from Booth's U.K. context, but his three-level schema still seems to hold for EBL practice in North America. The practitioner level involves reflecting honestly on whether one practices the EBL process in making important decisions. At the institutional level, librarians need to ask themselves collectively if they are practicing and promoting EBL for their most important decisions. Additionally, are they ensuring that each professional within their libraries has the resources, including the skills set, to practice EBL? On the professional level, are associations ensuring that EBL occurs? MLA, primarily in its Research Section and its Task Force on Research Policy Revision, has championed the practice of EBL in many respects over the past few years.

The EBL Process in Perspective

Apocryphal accounts from the management literature suggest that chief executive officers and other high-level corporate managers engage in mysterious, almost occult processes when making important decisions. Since much, if not all, of these management leaders' approaches remain ostensibly shrouded in the realm of proprietary information, professionals such as librarians instead need a reliable process for making their own important decisions. EBP enables librarians and other professionals to identify questions related to their important decisions, find relevant evidence, critically appraise that evidence, and then, while fully cognizant of potential biases, make sound decisions.

Future Directions for EBL

EBL has evolved so dramatically over the past decade that it seems risky to even attempt to predict to where it might evolve within the next decade. The core principles of EBL, such as the EBL process and the Levels of Evidence, have endured, and they most likely will remain essentially the same. The diffusion of EBL into other types of libraries probably will increase the diversification of EBL, but hopefully not to the extent that EBL becomes an empty slogan to describe any use of any form of evidence to justify any action. To make EBL a reality, professionals need to acquire a useful set of professional skills centered upon the EBL process. Health sciences librarians most definitely will be needed to provide this training to other types of librarians who have no ready access to these skills sets.

Heather Morrison recently has noted the need for librarians to publish EBL-related publications in open access venues as much as possible,[99] and this alone will greatly ensure the successful and accurate diffusion of EBL skills. This diffusion would reach, not only librarians in different types of libraries, but also librarians around the world. The three principal outlets for EBL skills training and the evidence itself in North America are open access journals: *Evidence Based Library and Information Practice; EBLIP* <http://ejournals.library.ualberta.ca/index.php/EBLIP>, *Hypothesis: Journal of the MLA Research Section* <http://research.mlanet.org>, and *Journal of the Medical Library Association* <http://www.mlanet.org/publications/jmla/index.html>. In the past, the pioneers of the EBL movement have come from North America and the United Kingdom primarily, but who knows where the next generation of pioneers will emerge, or from what types of libraries they will originate? Open access will facilitate the accurate and more complete diffusion to increase the probability of cultivating such leaders.

Training and graduate education will enhance the smooth diffusion of EBL. Andrew Booth and Anne Brice in the United Kingdom have been tireless trainers on EBL skills, particularly critical appraisal. MLA's continuing education course on EBL, taught twenty times only in face-to-face venues since 1998, became available to all librarians everywhere online during 2007. The National Library for Health Librarian Development Programme in the United Kingdom provides EBL training, but only for librarians in the United Kingdom.[100] Graduate education will be another major nexus for the diffusion of EBL.[101, 102] The University of North Texas, University of North Carolina, Wayne State University,[103] and Queensland University of Technology in Australia have taught EBL as part of their library and information graduate programs. Informal methods for enhancing diffusion of EBL include journal clubs and one-on-one collaborative or mentoring relationships.

A collaborative project at California Polytechnic State University in San Luis Obispo among colleagues from the United States, Australia, and Sweden offers a glimpse of where EBL might be headed next. This project involved librarian and teaching faculty members' oversight of student-conducted service learning research to produce EBL evidence for decisions at that library.[52] This arrangement might help reduce the workload of the producers of EBL evidence. The practical dimension of the situation suggests, however, that the consumers of EBL evidence will need to support the efforts of the producers of EBL evidence through institutional incentives and professional association advocacy of funding for the research needed to answer the most important EBL questions as a direct means to ensure informed decisions can occur within libraries.

CONCLUSION

Evidence-based practice has become a widespread approach to making informed decisions for many professions. Librarians can play essential roles in EBP as currently practiced by most professions. This chapter has focused upon the health science librarian's roles in evidence-based medicine, but many similar roles also exist in other professional contexts. Evidence-based librarianship provides a sequential process for making important decisions within the profession. While an assortment of biases might threaten to distort the EBL decision-making process, librarians' awareness of these biases can prevent such distortions and thereby ensure that informed decisions indeed do occur.

REFERENCES

1. Guyatt, G. "Evidence-Based Medicine." *ACP Journal Club* 114(Suppl 2, March/April 1991): A-16.

2. Rogers, E.M. *Diffusion of Innovation.* 4th ed. New York: The Free Press, 1995.

3. Goldberg, J. "The Starting Gate: Foreign Policy Divides the Democrats." *New Yorker* 82(January 15, 2007): 26-36.

4. Sackett, D.L.; Straus, S.E.; Richardson, W.S.; Rosenberg, W; and Haynes, R.B. *Evidence-Based Medicine: How to Practice and Teach EBM.* 2nd ed. Edinburgh: Churchill Livingstone, 2000.

5. Nollan, R.; Fineout-Overholt, E.; and Stephenson, P. "Asking Compelling Clinical Questions." In: *Evidence-Based Practice in Nursing and Healthcare: A Guide to Best Practice,* edited by B.M. Melnyk and E. Fineout-Overholt, 29-35. Philadelphia: Lippincott Williams & Wilkins, 2005.

6. Eldredge, J. "Evidence-Based Librarianship: Levels of Evidence." *Hypothesis; The Journal of the Research Section of MLA* 16, no 3 (Fall 2002): 10-3. Available: <http://research.mlanet.org>. Accessed: November 14, 2006.

7. Carr, R., and Eldredge, J. "A Content Analysis of Questions Generated by Public Health Practitioners in New Mexico." Poster presented at the Medical Library Association Annual Meeting, Phoenix, AZ, May 16, 2006.

8. Sackett, D.L.; Rosenberg, W.M.C.; Muir Gray, J.A.; Haynes, R.B.; and Richardson, W.S. "Evidence Based Medicine: What It Is and What It Isn't." *BMJ; British Medical Journal* 312(January 13, 1996): 71-2.

9. Del Mar, C.; Glasziou, P.; and Mayer, D. "Teaching Evidence Based Medicine." *BMJ; British Medical Journal* 329(October 30, 2004): 989-90.

10. Evidence-Based Medicine Working Group. "Evidence-Based Medicine: A New Approach to Teaching the Practice of Medicine." *JAMA; Journal of the American Medical Association* 268(November 4, 1992): 2420-5.

11. Centre for Evidence Based Medicine. Oxford, England. Available: <http://www.cebm.net/levels_of_evidence.asp>. Accessed: January 25, 2007.

12. *Systematic Reviews: Synthesis of Best Evidence for Health Care Decisions*, edited by C. Mulrow and D. Cook. Philadelphia: American College of Physicians, 1998.

13. Harris, M.R. "The Librarian's Roles in the Systematic Review Process: A Case Study." *Journal of the Medical Library Association* 93(January 2005): 81-7.

14. Patrick, T.B.; Demiris, G.; Folk, L.C.; Moxley, D.E.; Mitchell, J.A.; and Tao, D.H.. "Evidence-Based Retrieval in Evidence-Based Medicine." *Journal of the Medical Library Association* 92(April 2004): 196-9.

15. Weller, A.C. "Mounting Evidence That Librarians Are Essential for Comprehensive Literature Searches for Meta-Analyses and Cochrane Reports." *Journal of the Medical Library Association* 92(April 2004): 163-4.

16. Santesso N. "Emphasis on the Need for Guidelines for Documentation of Search Strategy and Results Was Needed, Criticism of a Cochrane Review Was Not." *Journal of the Medical Library Association* 92(October 2004): 393-4; author reply: 394.

17. Booth, A. "'Brimful of STARLITE': Toward Standards for Reporting Literature Searches." *Journal of the Medical Library Association* 94(October 2006): 421-9.

18. Crumley, E.T.; Wiebe, N.; Cramer, K.; Klassen, T.P.; and Hartling, L. "Which Resources Should Be Used to Identify RCT/CCTs for Systematic Reviews: A Systematic Review." *BMC Medical Research Methodology* 5(August 10, 2005): 13 pages

19. Zhang, L.; Sampson, M.; and McGowan, J. "Reporting on the Role of the Expert Searcher in Cochrane Reviews." *Evidence Based Library and Information Practice* 1(July 14, 2006): 3-16. Available: <http://ejournals.library.ualberta.ca/index.php/EBLIP>. Accessed: November 19, 2006.

20. Kaska, S.C., and Weinstein, J.N. "Ernest Amory Codman, 1869-1940: A Pioneer of Evidence-Based Medicine: The End Result Idea." *Spine* 23(March 1, 1998): 629-33.

21. Allemann, A. "Foreword." *Medical Interpreter* 1 (1928): unnumbered [2 pages].

22. Chapman, C.B. *Order Out of Chaos: John Shaw Billings and America's Coming of Age.* Boston: Boston Medical Library, 1994.

23. *Informatics in Health Sciences Curricula.* Rev. ed., edited by R.R. Sewell; J.F. Brown; and G.G. Hannigan. MLA DocKit. Chicago: Medical Library Association, 2005; unnumbered.

24. Coomarasamy, A., and Khan, K. S. "What Is the Evidence That Postgraduate Teaching in Evidence Based Medicine Changes Anything? A Systematic Review." *BMJ; British Medical Journal* 329(October 30, 2004): 1017-21.

25. Eldredge, J.D. "Search Strategies for Population and Social Subjects in a Medical School Curriculum." *Medical Reference Services Quarterly* 23, no. 4 (Winter 2004): 35-47.

26. Davidoff, F., and Florance, V. "The Informationist: A New Health Profession?" *Annals of Internal Medicine* 132(June 20, 2000): 996-8.

27. Plutchak, T.S. "The Informationist—Two Years Later." *Journal of the Medical Library Association* 90(October 2002): 367-9.

28. Shipman, J.P.; Cunningham, D.J.; Holst, R.; and Watson, L.A. "The Informationist Conference: Report." *Journal of the Medical Library Association* 90(October 2002): 458-64.

29. Byrd, G.D. "Can the Profession of Pharmacy Serve As a Model for Health Informationist Professionals?" *Journal of the Medical Library Association* 90(January 2002): 68-75.

30. Banks, M.A. "Defining the Informationist: A Case Study from the Frederick L. Ehrman Medical Library." *Journal of the Medical Library Association* 94(January 2006): 5-7.

31. Vanderbilt Center for Evidence-Based Medicine. Available: <http://ebm.vanderbilt.edu>. Accessed: January 24, 2007.

32. Jerome, R.N.; Giuse, N.B.; Gish, K.W.; Sathe, N.A.; and Dietrich, M.S. "Information Needs of Clinical Teams: Analysis of Questions Received by the Clinical Informatics Consult Service." *Bulletin of the Medical Library Association* 89(April 2001): 177-84.

33. McKibbon, A.; Eady, A.; and Marks, S. *PDQ: Evidence-Based Principles and Practice.* Hamilton, Ontario: B.C. Decker, 1999.

34. National Library of Medicine. *"Medical Subject Headings 2007.* MeSH Qualifier Data: Therapy." Available: <http://www.nlm.nih.gov/cgi/mesh/2007/MB_cgi?mode=&term==THERAPY&field=qual>. Accessed: February 25, 2007.

35. Strauss, S.E.; Richardson, W.S.; Glasziou, P.; and Haynes, R.B. *Evidence-Based Medicine: How to Practice and Teach EBM.* 3rd ed. New York: Elsevier/Churchill Livingstone, 2005.

36. National Library of Medicine. "PubMed. Clinical Queries. Clinical Queries Filter Table." Available: <http://www.ncbi.nlm.nih.gov/entrez/query/static/clinicaltable.html>. Accessed: February 25, 2007.

37. Eldredge, J.D. "The Randomized Controlled Trial Design: Unrecognized Opportunities for Health Sciences Librarianship." *Health Information and Library Journal* 20(Suppl 1, June 2003): 34-44.

38. Eldredge, J. "Cohort Studies in Health Sciences Librarianship." *Journal of the Medical Library Association* 90(October 2002): 380-92. Available: <http://www.pubmedcentral.nih.gov/articlerender.fcgi?tool=pubmed&pubmedid=12398244>. Accessed: February 26, 2007.

39. Bennett, M.D., and Gibson, J.M. *A Field Guide to Good Decisions.* Westport, CT: Praeger, 2006: xii.

40. Eldredge, J. "Evidence-Based Information Practice: A Prehistory." In: *Evidence-Based Practice for Information Professionals,* edited by A. Booth and A. Brice, 24-35. London: Facet Publishing, 2004.

41. Eldredge, J. "Evidence-Based Librarianship." *Hypothesis; The Journal of the Research Section of MLA* 11, no. 3 (Fall 1997): 4-7. Available: <http://www.mlanet.org/research>. Accessed: November 19, 2006.

42. Bayley, L., and McKibbon, A. "Evidence-Based Librarianship: A Personal Perspective from the Medical/Nursing Realm." *Library Hi Tech* 24(2006): 317-23.

43. Eldredge, J. "First International Evidence-Based Librarianship (EBL) Conference." *Hypothesis; The Journal of the Research Section of MLA* 15, no. 3 (Fall 2001): 1, 3, 8-11. Available: <http://www.mlanet.org/research>. Accessed: December 1, 2006.

44. Booth, A. "Evidence Based Librarianship Conference: The Award Winners." *Hypothesis; The Journal of the Research Section of MLA* 17, no. 3 (Fall 2003): 1, 4-5. Available: <http://www.mlanet.org/research>. Accessed: December 1, 2006.

45. West, K. "The Librarianship Conference Report: Convincing Evidence." *Information Outlook* 7, no 12 (December 2003): 12-4.

46. Eldredge, J. "Report from Brisbane: Third International Evidence Based Librarianship (EBL) Conference." *Hypothesis; The Journal of the Research Section of MLA* 20, no. 1 (Spring 2006): 4-5. Available: <http://www.mlanet.org/research>. Accessed: November 19, 2006.

47. University of North Carolina. School of Information and Library Science. 4th International Evidence Based Library & Information Practice Conference. May 6-11, 2007. Available: <http://www.eblip4.unc.edu>. Accessed: November 14, 2006.

48. Naylor, B. "The Evidence-Based Academic Library: Maurice Line and the Parry Report." *Interlending & Document Supply* 33, no. 2 (2005): 95-9.

49. Baker, L. "Library Instruction in the Rearview Mirror: A Reflective Look at the Evolution of a First-Year Library Program Using Evidence-Based Practice." *College & Undergraduate Libraries* 13, no. 2 (2006): 1-20.

50. Brooks, C.; Irwin, K.M.; Kriigel, B.J.; Richards, T.F.; and Taylor, E.J. "What, So What, Now What." In: *Evidence-Based Librarianship: Case Studies and Active Learning Exercises,* edited by E. Connor, 63-84. London: Chandos Publishing, 2007.

51. Vezzosi, M. "Action Research and Information Literacy: A Case Study at the University of Parma." In: *Evidence-Based Librarianship: Case Studies and Active Learning Exercises,* edited by E. Connor, 19-40. London: Chandos Publishing, 2007.

52. Somerville, M.M.; Rogers, E.; Mirijamdotter, A.; and Partridge, H. "The Cal Poly Digital Learning Initiative." In: *Evidence-Based Librarianship: Case Studies and Active Learning Exercises,* edited by E. Connor, 141-61. London: Chandos Publishing, 2007.

53. Missingham, R. "Evidence-Based Librarianship Down Under: Improving a Nation's Resource-Sharing." In: *Evidence-Based Librarianship: Case Studies and Active Learning Exercises,* edited by E. Connor, 85-101. London: Chandos Publishing, 2007.

54. Lerdal, S.N. "Evidence-Based Librarianship: Opportunity for Law Librarians?" *Law Library Journal* 98(2006): 33-60.

55. Asselin, M. "Evidence-Based Practice." *Teacher Librarian* 30, no. 1 (October 2002): 53-4.

56. Todd, R.J. "Irrefutable Evidence." *School Library Journal* 49, no. 4 (April 2003): 52-4.

57. Oberg, D. "Looking for the Evidence: Do School Libraries Improve Student Achievement?" *School Libraries in Canada* 22, no. 2 (2002): 10-3, 44.

58. Langhorne, M.J. "Evidence-Based Practice: Show Me the Evidence!" *Knowledge Quest* 33, no. 5 (May/June 2005): 35-7.

59. Marshall, J.G. "A Look at SLA's Evidence-Based Practices." *Information Outlook* 7(January 2003): 42-3.

60. Special Libraries Association. Research Committee. "Influencing Our Professional Practice by Putting Our Knowledge to Work." *Information Outlook* 7(January 2003): 40-1.

61. Eldredge, J. "Evidence-Based Librarianship: The EBL Process." *Library Hi Tech* 24(2006): 341-54.

62. Powell, R.R.; Baker, L.M.; and Mika, J.J. "Library and Information Science Practitioners and Research." *Library & Information Science Research* 24, no. 1 (2002): 49-72.

63. Zona, G.A. *The Soul Would Have No Rainbow If the Eyes Had No Tears.* New York: Simon & Schuster, 1994: 63.

64. Dewey, J. *How We Think.* Boston: D.C. Heath and Company, 1933: 108.

65. Cole, K.C. "Weird Science." *Columbia Journalism Review* 45(July/August 2006): 10-1.

66. Medical Library Association. Research Section. Evidence-Based Librarianship Implementation Committee. "The Most Relevant and Answerable Research Questions Facing the Practice of Health Sciences Librarianship." *Hypothesis; The Journal of the Research Section of MLA* 15, no. 1 (Spring 2001): 9-15. Available: <http://www.mlanet.org/research>. Accessed: October 20, 2006.

67. Eldredge, J.D. "Evidence-Based Librarianship: Formulating EBL Questions." *Bibliotheca Medica Canadiana; BMC* 22, no. 2 (Winter 2000): 74-7.

68. Booth, A. "Turning Research Priorities into Answerable Questions." *Health Information and Libraries Journal* 18(June 2001): 130-2.

69. Richardson, W.S., and Mulrow, C.D. "Lifelong Learning and Evidence-Based Medicine for Primary Care." In: *Textbook of Primary Care Medicine.* 3rd ed., edited by J. Noble, 2-9. New York: Mosby, 2001.

70. Booth, A. "Clear and Present Questions: Formulating Questions for Evidence Based Practice." *Library Hi Tech* 24(2006): 355-68.

71. Eldredge, J.D. "Evidence-Based Librarianship: Searching for the Needed EBL Evidence." *Medical Reference Services Quarterly* 19, no. 3 (Fall 2000): 1-18.

72. Eldredge, J. "How Good Is the Evidence Base?" In: *Evidence-Based Practice for Information Professionals,* edited by A. Booth and A. Brice, 36-48. London: Facet Publishing, 2004.

73. Perryman, C., and Lu, D. "Finding Our Foundation: Analysis of the Library and Information Science Abstracts Database for Research Article Retrievability." Presented at the Medical Library Association Annual Meeting, Phoenix, AZ, May 23, 2006.

74. Crumley, E., and Koufogiannakis, D. "Developing Evidence-Based Librarianship: Practical Steps for Implementation." *Health Information and Libraries Journal* 19, no. 2 (2002): 61-70.

75. Koufogiannakis, D., and Crumley, E. "A Content Analysis of Librarianship Research." *Journal of Information Science* 30(2004): 227-39.

76. Winning, A. "Identifying Sources of Evidence." In: *Evidence-Based Practice for Information Professionals,* edited by A. Booth and A. Brice, 71-88. London: Facet Publishing, 2004.

77. Beverly, C. "Searching the Library and Information Science Literature." In: *Evidence-Based Practice for Information Professionals,* edited by A. Booth and A. Brice, 89-103. London: Facet Publishing, 2004.

78. Information for the Management of Healthcare. "Research in the Workplace Award." Available: <http://ifmh.org.uk/RIWA.html>. Accessed: March 2, 2007.

79. Bayley, L., and Eldredge, J. "The Structured Abstract: An Essential Tool for Researchers." *Hypothesis; The Journal of the Research Section of MLA* 17, no 1 (Spring 2003): 1, 11-13. Available: <http://www.mlanet.org/research>. Accessed: January 3, 2006.

80. Baron, J. *Thinking and Deciding.* Cambridge: Cambridge University Press, 1988: 259-61.

81. Koufogiannakis, D., and Crumley, E. "Research in Librarianship: Issues to Consider." *Library Hi Tech* 24(2006): 324-40.

82. Yin, R.K. *Case Study Research: Design and Methods.* 2nd ed. Newbury Park, CA: Sage Publications, 1994.

83. Baumeister, R.F., and Newman, L.S. "The Primacy of Stories, the Primacy of Roles, and the Polarizing Effects of Interpretive Motives: Some Propositions About Narratives." *Advances in Social Cognition* 8(1995): 97-108.

84. Pennington, N., and Hastie, R. "Explaining the Evidence: Tests of the Story Model for Juror Decision Making." *Journal of Personality and Social Psychology* 62(1992): 189-206.

85. Baumeister, A.S., and Wotman, S.R. "Victim and Perpetrator Accounts of Interpersonal Conflict: Autobiographical Narratives About Anger." *Journal of Personality and Social Psychology* 59(1990): 994-1005.

86. McGregor, I., and Holmes, J.G. "How Storytelling Shapes Memory and Impressions of Relationship Events Over Time." *Journal of Personality and Social Psychology* 76(1999): 403-19.

87. McAdams, D.P. *Power, Intimacy, and the Life Story: Personological Inquiries into Identity.* Homewood, IL: The Dorsey Press, 1985.

88. Given, L. "Qualitative Research in Evidence-Based Practice: A Valuable Partnership." *Library Hi Tech* 24(2006): 376-86.

89. Booth, A., and Brice, A. "Appraising the Evidence." In: *Evidence Based Practice for Information Professionals,* edited by A. Booth and A. Brice, 104-18. London: Facet Publishing, 2004.

90. Glynn, L. "A Critical Appraisal Tool for Library and Information Research." *Library Hi Tech* 24(2006): 387-99.

91. Glynn, L. E-mail correspondence with J. Eldredge. January 29, 2007.

92. Milgram, S. *Obedience to Authority: An Experimental View.* New York: Perennial Classics Editions, 2004, 1974.

93. Fearnside, W.W., and Holther, W.B. *Fallacy: The Counterfeit of Argument.* Englewood Cliffs, NJ: Prentice-Hall, 1959: 84-9.

94. Copi, I.M. *Introduction to Logic.* 7th ed. New York: Macmillan Publishing Company, 1986: 98-9.

95. Kilgore, W.J. *An Introductory Logic.* 2nd ed. New York: Holt, Rinehart and Winston, 1979: 22-4.

96. Webster, D.M., and Kruglanski, A.W. "Individual Differences in Need for Cognitive Closure." *Journal of Personality and Social Psychology* 67(1994): 1049-62.

97. Dobrow, M.J.; Goel, V.; Lemieux-Charles, L.; and Black, N.A. "The Impact of Context on Evidence Utilization: A Framework for Expert Groups Developing Health Policy Recommendations." *Social Sciences & Medicine* 63(2006): 1811-24.

98. Booth, A. "Evaluating Your Performance." In: *Evidence-Based Practice for Information Professionals,* edited by A. Booth and A. Brice, 127-37. London: Facet Publishing, 2004.

99. Morrison, H. "Evidence Based Librarianship and Open Access." *Evidence Based Library and Information Practice* 1(2006): 46-50. Available: <http://ejournals.library.ualberta.ca/index.php/EBLIP>. Accessed: December 21, 2006.

100. Booth, A. E-mail LISTSERV communication. Evidence-based-libraries@JISCMAIL.ACUK. February 5, 2007.

101. Partridge, H., and Hallam, G. "Educating the Millennial Generation for Evidence Based Information Practice." *Library Hi Tech* 24(2006): 400-19.

102. Hallam, G., and Partridge, H. "Evidence Based Library and Information Practice: Whose Responsibility Is It Anyway?" *Evidence Based Library and Information Practice* 1(2006): 88-94. Available: <http://ejournals.library.ualberta.ca/index.php/EBLIP>. Accessed: November 19, 2006.

103. Baker, L.M. Personal e-mail correspondence with M.S. Wood. January 19, 2007.

Chapter 12

Health Informatics

K. Ann McKibbon
Ellen Gay Detlefsen

SUMMARY. Health informatics and health sciences librarianship are separate disciplines, although both embrace computers and information. This chapter provides a basic framework for health informatics, including definitions and history. Specific divisions of health informatics include bioinformatics, imaging, clinical informatics, and public health informatics; these are discussed as well as overarching issues of standards and vocabularies, information retrieval and automatic classification, education in informatics, and privacy, confidentiality, and security. The chapter ends with a brief look at the future of health informatics, a discussion of the overlap between health sciences librarianship and health informatics, and potential roles for health sciences librarians.

INTRODUCTION

Medical or **health informatics** is an emerging field that has substantial overlap with health sciences librarianship. Knowing what constitutes the fields of informatics and librarianship along with their common ground can enhance health sciences librarians' roles and abilities to function as health professionals. Health informatics has many definitions. This chapter discusses several standard definitions and develops the one used throughout. After a short history of informatics the chapter describes the most important divisions of health informatics (bioinformatics, imaging informatics, clinical informatics, and public health informatics) with brief discussion of consumer informatics. Sections of the chapter will deal with topics in informatics that have applicability to all of these domains (e.g., confidentiality, education, and standard vocabularies).

The chapter ends with some future directions in health informatics and a summary discussing health sciences librarians' potential roles in health informatics. By obtaining additional training or an understanding of health informatics, health sciences librarians can strengthen and build their profession and collaborate with others interested in using technology to harness health care information. The chapter is designed to provide an introduction and a broad general coverage of

Authors' note: Much of the material in this chapter comes from an eight-hour workshop developed by the chapter authors for use as a continuing education course by the Medical Library Association. They have given this workshop several times to librarian audiences and each time have been impressed by the interest and commitment that health sciences librarians have for informatics and their own profession. Both authors state that they are not associated with any of the products or services listed in the chapter and do not stand to gain financially in the use of any of them. The authors also wish to thank their colleague Jonathan Eldredge at the University of New Mexico for his input on the outline and later for his critical review of this chapter.

important topics in health informatics. Additional sources of information can be found in Appendix 12.A.

DEFINITIONS

The American Medical Informatics Association (AMIA), one of the major professional groups in health informatics, defines the discipline as a field that has "to do with all aspects of understanding and promoting the effective organization, analysis, management, and use of information in health care."[1] Other definitions emphasize the role of technology. For example, the U.S. **National Library of Medicine (NLM)** defines informatics as the "field of information science concerned with the analysis and dissemination of medical data through the application of computers to various aspects of health care and medicine."[2] A practical working definition can be stated as follows: applications of advanced computer and communications technologies to health care and specifically to information in health care. A more graphic definition comes from Friedman,[3] who states that successful informatics occurs when a person interested in health interacts with a computer and the results are better than either the person or computer acting alone.

Two schools of thought exist in defining health informatics. One school feels that the "computer" or "technology" aspect is paramount while the second stresses that the "health information" component of informatics is the prime factor. Whatever definition one adopts must be broad enough to include technology *and* health information. This chapter acknowledges the importance of the technology aspects of informatics but emphasizes the prominence of health information in health informatics domains.

HISTORY

The history of health informatics (or **computers and technology in medicine,** as the discipline was once called) is interesting and sets the stage for the rest of the chapter. The spread of mainframe computers, which started in earnest in the 1950s and quickly moved into health care, paved the way for health informatics.[1] Early advances in health care were centered on programming large computers to guide diagnosis or treatment. For example, ELIZA, a simple computer program that is still working today, was developed by Weitzenbaum at the Massachusetts Institute of Technology in 1966.[4] It "interviewed" people based on Rogerian therapeutic principles, using a simple analysis of sentences and reflecting back the content by asking further questions. Testing showed that, in some cases, ELIZA helped individuals gain insight into their mental health situations.[4] ELIZA is still available online.[5]

One early, effective diagnostic application was developed by de Dombal and colleagues. His 1972 computer program predicted the need for surgery in patients with stomach complaints when clinicians fed information about the patient into the system.[6] Accuracy rates were 91.8 percent for the computer and 79.6 percent for the physicians. In 1975, Shortliffe, a pioneer in health informatics, developed an automated system that proposed appropriate choices of antibiotics in infections.[7] His MYCIN system proved to be equal to or better than physicians. In 1977, McDonald showed that a computerized **medical records system** providing advice to physicians (e.g., this patient is due for a tetanus vaccination) improved care.[8] The early efforts in the field were typically physician-led projects that studied hospitalized patients. This was because only hospitals were large enough to buy or lease the mainframe computers and hire the staff needed to develop and maintain large systems. The discipline soon became known as **medical informatics.**

Many of these prototype systems were developed locally and did not gain widespread application, probably because of the substantial amount of time needed to enter patient data, huge variability across hospitals, and technical requirements to maintain the programs. In spite of their failure to become widely used, the influence of these early systems is still being felt in informatics applications in the twenty-first century.

With the introduction of the computer chip and the ensuing spread of smaller computers, more readily available and robust programs, and the Internet, more people and more diverse groups started to use computers to manage health information. For example, nursing, pharmacy, and dentistry have made major strides in using computers to digitize and control their information. Patients have also started using computers and the Internet to seek health information. The label "medical informatics" became too limiting for the new discipline, so a more inclusive title has evolved—"health informatics" or "health care informatics."

This chapter uses the term "health informatics," with an emphasis on "information." The term **e-health,** often used when referring to the transfer of health information using computers, may be too restrictive. Some see eHealth as not broad enough to fully include the information that clinicians use when caring for patients.[9]

TYPES OF DATA USED IN HEALTH INFORMATICS

Understanding health informatics requires a consideration of the kinds of health information with which it deals. Health information is divided into two major categories. The first is information gathered about individuals. These data are collected and used in interactions between a health professional and the person seeking care—the typical office visit or hospital encounter where the patient interacts with health professionals. The data on that person are the basis for making decisions. Data from individuals can also be used in "aggregate" form. This compilation of data across groups of patients is often done in health care research. The second category is the information which is published in journals, books, and the Internet—the "knowledge-based" information that fills traditional and digital libraries. Both categories of information are important to health informatics and they have unique needs for handling, manipulation, and presentation.

The first category, information on individuals, ideally encompasses data from a person's family history, their genetic makeup, and past lifestyle. These three factors account for a substantial part of a person's current state of health. Additional patient-specific information includes the person's health care history as well as current conditions and treatments. Comprehensive personal health care information should also include records of immunizations, diagnostic test results (e.g., computerized axial tomography [CAT] scans to determine if recurring headaches are related to a brain tumor), routine screening tests (e.g., Pap smears to detect cervical cancer), individual preferences (e.g., religion), health insurance status, legal issues (e.g., power of attorney or living will information), and contact information. Health care professionals who provide care for patients should be able to get information about their patients quickly and effectively, while those not involved with care should be blocked from access.

An individual's data can also be used for research or administrative purposes. An example of research data is the Nurses' Health Study.[10] Since 1976, an incredible amount of data has been collected on 121,700 women who are nurses. These nurses are surveyed every other year and will continue to be studied for many more years. This project is the largest and most important study of women's health and acute and chronic diseases ever done. The currently available data have been analyzed and many important findings published. Two reports show the range of issues. Stampher and colleagues found that up to one drink of alcohol per day may be protective from cognitive decline.[11] Lee and colleagues discovered health-damaging and health-promoting changes in women after widowhood or divorce, while remarriage was associated with mostly health-promoting behaviors.[12]

The data in this and other longitudinal studies, such as the Framingham Health Project,[13] the Harvard Physicians Study,[14] the Nun Study,[15] and studies from Johns Hopkins,[16] are not intended to provide information about an individual registered in the project but to enable researchers to study the group as a whole using data aggregation. Analyses of studies with a large number of participants provide a strong foundation for understanding what causes disease (e.g., shift work and suicide); what happens to people after they are diagnosed with a disease or condition (e.g., how long the depression will last and whether it will come back); and what new treatments are beneficial.

The second type of health care information is the published literature—journal articles, conference abstracts, posters, presentations, and technical reports that often provide the results of health research. This information is handled differently from patient-specific data. The volume of published information is immense; **MEDLINE®** had over 16 million citations in early 2007. Books and materials made available on the Web also contribute to this proliferation of publicly accessible information.

Most health informatics applications use patient-specific information while many also incorporate published information in the form of electronic textbooks, information resources on the Web, and specific knowledge collections. One of the biggest challenges of informatics is effective integration of published information into electronic medical records systems—getting useful information to clinicians when and where they need it, at the point of care. Health sciences librarians are important partners in this work.

FORMATS OF HEALTH INFORMATION

Another way to view health information is to consider the formats in which it occurs. Health data from individuals and studies come in a variety of formats: images, numbers, and text. Much health data are captured and stored as images. Examples are X-rays of bones and organs, CAT scans which use X-ray techniques to produce films of normal and abnormal tissue structure, and magnetic resonance imaging (MRI), functional MRI, positron emission tomography (PET), single photon emission tomography (SPECT), and others that harness advanced computer power to produce and store images.

Much health care data also exist in numerical format. Examples are laboratory data, appointment and procedure dates, and history and physical examination material. These data can be discrete and limited, such as the number of pregnancies that a woman has had or her birth date or height. These pieces of information are easy to store electronically and do not often change. Health data can also be continuous. For example, heart rate and breathing monitors connected to hospitalized patients display data on the monitors and then store the data in the hospital's computer system. Data sets, especially those that store numerical information, as well as process the continuous data, can be huge.

Most of the data or information in published sources is text based, in paper or electronic form, although some data are numerical or in image format. Examples of numerical data are census reports. Images in libraries are often used in professional learning or patient education situations. A mix of text and numerical data is also found in electronic health records. To more easily understand health informatics projects or services, it is necessary to think of what kind of data are being collected and used. Are they patient related? Are they personally identifiable? Are they numerical, image, or text based?

Now that health informatics data types and formats have been presented, the chapter next describes the four major domains of health informatics. After discussion of these, the chapter considers a number of content areas that affect them: standards and vocabulary; information retrieval; **privacy, confidentiality,** and **security;** and education.

DOMAINS OF HEALTH INFORMATICS

Shortliffe provides a conceptual framework of health informatics in four hierarchical domains.[17] These domains reflect what kinds of health information are collected and processed and move from the cellular level to populations.

1. **Bioinformatics** focuses on health information at the molecular and cellular levels, concentrating on processes. Information discovered here will have likely substantial impacts on the health profession in the next decade. Many current bioinformatics discoveries are important but not ready for clinical application.
2. **Imaging informatics** involves information obtained from tissues, organs, and other body structures by trained technicians using sophisticated equipment and processes and evaluated by pathologists and radiologists who make diagnoses and treatment decisions.
3. **Clinical informatics** deals with health data on individuals that are collected and used by many health professionals. This is the biggest, oldest, and most practical domain of health informatics. Clinical informatics is also the domain in which health sciences librarians have the most potential to use their skills and knowledge.
4. **Public health informatics** encompasses the collection, analysis, and presentation of data based on populations and societies. This domain includes reporting and research related to groups of people or geographic areas, for example, bioterrorism, influenza immunizations, and food inspections of restaurants and suppliers.

BIOINFORMATICS

Bioinformatics is defined as the study of information related to cells, genes, and molecules. It integrates computer programming, statistical analyses, and biology. Many people feel that bioinformatics is a domain separate from health informatics; other proponents feel strongly that it belongs within health informatics. Maojo and Kulikowski provide a useful comparison of bioinformatics and health informatics.[18] Librarians should consider bioinformatics as part of health informatics for three major reasons. First, bioinformatics and health informatics share many of the same methods and technologies. Second, researchers in both domains readily share experience, research findings, and communication channels. Graduate training programs in informatics often train students in both domains in the same department or unit.[18] The third reason is more philosophical—both domains have the basic goal of improving health and health care through innovative uses and applications of health information.

Bioinformatics focuses on research and teaching on **genomics** (i.e., genes) and **proteomics** (i.e., proteins), which are the basic building blocks of life. Bioinformaticians produce and collect huge amounts of complex data using the techniques of computational biology to determine and analyze genetic information. Bioinformaticians also use techniques from many other fields, such as combinatorial and structural chemistry and biology, imaging, structural biology, and neurobiology. Their research will have huge implications in understanding health and directing care in coming generations.

A better understanding of the complexities of bioinformatics is obtained through observation of its tools and Web sites. The University of British Columbia Bioinformatics Training Centre maintains a Web site of common tools and techniques for those interested in bioinformatics[19];

Teufel and colleagues review how these tools can be used.[20] Bioinformatics researchers are even applying standard library science information retrieval methods to solve bioinformatics problems; the work of Sehgal and Srinivasan on gene query retrieval is typical.[21] Several large U.S. academic health sciences libraries have hired bioinformaticians, often with PhDs in molecular biology, as information specialists.[22] Librarians interested in bioinformatics need additional training in computer sciences, biology, or both, preferably at the PhD level, to function well in these positions.

IMAGING INFORMATICS

Images play a major role in modern health care. These images help clinicians primarily with diagnosis (the condition or disease that is causing the symptoms) or with determining the causes of disease. Images can also be used to guide and assess treatment and monitor recovery. Medical specialties such as pathology and radiology are almost completely image based. Nurses are also using images more often.[23, 24] For example, nurses can take serial pictures which are automatically analyzed to monitor diabetic wound healing in patients being seen at home. Physical therapists also rely on images in their choice of regimen and monitoring care.[24] Images play a major role in health professions education. Real and simulated pictures and images, especially ones that can be manipulated, are becoming increasingly important. Pictures of procedures and other audiovisual materials are also becoming more important to patients and consumers.

With advances in information and computer science, imaging capabilities, and the rapidly decreasing costs of storage, more images are being produced, their quality is improving, and capabilities for collection, assessment, and storage are increasing. Storage and control of images collected from individual patients occur via **PACS (picture archiving and communication system)** and **RIS (radiology information system)** technology, with each hospital or hospital system having its own PACS.

Librarians are involved in the areas of storage and retrieval of patient-specific images. They provide input into how the images can be indexed and described so that they are readily retrievable by health professionals involved with that patient's care. Finding and providing images of planned procedures or disease processes for patients and families is also an important role for librarians. Work pressures reduce the amount of time patients have with their clinicians, and procedures are becoming increasingly complex and mechanized. Many Web portals, such as **MedlinePlus®,** provide high-quality, accurate, and easy-to-understand images or video of procedures for patients and consumers. As an example, MedlinePlus includes a tutorial on CAT scans[25] as well as videos of actual operations performed at U.S. medical centers.[26] The RadiologyInfo site[27] is an industry-based site with high-quality and readily available images for patients and families, with special emphasis on diagnostic tests and procedures.

The examination of RadiologyInfo or MedlinePlus provides practical insight into the sort of images and issues involved in imaging informatics. NLM's research endeavor titled the Visible Human Project® provides additional examples of medical images for many different uses.[28] Important secondary resources from NLM are AnatLine[29] and AnatQuest.[30] Anatomy and pathology education are other areas where images and Web-delivered resources are particularly important; examples include WebAnatomy,[31] a free interactive anatomy and physiology Web tutorial from the University of Minnesota, and the Virtual Autopsy Web site from the University of Leicester in the United Kingdom.[32] Additionally, any consideration of images in health includes nonclinical, image-rich Web sites, ranging from historical sites such as NLM's "Turning the Pages" online exhibition[33] and their database of Images from the History of Medicine,[1] to the vast photography files of the Wellcome Trust,[34] and the U.S. Centers for Disease Control and Prevention's PHIL (Public Health Image Library) file.[35]

CLINICAL INFORMATICS

Introduction

Clinical informatics is the largest and most fully developed domain of health informatics. As described previously, clinical informatics concerns itself with patient-specific information and data collection related to health and wellness. Ideally this data collection would start before birth and continue until after the person has died (autopsy data) and be kept to provide historical data for other members of a family or for research. The perfect electronic collection of personal health and wellness data has not been built yet, although many existing and experimental systems are striving to accomplish the ultimate goal: a complete and useful collection of data available to an individual and all those concerned with his or her health and well-being over the full life span of the person.

This chapter section is divided up into several subsections that include computerized health records and their various components, information support systems and **clinical decision support systems (CDSSs),** and telemedicine (information communication systems and how they are used in health). Each section is a short overview and readers are encouraged to seek additional information to expand areas of special interest. For example, the Wikipedia entry on electronic health records is a good summary of the electronic health records with excellent links to further information.[36]

Computerized Health Records

Definitions

A person's accumulation of health data is a huge, complex, and ever-changing collection of text, numbers, and images. Once these data are made available on large computers or the Internet, the label "computerized" or "electronic" health records comes into play. Electronic health records have many names. It is important to note the names, as variants of the concept exist, and each has its own limits and boundaries. For example, the electronic records of hospitalized patients are often called electronic medical or patient records. This "medical" or "patient" emphasis reflects that hospital care is physician-directed summaries of discrete admissions rather than long-term health of an individual.

Moving from an electronic medical records system to a system that includes more than hospital-based data, one goes to a system with the label electronic **health records system.** This label is broader than hospital-based electronic medical records system. Primary care clinicians in clinical settings (e.g., doctors' offices) use these electronic health records systems. Much of the care given by primary care physicians and nurses is centered on a person's health and wellness care over time rather than having an emphasis on discrete hospital admissions. Unfortunately at present, many of these clinic-based electronic health records systems have not been integrated with hospital systems.

The concept of **clinical information systems** is broader and newer. Clinical information systems were developed to encompass a broad array of health information on a person, and they often integrate data from clinics and hospitals. Some systems may also include data from pharmacies and other health professionals (e.g., physiotherapists and ophthalmologists). Health information system is a synonym for these systems.

A well-known example of a fully functioning clinical or health information system is the U.S. Veterans Affairs (VA) Vista system.[37] It is a single information system that integrates health data from 128 VA hospitals and clinics and 99 different applications (2003 data). Many non-VA centers have adopted the VA system. Care is streamlined and has improved with the use of Vista.

For example, medication mistakes decreased from 2/1,000 prescriptions to 5/100,000 after implementation—a huge reduction. A demonstration site is available.[38] More of these broad all-encompassing systems will likely evolve. Governments in many countries are seeking to implement broad-based systems that have the same control of health care information that aviation and banking have over their information.

Individuals are also seeking greater access to, and control over, their own health and wellness data. They want to contribute information to build a more complete picture of their health and well-being. Most of the currently-available health care information systems do not allow individuals easy access to their own information. However, with the spread and maturing of computers and the Internet, the ability to have access and contribute to one's own health data may become more common. Systems that allow people to control their own data either on the Internet or on their own computer are referred to as "personal health systems." Two examples of the integration of personal access and control of health information and hospital and clinic data are the Guardian Angel system from Harvard University and Massachusetts Institute of Technology[39] and the VA My Health*e*Vet system.[40] The Guardian Angel system allows data contained within the system to be transferable across institutions and insurance providers.

Components of an Electronic Health Record

Electronic health records are more than just the digitized equivalent of the traditional paper-based records of one's care. They integrate and process health information from many sources: family and medical history, current and past medications, laboratory test results, monitoring data, images, insurance provider data (e.g., what medication classes are covered), preferences (e.g., living wills), and a growing number of other data elements. This huge amount of data for each person is not maintained on one large computer but "distributed" across many computers. For example, a hospital-based medical records system links the pharmacy database with clinical, laboratory, billing, and nutrition services; radiology and other diagnostic services; and other systems such as scheduling for operations or consultations.

Comprehensive **personal health records** may contain more information, such as preferred appointment times as well as data added by the patient (e.g., weight loss and exercise diaries). Over time, Internet applications are probably the only feasible method of maintaining access to all of a person's health data in one system for use by multiple organizations and individuals.

One of the more exciting and powerful aspects of electronic health records is that computers can process information across time and settings and provide summaries in useful formats. For example an electronic system can provide patients and caregivers with detailed trends on changing cholesterol levels, guidance on dose adjustments to maximize the effectiveness of treatments, automatic reminders, or booking appointments.

Alerting Capabilities

Electronic health systems have the ability to provide **alerts** or decision support for clinicians. At the simplest level, computer systems can alert a physician or nurse practitioner that, for example, the patient smokes or has not received an influenza vaccination. The system suggests that these issues be addressed by setting flags or sending e-mail to clinicians. These flags or "ticklers" can trigger actions in that office visit or arrange for the patient to set up an appointment for counseling or further work. Advanced systems provide warning of inaccurate drug doses or patient allergies to certain drugs, as well as suggestions for improvements in care, such as timing of medication before surgery or rehabilitation sessions after stroke. In some instances these alerting services have been developed to provide information or direction to make or change clinical decisions. Advanced alerting systems are called clinical decision support systems.

Clinical Decision Support Systems

CDSSs are advanced computer programs or applications that are often built into electronic health records systems. Wyatt and Spiegelhalter define CDSSs as "active knowledge systems which use two or more items of patient data to generate case-specific advice."[41] Patient-specific data (e.g., the patient's age, disease status, and current medications) are assembled by the CDSS programs and then analyzed against a built-in knowledge base (e.g., if the patient has had high blood pressure for at least six months and is not taking antihypertensive medication, then consider starting one medication). The CDSS synthesizes information from the knowledge base and patient and presents suggestions so that the clinicians can make decisions more easily and effectively.

CDSSs have been widely used in business and industry. The Open Clinical Web site[42] describes the function and history of CDSSs and contains a comprehensive bibliography of successful systems. (The Open Clinical site has good sections on many informatics topics in health care.) CDSSs date back to the early 1970s when computer-guided systems showed improved assessment of stomach pain and surgery,[6] as well as improved antibiotic prescribing for infections,[7] and helped guide the choice of cancer chemotherapy regimens.[43]

CDSSs fulfill four basic functions in health care. First, they support administrative processes such as coding, documentation, authorization of procedures, making referrals, and summarizing data. Second, these systems help manage clinical complexity (e.g., keeping patients on the correct chemotherapy protocols) and ensure timely preventive care. Third, they are used in cost and quality control, managing orders, and avoiding duplication and unnecessary tests or procedures. Fourth, these systems are used in encouraging and enabling (and at times enforcing) the best possible care for patients—helping clinicians make decisions based on the best possible evidence from published studies (evidence-based practice).

Garg and colleagues[44] summarize the effectiveness of CDSS in clinical care: approximately 60 percent improve the care process and about one in six improve patient outcomes. Their review identified formal assessments of 100 CDSSs. Ten were diagnostic systems, twenty-one were reminder systems, thirty-seven aided in disease management, and twenty-nine assessed drug-dosing or prescribing systems. One promising arena of care for CDSS is in diagnosis, that is, identifying which disease or condition is causing the patient's symptoms. A relatively new Web-based application called Isabel analyzes symptoms entered by users and suggests diagnoses.[45] In the future these symptoms could easily be entered by an electronic medical records system. Although Isabel is a fee-based system, it allows trial access. To fully understand CDSSs, readers are encouraged to try Isabel.

The knowledge base of a CDSS is ideally built using data from published studies and other evidence sources. Building this knowledge base requires the skills of clinicians, computer scientists, and librarians. Because of the power of computers, the knowledge base can be quite complex. For example Ridker and colleagues developed a complex, useful scoring system to predict how likely a given woman will have a stroke or myocardial infarction. The data elements in the scoring system include age, smoking and diabetes status, blood pressure, and multiple cholesterol levels, which are given numerical scores that are summed.[46] This scoring can only be realistically done with a clinical information system. More CDSSs will be built, and they will be increasingly more complex as health care research expands and technology matures. Librarian input is important in the initial production of a CDSS and in keeping it current.

Information Resources in Electronic Health Records Systems

One area of value for librarians is the integration of information resources into the electronic health records. Chen,[47] Cimino,[48] and Magrabi and colleagues[49] and other groups have done much work in this area, but much remains to be done. The dream of health informaticians is to provide a system that can quickly and accurately assess when a clinician needs information and quickly provide what he or she needs. This information can be a pop-up or link to an electronic textbook or another information resource that can help the clinician make a specific decision. Standard textbooks may not be current enough, or provide enough detail so that care for a specific patient can be readily or accurately determined. Further research is needed to produce a system that can supply an appropriate answer to a question, before the question is asked. This area of harnessing external information resources to an electronic health records system can be thought of as an extension of CDSSs discussed in the previous section.

One indication of the need for these information support systems is that clinicians have been observed to need patient care information about twice for every three patients they encounter.[50] Information is needed more often for hospitalized patients and by clinicians early in their careers. The number of times clinicians need information has remained fairly constant since it was first measured in the early 1980s.[51] Not all information resources, however, are equally accurate or even helpful in clinical settings—in fact, four studies provide data showing some resources can change an initially correct answer to one that is wrong.[52-55] Librarians can provide valuable research in this complex area of intelligent integration of information resources into electronic health records systems.

Telemedicine

Telemedicine is the use of telecommunications technology for medical diagnoses (e.g., determining whether a mole is cancerous) and patient care (e.g., psychotherapy provided by a trained counselor), and for delivering medical services (e.g., reading radiology images) to sites that are at a distance from the provider. "Tele" comes from the Greek *telos* meaning "distance." Adding in the Latin root *medicus,* the term translates to "healing at a distance."[56] Telemedicine is a diverse collection of technologies and clinical applications used to transfer information from one site to another. The term **telehealth** is generally used to cover educational and consultative activities, while the term **telemedicine** encompasses direct patient care activities. In some situations, however, telehealth is a broader term that includes telemedicine. Both encompass everything from the use of standard landlines or mobile and cell telephone service for advice, to high-speed, wide-bandwidth transmission of digitized signals using computers, fiber optics, satellites, and other sophisticated peripheral equipment and software.

Telehealth started with telegraphy in the American Civil War and early consultations and data transmission using telephone lines,[56] radio communication in World War II, and the use of closed-circuit television. Almost every new communication method, major war, or health professional shortage has facilitated the development of new telemedicine services. As telemedicine has taken advantage of new communication technologies, it has become used more heavily. Once telemedicine was a domain separate from health informatics, but now it is now considered part of it because of its reliance on communication technology, digital information transfer, and computers.

Telemedicine or telehealth is useful for situations when or where physical barriers prevent transfer of information between patients and health care providers and the availability of information is vital to proper care decisions. The distance can be within the same building or health care complex but can also be across oceans and continents, or in outer space. Telehealth can be still (one picture), live, or voice only and occur either in real time or in a "store and forward" data mode.

Many groups of people use telehealth capabilities: clinically oriented specialties such as radiology, where trained professionals read electronic images to detect disease; laboratory personnel who transmit specialized data and images from tests such as electrocardiograms or pathology reports; and mental health professionals dealing with remote populations. Telemedicine will likely expand to surgeons and emergency physicians, who will perform or direct remote or robotic procedures.

Real-time transmission of vital sign data from patients in ambulances to a hospital trauma center can improve the quality and timeliness of care. Many conditions, such as stroke, must be treated early to prevent severe damage. Providing patient-specific information to clinicians in the emergency department allows care to be given in the ambulance and supplies information that the staff will use to become fully apprised of the situation and prepared for the arrival of the patient.

An international example of telemedicine comes from Bahrain. Its population has the highest national rate of diabetes (25 percent) with an additional 40 percent of the population at risk. The country has limited health care resources, especially trained health professionals. The Bahraini health professionals rely on telemedicine (twenty-two hospitals with satellite links) to link with Joslin Diabetes Center (Harvard Medical School) specialists in Boston, who, among other tasks related to diabetes, assess images of the retinas of patients (vision assessment is crucial in patients with diabetes) in Bahrain. Digital retinal evaluation tools are used for diagnosis and treatment of diabetic retinopathy (vision problems). Specialists in Boston also provide electronic consultations on many other diabetes-related issues for Bahraini clinicians and patients.[57]

Another example of telemedicine in action is sending X-rays and other similar images electronically to foreign sites so that the radiologist can read the images and provide diagnoses and treatment decisions. Small hospitals often see only a few cases at night that need radiologist input. They find it less expensive to pay someone $50 to evaluate one X-ray or other image than to spend $200,000 per year to employ a radiologist. Thus, an increasing number of hospitals are relying on "nighthawking" services to read and report on their images. Using this type of service, a hospital sends X-rays, CAT scans, and MRI images to Israel, India, and Australia, in time zones seven to fourteen hours ahead of the sending hospital. These images are read by fully trained and certified radiologists during their regular daytime hours.[58, 59] If the scan is top priority, it is flagged and read immediately, often in less than ten minutes. Otherwise, doctors read the scan, dictate a report, and send it back to the hospital, usually in less than thirty minutes.

Psychiatrists, other health professionals, and peers can provide high-quality care using the Internet.[60-62] Hospices, airplanes during flight, educational institutions, and patient education benefit from telemedicine applications. A substantial amount of professional education at all levels uses telehealth applications. For those interested in learning more about telemedicine, an online bibliography is available.[63]

In summary, many exciting and important advances of using technology to collect, analyze, and present health care information on individual patients are in place. Health care is changing constantly, with technology becoming a vital component of modern care. Computers and information technology are also revolutionizing the way public health professionals are working, providing faster and better ways of accomplishing routine tasks and providing new ways of practice.

PUBLIC HEALTH INFORMATICS

Public health informatics is the application of information collection, analysis, and presentation to public health practice, research, and education. Public health concentrates on the health and wellness of communities rather than individual patients. Examples of major public health advances include vaccinations, motor vehicle safety (e.g., legislation on infant seats, seatbelts, drinking and driving, and motorcycle helmets), control of infectious diseases, safer foods (restaurant and food service inspections), more effective family planning, and fluoridation of water. Public health informatics concerns itself with the flow of information around these and other community issues. Informatics is central to the ten essential services of public health:

1. Monitor health status of individuals to identify community health problems (e.g., high rates of teen pregnancy).
2. Diagnose and investigate health problems and health hazards in the community (e.g., industry-related particulate emissions).
3. Inform, educate, and empower people about health issues (e.g., prenatal classes).
4. Mobilize community partnerships to identify and solve health problems (e.g., outbreaks of food-borne illnesses in fast food restaurants or nursing homes).
5. Develop policies and plans that support individual and community health efforts (e.g., breakfast programs for young children in lower-income neighborhoods).
6. Enforce federal, state or provincial, and municipality laws and regulations that protect health and ensure safety.
7. Link people to needed personal health services and assure the provision of health care when otherwise unavailable.
8. Assure a competent public health and personal health care workforce fully equipped with the necessary equipment, tools, and services.
9. Evaluate effectiveness, accessibility, and quality of personal and population-based health services (e.g., early childhood education and mothers-at-risk programs).
10. Discover, through research, new insights and innovative solutions to existing and potential health problems (e.g., screening for lead poisoning in poor children).

Librarians have built effective partnerships with many public health agencies at the local, state, national, and international levels and fostered links with many schools of public health.[64] These partnerships will continue to grow and develop especially as concerns such as biosurveillance monitoring or pandemic influenza tracking are tackled.

Public health practitioners primarily operate on a community level but are also concerned with international and global issues (e.g., eradication of smallpox). The word "international" is defined in terms of national borders, whereas the word "global" encompasses the entire world. As it becomes increasingly clear that countries share many of the same health problems (pollution and infectious agents do not respect legal boundaries), the term "global health" becomes more aligned with current realities.

The future of public health informatics centers on the ability of technology to rapidly integrate data. Examples of data that can be successfully integrated are the reasons for emergency department visits; grocery store and drugstore purchases of over-the-counter medications; postal codes and local community locations of these occurrences; GIS (geographic information system) and GoogleEarth™ data; and school absences. Successful integration of these data suggests locations and types of outbreaks of disease, bioterrorism activity, or effectiveness of targeted prevention programs. A recent successful example of data integration is the public health preparedness planning that was done for the Salt Lake City Winter Olympics in 2002.[65]

Public health informatics is a rapidly growing and expanding area of health and wellness with promise for much expansion and need for trained information specialists. Public health informatics is the final domain of informatics. The next section of this chapter deals with informatics applications common to all four domains.

STANDARDS AND VOCABULARY

All disciplines have their own established standards and vocabularies to enhance communication and interoperability in their own and other disciplines. Standards become more important when a discipline is large, diverse, and complex; requires precision; and relies on computers and telecommunications. Their importance also grows if a discipline is international in scope, as differences across nations and languages are reflected in a range of terms and definitions. Health informatics has all of these characteristics, making standards and vocabulary especially vital to the function of health informatics products and services. Hammond and Cimino provide a broad in-depth coverage of standards and vocabulary issues in informatics that expands this section.[66]

Standardization is important for the collection, analysis, and transmission of data among systems within an institution and becomes more important when the transmission is across institutions. Examples of the kinds of transmission that occur in a health care setting would be knowing where a hospitalized patient is at all times (e.g., in surgery or rehabilitation), sending timely results of diagnostic tests from the hospital laboratory to the physicians caring for the patient, prescribing drugs that are covered by the patient's insurance benefits, or planning for hospital discharge of a mother and newborn infant. With respect to prescribing medication, an effective online system can check the patient's allergies, dosage, and duration, and if it is covered by the patient's health insurance. Once these issues are verified, the system can route the prescribing data to the patient's chosen pharmacy to ensure timely access to the drug and any patient educational material.

Several communication standards exist that enable different systems to transfer data back and forth, but North American standards are often different from European standards. Most North American health systems use a communication standard called **HL7 (Health Level 7)**.[67] HL7 sets stringent format and tagging criteria so that different computer applications can communicate effectively. For example, a hospital with a patient information system that is HL7 compliant will allow its electronic medical records system components to record, accept, send, integrate, and act upon information from nursing notes; physician orders; laboratory test sample scheduling, acquisition, and results reporting; pharmacy; discharge planning; and the patient's personal data. With effective communication, health care is improved for individuals, streamlined and simplified for clinicians, and easier to monitor and manage for hospital administrators. Often both costs and errors decrease when systems communicate flawlessly.

An important component of good communication across electronic systems is vocabulary control. Standard vocabularies label and describe items and actions. An effective vocabulary system deals with preferred terms, synonyms, antonyms, and relations among terms, in text or numerical format. Health care vocabularies are used to

- provide precise, concise, and accurate data to clinicians who use this information to make health care decisions;
- ensure uniform and consistent reporting of data (e.g., census data);
- enhance information retrieval (e.g., when this patient had an appendectomy) and streamline administrative functions such as billing or scheduling; and
- enable good data collection and analyses for research purposes (e.g., for patients with a specific disease, the factors that predict a successful recovery or death).

Many standard vocabularies exist in health informatics. The **Medical Subject Headings (MeSH®)** from NLM is probably the vocabulary best known by health sciences librarians.[68] This vocabulary is used for cataloguing and similar functions in libraries, indexing MEDLINE citations, and in many health informatics applications. MeSH will also likely play a major role in the integration of knowledge sources, such as textbooks, into electronic medical records systems.[5] Two other important vocabularies for informatics applications that are used more often than MeSH are the *International Classification of Diseases (ICD)* and the Systematized Nomenclature of Medicine (SNOMED®). Because so many different vocabularies exist, NLM developed its **Unified Medical Language System (UMLS®)** project, designed to bring together or interweave the vocabularies so systems can work together regardless of their structure.

The *ICD,* in its tenth edition *(ICD-10),*[69] is published by the World Health Organization. First developed in the 1850s, *ICD* has been used internationally for more than 150 years to report summaries of diseases and conditions, especially those that appear in health records and death certificates. Librarians often think of *ICD* as the "Dewey Decimal System" of health care because of its decimal presentation format. The Internet site <http://icd9cm.chrisendres.com/index.php> provides a searchable index to the *ICD-9* vocabulary. Readers are encouraged to look at this site to increase their knowledge of this vocabulary and its numbering system. Because of its use in broad standardized reporting of diseases and conditions in populations, *ICD* is not heavily used in nonhospital patient care settings (e.g., family physician's offices and nursing homes). *ICD* is considered to be weak in such prevention issues as well-baby visits or procedures and screening tests and may be too broad to cover health topics in enough detail to be useful in all clinical settings. The *ICD* classification system has been used as a foundation for other vocabularies because of its age and broad foundation. Work still needs to be done to make *ICD* into a truly clinically useful system—work that may need librarian input.

Many people working in informatics use adaptations of SNOMED and SNOMED CT® (Clinical Terms), the clinical arm of SNOMED.[70] This widespread use is especially true in the United States, as the Department of Health and Human Services (DHHS) signed legislation and contracts that allow anyone in the United States to use SNOMED.

SNOMED, developed by the College of American Pathologists, was started in 1964 as a list of procedures, laboratory samples, and outcomes used by pathologists. With the addition of the Read Codes (clinical codes used in informatics projects in the United Kingdom), SNOMED became an important vocabulary for broad-based clinical and health use.[71] One of SNOMED's major criticisms is that, in contrast with *ICD,* it is almost too comprehensive for clinical application. SNOMED has more than 364,000 codes with 1.45 million inter-relationships. Work, probably involving librarians, still needs to be done to make SNOMED more useful clinically.

Hundreds of other codes, vocabularies, and lists of terms exist in health care. This plethora of terminologies produces a "Tower of Babel" situation for those interested in high-quality and accurate data sharing. One way to remedy this multiplicity of terminologies would be to standardize and adopt one or two vocabularies. This is not practical, especially when considering the unique needs of clinical specialties, nations, and professional groups, and the number of existing vocabularies. To overcome the diversity of existing vocabularies and needs, NLM implemented the UMLS project in 1986. UMLS staff seek to take as many of the codes and vocabularies as possible and map them together in a complex system that is understood by both humans and computers.[72]

More than 120 separate source codes (term lists or vocabularies) that include 1.35 million terms in seventeen languages are analyzed and interlinked in the current version of UMLS. This list of vocabularies is available.[73] UMLS has three basic components: the Metathesaurus® (the terms), semantic net (the interconnections between the terms), and specialist lexical and other tools that make the system understandable. Figure 12.1 provides a brief piece of the semantic net.

The UMLS project is best described as an integrator of existing vocabularies and term lists rather than being a stand-alone vocabulary. Its major purpose is to allow different information systems to "understand" one another even if the systems use a different vocabulary base. It interconnects multiple vocabularies and codes so that online systems behave as if they understand the data each is processing and sharing.

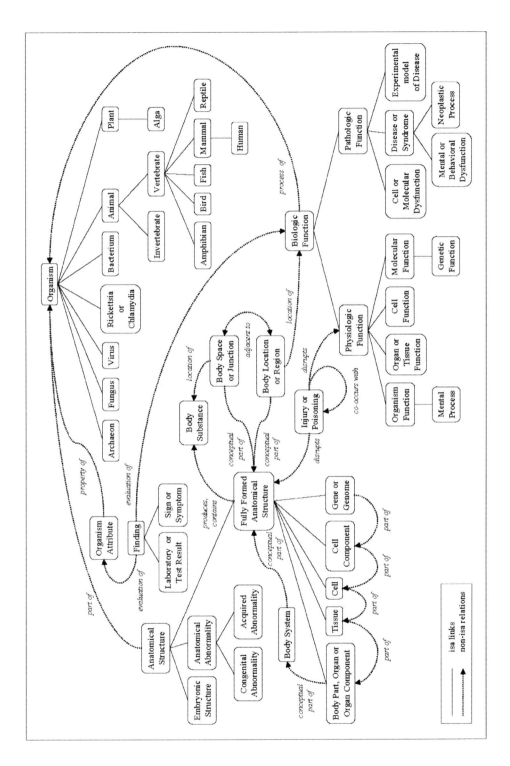

FIGURE 12.1. Part of the Semantic Net from UMLS. *Source:* From McCray, A.T., and Bodenreider, O. "A Conceptual Framework for the Bio-medical Domain." In: *The Semantics of Relationships: An Interdisciplinary Perspective,* edited by R. Green; C.A. Bean; and S.H. Myaeng, 189. Dordrecht; Boston: Kluwer Academic Publishers. © 2002 Kluwer Academic Publishers. Reproduced with kind permission of Springer Science and Business Media.

One example of using UMLS is a study by Robinson and colleagues at St. George's Hospital in London. They used UMLS to map their Primary Care Electronic Library resources, which are classified using MeSH, into their electronic medical records system that is based on SNOMED codes.[74] Their goal was to enhance retrieval of library information by the clinicians while working in the hospital. Although the task was difficult (MeSH has less than 10 percent of SNOMED codes), the researchers reported that their project was successful and increased the use of their electronic library.

The best way to learn more about UMLS beyond this limited introduction is to go to the UMLS Web site and either explore its components or take the online tutorial.[75] One of the applications of the project, and one important to librarians, is the possibility of UMLS to become a major component of seamless integration of patient records and the research literature, building on work already started. In summary, health informatics applications rely on standards and vocabularies. This reliance will only increase. Librarian input is vital. Another area of librarian expertise important to informatics applications is information retrieval.

INFORMATION RETRIEVAL AND AUTOMATIC CLASSIFICATION

Information retrieval is tremendously important in health informatics for two major reasons. Information retrieval allows for unique retrieval of desired material *and* automatic tagging (or indexing) of existing content.[76] Accurate storage and retrieval of information is important for clinicians, researchers, and administrators. Efficient, cost-effective retrieval is difficult in health because of the volume of information, its constant accrual, and the increasing complexities of modern health care. Tagging and retrieval of documents and information are important in almost all areas of health informatics; they are absolutely essential for electronic health records and clinical information systems.

Because clinical information systems are comprised of many interconnected systems or components, information tagging and retrieval methods ensure that all laboratory values, drug prescriptions, family history, previous hospital admissions, and other health or demographic data are available to health professionals regardless of changed names, different addresses, variation in health insurer, and care from different hospitals, clinicians, laboratories, and clinics. Good information retrieval also ensures that no information from other people or inappropriate situations is integrated (e.g., siblings or previous pregnancies). Information retrieval is also complicated by ethical and logistic considerations. For example, a physician should know that a person is HIV positive, but the clerk assembling hospital stay data for billing needs to be blocked from health status information. Some institutions refer to this restriction as "data hygiene."

Information retrieval is also important beyond good control within an individual's electronic health record and the systems in which it resides. Data from many records can be combined to provide useful information for researchers and administrators. For example, an assessment of data from hospital wards can determine if a specific hand-washing program decreased the infection rate of surgical patients or if more children with asthma came to the emergency department in the early fall than in the spring or summer. If seasonality in asthma was identified, staffing for pediatric pulmonologists and appropriate support staff could be adjusted for periods of differing needs. A Canadian research study using patient data showed that Sundays and Mondays in October and December have high rates of emergency department visits for asthma.[77] Emergency department administrators now adjust professional staffing according to the calendar.

Legal standards dictate that both administrative and research data must be viewed in a blinded manner; no personally identifying information can be allowed for legal, ethical, and societal reasons. Good information retrieval procedures allow for "de-identification" of records by detecting personal names of patients and care providers, addresses, birth dates, insurance numbers, dates of admissions and surgeries, and other possible identifying features. Once these identifying features are determined, they can be changed or deleted electronically so that the privacy of all concerned is respected while ensuring accuracy of the data. This de-identifying process is complex. For example, in the asthma visits study, the exact date of the visit must be changed for complete blinding, but if this date was changed to a random date in the year, the ability to determine the true seasonality of the asthma data would be lost.

Information retrieval is also vital for administration, billing, supply ordering, and insurance reporting. In addition, hospitals and other health groups, such as public health departments, have legal obligations to report statistical data on use of resources and diseases and conditions encountered. Local hospitals, cities, states or provinces, national and international bodies report these data, often on an annual basis. For example, all countries must report number and causes of deaths. In addition, approximately thirty to forty other conditions, such as infectious diseases, must be reported to various governmental agencies. These reportable conditions are fairly consistent across nations, although each country has its own reporting regulations. The Centers for Disease Control and Prevention maintain and report data on these conditions in the United States.[78]

Traditional information retrieval techniques are classified into three basic types:

1. Those based on set theory such as Boolean operators
2. Those based on algebraic methods (e.g., vector space models, cosine measures)
3. Those using probabilistic methods (e.g., fuzzy logic)

Database querying, standard mark-up languages (XML), and metadata systems can also be considered information retrieval processes for informatics applications. Several newer methodologies that enhance information retrieval systems include natural language processing, machine-learning algorithms, relevance feedback, term proximity, and combinations of methods (e.g., Boolean searching with terms processed for synonyms using UMLS or using semantic or meaning-based term mappings).

Much of the material that needs to be processed in health informatics is in full-text format that is not manually indexed or tagged. The most inaccurate of any of the retrieval processes is full-text information retrieval of unindexed documents. Searching for data in traditional spread-sheets is almost 100 percent accurate (e.g., determining if this child lives in Toledo or how many surgeries started after 11:00 p.m. in 2006). Because of the difficulties with full-text information retrieval, computer and information scientists are studying automatic indexing programs, data mining techniques, and other potential methods to improve retrieval in informatics. One important activity is NLM's own Indexing Initiative (II), a research project exploring both semiautomatic and fully automated methods for indexing biomedical text, especially for MEDLINE.[79] The II team created the Medical Text Indexer (MTI), which has been in use by NLM's indexers since late 2002 to assist in assigning MeSH terms to MEDLINE citations.

Health data present special challenges in retrieval. Temporality (what happens over time) is tremendously important and hard to represent in indexing and retrieval systems. For example, physicians need to segregate data according to this pregnancy and not the other two previous pregnancies, or they want to see blood glucose levels for today and compare them with those of the previous month and year to assess time trends.

In addition, a substantial amount of information in medical charts is included as speculation—possible diagnoses for given symptoms. All of the possible diagnoses are often listed in physician notes, and this factor must be accounted for in information retrieval. For example, a person with a chronic cough might have a chart note that included the text "we ruled out tuberculosis, asthma, and lung cancer and came to the final diagnosis of esophageal reflux." A good retrieval program should be able to identify that this patient has only the reflux and not the conditions that were ruled out. Different languages, cultures, disciplines, and vocabulary also complicate retrieval, as does the sheer volume of material. Information classification and retrieval is important to those interested in clinical informatics, and it is also being studied seriously in bioinformatics research centers[80] and by public health informaticians.[75]

This chapter cannot cover all aspects of information classification and retrieval; this section just raises issues important to informatics and shows where librarians are needed. Many resources exist for expanding information retrieval knowledge.[81, 82]

PRIVACY, CONFIDENTIALITY, AND SECURITY

Privacy, confidentiality, and security are vitally important features of informatics applications. These features reflect ethical, legal, and societal considerations around information and data collected and maintained by computers.[83] Because of the nature of health and wellness, health informatics applications are and must be held to very high standards of privacy, confidentiality, and security.

Security deals with how robust the application is in relation to protecting its data from external tampering or access from unauthorized people or systems. Put another way, security is a system's ability to protect itself and its data. Health care applications must be very secure. Altered, inaccurate, or inappropriately disclosed health data can irrevocably change peoples' lives.

Confidentiality is defined as ensuring that only those people who are authorized have access to certain information. Health care organizations usually deal with this by assigning people function-based roles or permission levels. For example, physicians in certain clinics or wards of a hospital would be given access to most, but not necessarily all, parts of a patient's medical record during hospitalization. Nurses on the wards would have access to less information on that patient, and billing clerks would have very limited access, especially in relation to identities linked with diagnoses. Sorting out levels of permission becomes complex in large institutions. For example, a middle-aged man admitted to a psychiatric hospital to treat issues arising from a combination of syphilis, obsessive-compulsive disorder, and alcoholism would likely have his three diagnoses available to the psychiatrist, two to his internist and nurses, and one to his rehabilitation staff. The billing clerk would not know any diagnoses—just the resources used during his stay to produce final billing information and hospital statistics.

Privacy is the amount of control that an individual has over what data are collected on him or her, who has access to the data, how they are stored and used, to whom they are passed, and who maintains the data. This is probably the most difficult of the three ethical/legal issues.

Many issues arising from security, privacy, and confidentiality are governed by local, regional, *and* national legislation. Every hospital and state has regulations in place and enforces them. In addition, the U.S. **Health Insurance Portability and Accountability Act (HIPAA)** was designed to ensure health insurance portability across health systems and severely limit the use of pre-existing condition exclusions by group health plans to deny anyone coverage or preferential charging. In carrying out this mandate, HIPAA staff identified many privacy issues that needed to be addressed. To do this, the U.S. government brought in the second part of HIPAA, Title II, Administrative Simplification. Title II requires the DHHS to establish national standards for electronic health care transactions and national identifiers for providers, health plans, and employers. It also addresses the security and privacy of health data. Working out the details of HIPAA and Title II came to mean the creation of minimum standards for the process through which providers, clearinghouses, and payers communicate confidential information about patients. When multiple rules exist for any given situation, legal opinion states that usually the most stringent criteria must be met.

Most other nations have similar sorts of protective legislation. Some critics say that privacy, security, and confidentiality issues have gone too far and placed undue restrictions on administrators and researchers. Much work remains to be done to perfect informatics systems and applications and how they process, present, and protect health information. Because many issues in this area of information and ethics are similar to issues that librarians deal with in running their systems, librarians have a voice that needs to be heard in health informatics and the appropriate use of information.

EDUCATION IN HEALTH INFORMATICS

Those who are interested in working in health informatics need to obtain relevant training and experience. Although many established informaticians obtained their training while working on projects, formal education is now required for most informatics positions.[84, 85] Four education models provide training or credentialing in health informatics. The initial method is to obtain a first degree in a university-based program. Some institutions offer an undergraduate degree in health informatics. Other relevant degrees can be in health care, computer science, or computer engineering. The second method of informatics training is postgraduate (MSc and PhD degrees or diplomas) training programs based in universities with a medical or health informatics program, or through one of the NLM training grants or related programs. Approximately eighteen of these NLM training programs exist. Other nations, especially those in Europe, have their own national training programs. The third option is the route to education that many of those aspiring to careers in health informatics take: attending medical or health informatics short courses, continuing education activities at professional meetings, and seeking instruction via distance education from the health informatics community. The fourth option is on-the-job training, with personnel working in informatics domains.

Many organizations provide informatics training opportunities. Web sites provide detailed information on courses and workshops and degree-based educational programs. NLM not only provides training, it funds many students for certificates and MSc and PhD degrees.[86] NLM programs are open to everyone, although funding is often restricted to U.S. citizens or those with "resident alien" status. AMIA has a comprehensive listing of programs[87] which includes approximate fifty international universities that offer degrees. An example of this kind of university-based program comes from the Department of Medical Informatics and Clinical Epidemiology (DMICE) at the Oregon Health and Science University.[84] The Web site includes a discussion of choosing a program of informatics education based on personal needs, background, and career expectations. AMIA also has established its 10x10 Program that uses curricular content from existing informatics training programs with special emphasis toward those programs with a proven track record in distance learning. This program aims to provide 10,000 trained informaticians by the year 2010 to meet the projected shortage of trained professionals that now exists and will likely continue for many years. They emphasize training in bioinformatics and clinical and public health informatics. People from many backgrounds and careers are seeking informatics training. Librarians have graduated from many of these programs and are working on informatics projects in many settings, both inside and outside libraries.

Individuals who want to work in informatics areas or just wish to keep current on advances in informatics should consider a mix of educational opportunities, probably on a continuing basis because of the ever-changing nature of the field. They also need to note that because health informatics is such a broad-based, multidisciplinary field, educational opportunities in many other domains outside informatics would enhance personal education and job readiness in informatics arenas.

FUTURE

These are exciting times for all, especially those who work with information management and technology. This section on the future could be the longest of the chapter, but it will only briefly mention some near-future developments in health care informatics. Wireless technologies are already bringing handheld resources for medical decision-making to the point of care. Fast-paced practice areas, such as emergency departments and intensive care units where clinicians and technicians must quickly deal with many potential conditions, will derive great benefit from use of these handheld applications to enhance care decisions. Voice technology will also improve abilities to provide high-quality care. For example, voice-activated data collection and manipulation of health information will improve the care process for those who gather substantial amounts of information from patients or those who cannot easily use keyboards (e.g., surgeons during surgery). Technology will also play an increasing role in computerized interviewing.[88] Education for consumers and health professionals at all levels will benefit from intelligent, computer-assisted tutoring and testing,[89] virtual reality and simulations,[90] and video games for health instruction and preparation for procedures.[91]

In the diagnostic area, people will request and receive full-body scans, including ones when they are still well, looking for potential problems. Pill cameras that can be swallowed and virtual colonoscopies will be routinely used. Robots will provide or enhance personal care and monitoring for the elderly and those needing rehabilitation.[92] Brain implants will be available for some conditions, including artificial vision and computer-assisted movement. Smart technologies will provide truly portable health records, automated furniture and clothing will help us stay mobile, toilets will analyze body fluids and record weight changes to monitor potential problems, and entire homes will have informatics applications to help and monitor those who need special care.[93] Wristwatches and implants with geographical information systems (GISs) will allow monitoring of adults with dementia and locate children before and after school. The pill bottle itself will notify people how and when to take their medications, initiate contact with physicians and pharmacies when refills are needed, and allow monitoring of medication adherence at a distance, a particularly attractive option for families concerned with elderly parents who are living alone.[94]

In addition, almost all areas of human involvement will have their own informatics applications. For example, such disciplines as chemistry, music, and social sciences already have strong informatics programs. The premise of this chapter is that librarians have much to learn from health informaticians. Other areas of informatics, such as nursing informatics and **social informatics**,[95-99] possess great relevance both to health informatics and librarianship. All of these advances in health informatics, and many more, will affect the lives of many people. The next section will discuss the areas of health informatics that influence the jobs and profession of health sciences librarians.

HEALTH SCIENCES LIBRARIANS AND HEALTH INFORMATICS

Health informaticians and health sciences librarians deal with computers and health information. Librarians have typically concentrated more on published health information such as books, journals, and reports, with health informaticians dealing more with patient-specific information. Librarians can contribute to both professions in three broad areas: sharing existing expertise; working collaboratively with informaticians on research and implementation projects and developing tools and services; and educating health professionals and consumers.

Librarians have expertise to share in developing and controlling access to large databases of diverse content. Health information systems in hospital and clinic settings share many of the characteristics and challenges of online catalogues, including issues of privacy, confidentiality, and security; ever-expanding volume of information; multiplicity of user groups; and tremendous size and complexities. Librarians working with computer scientists have been in the forefront of manual and automated indexing content, setting standards and vocabularies, and improving information retrieval. This expertise and these skills sets are needed to develop effective and comprehensive clinical information systems.

Librarians will also play roles in the development of new information products and services. Much work is being done by librarians and others to produce useful resources that can be implemented into clinical information systems to provide clinicians with evidence-based decision support. An example of the work of librarians who are collaborating with clinicians to build high-quality information resources is the product *BMJ Clinical Evidence,* a new-generation, textbook-like clinical resource from BMJ Publishing Group.[100] These new information resources may resemble a comprehensive electronic textbook or be the knowledge base that drives CDSSs.

As well as working on teams to develop new tools, librarians will continue to produce informatics research. For example, librarians played a major role in developing the Clinical Queries in PubMed, designing the embedded search strategies that retrieve only clinically-relevant studies that are appropriate for clinical care decision-making.[86, 101] Many other examples of librarian-assisted implementations exist, including the work of Duke University librarians, who have produced high-quality informatics research working with clinicians.[102]

The final informatics area that is rich for librarians is the education of health professionals. Librarians have long been strong teachers in information literacy skills and in tools for information management by health professionals. This teaching may be in formal face-to-face classes, or in support of problem-based learning, or simply at a teachable moment; it may also be provided in Web-based formats or via online tutorials. Health sciences librarians working in academic centers provide a number of excellent teaching examples, including those at Indiana University[103] and the University of Chicago.[104] Many other examples of librarian involvement in health professional education exist. Librarians are also educating consumers in areas of health informatics, especially in public and consumer libraries. Health sciences librarians need to realize that public librarians provide more health reference service than they do and work to build partnerships among groups of librarians and health informaticians.[105]

The challenge for librarians interested in working in the area of informatics is twofold. First, librarians need to enhance their training in informatics. Health sciences librarians come to the profession with many skills and abilities, but they almost always need to seek more training and experience to be able to function effectively in modern health care settings. Second, librarians must actively seek opportunities to collaborate with health informatics researchers and educators. These two challenges are not unique to health care. These same challenges are often brought forth in any discussion of professional advancement for librarians. Health informatics provides special, unique, and important rewards for those health sciences librarians who want to build their skills and abilities and work in this exciting and growing area.

CONCLUSION

This chapter has sought to provide an introduction to health informatics for librarians interested in careers in health sciences. Many exciting possibilities of collaboration, service, and education exist. Health informatics is a vital and growing field that influences and learns from many disciplines. Librarians have been involved in health informatics since its inception and will continue to play important roles in the future. Both health informatics and health sciences librarianship are changing and exciting fields and hold the promise of improving health and well-being. Working collaboratively on informatics teams will only enhance the benefits.

APPENDIX 12.A. HEALTH INFORMATICS ASSOCIATIONS AND JOURNALS

Health Informatics Associations

ACMI: Amcrican College of Medical Informatics *(honor society)*
<http://www.amia.org/college/>; <http://www.amia.org/college/fellows.asp>

AHIMA: American Health Information Management Association
<http://www.ahima.org/about/>

AHRQ: Agency for Healthcare Research and Quality (formerly AHCPR—Agency for Healthcare Policy & Research)
<http://www.ahrq.gov>; <http://www.ahrq.gov/about/profile.htm>

AMIA: American Medical Informatics Association
<http://www.amia.org/inside/faq/>; <http://www.amia.org/mbrcenter/wg/>

ANIA: American Nursing Informatics Association
<http://www.ania.org/Resources.htm>

ASIST: American Society for Information Science and Technology; SIG MED Medical Information Systems
<http://www.asis.org/AboutASIS/asis-sigs.html#SIGMED>

HIMSS: Healthcare Information and Management Systems Society
<http://www.himss.org/ASP/index.asp>; <http://www.himss.org/ASP/sigsHome.asp>

HRSA: Health Resources and Services Administration (DHHS)
<http://www.hrsa.gov/about.htm>

IMIA: International Medical Informatics Association
<http://www.imia.org/about.html>; <http://www.imia.org/member_societies.html>

LHNCBC: Lister Hill National Center for Biomedical Communications (NLM)
<http://lhncbc.nlm.nih.gov/lhc/servlet/Turbine>

MLA: Medical Library Association; Medical Informatics Section
<http://www.medinfo.mlanet.org/>

NCBI: National Center for Biotechnology Information
<http://www.ncbi.nlm.nih.gov/>

NICHSR: National Information Center on Health Services Research and Health Care Technology
<http://www.nlm.nih.gov/hsrinfo/hsrsites.html>

NLM: National Library of Medicine; NLM Research Programs
<http://www.nlm.nih.gov/biomedical.html>

SMDM: Society for Medical Decision Making
<http://www.smdm.org/>

Partial List of Health Informatics Journals

Artificial Intelligence in Medicine
Bioinformatics
BMC (BioMed Central) *Bioinformatics*

BMC Medical Informatics and Decision Making
Computers in Biology and Medicine
CIN: Computers, Informatics, Nursing
Health Informatics Journal
Healthcare Informatics
IEEE (Institute of Electrical and Electronics Engineers) *Transactions on Information Technology in Biomedicine*
Informatics in Primary Care
International Journal of Medical Informatics
Journal of Biomedical Informatics
Journal of Healthcare Information Management
Journal of Medical Internet Research
Journal of Telemedicine and Telecare
JAMIA: Journal of the American Medical Informatics Association
Medical Decision Making
Medical Informatics and the Internet
Online Journal of Nursing Informatics
Telemedicine Journal and eHealth

REFERENCES

1. American Medical Informatics Association. "History of Medical Informatics." (2003). Available: <http://www.amia.org/history/>. Accessed: January 19, 2007.

2. U.S. National Library of Medicine. MeSH Browser. "Medical Subject Headings." (2007). Available: <http://www.nlm.nih.gov/mesh/MBrowser.html>. Accessed: January 20, 2007.

3. Friedman, C.P., and Wyatt, J.C. *Evaluation Methods in Biomedical Informatics.* 2nd ed. New York: Springer, 2006.

4. Wikipedia. "ELIZA." (2006). Available: <http://en.wikipedia.org/wiki/ELIZA>. Accessed: February 5, 2007.

5. "ELIZA—A Friend You Could Never Have Before." Available: <http://www-ai.ijs.si/eliza/eliza.html>. Accessed: March 15, 2007.

6. de Dombal, F.T.; Leaper, D.J.; Staniland, J.R.; McCann, A.P.; and Horrocks, J.C. "Computer-Aided Diagnosis of Acute Abdominal Pain." *BMJ; British Medical Journal* 2, no. 5804 (April 1, 1972): 9-13.

7. Shortliffe, E.H.; Davis, R.; Axline, S.G.; Buchanan, B.G.; Green, C.C.; and Cohen, S.N. "Computer-Based Consultations in Clinical Therapeutics: Explanation and Rule Acquisition Capabilities of the MYCIN System." *Computers in Biomedical Research* 8, no. 4 (August 1975): 303-20.

8. McDonald, C.J.; Murray, R.; Jeris, D.; Bhargava, B.; Seeger, J.; and Blevins, L. "A Computer-Based Record and Clinical Monitoring System for Ambulatory Care." *American Journal of Public Health* 67, no. 3 (March 1977): 240-5.

9. Oh, H.; Rizo, C.; Enkin, M.; and Jadad, A. "What Is eHealth (3): A Systematic Review of Published Definitions." *Journal of Medical Internet Research* 7, no. 1 (February 24, 2005): e1. Available: <http://www.jmir.org/2005/1/e1/>. Accessed: March 23, 2007.

10. Field, A.E.; Byers, T.; Hunter, D.J.; et al. "Weight Cycling, Weight Gain, and Risk of Hypertension in Women." *American Journal of Epidemiology* 150, no. 6 (September 15, 1999): 573-9.

11. Stampfer, M.J.; Kang, J.H.; Chen, J.; Cherry, R.; and Grodstein, F. "Effects of Moderate Alcohol Consumption on Cognitive Function in Women." *New England Journal of Medicine* 352, no. 3 (January 20, 2005): 245-53.

12. Lee, S.; Cho, E.; Grodstein, F.; Kawachi, I.; Hu, F.B.; and Colditz, G.A. "Effects of Marital Transitions on Changes in Dietary and Other Health Behaviours in U.S. Women." *International Journal of Epidemiology* 34, no. 1 (February 2005): 69-78.

13. Jonker, J.T.; De Laet, C.; Franco, O.H.; Peeters, A.; Mackenbach, J.; and Nusselder, W.J. "Physical Activity and Life Expectancy With and Without Diabetes: Life Table Analysis of the Framingham Heart Study." *Diabetes Care* 29, no. 1 (January 2006): 38-43.

14. Djousse, L., and Gaziano, J.M. "Alcohol Consumption and Risk of Heart Failure in the Physicians' Health Study I." *Circulation* 115, no. 1 (January 2, 2007): 34-9.

15. Snowdon, D.A. "Healthy Aging and Dementia: Findings from the Nun Study." *Annals of Internal Medicine* 139, no. 5, pt. 2 (September 2, 2003): 450-4.

16. Kuo, W.H.; Gallo, J.J.; and Eaton, W.W. "Hopelessness, Depression, Substance Disorder, and Suicidality—A 13-Year Community-Based Study." *Social Psychiatry and Psychiatric Epidemiology* 39, no. 6 (June 2004): 497-501.

17. Shortliffe, E.H. "Overview of Biomedical Informatics." New York: Columbia University, 2006. Available: <http://bmi.asu.edu/symposium/downloads/EdwardShortliffe_presentation.pdf>. Accessed: January 23, 2007.

18. Maojo, V., and Kulikowski, G.A. "Bioinformatics and Medical Informatics: Collaborations on the Road to Genomic Medicine?" *Journal of the American Medical Informatics Association* 10, no. 6 (December 2003): 515-22.

19. University of British Columbia Bioinformatics Centre. "Bioinformatics Links Directory." (2007). Available: <http://bioinformatics.ubc.ca/resources/links_directory/>. Accessed: February 6, 2007.

20. Teufel, A.; Krupp, M.; Weinmann, A.; and Galle, P. R. "Current Bioinformatics Tools in Genomic Biomedical Research." *International Journal of Molecular Medicine* 17, no. 6 (June 2006): 967-73.

21. Sehgal, A.K., and Srinivasan, P. "Retrieval with Gene Queries." *BMC Bioinformatics* 7 (April 21, 2006): 220. Available: <http://www.biomedcentral.com/1471-2105/7/220>. Accessed: March 23, 2007.

22. Helms, A.J.; Bradford, K.D.; Warren, N.J.; and Schwartz, D.G. "Bioinformatics Opportunities for Health Sciences Librarians and Information Professionals." *Journal of the Medical Library Association* 92, no. 4 (October 2004): 489-93.

23. McCartney, P.R. "Leadership in Nursing Informatics." *Journal of Obstetrics and Gynecological Neonatal Nursing* 33, no. 3 (May-June 2004): 371-80.

24. Royal College of Nursing. "Clinical Image Requests from Non-Medically Qualified Professionals." (2006). Available: <http://www.rcn.org.uk/publications/pdf/clinical_imaging.pdf>. Accessed: February 5, 2007.

25. U.S. National Library of Medicine. MedlinePlus. "CT Scan." (2004). Available: <http://www.nlm.nih.gov/medlineplus/tutorials/ctscan/htm/index.htm>. Accessed: March 9, 2007.

26. U.S. National Library of Medicine. MedlinePlus. "Videos of Surgical Procedures." (2007). Available: <http://www.nlm.nih.gov/medlineplus/surgeryvideos.html>. Accessed: March 9, 2007.

27. American College of Radiology and the Radiological Society of North America. "RadiologyInfo: The Radiology Information Resource for Patients." (2007). Available: <http://www.radiologyinfo.org/index.cfm?bhcp=1>. Accessed: January 21, 2007.

28. U.S. National Library of Medicine. "The Visible Human Projects: Overview." (2006). Available: <http://www.nlm.nih.gov/research/visible/visible_human.html>. Accessed: March 9, 2007.

29. U.S. National Library of Medicine. "AnatLine." (2004). Available: <http://anatquest.nlm.nih.gov/Anatline/index.html>. Accessed: March 9, 2007.

30. U.S. National Library of Medicine. "AnatQuest." (2004). Available: <http://anatquest.nlm.nih.gov/>. Accessed: March 9, 2007.

31. University of Minnesota. "WebAnatomy." (2006). Available: <http://msjensen.education.umn.edu/Webanatomy/>. Accessed: March 9, 2007.

32. University of Leicester, UK. "Virtual Autopsy." (2001). Available: <http://www.le.ac.uk/pathology/teach/va/titlpag1.html>. Accessed: March 9, 2007.

33. U.S. National Library of Medicine. "Turning the Pages Information System." (2005). Available: <http://archive.nlm.nih.gov/proj/ttp.php>. Accessed: February 16, 2007.

34. Wellcome Trust. "Medical Photographic Library: Wellcome Trust." (2007). Available: <http://medphoto.wellcome.ac.uk/ixbin/hixclient.exe?_IXDB_=wellcome&_IXSESSION_=&search-form=main/home.html&submit-button=search>. Accessed: February 16, 2007.

35. Centers for Disease Control and Prevention. "Public Health Image Library." (2005). Available: <http://phil.cdc.gov/phil/home.asp>. Accessed: February 16, 2007.

36. Wikipedia. "Electronic Health Record." (2007). Available: <http://en.wikipedia.org/wiki/Electronic_health_record#_note-25>. Accessed: February 16, 2007.

37. Brown, S.H.; Lincoln, M.J.; Groen, P.J.; and Kolodner, R.M. "VistA—U.S. Department of Veterans Affairs national-scale HIS." *International Journal of Medical Informatics* 69, no. 2-3 (March 2003): 135-56. Available: <http://www1.va.gov/cprsdemo/docs/VistA_Int_Jrnl_Article.pdf>. Accessed: March 23, 2007.

38. U.S. Department of Veteran Affairs. "VHS Office of Information: VISTA®/CPRS Demo Site." (2006). Available: <http://www1.va.gov/CPRSdemo/>. Accessed: March 8, 2007.

39. "Personally Controlled Health Records: Are They the Next Big Thing?" *Focus Online.* (2006). Available: <http://focus.hms.harvard.edu/2006/102706/information_technology.shtml> Accessed: February 16, 2007.

40. U.S. Department of Veterans Affairs. "My Health*e*Vet: VA and DoD Sharing Medical Histories." (2006). Available: <https://www.myhealth.va.gov/mhvPortal/anonymous.portal?_nfpb=true&_nfto=false&_pageLabel=mhvHome>. Accessed: February 16, 2007.

41. Wyatt, J., and Spiegelhalter, D. "Field Trials of Medical Decision-Aids: Potential Problems and Solutions." *Proceedings of the Annual Symposium on Computer Applications in Medical Care* (November 1991): 3-7.

42. Open Clinical. Knowledge Management for Medical Care. "Decision Support Systems." (2006). Available: <http://www.openclinical.org/dss.html>. Accessed: January 21, 2007.

43. Hickam, D.H.; Shortliffe, E.H.; Bischoff, M.B.; Scott, A.C.; and Jacobs, C.D. "The Treatment Advice of a Computer-Based Cancer Chemotherapy Protocol Advisor." *Annals of Internal Medicine* 103, no. 6, pt. 1 (December 1985): 928-36.

44. Garg, A.X.; Adhikari, N.K.; McDonald, H.; et al. "Effects of Computerized Clinical Decision Support Systems on Practitioner Performance and Patient Outcomes: A Systematic Review." *JAMA; Journal of the American Medical Association* 293, no. 10 (March 9, 2005): 1223-38.

45. "Isabel." Srishti Software, Bangalore, India. (2007). Available: <http://www.isabelhealthcare.com/>. Accessed: January 21, 2007.

46. Ridker, P.M.; Buring, J.E.; Rifai, N.; and Cook, N.R. "Development and Validation of Improved Algorithms for the Assessment of Global Cardiovascular Risk in Women: The Reynolds Risk Score." *JAMA; Journal of the American Medical Association* 297, no. 6 (February 14, 2007): 611-9.

47. Chen, E.S.; Bakken, S.; Currie, L.M.; Patel, V.L.; and Cimino, J.J. "An Automated Approach to Studying Health Resource and Infobutton Use." *Studies in Health Technologies and Information* 122(2006): 273-8.

48. Cimino, J.; Johnson, S.; Agurirre, A.; Roderer, N.; and Clayton, P. "The MEDLINE Button." *Proceedings of the Annual Symposium on Computer Applications in Medical Care* (November 1992): 81-5.

49. Magrabi, F., Westbrook, J.I., and Coiera, E.W. "What Factors Are Associated with the Integration of Evidence Retrieval Technology into Routine General Practice Settings?" *International Journal of Medical Informatics* 76, no. 10 (October 2007): 70-109.

50. Dawes, M., and Sampson, U. "Knowledge Management in Clinical Practice: A Systematic Review of Information Seeking Behavior in Physicians." *International Journal of Medical Informatics* 71, no. 1 (August 2003): 9-15.

51. Covell, D.G.; Uman, G.C.; and Manning, P.R. "Information Needs in Office Practice: Are They Being Met?" *Annals of Internal Medicine* 103, no. 4 (October 1985): 596-9.

52. McKibbon, K.A., and Fridsma, D.B. "Effectiveness of Clinician-Selected Electronic Information Resources for Answering Primary Care Physicians' Information Needs." *Journal of the American Medical Informatics Association* 13, no. 6 (November-December 2006): 653-9.

53. Hersh, W.R.; Crabtree, M.K.; Hickam, D.H.; et al. "Factors Associated with Success in Searching MEDLINE and Applying Evidence to Answer Clinical Questions." *Journal of the American Medical Informatics Association* 9, no. 3 (May-June 2002): 283-93.

54. Tsai, T.L.; Fridsma, D.B.; and Gatti, G. "Computer Decision Support As a Source of Interpretation Error: The Case of Electrocardiograms." *Journal of the American Medical Informatics Association* 10, no. 5 (September-October 2003): 478-83.

55. Westbrook, J.I.; Coiera, E.W.; and Gosling, A.S. "Do Online Information Retrieval Systems Help Experienced Clinicians Answer Clinical Questions?" *Journal of the American Medical Informatics Association* 12, no. 3 (May-June 2005): 315-21.

56. Strehle, E.M., and Shabde, N. "One Hundred Years of Telemedicine: Does This New Technology Have a Place in Paediatrics?" *Archives of Disease in Childhood* 91, no. 12 (December 2006): 956-9.

57. Joslin Diabetes Center. Harvard Medical School. "Joslin Diabetes Center Affiliate—Bahrain." (2006). Available: <http://www.joslin.org/International_Programs_2232.asp>. Accessed: February 21, 2007.

58. Larson, P.A., and Janower, J.M. "The Nighthawk: Bird of Paradise or Albatross?" *American Journal of Radiology* 2, no. 12 (December 2005): 967-70.

59. Mun, S.K.; Tohme, W.G.; Platenberg, R.C.; and Choi, I. "Teleradiology and Emerging Business Models." *Journal of Telemedicine and Telecare* 11, no. 6 (September 2005): 271-5.

60. Christensen, H.; Griffiths, K.M.; and Jorm, A.F. "Delivering Interventions for Depression by Using the Internet: Randomised Controlled Trial." *BMJ; British Medical Journal* 328, no. 7434 (January 31, 2004): 265.

61. Eysenbach, G.; Powell, J.; Englesakis, M.; Rizo, C.; and Stern, A. "Health Related Virtual Communities and Electronic Support Groups: Systematic Review of the Effects of Online Peer to Peer Interactions." *BMJ; British Medical Journal* 328, no. 7449 (May 15, 2004): 1166.

62. Griffiths, K.M.; Christensen, H.; Jorm, A.F.; Evans, K.; and Groves, C. "Effect of Web-Based Depression Literacy and Cognitive-Behavioural Therapy Interventions on Stigmatising Attitudes to Depression: Randomised Controlled Trial." *British Journal of Psychiatry* 185(October 2004): 342-9. Available: <http://bjp.rcpsych.org/cgi/content/full/185/4/342>. Accessed: March 23, 2007.

63. Telemedicine Research Center. "Telemedicine Information Exchange. Bibliographic Citations for Telemedicine." (2007). Available: <http://tie.telemed.org/default.asp>. Accessed: January 22, 2007.

64. Telleen, S., and Martin, E. "Improving Information Access for Public Health Professionals." *Journal of Medical Systems* 26, no. 6 (December 2002): 529-43.

65. Utah Department of Health, Salt Lake City, UT. "Managing the Public Health Impacts of Housing the 2002 Winter Olympics" (2002). Available: <http://phs.os.dhhs.gov/ophs/BestPractice/UT_olympics.htm>. Accessed: March 7, 2007.

66. Hammond, H.E., and Cimino, J.J. "Standards in Biomedical Informatics." In *Biomedical Informatics: Computer Applications in Health Care and Biomedicine (Health Informatics),* edited by E.H. Shortliffe and J.J. Cimino, 265-311. New York: Springer Science, 2006.

67. Beeler, G.W. "HL7 Version 3—An Object Oriented Methodology for Collaborative Standards Development." *International Journal of Medical Informatics* 48, no. 1-3 (February 1998): 151-61.

68. U.S. National Library of Medicine. *Medical Subject Headings.* Bethesda, MD: National Library of Medicine, 2006. Available: <http://www.nlm.nih.gov/mesh/meshhome.html>. Accessed: January 21, 2007.

69. World Health Organization. *International Classification of Diseases.* Geneva, Switzerland: World Health Organization, 2007. Available: <http://www.who.int/classifications/icd/en/>. Accessed: January 21, 2007.

70. College of American Pathologists. SNOMED. (2007). Available: <http://www.snomed.org/index.html>. Accessed: January 21, 2007.

71. Health Data Management. "New Clinical Terminology Available from SNOMED." (2002). Available: <http://www.healthdatamanagement.com/html/PortalStory.cfm?type=newprod&DID=7841>. Accessed: February 23, 2007.

72. U.S. National Library of Medicine. "Unified Medical Language Fact Sheet." (2006). Available: <http://www.nlm.nih.gov/pubs/factsheets/umls.html>. Accessed: January 21, 2007.

73. U.S. National Library of Medicine. "Unified Medical Language System. Appendix A.1 UMLA Metathesaurus Source Vocabularies. 2007AB edition" Available: <http://www.nlm.nih.gov/research/umls/metaa1.html>. Accessed: August 6, 2007.

74. Robinson, J.; de Lusignan, S.; Kostkova, P.; and Madge, B. "Using UMLS to Map from a Library to a Clinical Classification: Improving the Functionality of a Digital Library." *Studies in Health Technology and Informatics* 121(2006): 86-95.

75. U.S. National Library of Medicine. "Unified Medical Language System (UMLS) Tutorial." (2006). Available: <http://www.nlm.nih.gov/research/umls/pdf/UMLS_Basics.pdf>. Accessed: February 23, 2007.

76. Lloyd, S.S., and Layman, E. "The Effects of Automated Encoders on Coding Accuracy and Coding Speed." *Topics in Health Information Management* 17, no. 3 (February 1997): 72-9.

77. Baibergenova, A.; Thabane, L.; Akhtar-Danesh, N.; Levine, M.; Gafni, A.; Moineddin, R.; and Pulcins, I. "Effect of gender, age, and severity of asthma attack on patterns of emergency department visits due to asthma by month and day of the week." *European Journal of Epidemiology* 20, no. 11 (2005): 947-56.

78. "Case Definitions for Infectious Conditions Under Public Health Surveillance. Centers for Disease Control and Prevention." *MMWR Recommendations and Reports* 46, no. RR-10 (May 2, 1997): 1-55.

79. Aronson, A.R.; Mork, J.G.; Gay, C.W.; Humphrey, S.M.; and Rogers, W.J. "The NLM Indexing Initiative's Medical Text Indexer." *Medinfo Proceedings* 11, pt. 1 (2004): 268-72.

80. Cohen, A.M., and Hersh, W.R. "The TREC 2004 Genomics Track Categorization Task: Classifying Full Text Biomedical Documents." *Journal of Biomedical Discovery and Collaboration* 14, no. 1 (March 14, 2006): 4. Available: <http://www.j-biomed-discovery.com/content/1/1/4>. Accessed: March 23, 2007.

81. Baeza-Yates, R., and Ribeiro-Neto, R. *Modern Information Retrieval.* Harlow, Essex, UK: ACM Press, 1999.

82. Hersh, W.R.; Stavri, P.Z.; and Detmer, W.M. "Information Retrieval and Digital Libraries." In *Biomedical Informatics: Computer Applications in Health Care and Biomedicine (Health Informatics),* edited by E.H. Shortliffe and J.J. Cimino, 660-697. New York: Springer Scientific, 2006.

83. Stanford University. "Computer Ethics." (2001). Available: <http://plato.stanford.edu/entries/ethics-computer/>. Accessed: January 24, 2007.

84. Murphy, J. "UK Health Informatics Today: Introducing a UK HIT Special Issue: Education and Training." *Newsletter of the UK Health Informatics Society* no. 51 (Autumn 2006): 1-11. Available: <http://www.bmis.org/ebmit/2007_53_spring.pdf>. Accessed: March 23, 2007.

85. Hersh, W.R. "Medical Informatics Education: An Alternative Pathway for Training Informationists." *Journal of the Medical Library Association* 90, no. 1 (January 2002): 76-9.

86. U.S. National Library of Medicine. "Fact Sheet: Opportunities for Training and Education Sponsored by the National Library of Medicine." (2006). Available: <http://www.nlm.nih.gov/pubs/factsheets/trainedu.html>. Accessed: February 23, 2007.

87. American Medical Informatics Association. "About Informatics Academic and Training Programs." (2007). Available: <http://www.amia.org/informatics/acad&training/>. Accessed: February 23, 2007.

88. Perlis, T.E.; Des Jarlais, D.C.; Friedman, S.R.; Arasteh, K.; and Turner, C.F. "Audio-Computerized Self-Interviewing versus Face-to-Face Interviewing for Research Data Collection at Drug Abuse Treatment Programs." *Addiction* 99, no. 7 (July 2004): 895-7.

89. Crowley, R.S.; Legowski, E.; Medvedeva, O.; ,Tseytlin, E.; Roh, E.; and Jukic, D. "Evaluation of an Intelligent Tutoring System in Pathology—Effects of External Representation on Performance Gains, Metacognition and Acceptance." *Journal of the American Medical Informatics Association* 14, no.2 (March-April 2007): 182-190.

90. Hilty, D.M.; Alverson, D.C.; Alpert, J.E.; et al. "Virtual Reality, Telemedicine, Web and Data Processing Innovations in Medical and Psychiatric Education and Clinical Care." *Academic Psychiatry* 30, no. 6 (November-December 2006): 528-33.

91. Griffiths, M. "Video Games and Health." *BMJ; British Medical Journal* 331, no. 7509 (July 16, 2005): 122-3.

92. Colombo, R.; Pisano, F.; Mazzone, A.; et al. "Design Strategies to Improve Patient Motivation During Robot-Aided Rehabilitation." *Journal of Neuroengineering and Rehabilitation* 4, no. 1 (February 19, 2007): 3.

93. Noury, N.; Virone, G.; Barralon, P.; Ye, J.; Rialle, V.; and Demongeot, J. "New Trends in Health Smart Homes." (2003). Available: <http://ieeexplore.ieee.org/xpls/abs_all.jsp?arnumber=1218728>. Accessed: January 23, 2007.

94. Cohen, B. "Talking Pill Bottles." National Public Radio. (2005). Available: <http://www.npr.org/templates/story/story.php?storyId=4779825&sourceCode=RSS>. Accessed: February 23, 2007.

95. Kling, R. "Learning About Information Technologies and Social Change: The Contribution of Social Informatics." *The Information Society* 16(July 1, 2000): 217-32.

96. Eldredge, J.D., and Karcher, C.T. "Does Face-to-Face Interaction of a Library Liaison with Faculty Change Faculty Perceptions of or Use of a Library?" Poster presented at the Medical Library Association Annual Meeting, Dallas, TX, May 17-23, 2002.

97. Eldredge, J.D., and Hendrix, I. "Determinants of Effective Library-Faculty Communications: A Randomized Controlled Trial." Contributed paper presented at the Second International Evidence-Based Librarianship Conference, University of Alberta, Alberta, Canada, June 5, 2003.

98. O'Neil, D. "Assessing Community Informatics: A Review of Methodological Approaches for Evaluating Community Networks and Community Technology Centers." *Internet Research* 12(2002): 76-102. Available: <http://www.emeraldinsight.com/Insight/ViewContentServlet?Filename=Published/EmeraldFullTextArticle/Pdf/17201 20107.pdf>. Accessed: March 23, 2007.

99. Kavanaugh, A.L.; Reese, D.D.; Carroll, J.M.; and Rosson, M.B. "Weak Ties in Networked Communities." *The Information Society* 21(2005): 119-31.

100. BMJ Publishing Group. "BMJ Clinical Evidence: About Us." (2007). Available: <http://www.clinicalevidence.com/ceweb/about/index.jsp>. Accessed: March 7, 2007.

101. Health Information Research Unit. "Health Information Research Unit: Evidence Based Health Informatics: The 'Hedges' Project." (2007). Available: <http://hiru.mcmaster.ca/hedges/indexhiru.htm>. Accessed: March 7, 2007.

102. Patel, R.; Schardt, C.M.; Sanders, L.L.; and Keitz, S.A. "Randomized Trial for Answers to Clinical Questions: Evaluating a Pre-Appraised versus a MEDLINE Search Protocol." *Journal of the Medical Library Association* 94, no. 4 (October 2006): 382-7.

103. Hatfield, A.J., and Brahmi, F. "Angel: Post-Implementation Evaluation at the Indiana University School of Medicine." *Medical Reference Services Quarterly* 23, no. 3 (Fall 2004): 1-15.

104. Scherrer, C.S., Dorsch, J.L., and Weller, A.C. "An Evaluation of a Collaborative Model for Preparing Evidence-Based Medicine Teachers." *Journal of the Medical Library Association* 94, no. 2 (April 2006): 159-64.

105. Stephenson, P.L.; Green, B.F.; Wallace, R.L.; Earl, M.F.; Orick, J.T.; and Taylor, M.V. "Community Partnerships for Health Information Training: Medical Librarians Working with Health-Care Professionals and Consumers in Tennessee." *Health Information and Libraries Journal* 21, Suppl. 1 (June 2004): 20-6.

SECTION IV: ADMINISTRATION

Chapter 13

Management in Academic Health Sciences Libraries

Francesca Allegri
Martha Bedard

SUMMARY. This chapter reviews the various roles of academic health sciences library administrators. Also covered are the expectations and skills needed to manage and lead academic health sciences libraries now and in the future. Included are operating in the academic health sciences environment; leading and managing change; choosing management styles; planning; creating a vision and mission; performing assessment, evaluation, and measurement; marketing and promoting the library; advocating policy and legislative issues; overseeing fiscal responsibilities; managing personnel; and managing facilities. Topics such as marketing and promoting the library and planning facilities are addressed from the administrator's viewpoint. These are covered in more depth in other chapters.

INTRODUCTION

Modern academic health sciences libraries reflect the changes taking place in the teaching, research, and clinical arenas of health sciences as well as those taking place within libraries in general. While academic health sciences librarians are typically agile in developing service models to respond rapidly to patient care situations, they face new challenges. These challenges include health care–related curricula moving away from lecture toward self-directed learning and hands-on experiences, complex interdisciplinary research projects that use sophisticated informatics tools and data sets, expectations for ubiquitous desktop delivery of information and knowledge management support, as well as the rapid expansion of academic programs to meet the health manpower shortage.

At the same time, the information resource environment has transformed from one largely based in print to one primarily electronic. With this transformation come the administrative challenges of negotiating licenses, managing authorizations, preserving digital content while maintaining print, and creating Web-based access points and instruction. Another challenge is understanding the variety of new models of scholarly communications, such as open access and local repositories. These challenges require today's managers and leaders in academic health sciences libraries to develop a high level of expertise in communicating with their users and upper-level health sciences administrators, assessing their collections, evaluating their services, reconfiguring their facilities, and updating the skills of library personnel.

MANAGING IN THE ACADEMIC HEALTH SCIENCES ENVIRONMENT

Each library operates in the environment of its parent institution, whether that is a hospital, pharmaceutical company, or educational institution.[1] The academic health sciences center or

Introduction to Health Sciences Librarianship
doi:10.1300/6041_13

university is the institutional parent of the academic health sciences library. Typically, it has many schools, programs, and institutes that may or may not be part of a larger university. The **Association of Academic Health Centers (AAHC)** addresses many of the cross-institutional issues affecting these centers.[2] The kinds of programs, administrative structure, and institutional complexity of the organization influence how involved a library administrator can be and at what level. For example, in some organizations library administrators have other departments besides the library reporting to them, such as technology support; the administrator may then have the title of **chief information officer (CIO).** The size of the parent organization can also affect funding and how much time the administrator spends in direct service, management, and leadership roles. Public and private institutions may operate differently, especially when it comes to funding sources, how funds are allocated, information disclosure policies, and personnel practices.

Library administrators' reporting relationships vary from institution to institution and can change with upper-level reorganizations. Some library administrators report to a dean or associate dean of a college. Others at large health sciences centers report to a health sciences president or vice president, chancellor, health systems **chief executive officer (CEO),** or to a university librarian. These reporting relationships can change frequently. There is no "best" reporting relationship in terms of organizational effectiveness. Generally, the higher up in the organization one can report, the fewer levels there are to go through to make a case for resources and to integrate the library into key institutional initiatives. Whatever the reporting line, learning the politics of the organization and building strong working relationships are the critical components. A productive relationship with one's supervisor cannot be overestimated in order to further the role of the library.

In today's academic health sciences libraries, there are an increasing number of other important relationships to cultivate. This seems to be the result of increasing interdependence as academic institutions respond to complex issues, relatively static or declining resources, and accountability initiatives. Other important types of relationships to cultivate are those with peer administrators, with university libraries (where applicable), with computing centers and other information technology units, with leaders of special campus projects, and others.

Another valuable relationship is that between the library administrator and the library committee or governing board. If there is no formally charged library board or advisory committee, bringing together a group of interested individuals from constituent groups outside the library can be very helpful in sharing ideas and feedback and for building advocacy support for programs and resources.

THE ROLES OF LIBRARY ADMINISTRATORS

People in charge of academic health sciences libraries have varied titles: director, manager, librarian, vice president, associate dean, department chair, knowledge manager, and others. These titles reflect the size, organizational structure, and culture of the parent institution. Whatever the title, effective administrators recognize two key intersecting roles: managing the resources of the library and assuming a leadership role within the institution and the profession. A good administrator combines both management and leadership traits.

Management

Management includes responsibility for day-to-day operations. Managers understand existing library operations enough to recognize when they work effectively and when they need improvement. Internally, effective managers make decisions and create policy based on knowledge

A Day in the Life of an Academic Health Sciences Library Director

Name: Julia F. Sollenberger, MLS, AHIP, FMLA
Position: Director, Health Science Libraries and Technologies, University of Rochester Medical Center, New York

Job description: Direct and coordinate the resources, programs, and services that support (1) the knowledge-based information needs of the education, research, and clinical enterprises at the University of Rochester Medical Center; and (2) the instructional computing needs of students in the School of Medicine. Responsible for overseeing staff (thirty FTEs), planning and evaluating the programs and services, and guiding and monitoring the budget and expenditures of the main health sciences library and two branch libraries.

Sample Day

7:30 a.m.–9:00 a.m.
- Attend biweekly meeting of the "Medical Center Leadership—Large" group, convened by the Medical Center CEO, with approximately twenty-five attendees; discussed the state health care budget "crisis," smoke-free campus implementation, and university branding and logo.

9:00 a.m.–10:00 a.m.
- Interview candidate for part-time Outreach Librarian position.

10:00 a.m.–11:00 a.m.
- Attend weekly meeting with Library Administrator; discuss ongoing personnel, facilities, and budget issues.

11:00 a.m.–Noon
- Attend presentation given by Outreach Librarian candidate, followed by Q&A.

Noon–1 p.m.
- Eat lunch at my desk while doing e-mail and working on performance review for Department Head (needs to be completed for tomorrow).

1:00 p.m.–2 p.m.
- Attend Medical Center Web Operations Committee meeting.

2:00 p.m.–3:00 p.m.
- Attend meeting with three librarian staff members to discuss marketing our patient/family Information Prescription program.

3:00 p.m.–3:30 p.m.
- Catch up on e-mail.

3:30 p.m.–4:00 p.m.
- Monthly conference call with Director of Major Gifts at UR Development office, to discuss fundraising for library renovation project

4:00 p.m.–5:00 p.m.
- Attend meeting with all library instructors to discuss Fall 2007 curriculum for "Mastering Medical Information" course.

5:00 p.m.–5:30 p.m.
- Catch up on more e-mail, then leave for home (finish performance review from 8:00-9:00 p.m.).

Summary statement: This is one of those "back-to-back" days that provides little time for completing tangible work. To get this done, I must block off time on my schedule—to write, plan, read, and strategize. *Every* day cannot look like this one (though many do)!

and evidence-based information. They carry out directives and share bad news, communicating them honestly to staff. Managers create an organizational structure, often designing workflows and staffing patterns. Managers are responsible for budget justification and allocation. Good managers involve staff in all of these activities, taking responsibility for mistakes and giving credit for successes. Holt states, "Good bosses are, first of all, effective bosses who get things done. They get things done because they either bring or acquire on the job the skills that make the organization more effective while helping all staff toward greater self-actualization, even as they complete assigned work tasks."[3]

Effective managers display other attributes and skills. A select list includes these abilities:

- Be available for and encourage questions.
- Analyze problems for root causes.
- Hire and trust those they hire.
- Organize and use their time well.
- Motivate, prepare, and delegate work to staff.
- Manage projects efficiently.
- Establish priorities.
- Make choices in an atmosphere of ambiguity.

Leadership

Leadership includes developing the relationships that keep the library relevant and central to the institution. Leaders understand and communicate directions and roles for the library. They champion a vision of how the library can serve its users better. Leaders create a sense of urgency around that vision and help make the necessary changes to achieve it. Effective leaders need to be externally focused and seize or create opportunities. Examples of opportunities are including the library in the preparation of a major grant proposal, offering to partner on multidisciplinary projects, managing biomedical communications or informatics centers, and cosponsoring important events. Leaders create visibility and gain leverage for their libraries by being active outside the library, working with executive groups, campus committees, the local community, consortia, and professional associations. They are often involved with fundraising and **development.** They set the tone and model the values of their organization and take a role in many ceremonial duties, such as convocation, graduation, **white coat ceremonies (WCCs),** and opening new services and facilities across the health sciences center.

In order to be effective in the dynamic health sciences environment, library administrators need to recognize the core responsibilities of libraries. No matter what the future holds, the following list represents those that are likely to remain the purview of libraries:

- Engaging in setting and attaining the priorities of the parent institution
- Understanding and responding to users
- Developing and communicating the library's mission, one that is aligned with that of the parent institution
- Providing information and knowledge management services
- Collecting, preserving, archiving, and making content accessible
- Providing physical spaces for common and special use
- Contributing unique resources, skills, and knowledge
- Communicating value by integrating into all aspects of the parent institution
- Assuring wise use of resources
- Continuously anticipating and planning for the future

The list of additional readings at the end of this chapter contains several good references to explore further the topics of management and leadership (see Appendix 13.A).

Leading and Managing Change

The leadership and management roles of a library administrator are critical in times of change. Sometimes administrators are agents of change and sometimes managers of change. As an agent of change, the library administrator must be proficient in **environmental scanning.** This means being aware of major trends, driving forces, and changes in the constituent communities, as well as in the library profession. There are numerous lists of trends and opinions about them from experts in technology and higher education. An excellent example is the New Media Consortium and EDUCAUSE Learning Initiative Horizon Report. The 2007 report highlights six trends that the underlying research suggests will become very important to higher education over the next one to five years. The report presents these as key trends, critical challenges, technologies to watch, and the time to adoption. A few examples from the report follow:

- Rapid changes are occurring in higher education economics, enrollments, and students.
- Globalization is changing learning and communication in significant ways.
- Assessment of scholarship is lagging behind the new formats in which work is conducted, such as games, simulations, and **blogs.**
- The information literacy skills of new students are not improving while the skills needed, for example, critical thinking, are increasingly important.
- Open source **gaming engines** will make it easier to develop interesting, multiplayer educational counterparts to commercial games.[4]

A leader would bring knowledge of these trends to the parent organization for consideration in planning. Awareness of trends and other critical reports, such as the **National Library of Medicine**'s long-range plan, is also important for preparing the library staff to respond to their impact on operations and constituents.[5] See Appendix 13.B for a description of the most influential trend reports relevant to health sciences libraries.

The administrator must also be cognizant of the potential impact of trends and specific changes on the institution, the library, and the user community. As a manager of change, leaders help their staff and superiors understand the need for change and lead the library and organization through a change process. Curzon outlines a change management cycle that includes conceptualization, preparing the organization for change, organizing the planning group, planning the change, deciding what needs to change, managing individuals during change, controlling resistance, implementing change, and evaluating the process.[6]

A leader needs to carefully assess the need for change because resistance to change is a common reaction. Effective managers of change clearly communicate the benefits and anticipated impacts of change and assist others to adjust and embrace the change. Other skills required include planning, project management, and evaluation. Evaluation includes looking at both the change process and the results of change.

Choosing Management Styles

There are many styles of management and many perspectives about which ones are most effective. Understanding what is expected and needed by library staff and upper administration, technical knowledge of library operations, hands-on problem-solving, open discussion of issues, and a manager's own personal philosophy and personality will define one's "style." An administrator's style determines how decisions are made and communicated. This can be represented in many ways: how input from staff and users is heard, whether there is an "open door policy" or many scheduled meetings, and whether authority and accountability for decisions such as hours of operations or selection of resources are delegated. Also, style determines how input is gathered and used, how librarians with faculty status share governance responsibility, and the degree to which collaboration and teamwork in decision-making occur in the library.

Numerous articles and books describing various styles are available to help one decide how best to manage and lead in an organization, each with advantages, disadvantages, and recommendations. One example comes from Daniel Goleman, who lists six leadership styles, paraphrased here.[7] He suggests that a mix of styles, customized to the situation, is generally the most effective approach.

1. The *visionary leader* moves people toward a shared vision and tells them where to go but not how to get there.
2. The *coaching leader* connects staff "wants" to organizational goals, holds long conversations that reach beyond the workplace, helps people find their strengths and weaknesses, and ties these to career aspirations and actions.
3. The *affiliative leader* creates people connections and thus harmony within the organization. It is a very collaborative style, which focuses on emotional needs over work needs.
4. The *democratic leader* acts to value inputs and commitment through participation, listening to both the bad and the good news.
5. The *pace-setting leader* builds challenge and exciting goals for people, expects excellence, and often exemplifies it. This type of leader identifies poor performers and demands more of them.
6. The *commanding leader* soothes fears and gives clear directions through a powerful stance, commanding and expecting full compliance (agreement is not needed).

Whatever the style or combination of styles, clear communication about what is needed and expected is a key to success. Keeping library staff regularly informed of organizational priorities, decisions, and events that impact their work life is the responsibility of every manager. Keeping staff aware that what they are doing is important is also part of this essential communication.

Planning

Planning involves setting a direction and specifying concrete goals and steps for achieving them. Five-year **strategic plans,** complete with the components of vision, mission, goals, objectives, and actions, have been commonplace in libraries and academic settings. However, the accelerated rate of change makes shorter time frames and annual or biennial planning more realistic. Crafting the statements of vision, mission, and goals should be part of a collaborative strategic planning process that takes place with the guidance of the library's chief administrator. The components of a strategic plan are described later in this chapter.

The initiation of a planning process may be driven by a request from administrators above the library director, an upcoming accreditation visit, a change in library director or other key personnel, or significant change in the environment, such as a new library or academic building, new programs, or additional colleges to support. As indicated by these events, plans should be grounded in an understanding of the library's current and future environment. Some environmental changes have an impact so profound, such as the rapid adoption of digital-only resources, that they may necessitate changes throughout the entire organizational structure. It is important that the library administrator work to include the library in the planning process for the entire institution.

In 2003, the **Association of Academic Health Sciences Libraries (AAHSL)** published "Building on Success: Charting the Future of Knowledge Management Within the Academic Health Center." This publication describes a vision of the future to assist member libraries in achieving leadership in dramatically changing environments.[8] The document suggests directions and opportunities for libraries and provides information targeted to the leadership of academic health sciences centers. It is an invaluable tool for initiating discussion and prompting ideas about the future.

At times, some organizations and some administrators may also focus on particular types of planning. Two examples are technology planning and disaster planning. These are discussed briefly here. Staff planning is addressed in the Managing Personnel section of this chapter.

Technology Planning

This type of planning takes many forms and encompasses a variety of activities. These include the following:

- Identifying emerging technologies and anticipating their impact on users, staff functions, and services
- Creating or modifying the library's mission and goals to take advantage of the opportunities technologies provide
- Helping the parent institution see the potential applications of new technologies and helping integrate these into institutional planning
- Specifying a technology budget and implementation timeline
- Anticipating and budgeting for replacement of technologies as they age (**life-cycle replacement**)
- Ensuring the infrastructure is kept current and can handle growth in technology use
- Monitoring performance of wiring, power, wireless, server space, and other technical infrastructure for both staff and users
- Evaluating and deciding when to purchase software or design applications in-house
- Making decisions about which technologies to support and which require, or are better suited to, external support, for example, by a campus instructional technology unit or a vendor

At the time this chapter was written, no comprehensive resource addressed the many aspects of technology planning for academic health sciences libraries. However, some resources address particular subtopics, such as incorporating technology as part of a new facility or service.[9, 10] Also, the Medical Library Association (MLA) offers continuing education on technology planning.[11] More information about technology planning is provided in the additional readings list.

Disaster Planning

Planning in this area can be focused, for example, how to prevent and recover from damage to collections, communications, and services in the case of floods or hurricanes, or very broad, for example, how the library will fit into the campus's pandemic flu response. The National Library of Medicine, in its long-range plan, has recommended its objectives for disaster preparedness and response, one of which engages medical librarians and public librarians as early responders.[5] This may influence libraries to broaden their role in local or regional efforts in disaster management.

The purposes of disaster plans include these goals:

- Prepare and train staff/first responders.
- Ensure the safety of people.
- Minimize damage.
- Continue or resume service quickly.
- Recover and salvage resources.

The "Comprehensive Disaster Plan of the Claude Moore Health Sciences Library at the University of Virginia" gives a good example of the scope of disaster preparedness and response.[12] The plan covers procedures for evacuations, bioterrorism, earthquakes, hurricanes, bomb threats, biological agents, power outages, prevention, personal preparedness, salvage, recovery, service continuity, and other aspects of this subject. There are other excellent resources available through organizations such as the Southeastern Library Network (SOLINET).

Creating a Vision and Mission

A library's mission statement is often accompanied by statements of vision, core values, goals, and objectives. Typically, vision, mission, and values statements are written or revised as part of a **long-range planning** process.[13] Goals and objectives are generally developed as part of multiyear, annual, or ongoing planning and describe how the library will achieve its mission and vision.

The library's vision and mission statements should be consistent with those of the parent institution and developed with input from both external and internal stakeholders. Internal stakeholders include library staff and users, library committee members, and library donors. External stakeholders include community-based organizations, campus administrators, vendors, and government agencies.

Vision. Vision statements represent the epitome of what the library aspires to be. They often depict a future state and project ideals such as "advance education, research, and health care," "leader in a global partnership," "provide exceptional service," "an essential partner," and "leader committed to excellence and innovation."

Core values. Values statements are the enduring and underlying approaches to the work to be done. Common components of value statements are integrity, excellence, the importance of staff, innovation, user-focused services, collaboration, neutrality, trust, accountability, honesty, privacy of information, equal access to information, and the importance of information to health care.[14, 15]

Mission. The mission statement communicates concisely the purpose of the library, whom it serves, and what it does. See Appendix 13.C for an example of a vision, mission, and values statement.

Goals. These are the key strategies used to achieve the library's mission.

Objectives. Effective objectives are written with particular elements. While some of the descriptor words vary slightly, the acronym SMART captures these elements. Objectives should be *s*pecific, *m*easurable, *a*ttainable, *r*esults-focused, and *t*ime-bound.[16]

Activities. Also called action plans, these have time frames of a year or less and are used to achieve the objectives. Activities include assignment of responsibility for carrying out the activity and noting any resources needed to achieve the objectives.

Example of Goal, Objective, and Action Plans

Goal
The library will work with faculty to educate medical students in basic information competencies.

Objective (original version)
The education department will increase attendance at its programs.

Measurable Objective (Revised/SMART)
The education services librarians will increase attendance at this year's PubMed Basic Training workshops by at least 10 percent over last year.

Action Plan
The head of information and education services will meet with second-year school of medicine course directors by April of this year to discuss proposal for instruction for next academic year.

Action Plan
Beginning this fall, the education services librarians will offer at least one session a month in the evening to reach students unable to attend during the day.

A key role of the administrator is to support and advocate the library's vision, mission, and core values, which should be shared widely, both inside and outside the library. This sets the tone for the entire library and encompasses a wide range of advocacy responsibilities, such as expanding services, building partnerships, developing electronic collections, using space differently, achieving pay equity for library staff, and fundraising. Typically, the library administrator and senior library management lead development of vision, mission, and values statements while those who will carry out goals, objectives, and activities have the primary role in developing those statements.

Creating these various statements and plans is an ongoing effort. A plan works best as a living, continuously revisited document—not shelved, once written—rather, a guide for future activities. For example, a current issue for many academic health sciences libraries is the changing nature of the library as a physical space.[17] A defining feature of a health sciences library had been its journal collection, current issues of which were displayed in a prominent location for browsing. Now those shelves may be empty because the library has switched to online subscriptions. The traditional use of library space to store books, journals, microforms, and other publications has changed. That space may be better utilized by people who can access the library electronically on mobile devices, such as wireless tablet computers, personal digital assistants (PDAs), or cell phones with Internet and text capabilities. A library administrator, aware of the increasing importance of group learning, electronic learning, and interdisciplinary research may see opportunities to convert space into classrooms, group study spaces, teleconference suites, and other collaborative workspaces.

Performing Assessment, Evaluation, and Measurement

Careful assessment provides critical information for planning and making organizational changes to achieve goals. Having solid evidence of the need for change aids the staff's, clients', and administrators' acceptance of, and support for, those goals. In assessment and planning, the emphasis is on reporting meaningful data and making data-driven decisions that result in a wise use of resources. For example, if the expansion of electronic resources reduces serials check-in and binding activities, then staff resources should be reallocated to meet new needs, such as creating Web-based access points or helping users navigate electronic resources.

The terms "assessment," "evaluation," and "measurement" are often used interchangeably in the library literature. However, in this chapter, the terms have a hierarchical relationship.

Assessment is used to describe library administrators' efforts to determine the extent to which the library meets client needs, achieves quality standards, and conveys value to higher-level administrators and others who have an interest in the success of the library. Assessment is the cumulative analysis of various evaluations and measurements. Continuous assessment should lead to continuous improvement. Building a "culture of assessment" and an assessment program is the responsibility of administrators.[18]

Evaluation includes the various types of actions taken to monitor progress toward library goals and program objectives:

> Evaluation has several distinguishing characteristics relating to focus, methodology, and function. Evaluation (1) assesses the effectiveness of an ongoing program in achieving its objectives, (2) relies on the standards of project design to distinguish a program's effects from those of other forces, and (3) aims at program improvement through a modification of current operations.[19]

Measurement is the collection of qualitative and quantitative data through the use of various tools such as surveys, scales, interviews, observation, and transaction logs. In simple terms, it is a "procedure for assigning a number to an object or an event."[19] Applications of various measurement tools have been discussed in the literature.[20-25]

In this hierarchical relationship, assessment is the umbrella program that encompasses a variety of evaluation activities. Measurement provides the data to inform evaluations. Since the 1980s, authors have focused on defining assessment in terms of the client's experience.[26, 27] There has been an increasing interest in measuring **outcomes,** which the AAHSL Outcomes and Quality Assessment Committee defines as "end results, evidence or benefits to people as a result of programs and/or services."[28]

Measurable **indicators** and outcomes are important for defining and communicating value to those outside the library, chiefly campus administrators and external funding agencies. Marshall states that recent studies show that

> we can go beyond the traditional measures—how much we do (output), the resources with which we do it (input), and customer satisfaction—to include outcomes measures as part of the evolutionary process of determining our worth. Measuring outcomes, the most recently developed measure, helps us to deduce how the information we give our users has improved their job productivity or quality of life. We need to have all these measures in our evaluation toolkit, because determining value is in the eye of the beholder: your organization.[29]

As this book goes to press, the AAHSL Assessment and Statistics Committee is conducting an exploratory survey of academic health sciences libraries' senior leadership to determine the state of readiness to move more aggressively toward outcome measures.

External Reporting

Academic health sciences libraries have been collecting statistics for comparison and other purposes since the mid-1970s.[30] Statistics are reported through the AAHSL annual survey. Libraries at large universities may also report statistics to the **Association of Research Libraries (ARL).** The library may also be involved occasionally in studies to determine the **federal overhead (facilities and administration)** percentage allowed in federal grants. In these studies, more use of the library attributed to sponsored research purposes raises the reimbursement rate

Selected Examples of Library Measurement Tools

Purpose	Example
Benchmarking	The MLA BENCHMARKING NETWORK offers hospital, academic, and specialty health libraries an opportunity to learn more about benchmarking, compare data, establish best practices, and identify and work with a benchmarking partner. From: <http://www.mlanet.org/members/benchmark>. ASSOCIATION OF RESEARCH LIBRARIES STATISTICS is a series of annual publications that describe the collections, expenditures, staffing, and service activities for ARL member libraries. Statistics have been collected and published annually for the members of the association since 1961-1962. From: <http://www.arl.org/stats/annualsurveys/arlstats>. The *ANNUAL STATISTICS OF MEDICAL SCHOOL LIBRARIES IN THE UNITED STATES AND CANADA* is a publication of the Association of Academic Health Sciences Libraries. Published since 1978, the *Annual Statistics* provides comparative data on significant characteristics of collections, expenditures, personnel, and services in medical school libraries in the United States and Canada. From: <http://www.aahsl.org/new/display_page.cfm?file_id=78>.
Assessing User Satisfaction and Expectations	LibQUAL+™ is a suite of services that libraries use to solicit, track, understand, and act upon users' opinions of service quality. These services are offered to the library community by the Association of Research Libraries (ARL). The program's centerpiece is a rigorously tested Web-based survey bundled with training that helps libraries assess and improve library services, change organizational culture, and market the library. From: <http://www.libqual.org>.
Identifying Information and Technology Competencies or Literacy	Association of College and Research Libraries *INFORMATION LITERACY COMPETENCY STANDARDS FOR HIGHER EDUCATION.* From: <http://www.ala.org/ala/acrl/acrlstandards/informationliteracycompetency.htm>. Project SAILS is a standardized test of information literacy skills based on the ACRL standards. This Web-based tool allows libraries to document information literacy skill levels for groups of students and to pinpoint areas for improvement. From: <https://www.projectsails.org>. Association of American Medical Colleges Medical School Objectives Project. MEDICAL INFORMATICS AND POPULATION HEALTH. From: <http://www.aamc.org/meded/msop/start.htm>. NURSING INFORMATICS COMPETENCIES: SELF-ASSESSMENT. From: <http://www.nursing-informatics.com/niassess/index.html>.
Conducting Needs and Outcomes Assessment	Association of Academic Health Sciences Libraries. OUTCOMES ASSESSMENT STANDARDS AND TOOLS. From: <http://www.aahsl.org/new/display_page.cfm?file_id=235>. National Network of Libraries of Medicine. EVALUATION GUIDES FROM THE OUTREACH EVALUATION RESOURCE CENTER. From: <http://nnlm.gov/evaluation/guide>.

Example Outcomes Questions for Instruction Programs

The important outcomes of an academic library program involve the answers to questions like these:

- Is the academic performance of students improved through their contact with the library?
- By using the library, do students improve their chances of having a successful career?
- Are undergraduates who used the library more likely to succeed in graduate school?
- Does the library's bibliographic instruction program result in a high level of "information literacy" among students?
- As a result of collaboration with the library's staff, are faculty members more likely to view use of the library as an integral part of their courses?
- Are students who use the library more likely to lead fuller and more satisfying lives?

Source: Task Force on Academic Library Outcomes Assessment Report, June 27, 1998. Available: <http://www.ala.org/ala/acrl/acrlpubs/whitepapers/taskforceacademic.htm>. Accessed: March 19, 2007.

to the institution. Publicly funded state institutions may also have reporting responsibilities to state higher education boards. At the present time, most of this reporting consists of input and output measures rather than outcomes. These data are useful for comparison purposes.

Preparation for institutional accreditation visits, usually preceded by an extensive self-study, is a common external reporting responsibility of academic health sciences library administrators. Most disciplines have their own accrediting agency, such as the **Liaison Committee for Medical Education (LCME)** and the **Council on Education for Public Health (CEPH).** Library administrators may also participate in their hospitals' or medical centers' response to the **Joint Commission on Accreditation of Healthcare Organizations (Joint Commision, formerly JCAHO)** and their regional higher education agencies' accreditation processes, such as the Southern Association of Colleges and Schools (SACS). These self-studies generally include the library and other campus units providing related information support services. Site visits present opportunities to highlight areas of excellence and deficiency. The results of self-studies and agency reports should be incorporated into any quality improvement or strategic planning activities.

Marketing and Promoting the Library

Libraries engage in a variety of marketing activities to determine what users need and how best to meet those needs, such as conducting user surveys. Libraries provide a variety of promotional materials (Web pages, brochures, flyers, tutorials) to highlight services for users or to assist them in using the library. Chapter 9, "Marketing, Public Relations, and Communication," gives more detail on these activities.

The library administrator oversees and provides direction and funding for these efforts, perhaps with the help of people with marketing, public relations, or fund development expertise. The library administrator may decide to "brand" the library's products and services. **Branding** is "selecting and blending tangible and intangible attributes to differentiate the product, service or corporation in an attractive, meaningful and compelling way."[31] Charbonneau and colleagues provide an example of branding health information services in the context of assessment, advocacy, and advertisement.[32]

The library administrator is the external public representative of the library and the most visible staff member to peers and upper-level administrators. However, it is important for the library administrator to ensure that every library staff member effectively represents the library and has a positive impact on users' library experiences. The personal interaction of library staff with library users, whether in-person or virtually, remains a critical aspect of marketing and promoting the role of the library and demonstrating visible and relevant services.

Advocating Policy and Legislative Issues

Academic health sciences library administrators are in positions to take active roles in policy development and legislation. Involvement in institutional information policy issues such as copyright, **intellectual property,** institutional repositories, and information technology priorities is in the best interest of the library and its users. This involvement enables the library administrator to advocate for information access and infrastructure within and beyond the institution. Beyond the institution, legislative or government relations groups, such as the Joint MLA/AAHSL Legislative Task Force, offer an administrator opportunity to actively participate. This task force develops and promotes a legislative agenda in the interest of members of both the Medical Library Association and the Association of Academic Health Sciences Libraries.[33] Examples of recent priorities include public access to government information, **National Library of Medicine (NLM)** funding and programs, open access, and multidisciplinary collaborative research. Annual reports of the task force contain that year's priorities and activities.

Overseeing Fiscal Responsibilities

Academic health sciences libraries are funded in various ways. Public institutions may receive an allocation for libraries directly or indirectly from the state. User fees in the form of service charges, such as for copying, printing, or document delivery, can provide income for the library.[34] Students may be charged a library or technology fee per semester or credit hour, which becomes part of the library's budget. Donations, endowments, and grants are also common sources of income. A portion of the parent institution's research overhead costs may be allocated for library resources. Regardless of the sources of income, it is important that the library's budget be based on what needs to be accomplished, with an agreed upon program plan, and the amount of money justified and negotiated to see that plan to fruition.

The parent institution generally determines the format of a budget, such as lump sum, line item, or programmatic. A line item budget is sometimes called an incremental budget if inflation or adjustments are made annually. Tables 13.1, 13.2, and 13.3 show partial views of line item, program, and performance budgets.

TABLE 13.1 Line Item Budget

	Last Year	**This Year**	**Next Year**
Salaries			
Journals			
Books			
Databases			
Miscellaneous			
TOTAL			

Source: Dossett, J. "Budgets and Financial Management in Special Libraries." CLIS 724 (April 28, 2004).

TABLE 13.2 Program Budget

	Pathology	**O&G**	**General Practice**	**TOTALS**
Salaries				
Materials				
Etc.				
Etc.				
Miscellaneous				
TOTALS				
%				100%

Source: Dossett, J. "Budgets and Financial Management in Special Libraries." CLIS 724 (April 28, 2004).

TABLE 13.3 Performance Budget, Function Budget

	Collections	**Reader Services**	**Outreach**	**TOTALS**
Salaries				
Materials				
Etc.				
Etc.				
Miscellaneous				
TOTALS				
%				100%

Source: Dossett, J. "Budgets and Financial Management in Special Libraries." CLIS 724 (April 28, 2004).

A typical budget is developed in accordance with the fiscal year schedule of the parent institution and divided into categories such as personnel, collections, operating, and capital costs. The personnel category is broken down into salaries and fringe benefits and may be further delineated by type of staff, such as professionals, support staff, student workers, and temporary staff. Staff development activities such as travel, continuing education, and professional meeting attendance may be included in the personnel portion of the budget. Collection budgets are usually broken down by type, such as serials, monographs, print or electronic, recurring or nonrecurring. Operating expenses represent infrastructure. Supplies, telecommunication costs, equipment and building maintenance, and small furniture or software purchases are typical in this category. Some libraries are expected to budget for heating, cooling, housekeeping, and insurance. Capital expenses are one-time costs over a certain dollar amount set by the institution, often for renovations or for new equipment. A manager may choose to further subdivide the budget based on internal needs, such as tracking new programs or services or to meet audit requirements. The institution may have policies on whether unspent funds can be carried over into the next fiscal year or used for purposes other than described in the original budget, for example, whether salaries accrued at the end of the year from vacant positions can be put on deposit with a vendor for collections.

The library director is ultimately responsible for managing the library's budget. In larger libraries, a business or administrative manager will perform most budget activities for the library director, for example, monitoring the budget and the performance of investments, approving purchases, gathering data, and preparing reports. In smaller academic libraries, the director and an administrative person may handle the budget, or the director may do this in consult with the parent organization's fiscal officer. In any case, frequent conversations between the administrator and the budget staff are critical to effective fiscal management.

MANAGING PERSONNEL

Excellent personnel practices help establish an environment that attracts and retains quality employees and helps employees perform at their best. Human resources practices are similar across libraries. The following discussion focuses on those that are most influenced by an academic health sciences environment or are most basic to an overview of this subject. Several good library personnel management texts exist and are listed in Appendix 13.A.

Preparing Staff for Health Sciences Work

Academic health sciences library work, particularly in teaching hospitals, encompasses certain characteristics that are different from work in other library settings. For example, staff who work in health sciences libraries, particularly staff who work directly with library users and health information resources, will encounter the emotional and urgent nature of personal health crises, the graphic and serious nature of the clinical content and situations, and the high-stress and high-stakes work of the clients served. In addition, staff need to be aware of the longer service hours with fewer days closed, the 24/7/365 nature of health care, and the fast pace of technological innovation and scientific discovery. Because of the intense nature of the work environment, managers should pay attention to building into the work ongoing training and enjoyable rituals, de-stressors, and ways for staff to come together as a community, for example, at coffee hours, at holiday parties, or through contests. Depending on the organizational culture, the library may invite users to join in these activities as well.

Other effective responses to this environment are to prepare and hire staff to be ready to change roles and jobs frequently and to engage in lifelong learning. For example, job descriptions, advertisements, and applicant interviews can be structured to request evidence of flexibility, creativity, early adoption of innovation, self-directed learning, and teamwork—critical skills and abilities in the academic health sciences environment. Applicants need to know that the job for which they are applying today may not be the one they have tomorrow.

Complying with Regulations

Institutional, state, and federal policies and procedures guide human resources activities, in addition to those that library management chooses to enact. For example, **hiring freezes** and merit raises can be set by external entities, while distribution of funds for professional activities is determined internally within the library. Compliance with external agencies' guidelines and regulations is a key component of human resources management.

Six Principal Types of Library Budgets

Type	Definition	Advantages	Disadvantages
Lump sum	Allocation by library's parent organization's upper-level management of a "lump sum" of budget resources to the library. Once lump-sum is allocated, library management allocates to lower-level library programs and services.	Can offer high level of flexibility and control within library itself	Since the lump sum method lacks specific ties to corporate goals and objectives, many library managers prefer other types of budgets.
Formula budget	Allocation tied to numeric value such as full-time-equivalents (FTEs), (i.e., FTE registered students multiplied by fixed amount).	Easier for funders to administer	Budget total calculated at a late point in time and intrudes on advance planning—especially for purchases and staffing increases—within the library. Does not link to organization's goals and objectives. Unpredictable, as formula is based on variables outside influence or control of special library.
Line-item budget (see Table 13.1)	Most commonly used budgeting method (Warner). Each category of activity has separate line. Facilitates low levels of detail for both planning and cost control purposes.	Ease of preparation. Useful for comparing performance from one fiscal period to another fiscal period.	Difficult to relate to goals of parent organization. May "perpetuate" a line (i.e., "once a line, always a line"). Miscellaneous line may become unwieldy as technologies and costs evolve. Comparing this year to last year is complex and represents variables unaccounted for within line-item budget (Warner).
Program budget (see Table 13.2)	Focuses on services library provides to its clients. Readily relates to overall organizational goals and objectives. Considered useful when establishing priority for library programs relative to parent organization.	Typically an extension of line-item budget method. Each program appears separately and is broken into categories similar to line-item budget (Robinson and Robinson). Easier to compare between multiple programs. Claimed to be easily understood and to minimize conflict and overlap between projects (Asantewa).	Forces staff members to think along program lines outside "comfort zone" associated with other methods. Some people are defensive when required to "analyze, report and justify how they spend their time."

Performance budget (see Table 13.3)	Some similarity with program budgets, but focuses primarily on what library staff members do or functions they perform in the library service. Tasks rather than programs are highlighted. Functions include technical services (i.e., cataloguing, materials processing); planning (budgeting, automation, employee selection, interviewing, development); patron contact (circulation desk, e-mail and telephone contacts).	Provides instrument for monitoring staff members and for developing unit costs.	Emphasizes quantity, not quality, of activity being monitored (Warner).
Zero-based budget (ZBB)	Starts from premise that "no costs or activities should be factored into the plans for the coming budget period, just because they figured in the costs or activities for the current or previous periods. Rather, everything that is to be included in the budget must be considered and justified" (CIPFA). Once value enhancing activities are identified, attendant costs are developed. May involve "decision packages" to examine each proposed program and rank its merits against parent organization's goals and objectives. Once top-ranking programs are identified, a program budget model is used to construct resource details.	Focuses on programs that will advance organization's goals for future. Challenges "way we've always done things." Is claimed to promote innovation, effectiveness and efficiency. "From scratch" approach appropriate for ranking programs by cost/importance to organizational goals. Also identifies and eliminates programs with minimal added value (Zach).	May prove time-intensive.

Source: Warner, Alice S. "Library Budget Primer." *Wilson Library Bulletin* 67, no. 9 (May 1993): 44-46; Facilitated Online Learning as an Interactive Opportunity (FOLIO). Financial Management: An Overview. Available: <http://exfiles.pbwiki.com/f/Financial%20Management%20briefing.doc>. Accessed: March 29, 2007; Dossett, Judith C. Budgets and Financial Management in Special Libraries 2/11/07. Prepared April 28, 2004, for CLIS 724 by Dr. Robert Williams. Available: <http://www.libsci.sc.edu/BOB/class/clis724/SpecialLibraries Handbook/Budgets%20and%20Financial%20Management.htm>. Accessed: March 29, 2007; Robinson, Barbara M., and Robinson, Sherman. "Strategic Planning and Program Budgeting for Libraries." *Library Trends* (Winter 1994): 420-8; Asantewa, D'Lle. "Holistic Budgeting: A Process: A Whole System Approach." *Information Outlook* 7, no. 8 (August 2003): 14-8; Chartered Institute of Public Finance and Accountancy. Zero-Based Budgeting. Available: <http://www.cipfa.org.uk/pt/download/zero_based_budgeting_briefing.pdf. Accessed: October 2, 2007; Zach, Lisl. "A Librarian's Guide to Speaking the Business Language (Tools of Budgeting)." *Information Outlook* 6, no. 6 (June 2002): 18-24.

Select List of Regulations in Human Resources

Affirmative Action Plans and Executive Order 11246
Age Discrimination in Employment Act
Americans with Disabilities Act
Civil Rights Act (Title VI, VII)
Equal Employment Opportunity Commission Guidelines
Equal Pay Act
Fair Credit and Reporting Act
Family and Medical Leave Act
Family Educational Rights and Privacy Act (FERPA)
Fair Labor Standards Act
Federal Work Study
Hatch Political Activities Act
Immigration Reform and Control Act
Jobs for Veterans Act
National Labor Relations Act
Occupational Safety and Health Act (OSHA)
Pregnancy Discrimination in Employment Act
Privacy Act
Rehabilitation Act

State and local legislation and guidelines:

"Employment at will doctrine"
Nondiscrimination
Sexual harassment
Diversity plans
Open records laws
Union and collective bargaining processes
Grievance processes
Political activities

Every library should have a human resources manual for employees, either provided by the parent institution or developed by the library, which explains pertinent policies, rules, and regulations. This "manual" can be part of an intranet site, also, to which all employees have ready access. In libraries with large numbers of employees, it is very beneficial to have someone on staff who knows the policies, procedures, and regulations that govern human resources. This knowledge and the ability to use it for the advantage of the library, combined with good external relationships, will make it likely that the library's workforce can adapt more rapidly to the needs of a changing environment.

Assessing Staffing Needs

In a broad context, human resources management is the allocation and oversight of a major resource, the library's employees, in order to accomplish the library and parent institution's vision, mission, goals, and objectives. Equally important is enabling people and the organization to perform at their greatest potential in a mutually fulfilling way. Salaries and wages comprise, on average, 40 percent of the health sciences library budget, almost as much as what the library spends on collections.[34] Staff planning is one tool that enables wise use of this major resource. In iterations of establishing a library's short- and long-range goals, attention should be paid to assessing staffing needs. The following are some aspects of staffing to consider:

- One-time, temporary, and long-term needs
- Adequate number of staff
- Roles to be performed at appropriate levels
- Boundaries between support staff, librarians, information technology specialists, and other staff's roles
- Expertise and skill sets needed and available (technical, subject, language, interpersonal)
- Diversity
- Organization structure and span of control (the number of employees supervised)
- Space, equipment, and other physical resources needed by staff
- Outsourcing or contracting services
- Learning contracts or class projects (field experience, independent study, internship, practicum, class assignment, research or graduate assistantship)

Three of these—roles, diversity, and learning contracts—are described in more detail to provide examples of their application in academic health sciences libraries.

Roles

Changing health care, information, and technological environments have had an impact on library staff roles. A widening continuum from novice to expert information competencies in library users also influences the roles of library staff. Changes in positions may mean new or additional roles for staff and training to help them perform optimally in these new roles.

Some examples of the changes are the increase in time spent troubleshooting electronic access issues (investigating and solving library, publisher, technical, and human errors), the increased use of evidence-based literature searching and evidence-based tools, the increased concern for safety of human subjects in research, and pressure to find alternatives to animals as research subjects. Several libraries have developed extensive roles for health sciences librarians within the users' environments. The Eskind Biomedical Library at Vanderbilt University Medical Center, the National Library of Medicine, and the National Institutes of Health (NIH) Library are three leaders in this area.[35-37] MLA and others have done work in defining the role of the **information specialist in context (ISIC),** who is an information specialist with subject expertise in health or research disciplines.[38, 39]

Diversity

Diversity is a work environment characteristic that enhances learning and decision-making.[40, 41] Different types of staff and perspectives are increasingly sought to better meet the needs of library users who are also becoming more diverse.[42, 43] Diversity is considered and addressed from several perspectives, such as race, gender, age, ethnicity, personality type, job type, disabilities, and career stage.

The important demographic, cultural, and learning style shifts that create the need for diversity have been discussed in the literature.[44, 45] These shifts affect human resources in academic health sciences libraries (and other settings) by motivating managers in these ways:

- Reexamine, update, and replace position descriptions to reflect new and higher-level skills required
- Adjust recruitment activities to actively seek applicants representing diverse backgrounds
- Plan for retirements and the capture or transfer of expertise and institutional history when new or less experienced staff are hired

- Develop, recruit, share, or contract for different expertise needed, for example, instructional design, systems analysis, fundraising, research experience, basic science, and other specialized subject knowledge
- Provide or obtain leadership and management training for the next generation of library directors
- Develop innovative approaches to career advancement, professional growth, and performance rewards
- Provide staff development programs that raise awareness and appreciation of diversity in its many forms

In academic settings, some of the ways libraries are addressing diversity include academic residency programs for minorities[46] and diversity training for staff.[40, 43] One of the roles administrators play is creating an environment that values diversity.[47-49] Library administrators may also be asked to respond to campus **diversity plans** or can use these as a guide for their own action plans in this area.[50]

Learning Contracts

Academic health sciences libraries, particularly those on a general academic campus, have access to help and expertise from faculty and students in statistics, **operations research,** planning, business, communications, marketing, or other fields. Providing projects for students may enable the library to accomplish something which could not be tackled otherwise due to lack of on-site expertise or time. The library provides the learning environment, project information, and on-site supervision in exchange for a product or service. One health sciences library provided projects for students in the field of operations research that resulted in studies and recommendations to improve interlibrary loan turnaround time, staffing a single service point, and copier service queues.[51]

Health sciences libraries near a library school can provide a research laboratory and job training through paid part-time positions, career guidance, and other contributions to the profession. In exchange, the library reaps the intellectual capital of library school students, particularly those interested in health sciences librarianship, archives, or public records management. Under the direction of the library administrator, a mutually beneficial learning atmosphere with meaningful experience for students can be established.

Establishing an Organizational Structure

The organizational structures within the library must respond to changes as priorities and needs in parent institutions evolve. At the same time, stability and continuity are needed in order to provide expected levels of service. Maureen Sullivan, a noted expert in organizational development, describes the key elements of an organization.[52] These are summarized here:

> *Organizational structure* is designed around the work processes. It has limited hierarchy and is focused on the coordination of work, not control. It encourages cooperation and collaboration and is easily understood and navigated by staff.
> *Organizational systems* include communication, decision-making, accountability, resource allocation, policy formulation, work design, culture, management practices, and climate.
> *Human resource systems* comprise position classification, compensation, benefits, performance feedback, learning and development, rewards and recognition, and competencies. These support people and the attainment of skills and abilities, and promote leadership.

Many books and articles describe various ways to organize library staff. The typical organizational structure is around functional areas such as administration, public services, technical services, and technology development and support. Traditional hierarchical structures in academic health sciences libraries determine the chain of command (who makes what decisions), the expectations for reporting and delegating, and who represents the library within the institution and in professional organizations. For example, large academic libraries may have the following:

- Director
- Deputy director or one or more associate directors
- Assistant directors, division heads, or department heads

Given the changes in the health sciences environment and in the way work is accomplished, these traditional organizational structures are being reconsidered.[53, 54] MLA publishes a series of DocKits, which are compilations of examples from the field. One describes a variety of organizational configurations, from the traditionally hierarchical to **matrix management.**[55] Another DocKit is available that provides examples of existing position descriptions, which are useful in thinking about job functions and how they relate to other positions in the organization.[56]

Issues Affecting Recruitment

Another distinguishing feature of managing personnel in academic health sciences libraries is that those working in these libraries are a relatively small professional community—only 160 libraries could have responded to the AAHSL 2004-2005 annual survey. The total number of **full-time equivalent (FTE)** staff was 4,550 for the 126 libraries that did respond. The median FTE staff for this same group of libraries was thirty-five, with a range from five FTEs to seventy-eight FTEs.[34] MLA lists 3,600 individual members from academic, corporate, hospital, and other health information settings combined.[57]

Some of the implications of this workforce characteristic are that applicant pools for specialized positions can be small and that managers may have to craft jobs, position descriptions, and advertisements to attract candidates from related disciplines or without a science- or health-related background or library experience.[58] For example, the "required" education, experience, and skills might concentrate on a few absolute essentials, putting others in the "desired" category in order to expand the pool of applicants. An advantage academic health sciences libraries have, particularly if the library is located on or close to an undergraduate college or university, is that the library is more likely to attract and employ students in part-time jobs.

Another unique aspect of academic health sciences libraries has been their tendency to be technologically advanced in relation to other types of libraries and in comparison to other parts of the parent institution. In the past, it was difficult to find library school graduates with high levels of technical skills to meet these libraries' needs. Continuing education programs had to catch up with practice as well. Fortunately, curricula have changed in graduate schools, and there are many opportunities for ongoing staff development. As a result, there is a larger pool of technologically savvy applicants for these library positions.

A Day in the Life of an Academic Health Sciences Library Associate Director

Name: Roberta Bronson Fitzpatrick, MLIS
Position: Associate Director, UMDNJ—George F. Smith Library of the Health Sciences

Job description: Serve as administrator for the state's flagship health sciences library, which is the health information resource for citizens of the state of New Jersey, as well as faculty, students, and staff of the UMDNJ. Responsible for daily operations of the following departments: information and education services, circulation, reserves, stacks maintenance, interlibrary loan (ILL) and photocopy services, acquisitions/collection development, serials, bibliographic search services, archives/special collections (2004-2007), library systems, and the computer-media center. Supervise twenty-nine FTEs.

Sample Day

8:30–9:00 a.m.
- Arrive at 8:30 a.m.
- Unlock administrative office suite, turning on lights.
- Check voicemail and note messages; return phone calls.

9:00–10:00 a.m.
- Check e-mail.
- Note appointments on electronic calendar; answer e-mails; place phone calls as needed.
- Go to Information Desk to discuss schedule with librarian on duty.

10:00–11:00 a.m.
- Meet with Head of Circulation to discuss staff disciplinary action and to review annual staff performance appraisals.
- Go over accounts of accumulated sick and vacation time.
- Discuss generic job descriptions for Circulation Department staff and position upgrades needed for two members of the department.
- Draft a generic job description with Head of Circulation and ask her to read it over, edit it, and return it by week's end.

11:00 a.m.–Noon
- Read through list of journal titles for possible subscription. These titles are part of a special offer from a vendor; most are out of scope for our collection.
- Give final list to E-Resources Librarian, who is collecting them to see if there are common requests among the UMDNJ campus libraries.

Noon–1:00 p.m.
- Lunch from 12:30–1:00 p.m.
- Read over draft minutes from last management meeting and review handouts.
- Review draft job description for new university-wide position to provide copyright support to faculty, students, and staff via in-person consultations, a Web page, and e-mail.

1:00–2:00 p.m.
- Check e-mail.
- Draft annual reports for the Public Services Section of the Medical Library Association (MLA) and for Chapter Council Representative/Alternate activities for the New York–New Jersey Chapter, MLA.

2:00–3:00 p.m.
- Meet with Head of Access Services and Head of Interlibrary Loan to discuss lease/purchase of color copier, to be networked to serve as a color laser printer.
- With salesman, visit other departments on the Newark campus having this equipment, to check copy and print quality.
- Ask salesman to prepare price quotes and send them via e-mail.

3:00–4:00 p.m.
- Meet with University Librarian to prepare agenda for upcoming Smith Library Committee meeting.
- Discuss color copier purchase, as well as effect of new scanning equipment on ILL department workflow.
- Return to office and make notes on agenda of talking points for meeting.

4:00–5:00 p.m.
- Work on Bioterrorism Webliography updates for NJ-PTC (New Jersey Preparedness Training Consortium) <http://www.nj-ptc.org/webliography/index.htm>. I am adding a list of full-text articles, freely available on the Internet, that discuss natural disasters, as well as a page in the Webliography which highlights the "best" sites on this topic.

5:00–6:00 p.m.
- Send out off-campus meeting request forms and travel reimbursement forms.
- Leave work.

A major study is underway to take an in-depth look at issues affecting the library workforce. The Institute for Museum and Library Science (IMLS) has funded a two-year study, "The Future of Librarians in the Workforce," that will achieve these goals:

- Identify the nature of anticipated labor shortages in the library and information science field over the next decade.
- Assess the number and types of library and information science jobs that will become available in the United States, either through retirement or new job creation.
- Determine the skills that will be required to fill such vacancies.
- Recommend effective approaches to recruiting and retaining workers to fill them.
- Provide better tools for workforce planning and management, a better match of demand and supply, and improved recruitment and retention of librarians.[59]

The Medical Library Association is one of the partnering organizations in the study. The results of this study should provide library administrators with valuable help in the areas of recruitment and retention. Because of the decreasing numbers of librarians—an impetus for this workforce study—library administrators may decide to focus greater attention on developing existing staff and becoming advocates for health librarianship as a career choice for young students, those changing careers, and support staff.

Hiring Process

Recruiting new staff varies by type and size of staff. Librarian recruitment includes multiple steps, as can be seen in Appendix 13.D, which is a modified checklist for recruiting librarians for a large university library. In smaller libraries, the process may be shorter and more informal. In larger libraries, a search committee, with administrative support, will handle most of the recruitment. For support staff recruitment, the steps are typically fewer; for example, the search committee may be the staff of the hiring unit, advertising may be local rather than national, and the approval process may be simplified.

The hiring library creates a significant impression on applicants by how it recruits employees. Immediate acknowledgment when applications are received, regular communications about the status of the search process (including delays), notification about interviews, and when candidates are no longer being considered, and communications with the candidate selected, and those not selected, are all important. As mentioned earlier, the health sciences community is relatively small and word gets around about applicants' experiences, both positive and negative.

Some of the steps in recruitment are listed here:

- Deciding or reviewing the work that the position needs to do
- Writing or revising the job description[56]
- Determining the appropriate salary range
- Advertising the job
- Reviewing applications and selecting candidates to interview
- Checking references
- Interviewing
- Hiring/making a job offer

These, and related steps, are described in more detail in articles in the additional readings at the end of this chapter.

Annotated Interview Schedule (Sample for Support Staff Position)

[Date]

8:15–8:45 a.m.
- Meet with supervisor: [name, title (location)].
- *Explain interview schedule, review job functions and organizational chart, answer questions.*

8:45–9:15 a.m.
- Tour the library.
- *Show work of the library, workspace, amenities.*

9:15–10:15 a.m.
- Meet with staff who will work most closely with position: [names, titles (location)].
- *Assess knowledge, training, experience related to job functions, answer questions.* **Tip:** Ask open-ended questions.

10:15–10:30 a.m.
- Break

10:30–11:15 a.m.
- **Optional:** Meet with staff from other areas of library: [names, titles (location)].
- *Assess knowledge, training, experience related to job functions, answer questions.* **Tip:** Let applicant do most of the talking.

11:15–11:30 a.m.
- **Optional:** Meet with human resources facilitator: [name, title (location)].
- *Explain other steps in hiring process: documentation required, background checks, who will contact applicant, approximate time frame, etc.*

11:30 a.m.–1:00 p.m.
- **Optional:** Lunch: [names, titles (location)].
- *Provide applicant with information about university and locale, if not from the area, and answer questions.*

1:00–1:30 p.m.
- Wrap up with supervisor: [name, title (location)].
- *Review job duties, hours, shift, deadlines, any planned program/organizational changes; explore inconsistencies or gaps in interview and application; assess interest in the position and possible start date if offered and accepted; confirm obtaining references.*

Overall Tips: Document applicant responses during or soon after the interview; evaluate applicant based on demonstrated knowledge, training, experience, and job requirements.

Developing Staff

Staff development can be defined broadly or narrowly. Here, it is defined broadly as encompassing the activities of orientation, professional development, job training and retraining, continuing education, and career planning and promotion. These activities can be a combination of formal and informal programs for groups or individuals. In an academic setting, there are typically many resources for staff development. Campus training departments within computing, research, human resources, and other departments often provide a wide range of programs. For example, there may be training for software applications, survey design, job skills such as résumé writing, grant writing, and many other topics. The educational policy statement of MLA, *Platform for Change,* outlines key areas of knowledge for health information professionals.[60] This policy is currently under review by MLA, but it is still a useful guide for staff development programs.

Orientation

New employee orientation is a key starting point for staff development and conveys the culture of the workplace to new staff. Some key elements of staff orientation follow:

- Tour of the facility and introduction to other employees
- Introductions to counterparts and key individuals in other parts of the institution
- Mission, goals, and objectives of the library and the parent institution
- Organization chart and governance
- Review of job expectations and how the new employee fits into the "big picture"
- Support services, for example, loaner equipment, technology, supplies, training
- Performance evaluation process
- Q&A opportunities

Professional Development

There are a few longstanding professional development programs aimed at new library professionals interested in health sciences librarianship. One that has been in existence for several years is the NLM Associate Fellowship Program.[61] NLM also provides training support through its informationist fellowships, medical informatics fellowships, and similar award programs.[36] There may also be regional training opportunities through professional organization chapters, formal coursework, consortia, and other groups.[35]

For managers, or those hoping to follow this career path, there are programs such as the NLM/AAHSL Leadership Fellows Program. This program selects five participants each year and is a significant credential for those wanting to become library directors.[62] Other excellent programs are the Association of Research Libraries Research Library Leadership Fellows (RLLF) Program; the University of California at Los Angeles (UCLA) Senior Fellows Program; MLA continuing education courses; and an AAHSL program begun in 2006 for recently appointed health sciences library directors.[63, 64] Administrators should also look at leadership programs that their own institutions offer for their academic managers.

The primary professional organization for health sciences librarians is the Medical Library Association. The Special Libraries Association has a Biomedical and Life Sciences Division that may be of interest to librarians. For support staff, the American Library Association (ALA) has organizations focused on support staff issues and a section for support staff resources.[65] The **Council on Library/Media Technicians (COLT)** is an affiliate of ALA focused on support staff issues such as "technical education, continuing education, certification, job description uniformity, and the more elusive goals of gaining recognition and respect for the very profes-sional work" done by support staff.[66]

While there is not a health sciences library license, there is professional recognition through MLA's **Academy of Health Information Professionals (AHIP).** This designation recognizes a professional's level of continuing education and professional contributions.[67]

Another key aspect of professional development for health sciences library staff at all levels is activities that support networking. The characteristics of the workforce described previously re-sult in a fairly close-knit profession. Administrators should encourage and financially assist staff attendance at conferences, participation in professional organizations, visits to other librar-ies, and formal and informal mentoring and peer relationships. These networking opportunities should be offered to both support staff and librarians.

Job Training

Job training is a continuous process from the time of hire until leaving the library. Job training encompasses those activities that expand the knowledge and skills needed by an employee to perform expected tasks. The supervisor is responsible for evaluating whether the necessary knowledge and skills have been obtained and for working to fill gaps in training. Good supervi-sors take on formal and informal mentoring roles with each employee, making sure that job training anticipates or keeps pace with change. The supervisor is also in a position to empower the employee to identify training needs and work as a team to meet them.

Performance Evaluation

The purposes of performance evaluation are threefold: to ensure that job expectations are be-ing met, that two-way feedback occurs between supervisor and employee, and that staff training and development occur. Different categories of staff have different required instruments, forms, and frequencies for evaluation. Administrative review for senior-level managers, such as the li-brary director, may be absent, based on a contract period, or based on an established cycle, such as every five years.

Various tools are available to evaluate performance, and the administrator may have some choice in the use of these. These can be used either as the primary instrument or in combination:

- Narrative/essay (self-assessment and supervisor assessment)
- Standard form (supervisor evaluation of staff)
- Peer performance appraisal (feedback from co-workers in a work unit or team)
- Reverse or upward performance review (evaluation of supervisors by their staff)
- Behavioral rating scales (numerical ratings on frequency or extent of desired behaviors)
- Competency-based reviews (MLA's *Platform for Change*, Special Libraries Association's *Competencies for Information Professionals of the 21st Century*)[60, 68]
- 360-degree assessment (self-assessment plus feedback from superiors, peers, subordi-nates, and possibly internal and external customers)

Regardless of the method, the library administrator needs to establish an environment in which regular informal and formal performance feedback happens. When performance prob-lems occur, they should be handled as quickly as possible. Another responsibility of the admin-istrator is to ensure that performance problems do not become chronic conditions affecting other staff's morale, productivity, or services to clients. If conflicts develop between staff that cannot be resolved internally, some academic institutions provide the services of a neutral third party, for example, an ombudsman. This position or office provides mediation, counseling, and support for a variety of workplace issues. In addition, these individuals or offices may promise confidentiality except when required by law.

Recognition, Motivation, and Retention

A key element of motivation and retention is having processes in place for gathering ideas, suggestions, and feedback from staff, for example, through discussions at all-staff meetings, anonymous suggestion boxes, and staff surveys. These are effective to the extent that staff receive responses or that follow-up action is taken based on the feedback received. If suggestions go into a "black hole," morale will soon follow.

Recognition

Recognition takes many forms and much is available on the subject.[69] In an academic setting, certain forms of staff recognition convey more meaning. Examples of these are professional contributions and activities through publishing; presenting papers or posters; attending professional meetings; obtaining faculty, adjunct, or clinical appointments in academic departments; and conducting research studies.

Administrators can submit, and encourage supervisors and other staff to submit, nominations for recognition awards offered by the parent institution. These can recognize excellent technological support, distinguished service, superior management, and other types of performance. Library administrators can also support the formation of formal library recognition programs. Parent institutions may provide guidelines and support for these, for example, paid time off as an award.

Career paths, or promotion from within, can be challenging, even in large libraries. Equal opportunity, affirmative action plans, and other regulations reduce flexibility in this area. Faculty status, or a similar academic promotional ladder, serves as a way for librarians to move up within the library or organization without necessarily moving into supervisory roles. However, the desirability of faculty status for librarians has been hotly debated for years.[70] Expanding one's subject knowledge and working in clients' environments have also been put forth as an alternative career path and form of recognition.[71]

Support staff's career paths may be governed by outdated position specifications and limited levels of advancement, many of which are no longer relevant to today's libraries. Promoting staff from within may be possible by moving appropriate positions from limited library tracks to information technology or administrative tracks, reclassifying positions, or abolishing and creating new positions, for which current staff can then apply. Administrators need creativity, commitment, and input from staff to find meaningful recognition for their employees' career growth.[72-74]

Motivation

An important, but not stand-alone, motivator is salary. The large proportion of the library's budget devoted to personnel makes salary administration a significant activity. The following aspects should be considered:

- Merit (extra pay given on the basis of performance)
- Equity (the requirement to pay staff, usually males and females, equal salary for work of equal value)
- Compression (new staff brought in at salaries equal to, or higher, than those of current staff)
- Market factors

- Cost of living
- Fringe benefits (the dollar amount or percent of salary for Social Security, retirement, health insurance, and other benefits paid by the organization)
- Bonuses and other one-time distributions
- Pay scales

Policies and procedures governing salary administration are, for the most part, provided by the parent institution. However, library management can have a positive influence on salaries by working with the parent institution to increase the pool of funds available for salaries from internal or external sources. For example, administrators can lobby for a portion of enrollment and tuition increases to address faculty salaries, particularly if librarians have academic status or appointments in academic departments. Another strategy is to make salary cost-sharing arrangements with departments. For example, a school may contribute to the salary of its assigned library liaison. Library managers may also be free to decide how to allocate a pool of funds across merit, equity, and compression. Other factors influencing motivation mentioned in the literature include clear communications, work relationships, involvement in decision-making, effective change management, and staff training and growth.[75-78]

Retention

Administrators need to determine what rate of staff **turnover** is desirable, acceptable, or manageable. Depending on the answer, strategies related to retention vary. Academic health sciences library directors tend to be concerned about excessive turnover rather than an insufficient level.

Because health sciences libraries are typically in the forefront of technology, they are often a training ground, particularly for those in information technology or systems support and administrative positions. Turnover in certain positions may be unacceptably high because of competition from other libraries or companies. These organizations may provide opportunities for compensation and advancement that the health sciences library does not have. Strategies for retention include building opportunities for growth and variety into the position, through cross-training and backup, for example. Academic health sciences library positions can also be constructed to provide more varied work through cross-functional teams, building the staff's breadth of experience, accomplishment, and skill. These efforts are known to encourage longer retention and job satisfaction.[79, 81]

Staff satisfaction and retention can also be enhanced by providing creature comforts such as the following:

- Vending machines and a break room
- Comfortable and attractive ergonomic furniture
- A budget for work tools that staff need to perform their jobs at the level expected
- Use of a ceremonial or comfortable space for staff events
- Catered food on occasion
- Staff social events or activities

Listening and responding in reasonable ways to staff requests along these lines is an important factor in job satisfaction, motivation, and retention.

Handling Personnel Records

The parent institution's human resources department will provide instruction on the retention, storage, and disposition of personnel records. Several of the steps mentioned in the recruitment process (see Appendix 13.D) help maintain the confidentiality of applicants and records generated by recruitment. While a great deal of communications can be handled by e-mail, some should not be; letters of references and candidate evaluations are examples.

Paper and electronic personnel records kept or accessed in the library must be secured from unauthorized access by means of locked file cabinets and network security procedures. Computer support personnel can suggest methods for protecting electronic systems and documents.

MANAGING FACILITIES

This role for library administrators includes activities such as space planning, facility maintenance, personal safety and building security, and use policies. This section provides a brief introduction to each of these aspects of facilities management.

Space Planning

A key question facing library administers is, "How much space does the library need?" The prevalent perception that "everything is electronic" has many library users no longer coming to the building and campus administrators questioning libraries' space needs. The AAHSL statistical reports cited earlier show continuing declines in library gate counts and circulation of materials. Universities and health centers are building on their remaining campus spaces while continuing to expand enrollments and research programs. In this situation, the competition for office, lab, classroom, meeting, and other kinds of space becomes intense.

The library administrator needs to examine the library's space needs and use space productively and wisely. Chapter 15, "Library Space Planning," discusses space planning in more detail. From the administrator's perspective, leading a process for planning is an important role. Ongoing identification of changing user needs and changing uses of library space is one step. There are several examples of the changes being made in academic library buildings.[17, 80-83] Some libraries are **repurposing** space rapidly and effectively to serve the institution. One strategy an administrator may choose is to explore mutually beneficial uses of space with fellow campus administrators. An advantage of sharing space can be more involvement in the hosted activity, for example, campus computing support, writing center programs, skills labs, or instructional media services.

In some cases, a reduction in space is dictated. Then, space planning becomes creative brainstorming on how to respond. The library administrator must manage staff and users' reactions to loss of space, as well as the effects on services, collections, and workspace. Use of compact shelving and off-site storage, large-scale digitization combined with storage or weeding, replacement of print back runs of journals with online **backfiles,** and other strategies can be considered.

Group use of the library's rooms and public areas demonstrates that the library is used for more than housing materials. Students use large screens and whiteboards to review for classes. They engage in discussion around anatomical and dental models and participate in faculty-led small group exercises. Visiting graduate school applicants and fellows may be interviewed in the library. These are examples of activities an administrator can decide to foster through space planning.

Building Maintenance

Managers are also responsible for care of the physical facilities. Library administrators typically delegate the day-to-day aspects of this work to administrative staff persons and their role becomes one of oversight or consulting. This part of management generally includes overseeing housekeeping, repairs, maintenance contracts, furnishings, telecommunications, equipment replacement, artwork inventory, and similar areas.

Building maintenance also includes surveying the building periodically for particular types of problems, for example, leaks, high humidity, mold and mildew, and insect or rodent problems. The particular problems one monitors regularly are tied to factors such as the age of the building and its environmental systems.

Another aspect of building maintenance is ensuring that users and staff have a clean, comfortable environment conducive to their work. This includes having a system in place for reporting and responding to building problems, whether they are related to housekeeping needs, furniture repairs, temperatures, equipment malfunctions, lighting, or plumbing.

Personal Safety and Facility Security

Ensuring the security and safety of library users, staff, the building, and contents is one of the most crucial areas of facilities management. Reliable and timely incident reporting and response systems (with backups) must be in place, as well as publicized and practiced emergency evacuation and response procedures. These should be evaluated periodically to make sure they continue to meet needs, particularly in the event of infrequently occurring emergencies, such as a fire, break-ins, leaks, or natural disasters.

In academic health sciences libraries, building access may be restricted because of factors such as crime rates, threatening client behaviors, animal research protection, or late-night hours. Security guards, card access, security cameras, staff identification badges, and similar systems may be used in these libraries.

Building Use Policies

Another management activity related to facilities is establishing use policies for users and staff. Clientele appreciate the availability of classrooms, computers, conference rooms, and other equipment or space in the library. Facilities use policies can create goodwill, as well as introduce potential users to the library. Policies that govern facilities use fall into the following categories:

- Food and drink
- Room reservations (eligibility, priorities, cancellations, fees)
- Room use support (equipment, setup, cleanup)
- Appropriate behavior and use of equipment and facilities
- **Americans with Disabilities Act (ADA)** accommodations and services (disability equipment, access, support services)
- Building access (particularly in private institutions)

Examples of use policies are easy to find by searching academic health sciences library Web sites. The administrator's role is to determine the types of use the library will encourage—or discourage—and advise the appropriate staff in establishing and evaluating use policies and procedures.

Shared Facilities Management

In an academic health sciences environment, responsibilities for facilities management are often shared by the campus, main library, medical school, and other agents. For example, the library may be responsible for distributing keys and enabling card access while the campus provides the keys, locks, locksmiths, card readers, and computer software for alarms, door controls, or other security systems.

Also, depending on the nature and severity of facilities issues, management will require coordination with service providers outside the library. There are usually experts on campus to assist with many aspects of facilities management. Examples include:

- Fire marshal
- Crime prevention officer
- Architecture and engineering staff
- Disability services office
- Health and safety staff
- Maintenance shops (electronics, carpentry, heating and air conditioning, plumbing)

These and others can be called upon for services or to perform audits and make recommendations for improvement.

CONCLUSION

Administration and management of academic health sciences libraries is, like many activities, a combination of art and science, theory and practice. This chapter has given an introduction to the roles of library administrators and an overview of each of their primary responsibilities. Continuous learning for administrators takes the form of conversations with colleagues, mentors, and staff; observation of exemplary leaders; reflection on personal experience; and reading and continuing education. Topics for further exploration include how to encourage staff to take risks, how to say "no" while providing excellent service, how to obtain grants and other new funding, how to make unpopular decisions, how to negotiate conflict between employees or between employees and users, balancing the safety of patrons and staff with the needs of challenging library users, and other topics. Fortunately, academic health sciences library directors have a strong and long-standing peer support network that can help with this ongoing learning. In addition, resources have been highlighted throughout this chapter and more are included in the additional readings. The rewards of effective leadership are well worth the learning endeavor.

APPENDIX 13.A. ADDITIONAL READINGS

Allan, Barbara. *Project Management: Tools and Techniques for Today's ILS Professional.* London: Facet Publishing, 2004.

American Research Libraries. "Salary Surveys." Available: <http://www.arl.org/stats/annualsurveys/salary/>. Accessed: March 26, 2007.

Avery, Beth; Dahlin, Terry; and Carver, Deborah A., eds. *Staff Development: A Practical Guide.* 3rd ed. Chicago: American Library Association, 2001.

Bell, Andrew. "Ten Steps to SMART Objectives." August 3, 2004. Available: <http://www.natpact.nhs.uk/uploads/Ten%20Steps%20to%20SMART%20objectives.pdf>. Accessed: March 14, 2007.

Bolan, Kimberly, and Cullin, Robert. *Technology Made Simple: An Improvement Guide for Small and Medium Libraries.* Chicago: American Library Association, 2007.

Breighner, Mary, and Payton, William. *Risk and Insurance Management Manual for Libraries.* Edited by Jeanne M. Drewes. Chicago: American Library Association, 2005.

Committee on the Status of Academic Libraries. "A Guideline for the Screening and Appointment of Academic Librarians Using a Search Committee: The Final Version." *College & Research Libraries News* 65, no. 4 (April 2004): 220-1.

Dugan, Robert E. "Information Technology Plans." *Journal of Academic Librarianship* 28, no. 3 (May 2002): 152-6.

Durrance, Joan C., and Fisher, Karen E. *How Libraries and Librarians Help: A Guide to Identifying User-Centered Outcomes.* With Marian Bouch Hinton. Chicago: American Library Association, 2004.

Eckert, Susan. *Intercultural Communication.* Mason, OH: Thomson South-Western, 2006.

Evans, G. Edward, and Ward, Patricia L. *Beyond the Basics: The Management Guide for Library and Information Professionals.* New York: Neal-Schuman, 2003.

Feiner, Michael. *The Feiner Points of Leadership: The Fifty Basic Laws That Will Make People Want to Perform Better for You.* New York: Warner Business Books, 2004.

Forsman, Rick B., ed. *Administration and Management in Health Sciences Libraries.* Vol. 8, Current Practice in Health Sciences Libraries. Lanham, MD: Scarecrow Press and Medical Library Association, 2000.

Gordon, Valerie S., and Higginbottom, Patricia C. *MLA DocKit #14. Staff Development.* Chicago: Medical Library Association, 2005.

Hallam, Arlita W., and Dalston, Teresa R. *Managing Budgets and Finance: A How-To-Do-It Manual for Librarians and Information Professionals.* New York: Neal Schuman, 2005.

Halsted, Deborah D.; Jasper, Richard P.; and Little, Felicia M. *Disaster Planning: A How-To-Do-It Manual for Libraries.* New York: Neal-Shuman, 2005.

Holst, Ruth, and Phillips, Sharon A., eds. *The Medical Library Association Guide to Managing Health Care Libraries.* New York: Neal-Schuman, 2000.

Joubert, Douglas J., and Lee, Tamara P. "Empowering Your Institution Through Assessment." *Journal of the Medical Library Association* 95, no. 1 (January 2007): 46-53.

Kuntz, Jennifer J.; Tennant, Michele R.; and Case, Ann C. "Staff-Driven Strategic Planning: Learning from the Past, Embracing the Future." *Journal of the Medical Library Association* 91, no. 1 (January 2003): 79-83.

Leonhardt, Thomas W. "Behind the Scenes: Hiring for Success." *Technicalities* 26, no. 4 (July/August 2006): 4-6.

Library Administration and Management Association. "Library Security Guidelines Document June 7, 2001." American Library Association. Available: <http://www.ala.org/ala/lama/lamapublications/librarysecurity.htm>. Accessed: February 11, 2007.

Lubans, John. "Coaching for Results." *Library Administration & Management* 20, no. 2. (Spring 2006): 86-9.

McKay, Richard. "Inspired Hiring: Tools for Success in Interviewing and Hiring Library Staff." *Library Administration & Management* 20, no. 3 (Summer 2006): 128-30.

Medical Library Association. "Hay Group/MLA 2005 Salary Survey." Available: <http://mlanet.org/publications/hay_mla_05ss.html>. Accessed: March 26, 2007.

Morgan, Arthur.; Cannan, Kath.; and Cullinane, Joanne. "360 Degree Feedback: A Critical Enquiry." *Personnel Review* 34, no. 6 (December 2005): 663-80.

Morris, Dilys E.; Bessler, Joanne M.; and Wilson, Flo. "Where Does the Time Go? The Staff Allocations Project." *Library Administration & Management* 20, no. 4 (Fall 2006): 177-91.

National Network of Libraries of Medicine. "Basic Medical Library Management: Administration." National Institutes of Health. Available: <http://nnlm.gov/management/admin.html>. Accessed: December 10, 2006.

Parrish, David. "Six Leadership Styles." Available: <http://www.davidparrish.com/leadership6styles.html>. Accessed: March 4, 2007.

Patkus, Ronald, and Rapple, Brendan A. "Changing the Culture of Libraries: The Role of Core Values." *Library Administration and Management* 14, no. 4 (Fall 2000): 197-204.

Schachter, Debbie. "How to Set Performance Goals: Employee Reviews Are More Than Annual Critiques." *Information Outlook* 8, no. 9 (September 2004): 26-9.

Scherrer, Carol S., and Jacobson, Susan. "New Measures for New Roles: Defining and Measuring the Current Practices of Health Sciences Librarians." *Journal of the Medical Library Association* 90, no. 2 (April 2002): 164-72.

Schwartz, Charles A., ed. *Restructuring Academic Libraries: Organizational Development in the Wake of Technological Change.* Chicago: American Library Association, 1997.

Schwartz, Peter. *The Art of the Long View: Planning for the Future in an Uncertain World.* New York: Doubleday, 1996.

Siess, Judith A. *Time Management, Planning, and Prioritization for Librarians.* Lanham, MD: Scarecrow Press, 2002.

Stueart, Robert D., and Sullivan, Maureen. *Performance Analysis and Appraisal: A How-To-Do-It Manual for Librarians.* New York: Neal-Schuman, 1991.

Tennant, Roy. "The Library Brand." LibraryJournal.com (January 15, 2006). Available: <http://library journal.com/article/CA6298452.html>. Accessed: March 26, 2007.

Trotta, Marcia. *Supervising Staff: A How-To-Do-It Manual for Librarians.* New York: Neal-Schuman, 2006.

Urquhart, Christine. *Solving Management Problems in Information Services.* Oxford: Chandos Publishing, 2006.

Winston, Mark D., and Dunkley, Lisa. "Leadership Competencies for Academic Librarians: The Importance of Development and Fund-Raising." *College and Research Libraries* 63, no. 2 (March 2002): 171-82.

Wittenborg, Karin. "Rocking the Boat." 2003. Available: <http://www.clir.org/PUBS/reports/pub123/wittenborg.html>. Accessed: December 11, 2006.

APPENDIX 13.B. SELECT LIST OF TREND REPORTS

This list highlights reports that are published on an annual or other recurring basis and are the most relevant to health sciences library administrators for strategic planning. Forecasting articles are also published and can provide examples of the use of trend information. See also more specialized trend reports, such as the Biomedical Journal Costs and Trends at <http://www.medlib.iupui.edu/rlml/bmjct.html>.

Library Trends

Title: Future of Libraries: Beginning the Great Transformation
Author: Thomas Frey, Executive Director and Senior Futurist at the DaVinci Institute
Web site: <http://www.davinciinstitute.com/page.php?ID=120>

Title: OCLC Membership Reports series
Source: OCLC
Web site: <http://www.oclc.org/reports/default.htm>

Title: National Library of Medicine planning documents
Source: National Library of Medicine
Web site: <http://www.nlm.nih.gov/pubs/plan/>

Technology Trends

Title: Pew Internet & American Life Project reports
Source: Pew Internet & American Life Project
Web site: <http://207.21.232.103/index.asp>

Title: Information and Communication Technology (ICT) Literacy Assessment
Source: Educational Testing Service (ETS)
Web site: Preliminary Results <http://www.ets.org/ictliteracy/prelimfindings.html>

Title: Library and Information Technology Association (LITA) Top Technology Trends
Source: LITA
Web site: <http://www.ala.org/ala/lita/litaresources/toptechtrends/toptechtrends.htm>

Title: Horizon Project Reports
Source: The New Media Consortium and the EDUCAUSE Learning Initiative (ELI)*
Web site: <http://www.nmc.org/pdf/2007_Horizon_Report.pdf> and <http://www.nmc.org/horizon/wiki/Main_Page>

Title: EDUCAUSE Current Issues Survey
Source: EDUCAUSE Current Issues Committee*
Web site: <http://www.educause.edu/CurrentIssues/875> (also published in summer issue of *EDUCAUSE Quarterly*)

Title: ECAR Research Studies
Source: EDUCAUSE Center for Applied Research (ECAR)*
Web site: <http://www.educause.edu/ResearchStudies/1010> (Latest materials require ECAR membership subscription or purchase; earlier ones are publicly available. All the survey instruments are available at <http://www.educause.edu/SurveyInstruments/1004>.) Other ECAR research publications are at <http://www.educause.edu/ResearchPublications/172>.

Health Care Trends

Title: California HealthCare Foundation reports
Source: California HealthCare Foundation
Web site: <http://www.chcf.org>

Title: Institute of Medicine reports
Source: Institute of Medicine
Web site: <http://www.iom.edu/CMS/2955.aspx>

Title: American Hospital Association research reports
Source: American Hospital Association
Web site: <http://www.aha.org/aha/research-and-trends/AHA-policy-research/2007.html>

Higher Education Trends

Title: CHEMA reports
Source: Council of Higher Education Management Associations (CHEMA)
Web site: <http://www.ala.org/ala/acrl/acrlissues/APPA39a_ScreenOpt.pdf>

Title: The Chronicle of Higher Education
Source: The Chronicle of Higher Education
Web site: <http://chronicle.com/>. Subscription required for complete publication.

APPENDIX 13.C. THE UNIVERSITY OF TENNESSEE GRADUATE SCHOOL OF MEDICINE, PRESTON MEDICAL LIBRARY & LEARNING RESOURCE CENTER

Mission Statement

The Preston Medical Library & Learning Resource Center's mission is to partner with the Graduate School of Medicine in providing excellence in education, patient care and research. The library is committed to ensuring access to clinical information through the acquisition, organization and management

---

*EDUCAUSE is a nonprofit association, of primarily U.S. colleges and universities, "whose mission is to advance higher education by promoting the intelligent use of information technology." Membership is by organization, with individuals designated as member representatives. Twelve percent of members are international (one-third Canadian).

of collections. We provide exceptional reference, research and instruction for faculty, residents, students and physicians and outreach to the community.

Vision Statement

Preston Medical Library & Learning Resource Center aspires to be an essential partner with the Graduate School of Medicine's endeavor to become a school of choice for graduate medical education and research through innovation, collaboration and providing exceptional, personalized services.

Values

We will actively seek to identify, meet and exceed client needs (in an accurate and timely manner).
We actively pursue new methods and the use of technologies in order to provide services essential to our clients.
We will be professional, conscientious and responsible and strive to exceed the expectations of our clients.
We are dedicated to providing quality service to our clients.
We believe in teamwork. We will work together both internally and externally to share knowledge, resources and ideas in order to fulfill our mission.
We will be positive in our interactions with each other and our clients.

Clientele

The primary clientele of the Preston Medical Library are the UTGSM faculty and staff, medical residents and students affiliated with the UTGSM, the UT Medical Center's staff, patients and area practicing physicians. Individuals with health questions may contact the library's Consumer & Patient Health Information Service.

The Library is open to everyone for in-house use of materials. Children under 18 are not permitted in the library without an adult. There is a one-hour time limit for computer use by patient families or general public. If all computers are occupied, preference is given to physicians, residents, and medical students. For more information on use of computers in the library, please read our Computer Use Statement.[84]

APPENDIX 13.D. CHECKLIST FOR LIBRARIAN RECRUITMENT (FOR PERMANENT POSITIONS)

_____ 1. Receive written resignation. Update all staff lists.
    ____a. Notify campus Affirmative Action Office of resignation.
_____ 2. Management reviews vacancy. Requests decision about recruitment from library EEO Officer. If recruitment is decided, proceed with these steps.
    ____a. Search Committee Chair requests position description from supervisor.
    ____b. Search Committee Chair drafts ad with EEO Officer.
    ____c. EEO Officer convenes Search Committee.
    ____d. EEO Officer announces beginning of search to library staff.
_____ 3. Search Committee reviews position description and advertisement.
    ____a. Determines recruitment plan (where to advertise). Can include journals, newsletters, newspapers, electronic job lines, library schools, minority schools, colleagues, placement services, library meetings, internal building locations, library intranet, and library Web site, as appropriate.
    ____b. Establishes time table.
_____ 4. Request review and approval of recruitment by designated campus administrator.
_____ 5. After campus administrator approval is received, get approval for recruitment plan and advertisement from campus Affirmative Action Office.
_____ 6. Submit copies to campus human resources for required minimum posting.
_____ 7. After recruitment plan is approved by Affirmative Action Office, place advertisements according to recruitment plan.

_____ 8. Receive applications; record on log.
     _____a. Date applications and send acknowledgment of receipt letter, along with standard application/request for additional information form to applicant, if required.
     _____b. Copy application letters and résumés for Search Committee members with alphabetic list of applicants.
     _____c. Copy the standard application/request for additional information form to the Search Committee Chair only.
_____ 9. Search Committee meets to review applications.
     _____a. Select list of candidates for whom to request references.
     _____b. Set date references are to be completed.
     _____c. Review/establish questions for references for this position.
_____ 10. Determine citizenship.
_____ 11. Contact references for selected candidates by telephone, e-mail, or letter.
     _____a. Thank references.
_____ 12. Submit Interim Affirmative Action statement to AAO. Receive approval before scheduling interviews with applicants.

If a deadline date for applications was set:

_____ 13. Send letters saying applications are no longer being considered to candidates not listed on Interim AA Statement.

If "review begins X date" was used:

_____ 14. Continue copying applications, etc., for Search Committee.
     _____a. Send status letters to those not selected for interviews.
_____ 15. Search Committee reviews references, new applications, and selects candidates for interviews.
     _____a. Select tentative dates for interviews.
     _____b. Select topic for interview presentation.
     _____c. Make faculty or similar rank recommendations to committee on appointments and promotion. After Library Director approves, schedule interviews.
_____ 16. Search Committee Chair invites candidates to interview (invitation by phone).
     _____a. Use candidate checklist and give to Administration.
_____ 17. Establish final interview schedule for each interviewee.
_____ 18. Send status letter to applicants who were not selected for interviews.
_____ 19. Send letter, interview packet, and interview schedule to candidates invited for interviews.
_____ 20. Announce interviews to library staff and send interview packets to library staff.
_____ 21. Reserve rooms and equipment for interviews.
_____ 22. Staff return written evaluations; send copies of evaluations to Search Committee.
_____ 23. Search Committee meets and makes selection.
_____ 24. Director calls successful candidate and makes conditional offer subject to approval of AAO.
_____ 25. Offer is accepted. Send letter of confirmation to successful candidate requesting library school transcript.
_____ 26. Director contacts other candidates who interviewed for position and notifies other unsuccessful candidates.
_____ 27. Submit Final Affirmative Action Plan. Update all staff lists.
_____ 28. Remind all Search Committee members to forward all applications, references, etc., relating to recruitment to Administration for shredding.
_____ 29. Request exception to policy, e.g., leave policies, from campus administrator, if needed.
_____ 30. Submit recommendation for appointment to campus administrator.
_____ 31. After approval, Library Director announces appointment to library staff.
_____ 32. Remove advertisement from Web page and other sources, as needed.
_____ 33. Send publicity on appointment to appropriate locations (Medical Library Association's *MLA News;* local, state, and regional library newsletters; campus publications).

____ 34. Send letter of appointment and conditions of employment to new staff member (after form received from Benefits Office).

____ 35. Notify Secretary of the Faculty office to add new person with rank to the faculty mailing and voting list and to delete name of person who resigned.

____ 36. Destroy all duplicate documents or material not maintained in the recruitment file.

REFERENCES

1. Thompson, Lora L. "Moving from a Hospital Library to an Academic Health Sciences Library: Advice from Those That Have." The Leading Edge 14, no. 3 (August 2002) Available: <http://www.library.umc.edu/lam/lam-14-3.html>. Accessed: January 22, 2007.

2. Wartman, Steven A. "Update from the President." The Association of Academic Health Centers. Available: <http://www.aahcdc.org/index.php>. Accessed: March 17, 2007.

3. Holt, Glen. "It's a Skill." *Public Libraries* 43, no. 4 (July/August 2004): 210.

4. New Media Consortium. "The Horizon Report 2007." Available: <http://www.nmc.org/pdf/2007_Horizon_Report.pdf>. Accessed: March 4, 2007.

5. National Network of Libraries of Medicine. "Charting the Course for the 21st Century: NLM's Long Range Plan 2005-2016." National Institutes of Health. Available: <http://www.nlm.nih.gov/pubs/plan/lrpdocs.html>. Accessed: March 16, 2007.

6. Curzon, Susan Carol. *Managing Change: A How-To-Do-It Manual for Librarians.* Rev. ed. New York: Neal-Schuman, 2005.

7. Goleman, Daniel; Boyatziz, Richard; and McKee, Annie. *Primal Leadership.* Boston: HBS Press, 2004.

8. Association of Academic Health Sciences Libraries. "Building on Success: Charting the Future of Knowledge Management Within the Academic Health Center." Available: <http://www.aahsl.org/document/CTFprint.pdf>. Accessed: March 16, 2007.

9. Barrentine, Jim. "Building the 21st Century Library: Planning for Technology in New Buildings." Available: <http://institute21.stanford.edu/programs/workshop/facilities/barrentine_tech.pdf>. Accessed: March 16, 2007.

10. Beagle, Donald Robert. *The Information Commons Handbook.* New York: Neal-Schuman Publishers, 2006.

11. McLendon, Wallace, and Ragon, Bart. "Technology Planning for Health Sciences Librarians, Medical Library Association Continuing Education Course." Available: <http://mlanet.org/education/cech/index.php3?mode=cdisplay&id=588>. Accessed: March 16, 2007.

12. Wilson, Daniel T., and Yowell, Susan. "Comprehensive Disaster Plan of the Claude Moore Health Sciences Library at the University of Virginia." Available: <http://www.healthsystem.virginia.edu/internet/library/admin/policy/disasterplan2006.pdf>. Accessed: February 10, 2007.

13. McNamara, Carter. "Basics of Developing Mission, Vision and Values Statements." Available: <http://www.managementhelp.org/plan_dec/str_plan/stmnts.htm#anchor519441>. Accessed: March 16, 2007.

14. Gorman, Michael. *Our Enduring Values: Librarianship in the 21st Century.* Chicago: American Library Association, 2000.

15. Medical Library Association. "Code of Ethics for Health Sciences Librarianship." Available: <http://www.mlanet.org/about/ethics.html>. Accessed: March 16, 2007.

16. Association of College and Research Libraries. "Writing Measurable Objectives: A Training Module." American Library Association. Available: <http://www.ala.org/ala/acrlbucket/is/organizationacrl/planningacrl/smartobjectives/writingmeasurable.htm>. Accessed: March 14, 2007.

17. Association of Academic Health Sciences Libraries. "The Library As Place: Symposium on Building and Revitalizing Health Sciences Libraries in the Digital Age." Available: <http://www.aahsl.org/building/index.html>. Accessed: March 16, 2007.

18. Lakos, Amos, and Phipps, Shelley. "Creating a Culture of Assessment: A Catalyst for Organizational Change." *Libraries and the Academy* 4, no. 3 (July 2004): 345-61. Available: <http://muse.jhu.edu/journals/portal_libraries_and_the_academy/v004/4.3lakos.pdf>. Accessed: March 16, 2007.

19. Bureau of Justice Assistance, Office of Justice Programs, U.S. Department of Justice, Center for Program Evaluation. "Glossary." Available: <http://www.ojp.usdoj.gov/BJA/evaluation/glossary/glossary_e.htm>. Accessed: March 16, 2007.

20. Foss, Michelle M.; Buhler, Amy; Rhine, Lenny; and Layton, Beth. "HSCL LibQUAL+ 2004: From Numbers and Graphs to Practical Application." *Medical Reference Services Quarterly* 25, no. 1 (Spring 2006): 1-15.

21. Dudden, Rosalind F. *Using Benchmarking, Needs Assessment, Quality Improvement, Outcome Measurement, and Library Standards: A How-To-Do-It Manual.* New York: Neal-Schuman, 2007.

22. Barton, Jane. "Measurement, Management and the Digital Library." *Library Review* 53, no. 3 (April 2004): 138-41.

23. Hiller, Steve, and Self, James. "From Measurement to Management: Using Data Wisely for Planning and Decision-Making." *Library Trends* 53, no. 1 (Summer 2004): 129-55.

24. Dudden, Rosalind F.; Corcoran, Kate; Kaplan, Janice; Magouirk, Jeff, Rand, Debra C.; and Smith, Bernie T. "The Medical Library Association Benchmarking Network: Results." *Journal of the American Library Association* 94, no. 2 (April 2006): 118-29.

25. Dudden, Rosalind F.; Corcoran, Kate; Kaplan, Janice; Magouirk, Jeff; Rand, Debra C.; and Smith, Bernie T. "The Medical Library Association Benchmarking Network: Development and Implementation." *Journal of the American Library Association* 94, no. 2 (April 2006): 107-17.

26. Dervin, Brenda, and Nilan, Michael S. "Information Needs and Uses." *Annual Review of Information Science and Technology* 21(1986): 3-33.

27. Dervin, Brenda. "From the Mind's Eye of the User: The Sense-Making Qualitative-Quantitative Methodology." In: *Qualitative Research in Information Management,* edited by Jack D. Glazier and Ronald R. Powell, 61-84. Englewood, CO: Libraries Unlimited, 1992.

28. Blackwelder, Mary; Cunningham, Diana; and Lee, Tamera. "Library Outcomes Assessment: A Selected Bibliography." Association of Academic Health Sciences Libraries. Available: <http://aahsl.org/new/display_page.cfm?file_id=234>. Accessed: February 19, 2007.

29. Marshall, Joanne G. "Determining Our Worth, Communicating Our Value." *Library Journal* 125, no. 19 (November 15, 2000): 28-30.

30. Shedlock, James, and Byrd, Gary D. "The Association of Academic Health Sciences Libraries Annual Statistics: A Thematic History." *Journal of the Medical Library Association* 91, no. 2 (April 2003): 178-85.

31. YellowPencil Brand Sharpening. "Glossary of Terms." Available: <http://www.yellowpencil.co.nz/brand%20sharpening/brand%20glossary>. Accessed: March 17, 2007.

32. Charbonneau, Deborah H.; Croatt-Moore, Carrie; and Ellis-Danquah, La Ventra. "Strategies for Planning and Promoting Library Services to New Users." *MLA Forum* 3, no. 2 (July 14, 2004). Available: <http://www.mlaforum.org/volumeIII/issue2/conf2.html>. Accessed: March 17, 2007.

33. Zenan, Joan S. "The Association of Academic Health Sciences Libraries' Legislative Activities and the Joint Medical Library Association/Association of Academic Health Sciences Libraries Legislative Task Force." *Journal of the Medical Library Association* 91, no. 2 (April 2003): 168-172.

34. Association of Academic Health Sciences Libraries. *2004-2005 Annual Statistics of Medical School Libraries in the United States and Canada.* 28th ed. Seattle, WA: Association of Academic Health Sciences Libraries, 2006.

35. Eskind Biomedical Library Vanderbilt Medical Center. Available: <http://www.mc.vanderbilt.edu/biolib/>. Accessed: March 17, 2007.

36. National Library of Medicine. "Grants and Funding: Extramural Support. Training Support." Available: <http://www.nlm.nih.gov/ep/Grants.html#training>. Accessed: March 17, 2007.

37. National Institutes of Health Library. "Informationists." Available: <http://nihlibrary.nih.gov/LibraryServices/Informationists.htm>. Accessed: March 13, 2007.

38. Duke University Medical Center Library Online. "Dual-Degree Program—MD/MSLS or MD/MSIS." Available: <http://www.mclibrary.duke.edu/about/dualdegree>. Accessed: March 17, 2007.

39. Shipman, Jean P. "Informationist or Information Specialist in Context: Who Is This?" 2006 IFLA Presentation. Available: <http://www.mlanet.org/research/informationist/pdf/shipman_ifla_isic.ppt>. Accessed: March 21, 2007.

40. Anti-Defamation League. Available: <http://www.adl.org/education/edu_awod/default_awod.asp>. Accessed: March 17, 2007.

41. South Metropolitan Higher Education Consortium. "Why Diversity Is Important on College Campuses." Connect to Higher Education. Available: <http://www.southmetroed.org/reports/SMRHEC%2002%2020%2006.pdf>. Accessed: March 17, 2007.

42. Hall, Tracie D. "Information 911: Increasing Diversity Makes Libraries More Important Than Ever." North Suburban Library System, August 3, 2006. Available: <http://www.nsls.info/articles/detail.aspx?articleID=83>. Accessed: March 17, 2007.

43. Hoxeng, Holly. "Addressing Diversity in the Public Library Community with Diversity on the Library Staff." *Colorado Libraries* 26, no.2 (Summer 2000): 14-5.

44. De Rosa, Cathy; Cantrell, Joanne; Cellentani, Diane; Hawk, Janet; Jenkins, Lillie; and Wilson, Alane. Perceptions of Libraries and Information Resources. Dublin, OH: OCLC Online Computer Center, 2005.

45. De Rosa, Cathy; Dempsey, Lorcan; and Wilson, Alane. The 2003 OCLC Environmental Scan: Pattern Recognition. Dublin, OH: OCLC Online Computer Library Center, 2004.

46. Cogell, Raquel V., and Gruwell, Cindy A., eds. *Diversity in Libraries: Academic Residency Programs.* Westport, CT: Greenwood, 2001.

47. Kathman, Jane M., and Kathman, Michael D. "What Difference Does Diversity Make in Managing Student Employees?" *College & Research Libraries* 59, no. 4 (July 1998): 378-89.

48. Owens, Irene. "A Managerial/Leadership Approach to Maintaining Diversity in Libraries: Accountability, Professionalism, Performance Evaluation, and Team-Building." *Texas Library Journal* 76, no. 1 (Spring 2000): 20-7.

49. National Coalition Building Institute, International. Available: <http://www.ncbi.org/home/index.cfm>. Accessed: March 17, 2007.

50. University of North Carolina at Chapel Hill. "Diversity Plan: Goals, Strategies and Responsibilities 2006-2010." Available: <http://www.unc.edu/diversity/diversityplan/diversityplan.pdf>. Accessed: March 16, 2007.

51. Tzenova, Elena. "An Analysis of Operations for the Health Sciences Library Photocopier Service." Department of Operations Research. June 1999 (internal document).

52. Sullivan, Maureen. "Organization Development in Libraries." *Library Administration and Management* 18, no. 4 (Fall 2004): 179-83.

53. Martin, Elaine R. "Team Effectiveness in Academic Medical Libraries: A Multiple Case Study." *Journal of the Medical Library Association* 94, no. 3 (July 2006): 271-8.

54. Higa, Mori L.; Bunnett, Brian; Maina, Bill. "Redesigning a Library's Organizational Structure." *College & Research Libraries* 66, no. 1 (January 2005): 41-58.

55. Norcross, Natalie. *MLA DocKit #13. Organization Charts of Academic Health Sciences Libraries.* Chicago: Medical Library Association, 2004.

56. Blumenthal, Jane; Murthy, Vani; Martinez, Ivonne; and Silver, Laura. *MLA DocKit #15. Position Descriptions in Health Sciences Libraries.* Chicago: Medical Library Association, 2006.

57. Medical Library Association. "About the Medical Library Association." Available: <http://mlanet.org/about/index.html>. Accessed: February 22, 2007.

58. Medical Library Association. "Tip Sheet for Graduate Students and Career Changers." Available: <http://mlanet.org/pdf/career/career_exp_graduate.pdf>. Accessed: March 17, 2007.

59. Griffiths, José-Marie, principal investigator. "The Future of Librarians in the Workforce." Study funded by the Institute for Museum and Library Science. Available: <http://libraryworkforce.org>. Accessed: March 26, 2007.

60. Medical Library Association. *Platform for Change: The Educational Policy Statement of the Medical Library Association.* Available: <http://www.mlanet.org/education/platform/index.html>. Accessed: March 17, 2007.

61. National Library of Medicine. "Associate Fellowship Program." National Institutes of Health. Available: <http://www.nlm.nih.gov/about/training/associate/index.html>. Accessed: March 17, 2007.

62. Association of Academic Health Sciences Libraries. "NLM/AAHSL Leadership Fellows Program." Available: <http://www.aahsl.org/new/display_page.cfm?file_id=65>. Accessed: March 17, 2007.

63. Medical Library Association. "Center of Research and Education (CORE)." Available: <http://mlanet.org/core/index.html>. Accessed: March 17, 2007.

64. Association of Academic Health Sciences Libraries. "Report of the AAHSL New Directors Development Symposium." Available: <http://www.aahsl.org/document/newdirectorssymposiumreportweb.doc?CFID=553759&CFTOKEN=10212227>. Accessed: March 17, 2007.

65. American Library Association. "Library Support Staff Resource Center." Available: <http://www.ala.org/ala/hrdr/librarysupportstaff/Library_Support_Staff_Resource_Center.htm>. Accessed: March 17, 2007.

66. Council on Library/Media Technicians. Available: <http://colt.ucr.edu/>. Accessed: March 17, 2007.

67. Medical Library Association. "Academy of Health Information Professionals." Available: <http://www.mlanet.org/academy/>. Accessed: March 17, 2007.

68. Special Libraries Association/Special Committee on Competencies for Special Librarians. *Competencies for Information Professionals of the 21st Century.* Revised edition (June 2003). Available: <http://www.sla.org/PDFs/Competencies2003_revised.pdf>. Accessed: March 21, 2007.

69. Association of Research Libraries/Office of Leadership and Management Services. "Online Lyceum. Motivation, Performance, and Commitment." Available: <http://mccoy.lib.siu.edu/arl/motivation/>. Accessed: March 17, 2007.

70. Hoggan, Danielle B. "Faculty Status for Librarians in Higher Education." *Libraries and the Academy* 3, no. 3 (July 2003): 431-45.

71. Giuse, Nunzia B. "The Next Challenge: Where Do We Go from Here?" *Journal of the Medical Library Association* 95, no. 1 (January 2007): 1-2.

72. Ransel, Kerry A. "Advancement at Last: Career-Ladder Opportunities for Library Support Staff." *Technical Services Quarterly* 19, no. 2 (December 2001): 17-26.

73. Huber, Jeffrey T.; Giuse, Nunzia B.; and Pfeiffer, John R. "Designing an Alternative Career Ladder for Library Assistants." *Bulletin of the Medical Library Association* 87, no. 1 (January 1999): 74-7.

74. Hurt, Tara L., and Sunday, Deborah S. "Career Paths for Paraprofessionals: Your Ladder to Success." *Library Mosaics: Magazine for Support Staff* 16, no. 1 (January/February 2005): 8-11.

75. Green, Jamie; Chivers, Barbara; and Mynott, Glen. "In the Librarian's Chair: An Analysis of Factors Which Influence the Motivation of Library Staff and Contribute to the Effective Delivery of Services." *Library Review* 49, no. 8. (2000): 380-6.

76. Oltmanns, Gail V. "Organization and Staff Renewal Using Assessment." *Library Trends* 53, no. 1 (Summer 2004): 156-71.

77. Plas, Jeanne. "Discover What Matters Most to Employees." *Library Personnel News* 13, no. 1-2 (Spring/ Summer 2000): 3.

78. Rockman, Ilene F. "Fun in the Workplace." Reference Services Review 31, no. 2 (June 2003): 109-10.

79. Musser, Linda R. "Effective Retention Strategies for Diverse Employees." *Journal of Library Administration* 33, no. 1-2 (January 2001): 63-72.

80. Dickinson, Gail K. "A New Look at Job Satisfaction." *Library Administration & Management* 16, no. 1 (Winter 2002): 28-33.

81. Shill, Harold B., and Tonner, Shawn. "Creating a Better Place: Physical Improvements in Academic Libraries, 1995-2002." *College & Research Libraries* 64, no. 6 (November 2003): 431-66.

82. Shill, Harold B., and Tonner, Shawn. "Does the Building Still Matter? Usage Patterns in New, Expanded, and Renovated Libraries, 1995-2002." *College & Research Libraries* 65, no. 2. (March 2004): 123-50.

83. Council on Library and Information Resources. *Library As Place: Rethinking Roles, Rethinking Space.* Washington DC: Council on Library and Information Resources, 2005.

84. Preston Medical Library and Learning Resource Center. Available: <http://gsm.utmck.edu/library/about/ mission.htm>. Accessed: August 17, 2007.

Chapter 14

Management of and Issues Specific to Hospital Libraries

Dixie A. Jones

SUMMARY. Hospital libraries share many commonalities with other health sciences libraries. However, they do have issues which are unique to them, and even those issues which are shared with other medical libraries sometimes have to be approached somewhat differently in hospital settings. This chapter discusses the many forms and roles that hospital libraries may have, as well as the standards which apply to them and the challenges faced by those who manage them.

INTRODUCTION

One hospital library can differ widely from another in size, collection, and scope of services depending on a number of variables, such as the type of institution, whether or not it is a **teaching hospital,** and whether or not it is independent or part of a health care system. Hospitals are not required by law or by the **Joint Commission on Accreditation of Healthcare Organizations (Joint Commission, formerly JCAHO)** to have on-site libraries or library staff. Hospitals affiliated with medical schools sometimes have their information needs served by academic health sciences libraries, which can make their resources available to hospital staff through extended licensing of electronic resources or other means of sharing resources. Some medical centers do not have in-house library staff but contract with external consultants to provide information services. That being said, the hospital staff are better served when professional library staff are available on-site to provide customized services and collections to meet the needs of patient care and research in that particular hospital. Teaching hospitals must also be able to meet the information needs of the students and the requirements of their accrediting bodies.

The health care environment is volatile and dynamic, with closings and mergers occurring regularly and medical centers being under pressure to cut costs. Many hospital libraries are thriving, but they do not always survive. One might assume that libraries in large, urban hospitals are less subject to closure than community hospitals in rural settings. However, oddly enough, the opposite may be true. The library in a small-town hospital may be "big and strong" because it is the only game in town, whereas in large cities with medical schools hospitals may rely on nearby academic medical libraries to be their providers of **knowledge-based information (KBI).**

While the phrase "hospital library" probably conjures a particular image in one's mind, there is no single concept that accurately portrays all hospital libraries. The term "library" is even somewhat controversial, as some administrators in medical centers with a small collection of books and a few journals in the residents' on-call room consider that to be a library. Others might believe that an Internet station and access to a full-text database or two comprise a library, even

Introduction to Health Sciences Librarianship
© 2008 by The Haworth Press, Taylor & Francis Group. All rights reserved.
doi:10.1300/6041_14

341

with no staff to provide any services. Regardless of one's opinion about the minimum of resources or staffing that defines a hospital library, there is great variation among them.

Hospitals themselves can be very different from one another. *The AHA Guide to the Healthcare Field* (a directory of hospitals produced by the American Hospital Association [AHA]) lists a facility as a hospital if it is accredited by the Joint Commission, is certified as a provider of acute services under Title 18 of the Social Security Act, or is state licensed as a hospital by an appropriate state agency and meets ten specified requirements.[1]

The kinds of library collections and services required depend on the type of hospital and its mission. The institution might be a large, metropolitan medical center, a small community hospital, or any size institution between. It can be a general facility or one with a narrower focus, such as pediatrics, orthopedics, cancer, rehabilitation, or some other specialty. It may be public or private, profit or nonprofit, part of a system or independent, teaching or nonteaching. It can even be in a prison setting. Health care systems may be investor owned, for profit (e.g., Universal Health Services); religious, nonprofit (e.g., Presbyterian Healthcare Services); other, nonprofit (e.g., Kaiser Foundation Hospitals); or government (e.g., Department of Veterans Affairs). The missions of these institutions will guide the kinds of library services provided and the populations served.

Libraries in particular health care systems often act as consortia, although such connectedness cannot be assumed. Independent hospital libraries sometimes form consortia for mutual benefits, such as reciprocal interlibrary loans, discounts on electronic resources, collection development agreements, and reference service coverage for one another.

REPORTING STRUCTURE

The library's place in a medical center's organizational chart is yet another example of how much difference there can be among hospital libraries. The library may report to the medical center's director/chief executive officer (CEO), several rungs down the ladder, or any level in between. To some extent, this placement depends on whether the library is a separate department of its own or a subdepartment of a larger one, such as information technology (IT), information management, or education. Organizational hierarchy placement can also depend on whether the library manager has additional responsibilities outside library services, such as continuing medical education, grants, or information technology. In a health care system setting, the hospital library manager may report to an administrative librarian who oversees several hospital libraries in the system. The Medical Library Association "Standards for Hospital Libraries 2002 with 2004 Revisions" (MLA Standards) stipulate that ideally the librarian should report to senior management, with the director of medical education being considered senior management in a large teaching hospital.[2]

An advantage of higher placement in the organizational hierarchy includes serving on top-level committees, thereby putting the library manager "in the know." Being in this position allows one to be proactive and able to prepare in advance for new institutional initiatives. The higher the library manager sits, the more likely he or she is to be in a position to directly make a case for budget requests and to advocate for funding, as well as to defend existing space or justify additional space. Funding, space, and personnel are the three things that generate the most competition among departments within hospitals. Being higher in the chain of command allows one to network more easily with top administrators. Having "friends in high places" is always a plus. Being farther down the chain is not necessarily a bad thing, but if the library is a subdepartment, the library manager might not have the opportunity to directly "make a case" to upper management and may be competing with other entities within the same department for scarce resources.

Many hospitals are divided into two administrative channels—clinical and nonclinical. In such hospitals, the clinical side is usually administered by the chief of staff or medical director, most often a physician, who oversees the departments that provide patient care. The nonclinical side is administered by an associate director or vice president or whatever nomenclature is used by the institution for the person who is responsible for departments that provide administrative support. The library may be placed on either side of the house and can fare well either way. However, some believe that being part of the clinical side is advantageous for funding—and even for survival when institutional **downsizing** occurs.

In some medical centers, there is a library committee. The role of this committee is different from one hospital to another. Often, the committee members can be political allies who champion library initiatives and serve as advocates for library services. Such committees are usually multidisciplinary and their members may include a mix of MDs, psychologists, RNs, pharmacists, dentists, physical therapists, speech pathologists, medical records professionals, dietitians or other allied health personnel, and administrators. Sometimes, these committees are tasked with making decisions about library collection purchases; this practice is to be discouraged, if at all possible. However, in hospitals where the library staff buy materials to be housed externally in other departments, the committee's help in prioritizing purchase selections for these departments can be very helpful and removes the librarian from the "hot seat" regarding such decisions. This committee, when it exists, usually reports to top management.

STAFFING

Size and composition of the staff comprise yet another variable among hospital libraries. Size ranges from one part-time person to a large staff serving in various aspects of librarianship, as in the academic model where library staff members specialize in areas such as cataloging, reference, interlibrary loan, systems, instruction, serials, and acquisitions. In hospital libraries with two librarians, the division of labor may be between patient services and employee services, rather than between public services and technical services. The one-person library may be staffed by a library technician or a health information professional or, in some cases, by a clerical person who serves as a secretary or administrative assistant who has been trained to provide rudimentary interlibrary loan services. The one-person library is sometimes referred to as an OPL. Librarians serving in OPLs often enjoy the variety of tasks they have to perform. They know the needs and preferences of their patrons, what is on order, what is being processed, and what the budget is because they handle all of these things, so internal communication is not a problem. Their lives can be stressful, however, with performing administrative duties of attending meetings, preparing reports, strategic planning, and managing budgets, while simultaneously providing both public services and technical services. In hospital libraries with only one librarian, having well-trained support staff eases the burden of multiple responsibilities.

MLA Standards provide a formula for determining the number of librarians and technical employees needed based on institutional **FTEs** and whether or not enhanced services are offered.[2] FTE is the **full-time equivalents** for employees, not the actual number of employees. For example, if two employees each work half time, they are equal to one FTE. According to the staffing formula, the minimum library FTEs is the total institution FTEs divided by 700 for a library that offers basic library services. Additional staffing is needed if enhanced services, such as responsibility for the hospital's Web site or consumer health services, are offered. Additional examples may be found in the MLA Standards.[2]

Some hospitals meet information needs by hiring a consultant librarian who is on-site on an occasional basis in lieu of a librarian being employed to work at the hospital on a regular basis. Whether or not such arrangements truly meet information needs of staff and patients is debatable, but on paper they satisfy external requirements, such as those of the Joint Commission,[3] and delineate the nature of a consulting agreement and the documentation that should be provided if such an agreement exists.[2]

Qualifications of library staff are determined by the institutions. Most hospitals require library-specific competencies, as well as competencies in customer service and communicating with people of highly variable literacy levels. MLA Standards indicate that a qualified librarian is

> [a] person who has earned a Master's degree from a program accredited by the American Library Association [ALA] or its successors , or from a master's [sic] level program in library and information studies accredited or recognized by the appropriate national body of another country.[2]

They also address competencies, stating that "Membership in the Medical Library Association's Academy of Health Information Professionals is one indication of a knowledgeable, capable medical librarian."[2] They further cite the Special Libraries Association's *Competencies for Special Librarians of the 21st Century*[4] and go on to list competencies unique to the hospital librarian, including "in-depth knowledge of print and electronic information resources in the health sciences and related fields, and the design and management of information services that meet the strategic information needs of the individual or group being served."[2] Competencies for health sciences librarians are also addressed in the *Educational Policy Statement of the Medical Library Association: Competencies for Lifelong Learning and Professional Success.*[5]

STANDARDS/ACCREDITATION

Within a given hospital, there may be many different organizations' standards that are applicable to various employment groups. The best-known standards that apply to the whole hospital are those of the Joint Commission. Its mission is to "continuously improve the safety and quality of care provided to the public through the provision of health care accreditation and related services that support performance improvement in health care organizations."[3] Many hospitals seek accreditation by the Joint Commission, even though accredited status is voluntary, not a legal requirement. A quick glance at the *AHA Guide to the Healthcare Field* shows that most hospitals are indeed accredited by the Joint Commission.[1] In the past, hospitals spent many hours preparing for Joint Commission surveyor visits to ensure that they would maintain their accreditation. Visits are no longer scheduled at regular intervals; they are unannounced, so hospitals must be prepared at all times for accreditation surveys. MLA has a representative to the Joint Commission who serves as a liaison between the two organizations. Librarians over the years have lobbied for a requirement in the Joint Commission's *Comprehensive Accreditation Manual for Hospitals* that hospitals must have libraries under supervision of professional medical librarians. This requirement has not made it into the standards, although not for lack of effort on the part of hospital librarians.

The Joint Commission Standard most applicable to hospital libraries is IM.5.10, found in the section Information Management: "Knowledge-based information resources are readily available, current, and authoritative."[3] The rationale in the manual explains why access to KBI is necessary for patient care, patient education, performance improvement, patient safety, educational needs, and research needs. KBI is the kind of information found in externally generated, authoritative resources traditionally provided by libraries to help employees better perform their duties and increase their knowledge of current standards of care and clinical guidelines, rather than the type of information generated by collection of in-house data pulled from patient records or performance measures. The elements of performance for IM.5.10 state that library services may be provided by cooperative or contractual arrangements with other institutions; they do not have to be available on-site. KBI may be in print, electronic, Internet, or audio formats. KBI must be available after hours for clinical staff either through electronic means or after-hours access to an in-house collection or some other method. Last, the hospital must have a process for providing access to KBI when electronic systems are not available.[3]

Another set of standards that may be applicable to some hospitals are those of the American Osteopathic Association whose revision became effective in July 2007 <http://www.osteopathic .org/pdf/acc_predoccom2007.pdf>. MLA had provided recommended language for the library-related elements of the osteopathic standards that included mention of a "qualified professional medical librarian," but these recommendations were not incorporated into the revision.[6]

An increasing number of hospitals are seeking recognition as **magnet hospitals** in order to recruit and retain nurses. The Magnet Recognition Program® was developed by the American Nurses Credentialing Center (ANCC) to recognize health care organizations that provide nursing excellence. ANCC is the credentialing arm of the American Nurses Association. Originally, there were forty-one magnet hospitals. As of this writing, there are 256 health care organizations in forty-five states plus facilities in Australia and New Zealand that have achieved this status conferred by the Commission on Magnet Recognition Program®.[7] This phenomenon is important to libraries because hospitals which seek magnet status must demonstrate that current literature is "available, disseminated, and used to change administrative and clinical practices in their facilities."[8] They must also describe resources available to nursing staff for support of nursing research. Additionally, they must demonstrate how nurses involved in direct patient care "use available professional standards, literature, and research findings to support control over nursing practice, independent decision-making, and assertiveness/leadership in patient care management and practice."[8] Plus, they must provide evidence that nurses have "access to the Internet, library, and/or other appropriate literature/data sources."[8] Obviously, the likelihood of meeting these requirements would be greatly enhanced by the presence of a full-service library! For more on implications of magnet status for hospital libraries, see Silver's article, listed in Appendix 14.A, Additional Readings.

MLA has standards for hospital libraries that were developed by a committee of the Hospital Libraries Section. While the Joint Commission does not require that hospitals meet MLA Standards, the standards can still be used to justify library staff, space, and resources. Some grassroots efforts to put "teeth" into these standards have been successful. For example, the Connecticut State Medical Society adopted MLA Standards as part of their accreditation process for **continuing medical education (CME)**.[2]

Teaching hospitals often must provide paperwork documenting that library services and resources are available to participants in their educational programs. In some cases, requirements can be satisfied through contractual agreements with a library outside the hospital, such as a medical school library. The exact requirements may vary from one educational program to another (e.g., nursing, radiologic technology, social work, medical technology), and from one residency specialty to another (e.g., internal medicine, surgery, psychiatry). MLA's Vital Pathways Project has been investigating library requirements in the many educational programs that may be affiliated with teaching hospitals. See MLA's Web site <http://www.mlanet.org> for additional information about this endeavor.

POPULATIONS SERVED

The mission of the hospital will drive which populations are served by its library. Historically, hospital libraries served clinical staff—sometimes only physicians. The consumer health movement and the evidence supporting the efficacy of **patient health education (PHE)** have driven the development of consumer health libraries. Today's medical center facilities may serve physicians, nurses, allied health staff, nonclinical employees, patients, patients' families and caregivers, affiliated students, and/or the public. In hospitals where information services are provided to both employees and patients, there might be one library used by all or there might be two separate libraries. In settings where one library serves all clientele, the library staff must be able to communicate well with people at all health literacy levels, be able to quickly assess clients' literacy levels, and have a knowledge of which materials are appropriate for a range of literacy levels.

If the hospital's mission does not include serving the public, the library staff must be prepared to offer alternatives to those who call, walk in, or e-mail the library with health-related questions. If the library has a public Web site, people are going to stumble upon it and contact the library even if the Web page indicates that services are provided only to the hospital's staff and/or patients. The public library's telephone number may be kept handy, as well as any other local libraries which provide consumer health services to the public.

In information centers where several populations are served, the staff must be able to triage requests. All types of clientele should be treated fairly, but the nature of their requests will vary in urgency. Ordinarily, patient care requests are handled before other types of requests, regardless of who is asking for the information—whether it be the chief of staff or a staff nurse. Information requests for updating procedures or for student papers are important, but information needed for emergent patient situations takes precedence.

SERVICES

Technical Services

Large hospital libraries may offer a full range of services, just as academic medical libraries do. As in any library, technical services include ordering materials in various formats, cataloging and classifying the materials, physically preparing the materials for shelving and circulation, checking in and claiming journals, and possibly binding journals. Binding of journals is becoming less common, even when print subscriptions are maintained. For libraries that do still bind journals in their collections, the added service of sending departments' or employees' personal materials to the bindery is sometimes considered a "perk" of institutional employment offered by the library on a cost recovery basis.

Acquiring, organizing, and providing materials in Web formats are now common in hospital libraries. Additional information regarding organization of resources may be found in Chapter 5, "Organizing Resources for Information Access." More and more hospital libraries are turning to electronic resources because of user convenience and demand, as well as the fact that these resources do not require shelf space. Space in most hospitals is a precious commodity, and many hospital libraries are pressured to reduce square footage. Most hospital libraries use **National Library of Medicine (NLM)** classification for organizing their physical collections, but those with consumer health collections sometimes use the **Planetree** system, which places materials in broad categories based on the ways that consumers approach health information. Libraries with small collections may just group books together by general categories determined locally, rather than actually classifying them and placing call numbers on the spines.

Integrated library systems are more common in hospital libraries these days than they formerly were, as certain vendors have begun providing affordable systems for smaller libraries, and some libraries have pooled financial resources to share advanced library systems that include not only online catalogs for the convenience of users but also modules for circulation, acquisitions, and serials.

Reference Service

Information Provision and Literature Searching

The range of reference service offered depends on qualifications of the staff and, to some extent, on FTEs of both the library and the hospital. Reference might consist solely of answering simple questions easily answered by authoritative Web sites or textbooks when there is only one staff member and that one person may not even be a librarian. Conversely, the library staff—size and expertise permitting—may offer extended reference service for complex questions, expert literature searching, and weekly or monthly alert service requested by clients.

Many databases relevant to hospital information needs, such as CINAHL® (*Cumulative Index to Nursing and Allied Health Information*) or PsycINFO®, require subscriptions, but NLM's extensive **PubMed®** database is free of charge and allows libraries to link their holdings from its citations through a utility called LinkOut®.[9] In addition to these forms of information supplied by librarians at a client's request, information may be "pushed" proactively through e-mail or the library Web site.

Reference service may be available through several different modes, such as in person, by telephone, by e-mail, through interactive Web sites, or through **virtual reference.** Virtual reference may consist of chat reference, which is very similar to instant messaging, or it may include a combination of chat and **co-browsing,** whereby the librarian actually pushes particular Web pages to the client's desktop. Librarians in hospital systems spread over large geographical areas may be able to take advantage of having staff at multiple locations to staff virtual reference for a broader range of hours. For further information about medical reference service, see Chapter 7, "Information Services in Health Sciences Libraries."

Hospital libraries may provide reference service using a corporate model rather than an academic model. Clinicians often just need an answer or a synthesis of the literature in order to make a patient care decision; they do not have time to go through the multistep process of reviewing citations from a search, then requesting the pertinent ones, and then reading through all of the articles requested. **Filtering information/literature** for library clients is considered controversial by some who think that librarians are not qualified to provide this service and/or that doing so puts them at legal risk. However, in clinical settings, having the librarian run the search, select the pertinent material, and package it may be exactly what the requester prefers and expects.

If a library serves patients and their families, the library staff must be familiar with consumer health resources. The staff may find information upon the request of patients, their caregivers, or their families under the broad umbrella of consumer health. If the staff are providing information for patients upon the specification of their clinicians, the service falls under the more tightly defined area of PHE. More information may be found regarding this distinction in Chapter 18, "Consumer Health Information." Hints for conducting reference interviews with consumers may be found in the article by Thomas, listed in Appendix 14.A.

Some hospitals use the **Information Rx** system in which providers write prescriptions for information. The prescription might be for information on a particular condition, procedure, or drug. NLM and the American College of Physicians Foundation have produced a tool kit for the Information Rx program which they jointly initiated. Materials available include a poster, information prescription pads, and bookmarks, all of which promote **MedlinePlus®,** NLM's consumer health Web site <http://medlineplus.gov>. Some libraries have adopted this idea and developed their own information prescription pads rather than ordering them from the NLM.

Depending on local policy, the library staff may document in the patient's record any information made available to the patient regarding diagnosis and treatment for his or her condition, instructions for aftercare, medication, or what to expect when undergoing procedures.

In a hospital that offers reference in a physical setting both to health care providers and to patients, the library may serve both types of users from one reference point or from two separate areas. More details on reference service are available in Chapter 7 and **consumer health information (CHI)** service is more fully described in Chapter 18.

Educational Services

Educational services may be offered in a number of ways to different types of clientele. Tutorials on using databases or finding particular types of information may be offered at the library's Web site. One-on-one instruction may be offered to patients and employees by appointment or on an ad hoc basis, in the library or at an employee's computer or even over the telephone. Libraries serving patients, their families, and their caregivers may also provide basic computer usage instruction in addition to instruction on finding health information.

Formal classes may be offered in the library or in a hospital computer lab. Classes may serve multiple purposes. In addition to teaching people to use resources to find the best health information, formal instruction in resources can have the added benefit of increasing usage of those resources, thereby decreasing the cost per usage and increasing hits on the library page as a launching spot for the resources. An unplanned benefit is the opportunity for the librarian to establish himself or herself as the expert. Expert status does not mean setting one's self above others in a superior way; the instructor should be able to admit if he or she cannot answer a question and offer to contact participants with the answer later. However, the librarian teaching a class should do his or her homework prior to a class to be as knowledgeable as possible about what is being taught, provide appropriate examples for the participants, bone up on techniques for adult learning, and inject humor into instruction, if possible. If perceived as an expert, the librarian's help is more likely to be called upon when employees are doing their own searches. Chapter 10, "Information Literacy Education in Health Sciences Libraries," provides a more comprehensive description of teaching **end users** in health care settings.

Document Delivery and Circulation

In small hospital libraries without professional staff, interlibrary loan (ILL) might be the only public service provided, and it is a very important one. Clients can buy their own materials and do their own searches, but they cannot deal directly with other libraries to borrow materials. Most hospital libraries participate in **DOCLINE®,** NLM's interlibrary loan program. Some hospital libraries also participate in other ILL systems, such as state document delivery programs or the national **OCLC (Online Computer Library Center)** system, which is used by many different types of libraries. In hospitals without libraries, health providers may use **Loansome Doc®,** but they must still contract with a library that serves as the intermediary who procures materials for them. (Loansome Doc is an NLM program in which a health provider who does not have direct access to a health sciences library's services can contract with a particular library for provision of document delivery service.) Some hospital libraries allow clinicians outside their hospitals to contract with them for Loansome Doc service; such arrangements again depend on the mission of the hospital as to whom it considers its customers. Offering Loansome Doc service to providers not affiliated with the hospital can be used to generate revenue for the library, if allowed.

The beauty of today's electronic environment is that entire ILL transactions may take place without the requester ever setting foot in the library. ILLs may be requested via e-mail or Web forms and can be delivered directly to the requesters' desktops. Hill describes the challenges for hospital libraries in providing digital document delivery and names "five areas of concern:

- equipment purchase or upgrading;
- software installation;
- learning and teaching new procedures;
- institutional interaction with information technology department;
- clinical/patient information security (hospital firewall)."[10]

One problem with trying to deliver materials electronically to busy clinicians is that their electronic mailboxes sometimes fill up and cannot accept ILL documents via e-mail. Once again, library staff must be familiar with their customers and tailor delivery to their stated preferences and known work patterns. Hospital libraries, even when woefully understaffed, must abide by ILL rules, copyright guidelines, and etiquette rules.

Circulation of materials in the collection is a traditional service. More and more hospital libraries are circulating nontraditional types of materials now, however. In the past, hospital libraries circulated print materials and audiovisuals, and sometimes audiovisual (AV) equipment. The current health care environment includes circulation of electronic items, such as CDs and DVDs, and can even include laptop computers. Materials may also be "circulated" via hospital computer systems or closed-circuit TV systems to patient rooms and to employees' offices.

Another traditional service is photocopying. Again, local policy dictates whether the library staff do the copying or the patrons do the copying or a combination, depending on the circumstances. Policy also dictates whether the patrons are charged for photocopying. A number of hospital libraries, unlike most academic libraries, offer free photocopying to all their library users. The smaller volume makes this service affordable. Photocopying supplies may come out of the library's budget or out of a different department's budget, another example of variance according to local policy or custom. Scanning service is similar to photocopying service in that it may be provided by library staff or may be "do-it-yourself." With both photocopying and scanning, copyright guidelines must be followed.

Online Services

Many hospital libraries are struggling to keep up with the changes brought about by today's electronic environment and the ensuing expectations of their customers. Younger generation physicians have been educated in medical schools whose libraries offer computer labs, wireless connections, and **personal digital assistant (PDA)** services. None of these come without cost or staffing needs. More hospital libraries are seeking ways to fund such services, either through increases in their budgets or through support from external sources.

Hospital library Web sites may function as service points for both employees and patients, depending on whether their sites are open to the public or not. Some hospital libraries are on their institutions' **intranets,** which may be accessed only by employees.

COLLECTION DEVELOPMENT AND MANAGEMENT

Decisions on the resources purchased for the library's in-house and online collections are dependent on funding, populations served, and ultimately the mission of the institution—factors which guide the library's collection development policy. To provide a simplified example, pediatric hospital libraries are not likely to collect materials on care of the aging, while veterans' hospitals are not likely to acquire neonatal resources. If a library provides consumer health materi-

A Day in the Life of a Hospital Librarian

Name: Carole M. Gilbert, MSLS, AHIP, FMLA

Position: Director, Helen L. DeRoy Medical Library, Providence Hospital and Medical Centers, Southfield, Michigan

Job description: The exciting thing about being a hospital librarian is that one never knows what the day will bring. Though I am the director of the library, I am first and foremost a librarian. The director tasks somehow get sandwiched in between the services that the DeRoy library staff (2.5 FTEs) provide. Typically, I work a ten-hour day. This allows us to provide library services to all three shifts.

Sample Day

6:00–6:30 a.m.
- Arrive at the library.
- Read e-mail.
- Talk with a resident about his research project, resulting in a literature search request.

6:30–8:00 a.m.
- Teach search class to three medical students.

8:00–9:00 a.m.
- Attend Research Committee meeting.

9:00–11:30 a.m.
- Today is my day to be on the Reference Desk from 9:00 a.m. to 4:00 p.m.
- Perform literature searches for Research Committee for drugs, protocols, and animal options for two research projects referred by the IRB.

11:30 a.m.–12:30 p.m.
- Catalog new books.

12:30–1:30 p.m.
- Meet with supervisor to go over proposed budget.

1:30–2:00 p.m.
- Attend working lunch: Staff meeting to choose next month's DOIT (Daily Ongoing Implementation Tactics) and report on progress of this month's DOIT for Service Excellence initiative.

2:00–2:30 p.m.
- Perform literature search for resident received this morning.

2:30–3:00 p.m.
- Work on acquisitions list for semiannual Book Fair.

3:00–3:30 p.m.
- Meet with architect and facilities director to review plans for the library at the new satellite hospital.

3:30–4:15 p.m.
- Attend Librarian's Journal Club discussion.

4:15–4:30 p.m.
- Wrap up the day.

4:30 p.m.
- Leave for the day.

Summary statement: All of these duties take place while manning (or at least keeping an eye on) the Reference Desk—fielding questions, answering the phone, checking out books, conducting orientation tours for new physicians, trouble-shooting computers, taking search requests, and making users feel welcome.

als, does the policy specify whether or not spiritual or inspirational materials are to be included? If certain subject areas are excluded from purchase, may they be added to the collection when donated? These kinds of issues need to be addressed by the collection development policy.

Finding and maintaining funding for collections that meet the needs of all populations served and a broad range of services can be a challenge. Materials in the medical field increase in price from year to year at a rate greater than that of general inflation. Most library budgets do not increase at the same rate every year, if at all. Tough decisions often have to be made regarding what can be eliminated in order to continue receiving and updating required resources and/or adding new resources that are in high demand. Consulting with users through surveys and other feedback methods can be valuable in making such decisions. If external funding is an option, librarians must learn how to obtain it.

One must also consider whether to pay for duplicating online resources in print formats. The Joint Commission requires that there be some sort of backup in case of electronic system unavailability.[3] Hospital libraries handle this requirement in different ways. Some have agreements with other libraries for providing information during these occurrences. Others maintain basic, updated print collections either in the library itself or in patient care areas, such as the emergency room and pharmacy. These collections do not have to duplicate the online resources in their entirety.

If a hospital librarian decides to offer journal subscriptions in online format only, whether because of user convenience and/or space, consideration needs to be given as to whether the **license agreement** offers **backfiles** of the title and whether or not access is provided to the actual years subscribed if a title is later dropped. That being said, however, many hospital libraries have not traditionally maintained extensive backfiles of journal collections, as information needs are mainly for clinical rather than academic purposes. Another consideration with online subscriptions is whether or not ILL is allowed and whether the number of concurrent users is adequate. Additionally, the extent of access must be considered. Is home access allowed, either through a **proxy server, virtual private network (VPN),** or password? Are **satellite clinics** allowed access? Is access allowed only in the building in which the library is housed? Licensing agreements are a very important part of the online world. Librarians must be careful not to sign agreements with which they cannot comply. Passwords may not be posted on publicly accessible Web sites. In some hospitals, the librarians may be required to run licensing agreements by the hospitals' legal counsel and/or IT management. Librarians can no longer simply place orders for subscriptions as they did in a solely print world. They must read any agreements and negotiate with the vendors on their terms—time-consuming activities for libraries with minimal staff.

Aside from print versus online, other formats may be considered for hospital library collections—audiocassettes, CDs, DVDs, videocassettes, or combination packages. Within these genres, the collection development policy may specify the audiences for these materials—whether it is the mission to provide materials for health professionals, nonclinical employees, administrators, researchers, students, patients, patients' families, patients' caregivers, and/or the general public. In some institutions, research materials must be paid for by the research department rather than by the library. If a hospital library serves all of these populations, the nonsubscription print materials acquired may range from pamphlets to multivolume textbooks. Literacy levels will need to be taken into account in acquiring materials for the various populations served. Materials for nonclinical employees may range from books on business etiquette to grounds-keeping. In some hospitals, recreational materials are provided. These materials may be distributed to waiting areas or to patients' rooms. They may also be maintained in the library. If PHE materials are purchased, they should be in a variety of formats and literacy levels in order to accommodate the learning styles and capabilities of individual patients.

Weeding guidelines should be included in the collection development policy. Some hospital libraries are very spacious, but most must weed their print collections regularly simply for space considerations. For those libraries which serve clinical needs only (i.e., do not have management/supervisory collections or recreational collections), weeding materials that are more than a few years old is an important task. If libraries supply clinical reference books to other departments, they must also weed out-of-date books from those departments. Joint Commission surveyors do look at the currency of materials such as drug reference books housed in patient care areas.

In recent years, hospital libraries along with other types of libraries, have been struggling with the best ways to handle books and journals that come with CDs. Decisions must be made for physical disposition of the CDs, as well as the types of notations made in the bibliographic records for these materials. Licensing issues can also come into play with these CDs, which may have restrictions on their use.

An additional consideration for some hospital library collections is that of censorship. In a library that collects only professional and consumer health materials, one does not usually worry about books that might have pornographic or hate content, so censorship is not an issue in that sense. However, some hospitals are run by organizations or systems which specifically forbid provision of information about topics such as abortion or embryonic stem cell research. Library staff must give some thought to whether such restrictions mesh with applicable ethical codes and whether or not they are comfortable with abiding by these restrictions.

NETWORKING AND VISIBILITY

Maintaining good relationships with fellow employees at all levels and in all departments as much as possible is important for the hospital librarian. Reasons for being on good terms with hospital administration are obvious, but other people should not be overlooked. Everyone is a potential friendly acquaintance, someone who may provide help someday or someone who will need the library one day. Peers who are on a collegial basis with library staff may attend meetings where the library is not represented and can act on the library's behalf by putting a bug in the librarian's ear about important changes in the wind. They can also act as champions to speak up for the library. Housekeeping staff may willingly come through with unscheduled vacuuming when there is a hole puncher spill or a **Jiffy bag** has exploded over the carpet if library staff members have established friendly working relationships with them.

Visibility may be maintained for library staff and the library itself through numerous avenues, for example, a library page on the hospital's Web site. The page should be as easy to find as possible and designed to be user friendly and informative in addition to offering links to the library's electronic resources. If library staff do not maintain the library's Web pages, a good relationship with the hospital's Webmaster is a must.

Visibility can also be heightened through offering classes, giving demonstrations of new library resources at meetings, e-mail announcements, newsletters, attendance at multidisciplinary meetings or hospital functions, and offering events in the library. Volunteering for hospital projects or teams identifies one as a team player, as well as providing another opportunity for networking and "being in the know." Additional hints for high visibility may be found in Bernal and Schneider's article, listed in Appendix 14.A.

Being in a position to know about upcoming events or initiatives allows one to seize opportunities where the library staff can step in to fill a niche. Preawareness of forthcoming actions that could have negative effects on the library gives the librarian a chance to act proactively before the proposed event becomes a fait accompli; the librarian can present statistics and facts which might prevent funding cuts or possibly save a staff person's position. Ideally, those in management make decisions based on all the facts, but, for any number of reasons, it is not uncommon for decisions to be made in the absence of complete information.

Networking with hospital librarians in other institutions is advantageous, especially for those in solo librarian settings. Casting the net even wider to include all health sciences librarians provides one with colleagues who can offer ideas and resources for handling areas in which they specialize, such as copyright, electronic licensing, or ILL regulations. Professional organizations offer wonderful networking opportunities. The Medical Library Association is the primary national organization for hospital librarians. MLA offers chapters in geographic regions and memberships in a number of sections relevant to hospital library work, with a couple of notable examples being the Hospital Libraries Section and the Consumer and Patient Health Information Section. Other organizations, such as the Special Libraries Association, have much to offer, also, in the way of relevant networking opportunities. The dividends of professional networking and involvement are well worth the effort in addition to often being enjoyable.

Having a presence in the **electronic health record (EHR)** is another niche for the library. The EHR, when fully implemented, eliminates the need for paper medical record charts and contains complete information about patients, including allergies, drug prescriptions, diagnoses, and providers' notes. If knowledge-based resources—preferably branded so that people recognize they are there because of the library—are accessible for quickly looking up patient information within the EHR system, people will find it easier to make the connection of the library's contribution to patient care. The EHR is well established in some medical centers but is far from being universal at this point. A number of commercial sources, as well as the federal government, have developed EHR systems. If a librarian is in an institution that is attempting to implement an EHR, he or she should get involved, if at all possible. Having the library involved from the outset can only be beneficial. The librarian can stress the importance of having electronic resources with drug, diagnostic, therapeutic and other knowledge-based information accessible from within the record system, truly at the point of patient care. The situation is even better if the resources are integrated through **information buttons** that provide topic-specific searches for the convenience of the provider seeking information applicable to a particular patient problem. The advent of the EHR also makes it easier for library staff members to document PHE that they have provided, since they can access patients' records at their desktops in those institutions which grant permission to do so.

MARKETING AND PROVING VALUE OF SERVICES

The library staff in a hospital can do a great job of selecting and acquiring resources that fit the needs of the institution, can make them accessible in convenient ways, and provide an array of services; but if administrators who make fiscal and space decisions are not aware of the library's contributions to education, research, and patient care, the library can be vulnerable to downsizing or, even worse, elimination. The library staff need to use whatever means are available to publicize what they are doing to serve the hospital's employees and to contribute to patient care. The librarian knows that he or she is

- providing information for the education of patients so that they can better understand their conditions and comply with self-care instructions;
- selecting resources and negotiating and complying with license agreements;
- quickly getting information from another library across the country if it is needed immediately in a critical patient situation; and
- doing expert searches which affect clinical decision-making and which guide the updating of institutional procedure manuals.

Clinicians and administrators need to be reminded of these library contributions and others through **branding** of electronic resources and various reporting mechanisms. The hospital librarian must be in constant communication with library users and potential users—seeking input and then acting upon it. The librarian must provide reports to management clearly illustrating the library's impact within the institution. These reports can stem from a number of sources, such as usage statistics, ILL statistics, customer surveys, and unsolicited customer feedback. The reports need to turn the data into **return on investment (ROI)** information.

If library staff members are serving on committees, they can use meetings as opportunities to volunteer looking up information about the issues that arise in meetings—serving as a reminder that answers and suggestions can often be found in the literature for administrative, public relations, personnel, and other issues, as well as clinical problems.

In addition to the traditional service of providing periodic literature alerts and **TACOs** (table of contents distributions) requested by customers, the library staff can proactively run searches for the latest information on certain topics and decide when to forward new literature. When something particularly good turns up, it can be "pushed" to the appropriate people. Care should be taken to use unsolicited information judiciously; library messages become part of the "junk" mail if they are received every day. Broadcast e-mails or targeted e-mails can be saved for the really "good stuff," which will be appreciated. In addition to having saved searches or alerts as a means of identifying new literature of interest, library staff can have selected Web sites which are viewed on a regular basis for information that might be worth sharing. If library staff members are the first ones to be aware of new facts or research, they should share them with the appropriate audiences within their institution.

Busy clinicians can be reminded that although they are capable of doing their own searches, the library staff can do them to save the time of the clinicians. Even when the library has a core of regular users, there are many more potential users out there—new employees, those who only occasionally need library service, and others. Creativity is needed to find new ways to keep the availability of library services and resources, as well as the expertise of library staff, on people's minds. Unlike academic health sciences libraries, which are required for school accreditation, hospital libraries are not required and so must constantly publicize their resources and services to justify their existence and use of scarce resources—FTEs, funds, and space.

The library can market its services in many traditional ways, such as the list of common marketing tools presented in this chapter. See also Chapter 9, "Marketing, Public Relations, and Communication," for additional information. Bridges' and Clemmons' articles, listed in Appendix 14.A, may be consulted for marketing information and tips geared specifically toward hospital librarians. Of course, librarians and library staff members themselves are the best marketing and public relations tools!

ROLES

Traditional roles for hospital library staff include the usual functions associated with overall library management, collection development and management, and services such as reference, document delivery (including ILL and photocopying), circulation of/access to materials, and alerts. Clinical reference has also been part of hospital library service in some settings for many years—attending rounds and/or morning report followed by provision of information relevant to the clinical cases. Gertrude Lamb "pioneered the concept" of the **clinical medical librarian** in 1971.[11] **LATCH (literature attached to chart)** was once part of the clinical medical librarian's role but has largely been replaced by literature in electronic formats (supplied either in response to rounds/morning report or available in the KBI portion of the electronic health record). For more about clinical medical librarianship programs, see the articles by Wagner and Byrd and

Marketing Tools

Branding of electronic resources
Testimonials of satisfied clients
Newsletters
Flyers
Announcements of
- Classes
- New resources
- New features of existing resources
- New services
Participation in new employee/student orientations
Demonstrations at
- Meetings
- Employee work areas
- The library
Sponsoring activities during
- National Medical Librarians Month
- National Library Week
- Medical Information Day
Hosting special events, such as TechnoFairs
Creating posters for hospital events
Promotional items, such as pencils, pens, Info Rx pads, and bookmarks

Note: Distribution mechanisms for readable materials may include Web pages and other Web technologies, e-mail, and print.

Burdick, listed in Appendix 14.A. The newest evolvement of the clinical medical librarian's role is the **informationist, or information specialist in context (ISIC)**—someone who has received education and training both in information science and clinical science. An informationist may be funded by a clinical department rather than the library. The concept of this role was first proposed by Davidoff and Florance in an article in *Annals of Internal Medicine*[12] and has been the subject of controversy among both clinicians and librarians. Time will tell whether or not educational programs, certification, and institutional demand, as well as funding support, for this career become well established and widely available.

Teaching of library resources is a role that is expected in hospital situations, even in hospitals not affiliated with educational programs. Database access has evolved from librarian-only access with the librarian acting as intermediary for searches, to in-library use by clients at workstations in the library with library staff at hand to help, to desktop access by clients. With the advent of desktop access to databases and to full-text information, the need to instruct users on the many platforms available has presented itself. Very few libraries offer information via one, unified interface. Savvy hospital librarians have been providing instruction for a number of years, but ways of delivering education on information retrieval have expanded to include, not only classes and one-on-one instruction in the library or computer lab and the old standby of printed handouts, but also one-on-one instruction at clients' work areas, programmed instruction via online tutorials, step-by-step guidance over the telephone while a client is in the midst of using an electronic resource, and virtual co-browsing of Web resources.

Some hospital librarians have nonlibrary roles, such as being responsible for CME. These librarians must be familiar with the Accreditation Council for Continuing Medical Education (ACCME) processes and criteria for approval of continuing education credits. Some hospital librarians administer and maintain the hospital's Web site, not just the library's Web site. Some hospitals are organized so that the head of the library is also the head of IT and/or medical records.

In many hospitals, librarians are serving on groups such as patient safety committees, **root cause analysis (RCA)** teams, or **failure modes and effects analysis (FMEA)** committees. RCA and FMEA are tools for quality improvement in patient safety and are employed to understand individual incidents such as medication errors so that they may be prevented in the future. Investigating the literature for these groups by library staff has not been unusual over the years, but for librarians to actually be standing members is becoming more common as their expertise and contributions are recognized. Those interested in librarians' involvement in patient safety may wish to consult the article by Zipperer and Sykes, in which they report results of a survey on the topic, or the newsletter piece with Gluck's tips on how to become part of the patient safety team, both listed in Appendix 14.A. A number of sources, such as MLA, the Joint Commission, and the National Patient Safety Foundation, offer information that librarians involved in patient safety can use.

Librarians have been at the forefront of IT in hospitals, being among the first to use technologies such as e-mail and Web applications. Because of this familiarity with the digital world, librarians have seen their roles, in some cases, evolve into their being responsible for IT departments. Even when the library and IT department are separate entities in the organization, the librarian must often be the troubleshooter for electronic resources.

Consumer health information has been offered by many hospital libraries over the years in response to questions from nonclinicians, but patient health education targeted specifically to the information needs of the individual patients is becoming a more common role for librarians. Librarians are now filling information prescriptions from clinicians. Once the information is provided, they may document the material viewed or presented in the patients' records. Along with this access to the medical record comes the duty to adhere to the **Health Insurance Portability and Accountability Act (HIPAA)** to ensure privacy. Hospital employees are required to receive HIPAA training so that they are fully aware of the legal requirement to ensure confidentiality and protection of patients' medical records and personal information. Librarians can sometimes find themselves being responsible for oversight of both departments in situations where libraries and medical records fall under the umbrella of information management.

Research is another area where hospital librarians' roles have expanded. Librarians have traditionally reviewed the literature and provided information for researchers preparing grant applications. Serving on **institutional review boards (IRBs)** which review and approve institutional research projects involving human subjects is an extension of this role. On the **MEDLIB-L** LISTSERV, an electronic discussion list of interest to medical librarians, Resnick, whose article is listed in Appendix 14.A, polled hospital librarians about their experiences with IRBs and reported the results informally in *National Network*. In some hospitals, librarians are even heading research departments and are responsible for administration of institutional grants.

An additional area of responsibility for some librarians is that of managing the hospital archive collection. A library science or information science degree does not necessarily prepare one to be an archivist! Librarians faced with this situation may find it helpful to become members, or at least consult the publications, of the Society of American Archivists.[13]

Library staff may also extend responsibilities into areas such as institutional newsletters, Web sites, and/or public relations. Librarians' skills lend themselves to many applications outside of traditional library duties and they are being tapped as hospitals become "leaner and meaner." Once independent departments within hospitals are being merged with and/or subsumed by other departments, and library staff members are taking on some of their roles as additional duties. MLA Standards provide a lengthy list of activities included in the role of the medical librarian.[2] This chapter also provides examples of some of the roles that librarians in clinical settings may have.

Potential Roles of Librarians in Clinical Settings

Clinical medical librarian—Providing information for patient cases
- Rounds
- Morning report

Informationist—Providing information for patient cases (person with clinical, as well as information, science background)

CME program responsibility:
- Committee member
- CME manager for the hospital

Information technology responsibility:
- Oversight of the whole IT department
- Management of the library's Web pages
- Troubleshooting of computers and/or electronic resources

Health information management responsibility:
- Oversight of the whole medical records department
- Management of KBI resources in the electronic health record
- Selection and purchase of coding/billing tools (print or electronic)

Patient safety responsibility:
- Providing literature searches regarding patient safety, as requested
- Serving on root cause analysis teams
- Serving on failure modes and effects analysis committees
- Serving on patient safety committee

Research responsibility:
- Oversight of the whole research department
- Serving on institutional review boards (IRBs)
- Running literature searches for researchers and IRBs
- Handling grants administration

Medical media responsibility:
- Oversight of the whole medical media department
- Management of parts of the department, such as graphics, photography, satellite coordination, or AV hardware

Hospital archives management

Consumer health services

Patient education services (not as actual educator, but as provider of information)*

Hospital newsletter responsibility:
- Committee member/contributor
- Editor of the whole publication

---

*Librarians are often educators for employees and students, particularly in information literacy, but as nonclinicians, they are not patient educators. They can provide information from the literature for patient education but cannot ethically interpret the information for patients or give them medical advice.

SPACE AND LIBRARY AS PLACE

Hospital settings can be very competitive for space. As libraries become increasingly virtual, facility planners eye library square footage as space that can be relinquished to other functions. Librarians must be extremely proactive in defending their space by ensuring that people are coming in and using that space, even though many resources and services are available in cyberspace. Being creative to ensure that people keep coming through the doors is a necessity. The library can be a working space, an educational space, a communal space, a meeting space, and/or a coffee break space. It can be the place where custodial staff or grounds-keeping staff who do not have access to computers in their work areas come for their continuing education needs. In a teaching hospital, it can be the place that offers computers and/or network connections for students to use. It can be the place where audiovisual materials for continuing education and patient education are viewed, the place where patients come for both educational and recreational materials. Many materials are still available only in video, not in digital, formats. Even when AV materials move to digital formats, there must be computers and/or DVD players for people to access the materials. Remote viewing throughout the hospital is possible on digital systems, but few hospitals can load absolutely everything into such a system.

Unlike many areas of hospitals, the library is often a public place and should therefore be attractive and comfortable. The location should be such that people can find it without having to first navigate a maze, especially if serving patients and their families. Ideally, it is on a low floor near the entrance and/or near the cafeteria where people can happen upon it without even looking for it. MLA Standard 10, which is printed in Chapter 15, "Library Space Planning," of this text, describes the space needed for a hospital library. The standards point out that a library with inadequate space is likely to be underutilized.[2]

LEGAL/ETHICAL ISSUES

With the advent of electronic resources, librarians have had to expand their knowledge of legal matters, such as licensing agreements. Such agreements must be carefully scrutinized and signed only if they can be upheld, so as not to expose the hospital to legal action. In shared systems such as multihospital intranets, care must be taken not to allow access to system members who are not under the single hospital library's licensing agreements. Librarians should negotiate licenses to include any branches of their hospital which they serve, if at all possible.

Adherence to copyright law and guidelines is important in hospitals, just as in academic institutions. Royalties must be paid for copying and for ILL items borrowed which are in excess of what is allowed by the guidelines. Hospital librarians must be knowledgeable about, and comply with, fair use guidelines and be able to explain them to clients who might not understand why the library cannot copy several chapters out of a book for them. Being in a small library is no excuse for noncompliance.

Confidentiality is an ethical as well as a legal issue in hospital libraries. Staff members have an ethical obligation to keep employees' and patients' circulation records and information requests private, according to ALA's Code of Ethics and MLA's "Code of Ethics for Health Sciences Librarianship."[14, 15] Library clients' transactions—literature searches, ILLs, circulation records—should be protected; both employees and patients are entitled to privacy. Many states have laws protecting library clients' privacy in state-owned facilities, although the **USA PATRIOT Act** and **Foreign Intelligence Security Act (FISA),** both pieces of federal legislation, can be invoked by federal authorities in order to obtain access to library records.

Patient information must never be revealed except to those on the treatment team. Conversations and computer printouts that reveal patient information should be closely guarded. No revelations in the cafeteria or elevator allowed! Shredders should be available for any patient record information printed out by librarians or clinicians on library computers. HIPAA, as previously mentioned, stipulates a federal, legal mandate to maintain privacy of patients' health information. Therefore, library staff members who are authorized to access patient records must take great care not to leave those records on their computer screens when they leave their desks. When librarians have the ability to pull up patient records at their desktops, they may do so only on a "need to know" basis. In other words, if a librarian is documenting provision of PHE information in the patient's record, it is fine to access the record. If the librarian is just curious about a neighbor or cousin who has been admitted as a patient, accessing the record is forbidden. Also, as patients become able to access their own records in some hospitals through computers in the libraries, library staff will have to be vigilant to ensure that patient-accessed computer screens are cleared and that printouts with confidential information are not sitting unattended at printers.

The **Americans with Disabilities Act (ADA)** requires that doorways and physical spaces be accessible to those with assistive devices for their mobility. Web sites should also be designed so that those with visual impairments can view the pages. Additionally, at least some materials in the print collection should be available in large print. Hospital libraries must comply with ADA, but they are not unique in this regard.

Is malpractice an issue for hospital librarians? If the librarian does not perform an adequate literature search and the clinician acts on inadequate information with poor results for a patient, potential is there. There is speculation that informationists or clinical medical librarians working on patient care teams may have more potential to be involved in lawsuits than reference librarians. A more common problem for librarians is the ethical issue of whether or not to provide information for those involved in two different sides of a malpractice case. In hospitals where the library provides service to the public and/or attorneys, a librarian may be asked to do a search for a malpractice case by both the litigator and the defendant. Should the librarian provide information to someone who is suing the hospital or one of its providers? Whether or not the librarian actually does the search for both sides or for only one side of a case, confidentiality is an issue. The request should not be revealed to either side.

Another ethical issue in providing health information is that of interpretation of the medical literature. If a client does not understand the information provided, the librarian may be tempted to explain it, but interpretation is under the purview of health professionals, not the librarian. This issue is addressed in more detail in Chapter 18, while ethical situations arising in reference transactions are discussed in Chapter 7. Censorship is another ethical issue which is discussed in the earlier section on collection management.

TIME MANAGEMENT

Time management can be a challenge for all librarians, but particularly for solo librarians. As roles expand in hospitals, the number of hours in a day does not likewise expand. Hospital librarians constantly find themselves reprioritizing. Demands are coming from several areas and there are many deadlines to meet.

A number of electronic calendars and task lists are available with features such as color coding or flagging or even alarms to help manage "to do" lists and meetings. Tasks can be sorted by due dates or urgency. Time-challenged librarians should take advantage of these tools. Old-fashioned paper lists can work, also. The main thing is to have everything documented somewhere and to check it faithfully so that no task is forgotten or ignored. In the fast pace of today's hospital environment, it is easy to feel overwhelmed. If the feeling arises that too much is undone, it can be helpful to take a moment to record the things that have been done. Even though everything is not getting accomplished, it can be surprising and gratifying to see that many things are indeed getting done. Psychologically, it is worth the effort to make at least a mental note of what has already been completed.

Some items on priority lists may stay there because they keep getting bumped from the top of a list by patient care requests or immediate deadlines imposed by management or technology emergencies. A way must be found to move these things to the top when there is a momentary lull in the ASAP items. The seemingly gargantuan tasks can be broken into smaller pieces. If one waits for a big chunk of time, it will never come.

Hospital librarians must strive for a balance between regular, mundane chores and urgent requests. If achieving any sort of balance is impossible and there is a constant barrage of rush items that prevents doing routine (but necessary) tasks, one needs to request additional staff! Staff can be expanded with use of volunteers, work-study students, library school students, or incentive therapy workers in hospitals which offer these possibilities. These supplementary staffers can photocopy, scan and deliver documents, serve as greeters, perform circulation duties, shelve items, shift shelves, make mail runs, and more, depending on their particular skills. Pros and cons regarding the use of volunteers can be found in the article by McDiarmid and Auster who did a survey. The most commonly listed benefit of having volunteers was "assistance with routine clerical tasks" while "unreliable attendance and commitment" was the most frequently listed pitfall.[16]

STRATEGIC PLANNING

Whether a strategic plan is a formal one presented to upper management or an informal one not seen by anyone other than library staff, it is good to think about changes and improvements and put them into a time frame. Planned change requires forethought and specific objectives to bring about short-term and long-term goals. The plan needs to be reassessed on an occasional basis to determine if the library is on track toward accomplishing these goals. If progress has not been made, it can be helpful simply to jot down a couple of things that are immediately doable toward the achievement of these goals. The first step may be "homework" in identifying the right person to talk to, for example, about what it takes to get the library on the schedule for new carpet. Once the library is on the hospital's schedule, the particulars can be worked out on how to handle services during the replacement process, how to move collections, and other considerations involved in such an endeavor. Big improvements (in facilities, services, or staffing) will not happen by accident. For more on strategic planning in hospital library settings, see the article by Siess, listed in Appendix 14.A.

Planning documentation should also include a disaster plan. Relying on the institution's emergency preparedness plan is not sufficient, as the library has specific needs which must be addressed. Emergencies can vary from localized water damage due to pipes bursting or smoke damage from a hospital fire to widespread destruction from tornadoes, hurricanes, floods, or bombs. Documentation needs to be in place for communication, recovery, continued access to electronic resources, and document delivery. Disaster planning is not unique to hospital libraries but is definitely a responsibility of their managers. For comprehensive information on this topic, see Halsted, Jasper, and Little's book, listed in Appendix 14.A.

PROFESSIONAL DEVELOPMENT

Librarians in hospital settings often need two different types of education. Like other librarians, they need to participate in professional continuing education to keep up with the latest developments in library and information science and to learn skills to fulfill new roles. They are also often required to participate in hospital-oriented training on topics such as safety, HIPAA, personnel management, computer security regulations, and more. Getting away for continuing education classes held at professional association meetings or any other off-site locations can be difficult in some hospital situations, especially for solo librarians. However, the beauty of the digital world is that librarians may participate in online courses and Web casts. Participation in continuing education may also be achieved through journal clubs and professional reading. The professional literature is available through personal subscriptions, subscriptions available with memberships, and library subscriptions. Some literature is also online at no charge or can be identified online and then acquired through ILL. The NLM-sponsored **National Network of Libraries of Medicine (NN/LM)** regional offices have professional continuing education materials that may be borrowed. Both special and medical library literature are of interest to hospital librarians. Periodicals of particular interest to those in hospitals include *National Network,* the newsletter of the Hospital Libraries Section of MLA, and the *Journal of Hospital Librarianship,* published by The Haworth Press.

Memberships in professional organizations, such as the Medical Library Association, the American Library Association, the Special Libraries Association, and others can be very beneficial because of the many resources they offer, such as publications, online information, professional meetings with opportunities for face-to-face networking with colleagues as well as vendor exhibits and demos, mentoring services, continuing education, and LISTSERVs.

Hospital librarians are the largest group in MLA but do not participate proportionally in the work of the association. The benefits of participation are worth the effort, even when it means having to do so on one's own time rather than during work hours. Hospital librarians can share their experience and help one another by teaching peer classes, presenting posters and papers, and contributing to the professional literature. If time is granted for professional meetings and continuing education but institutional funding is not forthcoming, grants and scholarships from organizations can make attendance possible.

TECHNOLOGY ISSUES

Large hospital libraries with large staff have systems personnel, but these are the exceptions. Most hospital libraries need the support of their medical center's IT staff for maintenance of computers, scanners, network connectivity, printers, and other IT equipment. Getting around hospital firewalls to participate in services such as document delivery via **Ariel®** requires IT support. Library staff may or may not have privileges to post pages on the hospital's Web site; if not, they need a good, working relationship with IT staff to ensure the library's presence on the Web. Computer security is tighter in some institutions than others; in a number of hospitals, librarians cannot even install software or upgrade their Web browsers because only IT staff members have administrative rights to perform these functions.

In medical center libraries that have computers for patients' use, privacy of Web sites visited must be protected, just as circulation records are protected. Privacy can be achieved through a number of methods—recessed monitor screens, individual carrels, or privacy screens placed over monitors. However, offering absolute privacy can create problems, such as making users think that they can access pornography or hate sites without being detected. Filtering software can be installed to prevent this sort of problem to some degree, although it should not be so restrictive that users are unable to visit legitimate health Web sites that discuss sexual health or diseases of sex organs. For libraries that have computers for employees' use, privacy of patient records must be protected if electronic records are available on the library's computers. Procedures must also be in place for quickly and properly disposing of printouts with patient information on them if the users have left them behind.

Regardless of the IT restrictions at any given institution, it behooves the librarian who does not have systems staff to learn as much as possible through online courses, offerings at local community colleges, extramural classes at local universities, or library and information science courses from universities that have such programs. Library staff members need to be knowledgeable enough to speak the lingo with IT staff and to be familiar with operating systems, have an understanding of **IP (Internet protocol) recognition,** and know how to do basic troubleshooting for common computer and connectivity problems.

New technologies are being developed every day. Various hospital libraries are offering PDA services and resources, as well as wireless connections, while others have not yet adopted these technologies. Technologies such as **wikis, blogs, podcasting,** and **RSS (really simple syndication)** feeds can be utilized but are generally less commonly found on hospital library Web pages at this point. Even when library staff have the expertise, there may be institutional restrictions prohibiting adoption of certain technologies. Certainly, the digital world is rapidly evolving and hospital librarians, with or without system staff, need to stay on top of developments with an eye toward implementation or adoption of new digital tools or delivery systems which would benefit their users.

SECURITY

Security of materials is an issue for any type of library. Hospital libraries are the same as others in their need to protect materials from theft, fire, mold, and other threats. What may be unique in hospitals is the need for twenty-four-hour access by clinicians—a requirement in both the Joint Commission Standards and the MLA Standards.[2, 3] Having electronic resources available 24/7 has generally lessened the need for after-hours access to the physical library space and meets the Joint Commission and MLA requirements for after-hours access to the literature for patient care. However, if the library does not have reliable electronic resources, it must provide after-hours access to its physical collection. The likelihood of a hospital library being staffed twenty-four hours, as are a few academic libraries here and there, is pretty slim. Therefore, security of materials from theft during unsupervised hours can be a problem.

Most hospital libraries that allow access after hours have records of those who have entered them—either through low-tech methods, such as signing for a key, or high-tech methods, like card-scanning entry. However, what library takes a complete inventory each morning to see what is missing?! Days or weeks might pass after the actual theft before an item is identified as missing. Night-entry records are not really useful without being able to pinpoint the date of disappearance. Security cameras can help but are certainly not a total solution. Systems that beep when materials pass through without being checked out are not effective when no staff members are present to hear the beeping. If security officers are willing to personally admit people to the library and stay with them, materials used after hours may be safer, but this is probably not a practical or acceptable procedure in many hospitals. Cuddy and Marchok chronicled their experience with controlling theft in an article in the *Journal of the Medical Library Association,* listed in Appendix 14.A.

Computer security is another matter. People who know how to tamper with settings will do so if at all possible. Software that locks down what users can do helps to prevent unwanted changes in computer settings to a large degree. If necessary, asking people to register to use computers can cut down on such mischief, although it does create more work for the library staff.

Security of employees can be an issue. This can vary from one situation to another, for example, a prison hospital library versus a pediatric hospital library versus a psychiatric hospital library. With many hospital libraries having only one staff member, there is no "safety in numbers" for the person working alone. No library is totally safe, as violence is often of a personal nature, for example, an irate spouse attacking an employee in the workplace. Again, a library located in a high-traffic area may be somewhat safer for employees than one located in a remote wing that is deserted at certain times. Having a panic button can bring help quickly, if necessary. Also, security cameras prominently placed may help deter some who enter library space with less than good intentions. For libraries that are used only by hospital employees, card entry can be a security measure for the protection of library staff, by keeping people on the street from wandering into the library. Glassed walls that allow passersby to see what is going on in the library might be considered a security measure of sorts.

DATA COLLECTION

Hospital libraries may collect various kinds of data. One type is the information gathered from conducting needs assessments, which is actually required both by element 6 of Joint Commission Standard IM.1.10 and MLA Standard 9.[2, 3] Libraries must stay in touch with the needs of their users, and the best way to find out what they think they need is to ask them! Collecting users' responses assures that the library is providing the materials and services they want and need; if their responses indicate that the library is not providing what they need, there is an opportunity to change in order to meet their needs. An example of a hospital library needs assessment survey may be found in Kennedy's article, listed in Appendix 14.A. Responses from such an assessment tool can be used to justify a larger budget if users are repeatedly requesting resources not supported by the current budget. If the library staff are doing a good job, the bonus of a formal needs assessment survey is that the library will receive praise which can be quoted on the occasions of performance analysis, budget hearings, and space utilization meetings. Including open-ended questions or space for comments on user surveys allows respondents to insert compliments, as well as suggestions which can be implemented for improved customer satisfaction.

Needs may also be assessed by analyzing ILL data. Libraries are required to maintain such data, anyway. If the data are reviewed to determine which titles are requested most often, this can be used to make future purchase decisions for collections and to demonstrate the need for an adequate resources budget. If a particular title is borrowed very often, the cost of ILL fees and copyright royalties may be more than the cost of an annual subscription. Another twist on ILL data is using it to illustrate what the cost for these materials would have been if the hospital had to use commercial services to obtain them. Libraries' ILL procurement methods, even when fees are charged, are usually much more cost-effective than having to purchase articles directly from publishers or online document delivery vendors.

Keeping circulation and usage statistics may be required in some hospital systems. Even when not required, it is a good idea to have these figures on hand. They can be used to justify the library's existence, providing proof that people are indeed using the library's resources. Statistics on print and AV resources can be used to show that hospital employees do not get all their information electronically. Statistics on electronic resources indicate that hospital employees do use information that the library subscribes to and that the staff provide through their expertise in dealing with publishers and other vendors to negotiate license agreements and set up appropriate means of access, for example, IP recognition and/or passwords for remote use. Usage statistics can be converted into cost per use. ILL statistics can be turned into dollars saved by acquiring through ILL versus acquiring through purchase or commercial document delivery services. Customer feedback can be used as anecdotal evidence of how the library staff have contributed to patient care in specific cases. Customer surveys can ask, and subsequently report, on how information from the library has resulted in earlier discharge (thus saving dollars), avoided complications (thus saving dollars), or saved time (thus saving dollars).

Even when not required to collect data, it is worth the time and effort to do so and to analyze the data collected. These data can be used proactively in written reports, in oral reports at meetings, in newsletters, and on the library's Web page. The data can also be ready to use reactively when the occasion calls for it. The unexpected can happen; plans for various hospital units can change seemingly overnight. Being prepared so that one can move swiftly if threatened is a recommended strategy. One might ask why library staff who are performing well would be placed in the position of having to defend themselves, but unless the library's contribution is very clear to decision makers or outside consultants, the library can be vulnerable. Hospitals themselves are subject to mergers, downsizing, and closing. The library is not immune to the effects of such events, which can trickle down throughout the organization. The best defense is a good offense. As Michael Schott says in his book on downsizing, "You need excellent information flowing in, but you also need excellent information flowing out. You are your own information ministry."[17]

Usage statistics are also helpful in knowing what to renew and what not to renew so that budget dollars can be spent wisely. Cost per usage can be determined from these statistics and is another way of illustrating the ROI of dollars spent for these resources. Recording the number of hits on the library Web pages can also be helpful in justifying staff time of library employees to maintain these pages.

Occasionally, library users may ask for an unreasonable amount of resources in their subject areas and claim that they do not have as many resources as other areas. Keeping a record of expenditures for each subject area can be useful in demonstrating that the library has been equitable in its use of funds.

Keeping a record of "thank you" notes (e-mails, formal letters, and handwritten notes) can be useful in demonstrating the contributions that library staff have made to the many departments within the hospital. The library staff probably do many things that others are not aware of; evidence of the cumulative effect of service provided to a great variety of people can be astounding. In addition to its traditional services, the library may be filling niches that no one else does. These little notes add up and can be used for performance appraisal and for proving the worth of the library. Anecdotal evidence on how the librarian helped with a particular patient case or a patient safety matter can be invaluable.

If the librarian is teaching classes, the evaluations should be maintained. Comments and ratings on these evaluations can also be used for both performance appraisal and for demonstrating the library's value. For similar purposes, library staff may wish to collect evaluations on literature searches or information packets provided to users. As in the Rochester study and subsequent similar studies, such data can clearly show the contribution of library services to clinical decision-making, patient safety, education, research, and the institution's bottom line.[18]

Patron counts can be useful. Security systems often provide "gate counts" of the number of people entering the library. If a small hospital library cannot afford a security system, it can acquire a relatively inexpensive electronic patron counter. Data on the number of people physically coming to the library again demonstrate the need for a physical library space and that people are not conducting all their information business electronically.

Hospital librarians can help one another by collecting and reporting data to MLA's Benchmarking Network survey, which originated in 2002. Types of **benchmarking** information reported include

- budget (e.g., salaries, monographs, serials, electronic resources);
- library staff (e.g., professional FTEs, support staff FTEs, total FTEs);
- additional responsibilities (e.g., archives, multimedia, clinical medical librarian);
- space;
- public services (e.g., reference questions, searches, circulation);

- technical services (e.g., print monographs, print serials titles, online serials titles); and
- special services (e.g., Internet library page, OPAC, consumer information).[19,20]

Analysis of survey results among comparable libraries can be used in a number of ways, such as performance improvement, justification of additional resources, and answering administrators' questions. "When hospital libraries benchmark or compare work processes with one another, best practices emerge."[21]

FISCAL MANAGEMENT

Budget control can vary from one hospital library to another. The best-case scenario is when the librarian is directly responsible for the library budget. Data collection mentioned in the previous section can be useful in justifying annual budget requests. Presenting literature regarding the inflation rate for medical and scientific publications can also be helpful. Additionally, the librarian needs to be aware of library requirements for any educational programs in teaching hospitals and information needs of nurses in magnet hospitals, as these requirements can be used as ammunition in fighting for an adequate budget to support resources for these programs. As with other types of libraries, funds may be more efficiently used when hospital libraries take advantage of consortia-related deals for resources or some of the package deals offered by vendors.

For hospital librarians who sometimes experience budget cuts before the end of the year, deposit accounts can be helpful. For example the **Electronic Fund Transfer System (EFTS),** used by medical libraries to pay ILL fees, uses a deposit account system. If sufficient funds are placed in the system early in the year, they can be used to pay ILL fees later in the year, even if the institution has cut off funding. Those interested in learning more about EFTS may wish to read the articles by Arcari and colleagues and Larson, listed in Appendix 14.A. To save paying ILL fees, hospital libraries may also participate in **Freeshare,** a "cross-regional DOCLINE® Library Group whose members agree to fill DOCLINE® requests free of charge on a reciprocal basis."[22]

The budget can be supplemented by donations. If allowed by the institution, the hospital librarian can solicit monetary gifts from interested groups, for example, grandparents (in a children's hospital), veterans' organizations (in a veterans' hospital), physicians' spouses' auxiliaries, former patients, faith-based groups, or pharmaceutical companies. The groups approached depend on the type of hospital and its clientele. Some libraries create "Friends of the Library" organizations for the purpose of receiving donations. Gorman describes an ongoing development plan that her library began in 1996 with the creation of a friends group. The effort was time-consuming but successful in soliciting donations from physicians and other library users.[23]

Regular funding can also be boosted by grants. Courses are available on writing grant proposals. Funding can stem from a variety of sources, such as community groups, NN/LM regions, the National Library of Medicine and other branches of the National Institutes of Health, and various organizations.

CONCLUSION

Hospital libraries are exciting places to work. They offer challenges and variety. There is never a dull day in administering a library in a hospital setting! People who like routine and/or who are resistant to change should probably not pursue hospital library work. While the library staff is often small, nonetheless, the challenges of managing a hospital library require excellent organizational, interpersonal, and leadership skills, as well as political savvy. The faint of heart need not apply.

APPENDIX 14.A. ADDITIONAL READINGS

Arcari, R.; Lewis, J.; and Donnald, E. "The Electronic Fund Transfer System (EFTS)." *Journal of the Medical Library Association* 92(October 2004): 493-5. Available: <http://www.pubmedcentral.nih.gov/articlerender.fcgi?tool=pubmed&pubmedid=15494765>. Accessed: February 19, 2007.

Bernal, N., and Schneider, J. "Hospital Librarianship: A Proactive Approach." *Medical Reference Services Quarterly* 21(Summer 2002): 65-73.

Bridges, J. "Marketing the Hospital Library." *Medical Reference Services Quarterly* 24(Fall 2005): 81-92.

Burdick, A. "Informationist? Internal Medicine Rounds with a Clinical Medical Librarian." *Journal of Hospital Librarianship* 4, no. 1 (2004): 17-27.

Clemmons, S.L. "Marketing Websites for Busy Hospital Librarians." *Journal of Hospital Librarianship* 5, no. 1 (2005): 83-90.

Cuddy, T.M., and Marchok, C. "Controlling Hospital Library Theft." *Journal of the Medical Library Association* 91(April 2003): 241-4.

Gluck, J. "Librarians As Members of the Patient Safety Team." *National Network* 29(April 2005): 17-8. Available: <http://www.hls.mlanet.org/NatNet/issues/v29n4.pdf>. Accessed: February 19, 2007.

Gorman, L. "Fundraising Efforts in Hospital Libraries." *Journal of Hospital Librarianship* 6, no. 2 (2006): 43-50.

Halsted, D.D.; Jasper, R.P.; and Little, F.M. Disaster Planning: A How-To-Do-It Manual for Librarians with Planning Templates on CD-ROM. New York: Neal-Schuman Publishers, 2005.

Kennedy, T. "Justification for the Library." *Journal of Hospital Librarianship* 2, no. 1 (2002): 63-76.

Larson, C. "Electronic Fund Transfer System—Making Your ILL Life Easier." *National Network* 29(July 2004): 16. Available: <http://www.hls.mlanet.org/NatNet/issues/v29n1.pdf>. Accessed: February 19, 2007.

Resnick, R. "IRB & You, the Hospital Librarian." *National Network* 26(October 2001): 5, 8. Available: <http://www.hls.mlanet.org/NatNet/issues/v26n2.pdf>. Accessed: February 19, 2007.

Siess, J.A. "Strategic Planning for Hospital Libraries." *Journal of Hospital Librarianship* 5, no. 4 (2005): 37-49.

Silver, J.I. "Implications for Librarians of Magnet Hospital Designation." *Journal of Hospital Librarianship* 4, no. 2 (2004): 37-42.

Thomas, D.A. "The Consumer Health Reference Interview." *Journal of Hospital Librarianship* 5, no. 2 (2005): 45-54.

Wagner, K., and Byrd, G. "Evaluating the Effectiveness of Clinical Medical Librarian Programs: A Systematic Review of the Literature." *Journal of the Medical Library Association* 92(January 2004): 14-33. Available: <http://www.pubmedcentral.nih.gov/articlerender.fcgi?tool=pubmed&pubmedid=14762460>. Accessed: February 19, 2007.

Zipperer, L., and Sykes, J. "The Role of Librarians in Patient Safety: Gaps and Strengths in the Current Culture." *Journal of the Medical Library Association* 92(October 2004): 498-500. Available: <http://www.pubmedcentral.nih.gov/articlerender.fcgi?tool=pubmed&pubmedid=15494767>. Accessed: February 19, 2007.

REFERENCES

1. American Hospital Association. *AHA Guide to the Health Care Field.* Chicago: AHA. Annual.

2. Medical Library Association, Hospital Libraries Section, Hospital Library Standards Committee. "Standards for Hospital Libraries 2002 with 2004 Revisions." *National Network* 29(January 2005): 11-7. Available: <http://www.hls.mlanet.org/otherresources/standards2004.pdf>. Accessed: December 31, 2006.

3. Joint Commission on Accreditation of Healthcare Organizations. *Comprehensive Accreditation Manual for Hospitals: The Official Handbook.* Oakbrook Terrace, IL: JCAHO, 2007.

4. Spiegelman, B.M.; Marshall, J.G.; and Special Libraries Association. Special Committee on Competencies for Special Librarians. *Competencies for Special Librarians of the 21st Century.* Washington, DC: Special Libraries Association, 1997.

5. Medical Library Association. *Educational Policy Statement of the Medical Library Association: Competencies for Lifelong Learning and Professional Success.* Available: www.mlanet.org/education/policy. Accessed: August 17, 2007.

6. Funk, C.J., and Shipman, J.P. Letter to George A. Reuther, Director, Healthcare Facilities Accreditation Program of the American Osteopathic Association. November 15, 2006.

7. American Nurses Credentialing Center. "Magnet-Designated Facility Information." Available: <http://www.nursecredentialing.org/magnet/searchmagnet.cfm>. Accessed: August 14, 2007.

8. American Nurses Credentialing Center. *The Magnet Recognition Program Application Manual.* Silver Spring, MD: ANCC, 2005.

9. Taylor, M.C. "LinkOut® for Libraries: Accessing Electronic Journals via PubMed." *Journal of Hospital Librarianship* 2, no. 1 (2002): 87-95.

10. Hill, T. "Document Delivery for the Hospital Library, 2005." *Journal of Hospital Librarianship* 6, no. 2 (2006): 85-94.

11. Guessferd, M. "The Clinical Librarian/Informationist: Past, Present, Future." *Journal of Hospital Librarianship* 6, no. 2 (2006): 65-73.

12. Davidoff, F., and Florance, V. "The Informationist: A New Health Profession?" *Annals of Internal Medicine* 132(June 20, 2000): 996-8. Available: <http://www.annals.org/cgi/reprint/132/12/996.pdf>. Accessed: February 17, 2007.

13. Sokolow, D. "You Want Me to Do What? Medical Librarians and the Management of Archival Collections." *Journal of Hospital Librarianship* 4, no. 4 (2004): 31-50.

14. American Library Association. "Code of Ethics of the American Library Association." 1995. Available: <http://www.ala.org/ala/oif/statementspols/codeofethics/codeethics.htm>. Accessed: December 31, 2006.

15. Medical Library Association. "Code of Ethics for Health Sciences Librarianship." 1994. Available: <http://www.mlanet.org/about/ethics.html>. Accessed: December 31, 2006.

16. McDiarmid, M., and Auster, E.W. "Volunteers@Your Library: Benefits and Pitfalls of Volunteers in Hospital Libraries." *Journal of the Canadian Health Libraries Association* 25(Winter 2004): 5-10.

17. Schott, M.J. *Medical Library Downsizing: Administrative, Professional, and Personal Strategies for Coping with Change.* Binghamton, NY: The Haworth Press, 2005.

18. Marshall, J.G. "The Impact of the Hospital Library on Clinical Decision Making: The Rochester Study." *Bulletin of the Medical Library Association* 80(April 1992): 169-78. Available: <http://www.pubmedcentral.nih.gov/articlerender.fcgi?tool=pubmed&pubmedid=1600426>. Accessed: February 19, 2007.

19. Dudden, R.F.; Corcoran, K.; Kaplan, J.; Magouirk, J.; Rand, D.C.; and Todd-Smith, B. "The Medical Library Association Benchmarking Network: Development and Implementation." *Journal of the Medical Library Association* 94(April 2006): 107-17. Available: <http://www.pubmedcentral.nih.gov/articlerender.fcgi?tool=pubmed&pubmedid=16636702>. Accessed: February 19, 2007.

20. Dudden, R.F.; Corcoran, K.; Kaplan, J.; Magouirk, J.; Rand, D.C.; and Todd-Smith, B. "The Medical Library Association Benchmarking Network: Results." *Journal of the Medical Library Association* 94(April 2006): 118-29. Available: <http://www.pubmedcentral.nih.gov/articlerender.fcgi?tool=pubmed&pubmedid=16636703>. Accessed: February 19, 2007.

21. Todd-Smith, B., and Markwell, L.G. "The Value of Hospital Library Benchmarking: An Overview and Annotated References." *Medical Reference Services Quarterly* 21(Fall 2002): 85-95.

22. National Network of Libraries of Medicine. "FreeShare—Free Reciprocal Interlibrary Loan Group." July 28, 2006. Available: <http://nnlm.gov/rsdd/freeshare/>. Accessed: March 6, 2007.

23. Gorman, Linda. "Fundraising Efforts in Hospital Libraries." *Journal of Hospital Librarianship* 6, no. 2 (2006): 43-50.

Chapter 15

Library Space Planning

Elizabeth Connor

SUMMARY. Library space planning can seem daunting to medical librarians unfamiliar with the complex processes involved. The design and usage of spaces that support collaborative, immersive, and social learning are dependent on how a particular library is perceived within the organization and how its constituents access, find, and use information. New learning environments are needed to engage born-digital learners and teachers. The chapter focuses on the importance of predesign, background research, and strategic planning approaches when participating in a renovation/construction project.

INTRODUCTION

Planning the renovation of an existing library or construction of a new facility is one of the most creative, demanding, and enduring contributions that a librarian can make to the institution and the field. A renovation/construction project requires a great deal of preparation, teamwork, stamina, and compromise. To a certain extent, this often protracted process is governed by strategic planning processes and politics at higher levels in the organization. Effective results are predicated on understanding and appreciating how the library is viewed within the organization and how a particular organization's clientele groups access and find information. As pointed out by Thomas,

> good planning and design require bringing both traditional collections and functions into harmony with new technology and new services. Before curtailing or radically reducing space for housing library collections and staff, reviewing both the actual pace of change and the emerging patterns of library usage is crucial.[1]

This chapter will address the concept of the health sciences library as space for teaching and learning; highlight some contemporary design trends; and ask readers to think about space in new and different ways that reflect changes in higher education and social computing.

BACKGROUND

The world over, research libraries symbolize the high value placed on thinking and the investment in future knowledge, expertise, and discoveries. The increasing proliferation of Web searching into daily work, educational, and recreational activities has "created perceived alternatives to libraries."[2] The flattening of time and distance barriers[3] has resulted in economic advantages and global relationships[4] that threaten to further marginalize libraries, especially in light of reportedly decreasing gate counts, instructional sessions, and circulation figures. Some

Introduction to Health Sciences Librarianship

academic librarians have predicted that digital collections will result in libraries that emphasize "social and learning space[s]"[5] over space for books and journals. "Library facilities . . . serve a social function, providing a common ground for users to interact or a neutral site for individuals from different disciplines to come together."[6] People go to the library to see and to be seen, although Ludwig and colleagues warned against touting a library as purely social space.[7] Technological advances continue to challenge the relevance of expensive facilities that house rarely used books or heavily used areas (computer labs and group study space) that could be located in buildings with lower overhead costs or situated on less valuable pieces of real estate.

John Seely Brown explained social learning environments that will appeal to generations of teachers and learners who were born digital.[8] He mentioned the typical architecture studio or **atelier** (see Figure 15.1, p. 389), which shows works in progress, and MIT's physics simulation and visualization studio[9] as examples of practice-based activities that help shift learning away from "learning about" toward "learning to be." Simulation labs and virtual reality technology allow "physicians at all levels the opportunity to refresh skills and learn new ones in a safe practice environment."[10] Librarians can readily support such activities and work with teaching colleagues to plan and incorporate immersive learning approaches into assigned space in the library or shared space across campus.

TRENDS IN LIBRARY DESIGN

Although most library renovation and construction project planners employ interior designers and architects to plan and execute their plans, it is important for librarians involved in these projects to understand basic principles related to composition (arranging or grouping of objects into a unified whole), proportion (dimensions or quantity of objects relative to each other or the whole), balance, scale (size of an object relative to other objects), style, perspective (point of view, particularly related to the illusion of depth), form (shape or structure of an object), light, and color. The golden mean refers to an aesthetically pleasing proportion, widely evident in nature and art, that is expressed mathematically as 1:1.618. According to this principle, a ten-foot-high wall is in proportion if its length is 16.18 feet. Familiar examples include the spiral of a Nautilus shell, the Parthenon in Athens, and Renaissance paintings such as Sandro Botticelli's *Venus.* The eye can be trained to detect the characteristics of well-designed spaces that are proportional and balanced, resulting in aesthetically pleasing facilities.

Library As Neutral Space

In many organizations, the library serves as neutral, somewhat cultural space. The evolving trend is toward imagining library spaces that support information needs and activities related to teaching and learning, rather than fitting an existing collection or series of departments into allotted or expanded space. How do people learn, where do they learn, and how can spaces be designed to promote learning? What do collaborative environments look like? Clifford Lynch remarked:

> Libraries must now turn their attention to defining their missions and activities in relationship to what is transforming them: the information technology revolution in teaching, learning, and research.[11]

Immersive Learning

In recent years, librarians have distributed their influence widely through the use of clusters and nodes, a concept that is far different from the departmental library model. The trend of situating or embedding librarians (liaison librarians, clinical librarians, informationists) in settings apart from the library has implications for future facility planning. The most dramatic example of this trend is evident at Johns Hopkins University's Welch Medical Library.[12-14] By designing and establishing touchdown suites[15] in several locations on the rather compact but burgeoning East Baltimore campus, librarians connect with basic science researchers, population health researchers, oncologists and cancer patients, and others by working among them. This important shift away from "location-centric to location-independent work"[14] is significant for how librarians work, and how library facilities will be designed, and was enabled by mobile technologies. Library space can be designed to attract transitional users without their own designated space on campus. For example, persons in between meetings, without offices, or awaiting results and visitors can use the library as a third place (not home, not work). Lougee stated:

> The transformations under way in teaching, learning, and research will require a far different conception of the library. At a minimum, structures for the acquisition and description of digital content need to be in place and services developed to respond to a more nomadic and virtual clientele. These minimal requirements, however, merely extrapolate existing roles for collections, access, and user support. Seizing opportunities for more diffuse roles will require investment in both tangible components and in intangible elements such as leadership and organizational development.[6]

Hinton used the term "third space" to denote multiuser online gaming environments[16] not entirely outside the realm of future library services as some academic and public libraries have started to schedule game events in their facilities. Libraries can regain their primacy in teaching and learning by using emerging technologies and social computing practices to their best advantage:

> The library is the only centralized location where new and emerging information technologies can be combined with traditional knowledge resources in a user-focused, service-rich environment that supports today's social and educational patterns of learning, teaching, and research. Whereas the Internet has tended to isolate people, the library, as a physical place, has done just the opposite. Within the institution, as a reinvigorated, dynamic learning resource, the library can once again become the centerpiece for establishing the intellectual community and scholarly enterprise.[17]

Reduced Need for Shelving

Changes in scholarly communication[18] have serious implications for librarians and library facilities alike. Apart from reducing the amount of floor space needed for collections, particularly in medical libraries, digital collections have transformed service and access expectations. Scott Bennett, Yale University Librarian Emeritus, referred to the World Wide Web and changes in teaching and learning as having profound implications for library design[19] and suggested that past space allocations were "tilted heavily toward library operations and away from systematic knowledge of how students learn."[20] A renewed focus on learning has inspired some organizations to situate nonlibrary services such as tutoring, writing, digital media, and language laboratories in library space. In some cases, these services had coexisted in library space in the past, were removed, and then reintroduced, as sharing space is now seen as a collegial advantage and not a drawback. Reduced print collections have allowed for the design and construction of group study rooms and other flexible areas that foster group work and collaboration.

Collaborative Learning Environments

New learning environments are needed to engage **born-digital** learners.[8] These places can be used to show work products,[8] similar to how works in progress are displayed in an artist's studio, or provide glimpses of work groups creating knowledge, such as in a war room, used for military or political strategizing. Biomedical research lends itself to intensive and immersive group work that benefits from the manipulation and display of digital images. Lougee noted that "libraries are becoming more deeply engaged in the creation and dissemination of knowledge and are becoming essential collaborators with the other stakeholders in these activities."[6] Notable examples of highly visible collaborative work spaces include Stanford Center for Innovations in Learning <http://scil.stanford.edu/>, Stanford University's visualization labs, and the Centers for Disease Control and Prevention's (CDC) **Collaboratory** Room (see Figure 15.2, p. 389), all designed by the DEGW architectural firm <http://www.degw.com/>. The Collaboratory Room at the CDC is situated at the front of the library and is intended to "stimulate creative thinking"[21] among researchers with its progressive and forward use of furnishings and technology. CDC researchers use this modern space's interactive displays to brainstorm and share data, developments, and images related to a disease outbreak, for example. Kirksville College of Osteopathic Medicine's Connell Information Technologies Center features a simulation lab, library, and laboratory space for osteopathic manipulative medicine (OMM). Bennett suggests "ask[ing] first how students learn and then …design[ing] environments, including seating, to foster that learning."[20] In medical and scientific settings, everyone is a learner given the exponential growth of research and discovery.

Imagining Library Space

One of the most challenging aspects of renovating or building a new facility is imagining future services and programs. It is tempting to request considerably more space especially if library resources, services, and staff have existed in inadequately designed and sized space for an extended period of time. By focusing on library strategies related to teaching and learning rather than specifying a bigger shoebox in which to place existing materials, equipment, furnishings, and staff, librarians can involve themselves in the more intellectually challenging process of determining *how* space is used and the *kinds* of spaces needed to foster collaboration, workplace productivity, and effective service provision. Librarians can prepare by gathering data, visualizing renovated or new space, and getting involved in institutional activities outside the library building and library organization.

Focus Groups, Surveys, and Observations

Several methods, such as focus groups, surveys, and informal observations, can be used to collect vital information about user perceptions and their behavior. For example, librarians at Swarthmore, Haverford, and Bryn Mawr (Tri-College Library Consortium) conducted focus group discussions in an effort to understand how faculty and students find, select, and access library materials within the context of consortial collection development.[22] Useful information included details about space needs for browsing, group viewing, group study, individual study, and social activities. Some libraries have used the LibQUAL+ instrument <http://www.libqual.org/> to survey user attitudes about a number of service issues, including perception of the library as place.[23, 24] More informal data gathering methods include walking around the facility and noting patterns of usage during specific times of the day, amount of group work, how furniture is used or rearranged, and other anecdotal evidence.

Mount Laurel Library staff in New Jersey use visual merchandising techniques to display library materials attractively in an effort to be customer focused and to help customers find materials easily.[25] Staff conduct regular facility walkthroughs and morning briefings to acknowledge hard-working staff and to detect problems that need to be addressed. Medical librarians can adapt this approach to improve navigation, note needed repairs, and observe how users interact with furniture and equipment.

Visualization Exercises

Depending on the organizational culture, reporting relationships, and the scope of the project planned, librarians may provide more input into the interior design planning than involvement in the selection of building site, architects and consultants, building materials, mechanical systems, and so forth, used in the project. To prepare thought processes to yield the most creative input, one or more of the following exercises can be used to visualize library space:

1. Imagine seeing a library space for the first time:
   a. What should be seen upon entering?
   b. What types of services are needed and which ones should be situated close to each other?
   c. Where should library space be situated relative to other buildings, departments, services, campus entrances?
2. Take a mental snapshot of each of the following (past or present) and write down at least three physical features of that image:
   a. Favorite library or museum (any type)
   b. Favorite retail space
   c. Favorite campus setting
   d. Favorite class session or classroom
3. Of the four mental snapshots (library/museum, retail space, campus, and classroom), are there any common elements?
4. Take photographs of the existing library and use these images to guide discussion and understand "existing conditions and the problems encountered by each target group,"[26] as suggested by Aaron Cohen Associates.
5. Take a piece of graph paper and sketch out a rectangular space that could be subdivided into sections depicting a library/museum, retail space, campus, or classroom.
6. List the three most important activities conducted by users and staff within a specific library. Compare this list with one or two colleagues in a work group or classroom setting.
7. Describe the furnishings (windows, lighting, acoustics, colors, textures, seating, work surfaces, artwork, etc.) preferred.
8. Request a set of drawings for an existing library and use tracing paper and graph paper to sketch out some alternative spaces, shapes, entrances, and so forth.

Getting Involved

The importance of being seen, getting involved, and representing the library in a wide range of institutional activities cannot be overstated. Some librarians make it a regular practice to have coffee or lunch with institutional colleagues; seek appointments or serve on key committees that place them in frequent contact with clinicians, educators, researchers, students, and other clientele; and remain acutely aware of societal, economic, educational, and health care changes, detailed in the next section, that affect libraries. These low-key but effective approaches can be used to stay informed and involved.

PREDESIGN PLANNING

Freeman pointed out that "the library must reflect the values, mission, and goals of the institution of which it is a part,"[17] now and in the future. In addition to aligning the library's mission with that of its parent organization, medical librarians involved in planning library facilities need to be acutely aware of forces and issues within higher education, health care, medical education, and librarianship that affect funding, enrollments, accreditation, and so forth. Key organizations to be aware of include these:

- Medical Library Association (MLA) <http://www.mlanet.org/>
- Council on Library and Information Resources (CLIR) <http://www.clir.org/>
- **National Library of Medicine (NLM)** <http://www.nlm.nih.gov/>
- Association of Academic Health Sciences Libraries (AAHSL) <http://www.aahsl.org/>
- Liaison Committee on Medical Education (LCME) <http://www.lcme.org/>
- Association of American Medical Colleges (AAMC) <http://www.aamc.org/>
- Accreditation Council for Graduate Medical Education (ACGME) <http://www.acgme.org/>
- National Resident Match Program (NRMP) <http://www.nrmp.org/>
- Joint Commission on Accreditation of Healthcare Organizations (Joint Commission, formerly JCAHO) <http://www.jointcommission.org/>
- Institute of Medicine (IOM) <http://www.iom.edu/>
- Agency for Healthcare Research and Quality (AHRQ) <http://www.ahrq.gov/>
- Health Resources and Services Administration (HRSA) <http://www.hrsa.gov/>

Medical librarians involved in design projects can look beyond medical library examples, in particular, and academic libraries, in general, to public libraries, museums, convention centers, and retail stores for creative ideas. Few articles or books offer a complete step-by-step or cookbook approach to planning or managing a building project, but a number of different works offer a wide range of information that can be useful (see Appendix 15.A, Suggested Readings). Because renovation/construction plans can take several years to complete, one needs to pay close attention to institutional changes and forces that can accelerate or delay the process, seemingly overnight. Even if a project seems doomed or derailed, it is important to keep thinking and planning about facility needs, collect information and user input, request furniture and equipment vendor catalogs, maintain accurate measurements and current drawings of existing space, and be prepared to move as quickly or as slowly as the project requires. Dykes Library at the University of Kansas Medical Center <http://library.kumc.edu/construction/index.html> has documented its renovations from 1984 to the present, indicative of the fact that effective facility design is an ongoing and continual process.

SITE VISITS, RESEARCH, AND READINGS

Site Visits

Librarians can benefit from visiting libraries that have been recently renovated or constructed[27] to get an insider's view of the processes involved, and to better understand building design. Library staff unable to travel widely can access facility renovation/construction sites that offer information about the project's program statement, drawings, and progress to date (see Table 15.1). These sites illustrate the complexity and duration of typical library renovation/construction projects, and the importance and value of documenting progress.

TABLE 15.1. Examples of Building Project Progress Sites

Project	Web Site
Claude Moore Health Sciences Library	
University of Virginia Health System	
2005-2006 Renovation	<http://www.healthsystem.virginia.edu/internet/library/admin/building/renov05_06.cfm>
1999-2002 Renovation	<http://www.healthsystem.virginia.edu/internet/library/admin/building/renov90s_project.cfm>
Expansion of David L. Rice Library	<http://www.usi.edu/library/buildproja.ASP>
University of Southern Indiana	
Renovation Central	<http://www.hsl.unc.edu/AboutLib/building/renovation.cfm>
Health Sciences Library	
University of North Carolina, Chapel Hill	
Renovation Information	<http://library.kumc.edu/construction/index.html>
Dykes Library	
The University of Kansas Medical Center	
Welch Medical Library Architectural Study	<http://cfweb.welch.jhmi.edu/welchweb/architecturalstudy/index.html>
Johns Hopkins University	
New Library Construction Update	<http://www.uflib.ufl.edu/pio/construction/default.htm>
George A. Smathers Libraries	
University of Florida	
Suzzallo Library Renovation Project	<http://www.lib.washington.edu/about/suzzren/>
University of Washington	
Herman Robbins Medical Library Renovation	<http://library.med.nyu.edu/HJD/renovation/Home.html>
New York University Medical Center	

Research

Several resources include features of interest and value to librarians planning renovation/building projects. Each April issue of *American Libraries* is devoted to photographs of recently constructed or renovated libraries. The Association of Academic Health Sciences Libraries maintains a list of planning resources <http://www.aahsl.org/building/planning.html> related to budgeting and fundraising, design and space issues, service points and library departments, storage, trends in library design, and much more. *Library Journal* publishes a yearly special supplement related to library interiors. Each year, the buildings editor of the *Journal of the Medical Library Association* describes recent building projects. The Coalition for Networked Information and Dartmouth College developed the Collaborative Facilities site <http://www.dartmouth.edu/~collab/info.html>, which collects and organizes planning documents and layouts of digital libraries, learning centers, multimedia production labs, information commons, and similar facilities. An edited collection of case studies features renovation/construction details about various medical libraries (ACOG [American College of Obstetricians and Gyne-cologists] Resource Center, Osler Library at McGill University, UMASS Medical School, University of New Mexico, University of Nebraska, University of Wisconsin at Madison, Welch Medical Library at Johns Hopkins University, and the University of Connecticut Health Center, among others).[28]

Hospital Libraries

Hospital librarians face space issues that are fundamentally different from their academic library counterparts. For example, hospital librarians may lose square footage to other hospital functions, move frequently within the same facility sometimes to less-desirable space or location, and/or combine with another library due to an institutional closure or merger. For example, ACOG Resource Center librarians doubled the size of their assigned space by moving to the basement and transformed the area by working closely with users, visiting other libraries, hiring a space planning consultant, and using a goals-based approach to communicate with the architects.[29] When Elizabeth General Medical Center and St. Elizabeth Hospital in Elizabeth, New Jersey, merged, the librarian took inventory of both collections to identify duplication; weeded materials; reconfigured the layout to accommodate more furniture, equipment, and shelving; and improved the library's Web presence as a means to provide essential services to clientele at both institutions, especially during the project's eighteen-month time period.[30] After occupying lower-level space distant from the main entrance for many years, the library at Greater Baltimore Medical Center in Baltimore, Maryland, relocated into a newly designed 3,000-square-foot space across from the main lobby gift shop (see Figures 15.3 and 15.4, p. 390).[31]

LIBRARY STANDARDS

Over time, accrediting agencies and library organizations have de-emphasized the relative size of library facilities. Previous versions (1979, 1989) of the Association of College & Research Libraries (ACRL) Standards for Libraries in Higher Education, for example, focused on prescriptive recommendations. Current ACRL standards refer to the adequate amount, distribution, and location of library space and the importance of "long-term planning," which are unique to each academic library.[32] These standards offer "suggested points of comparison," such as the ratio of square footage to student/faculty **full-time equivalents (FTEs),** ratio of seating to student/faculty FTEs, and ratio of computer workstations to student/faculty FTEs.[32]

Standards set forth by MLA, the Joint Commission, ACGME, and LCME are of particular interest and importance to medical librarians. MLA's Standards for Hospital Libraries 2002 are similarly and intentionally vague related to physical facilities, recognizing that institutional needs and resources vary:

STANDARD 10
The physical library will be large enough to accommodate the library staff, the in-house collection, and appropriate amount and selection of personal computers or other information technology hardware, and seating for an appropriate number of users. A separate office will be provided for at least the professional library staff.[33]

As with other accrediting bodies, over time, the Joint Commission's requirements for professional library services have evolved to emphasize access to knowledge management resources rather than collections of books and journal issues. MLA's Hospital Libraries Section has worked closely with the Joint Commission to help accreditors understand librarians and help librarians understand the accreditation process and prepare for site visits.[34] ACGME "evaluates and accredits medical residency programs in the United States,"[35] and in 2006, the organization revised the section of its 1994 standards that relates to library collections and services, to take effect July 1, 2007, as follows:

> There must be access to an on-site library or electronic access to a collection of appropriate texts and journals in each institution participating in the residency program. Residents must have ready access to a computerized literature search system and electronic medical databases. Access must be readily available at all times, including nights and weekends.[35]

LCME site visits are of vital interest and importance to academic health sciences librarians.[36] Essentially, LCME requires collections that support the missions of the institution, and, additionally, librarians and library staff are expected to be "responsive to the needs of the faculty, residents, and students of the medical school."[36] New and experienced medical librarians alike can consult MLANET's list of links <http://www.mlanet.org/resources/hospaccr.html> related to hospital accreditation, and note how these standards may or may not affect the quality and quantity of space assigned to the library.

Librarians involved in renovation and construction projects should be familiar with the standards that govern their organization in order to interact effectively with other members of the project team. Vague language in various standards and guidelines used by health care institutions may have the effect of de-emphasizing the need for square footage within an organization, while in other settings, such as colleges and universities, the reverse has been true, resulting in grand, flexible spaces that welcome learners to stay and linger. Younger generations of users who have been exposed to expansive, well-designed, beautifully furnished, and flexible libraries that accommodate a variety of activities, such as quiet study, group work, wireless and hard-wired computing, will expect these same accoutrements when studying science or medicine on a health sciences university campus, and future medical library building projects can take this into consideration.

HIRING CONSULTANTS AND ARCHITECTS

The American Institute of Architects (AIA) developed a helpful document[37] about choosing and working with an architect. The Library Administration and Management Association (LAMA) division of the American Library Association (ALA) maintains a list of building consultants <https://cs.ala.org/lbcl/search/> that can be searched for a modest fee for one time, thirty days, or a longer period of time. Library Consultants Directory Online <http://www .libraryconsultants.org/> is another useful resource, although many libraries rely on word-of-mouth recommendations. Librarians eligible to subscribe to the AAHSL LISTSERV can use the collective wisdom of academic health sciences library leaders to identify and recommend building consultants.

FACILITY PLANNING AS PART OF STRATEGIC PLANNING

Understanding how a library facility will function in the near and distant future is an important part of overall strategic planning. Adamson and Bunnett reported their experiences renovating the University of Texas Southwestern Medical Center at Dallas library as one of the "first team-based, customer-centered activities the library pursued."[38] In 2002, the University of Texas Health Science Center at San Antonio (UTHSCSA) initiated a strategic planning process that resulted in three views developed by different teams:

- Plan A—"A predominantly electronic repository of resource materials relevant to the missions of the Health Science Center offering rapid, convenient, 24-hour/7 day a week high speed electronic access on- and off-campus to all students, residents and faculty."[39]
- Plan B—"The Library is a center of excellence providing premier and innovative health sciences information services, programs, and information to customers when and where they need it and in the most appropriate format for their need."[39]
- Plan C—"The major missions of all the schools of our Health Science Center (HSC) are the creation of new knowledge, through research, and the dissemination of existing knowledge, by teaching and performing clinical services. . . . Libraries, though, are in a time of rapid and profound transition. The World Wide Web has altered how libraries deliver services. No longer are libraries primarily print repositories to which users must come physically. Rather, they are becoming gateways to electronic and network-accessible collections and services. We are in the midst of this change, which holds not only great promise but also significant challenges, particularly as our Library must not only serve our faculty, students and staff (at all their locations), but should also provide health information services to appropriate professionals in 43 counties of South Texas."[39]

Significant input, as generated by UTHSCSA's teams, for example, can be used to involve various constituencies before a project begins and to build the grassroots support needed as strategic planning and fundraising processes go forward. Being known, visible, and involved throughout the organization, as mentioned earlier, are important for librarians at all levels, as hallway conversations and formal meetings can yield valuable information about future initiatives, partnerships, and opportunities.

SIGNIFICANCE OF LIBRARY 2.0 ON DESIGN

Library 2.0 refers to a constellation of Web 2.0 technologies (blogs, wikis, podcasts, social networking sites, user-supplied tags and reviews) applied to library services.[40, 41] While it is still unclear as to whether these terms are hyperbole or indicative of true sea changes that will transform libraries, there have been some early reports of the usefulness of Web 2.0 tools for ubiquitous learning in clinical settings[42] and the potential of the read/write Web to understand, meet, and anticipate user expectations.[43] How will these changes affect library functions and facilities? When asked about the still nebulous concept of Library 2.0, blogger Edward Vielmetti said:

> Next-generation libraries are really cool. They are inviting physical spaces with good **signage** [emphasis added] and architecture that serves the collection and the patrons, websites that let patrons make comments and take notes on the collection to share with others, and where librarian recommendations are frequent and ubiquitous. But you can do all of that with paper, pencil, and old-fashioned card catalogs. So it's not so much about technology as about attitude.[44]

Several aspects of Web 2.0 tools may influence space planning. The examples given are outside medical settings because of the newness of the phenomenon, and age and habits of typical undergraduate patrons. For example, at St. Martin's College in Carlisle, United Kingdom, the Learning Gateway features social learning space, touchdown areas, flexi-rooms for collaborative work, and shows "how building design can potentially be used to influence user behaviour."[45] Informal and formal areas within the Learning Gateway complement library space, and both facilities are managed by the head of learning and information services. See Figures 15.5

and 15.6 (p. 391) for illustrations of the Learning Gateway's different "seating groupings, surfaces and layouts."[45]

Health sciences librarians can benefit from tracking Library 2.0 influences on the design of undergraduate libraries. David Adamany Undergraduate Library at Wayne State University features Windows on the Arts and Windows on the World, which take advantage of three-story-high atrial space to highlight art performances and televised current events, respectively.[46] Other undergraduate libraries are good sources of imaginative displays, study space, and work environments that appeal to younger generations of learners, teachers, and librarians. Librarians can develop a collection of catalogs, drawings, Web sites, journal articles, book chapters, and books related to the project at hand; make the materials available to all members of the project team to spark discussions and foster creative pollination of ideas; and note imaginative spaces in other libraries and public spaces.

ADVICE FOR NEWBIES

Librarians can also familiarize themselves with several aspects of planning that may vastly improve a library's interior design by understanding the amount of space required for library materials, equipment, and staff;[47] learning to read blueprints and schematic drawings;[48] understanding regulations regarding accessibility;[49, 50] learning about features and advantages of green and sustainable building design;[51] testing out innovative and ergonomic furniture; thinking about aspects of effective signage that help users navigate a space independently; considering high-density or off-site storage solutions; discussing the value of stand-alone versus shared space; and planning a computing infrastructure that addresses present and future requirements.

Space Concerns

Dahlgren uses a rule-of-thumb formula for estimating the amount of square footage needed for books, journals, workstations, seats, meeting space, and staff (see Table 15.2).[47] Although these calculations are normally used to plan space within a public library, particularly estimating "design population," which is dividing the "resident population by the percentage of resident borrowing,"[47] medical librarians can use these guidelines to roughly estimate the amount of square footage needed in a specific situation. This is a useful exercise when first starting a building project.

Blueprints

While it is not essential for librarians to understand every aspect of architectural and electrical drawings, the more an individual knows,[48] the easier it will be to communicate with architects, contractors, plumbers, electricians, engineers, and other project personnel, and to avoid misunderstandings that can be costly to correct. Typically, these documents include two-dimensional floor plans; elevation and landscape drawings; diagrams (electrical, plumbing, mechanical) with specialized symbols that denote placement of common features, such as electrical receptacles, light fixtures, lavatories, roof vents, and the like; and detailed information about dimensions, materials, and plumbing and mechanical systems. Librarians involved in renovation/building projects should request updated copies of these documents.

TABLE 15.2. Rough Example of Space Requirements for Library Materials, Furniture, and Staff

Type	Guideline	Example	Space Required
Books	10 vols./sq. ft. (shelving with aisles)	50,000 books	5,000 sq. ft. (normal 84-90-in.-high units with aisles)
	25 vols./sq. ft. (compact shelving)		2,000 sq. ft. (compact shelving)
Journals	divide number of current titles by 1.5	150 current titles	100 sq. ft.
	multiply backfile titles by .5 per title and multiply by number of years retained	10 years backfiles	750 sq. ft.
Computer workstations	50 sq. ft./workstation	computer area with 20 workstations	1,000 sq. ft.
Seats	30 sq. ft./seat	25 seats	750 sq. ft.
Staff			
	125-150 sq. ft./staff member (this figure can be used for staff assigned at service points, private and shared workspace)	10 FTE library staff	1,250-1,500 sq. ft.
Meeting room space	10 sq. ft./seat	15-seat space	150 sq. ft.
	plus 100 sq. ft. for podium area	with podium area	100 sq. ft.
Instructional space	50 sq. ft./workstation	20 workstations	1,000 sq. ft.
	80 sq. ft. for instructor	with space for instructor	80 sq. ft.
SUBTOTAL			7,180-11,930 sq. ft.
Unassignable space	~1/5 to 1/3 of total space		~1,400-~3,600 sq. ft.
TOTAL SPACE			~8,600-~15,500 sq. ft.

Source: Adapted from Dahlgren, Anders C. *Public Library Space Needs: A Planning Outline.* Available: <http://dpi.state.wi.us/pld/plspace.html>. Accessed: February 15, 2007.

Accessibility

The Americans with Disabilities Act (ADA) Accessibility Guidelines for Buildings and Facilities <http://www.access-board.gov/adaag/html/adaag.htm> provide specific standards for libraries, including aisle widths and height of the lowest card catalog drawer, as well as accessibility guidelines for public areas of the library building. Publications of interest to librarians include complying with the guidelines[48] and the use of adaptive technology to improve service to patrons with functional impairments.[49]

Sustainable Buildings

In this context, sustainability refers to the use of environmentally friendly and energy-saving design principles, building materials, and facility operations. The U.S. Green Building Council (USGBC) <http://www.usgbc.org/> is an organization that promotes healthy workplaces and homes. Architect Johanna Sands developed a useful document that outlines the qualities of sustainable libraries, including environmental impact of a building in terms of water efficiency, energy expenditures, energy-efficient building materials, environmental quality of indoor environments, and notable examples of sustainable libraries (Phoenix Central Library, Library at Mt. Angel Abbey, Delft University of Technology Library).[51] The USGBC's Leadership in Energy and Environmental Design (LEED®) is a set of standards for measuring the performance of sustainable buildings. Many architects are LEED-certified and are open to discussing the economic and environmental value of designing "green" buildings, but such conversations should take place rather early in the planning process.

Innovative Furniture

Some recent library projects reflect fundamental changes in higher education. Rensselaer Polytechnic Institute's Folsom Library features a Collaborative Learning Table (see Figure 15.7, p. 392) that can be used for individual and group work. The table has six workstations, three laptop ports, and three extra monitors. Although this table is intended for group work conducted by patrons, such a design could easily be adapted for small group teaching or reference transactions. Holberg suggests the use of shared space to conduct reference transactions,[52] while Bennett wonders whether situating reference services within a configuration of lounge seating would fundamentally change the learning experience.[20] In the Conservatory at North Carolina State University, an **Astral** Bench (see Figure 15.8, p. 392) serves as a focal point for reflection in the library. Valparaiso University's Christopher Center for Library and Information Resources features a linear grouping of six computer workstations on its first floor that resembles banquette seating (see Figure 15.9, p. 393). Librarians can collect furniture catalogs and consult with colleagues at other institutions about the popularity, comfort, and durability of specific types of chairs, tables, carrels, and so forth.

Combined Service Points

Some libraries have reduced the number of service desks throughout the library or combined circulation and reference functions to create a single service point. This approach requires a great deal of planning, training, and teamwork.[53-55] Mozenter and colleagues pointed out that "buildings and renovations are often designed based on factors of cost and available campus space. The placement of service desks often reflects building design rather than well-thought-out user-oriented service needs."[56]

Storage

Some architects familiar with designing library facilities recommend accommodating the live loads needed for compact shelving throughout the design, to allow greater flexibility in the use of space in the future.[57] For example, office space exerts a live load of 50 pounds per square foot, normal library shelving units require at least 150 pounds per square foot, and compact shelving units need 300 pounds per square foot. By specifying that library floors require 300 pounds per square foot throughout, future designs can feature standard or compact shelving anywhere in the library.

Valparaiso University uses robotic retrieval to optimize its use of high-density storage (see Figure 15.10, p. 393). While compact storage vendors state that libraries can double their capacity by eliminating aisle space between shelving units, libraries that utilize robotic technology can increase their capacity by as much as tenfold.[58]

Some medical libraries have built or leased off-site space to store older and lesser-used materials and provide courier or document delivery services from those collections. In some situations, the storage was initiated during a renovation process, as in the case of the Health Sciences Library at the University of North Carolina at Chapel Hill (UNC-CH).[59] Interestingly, UNC-CH library staff anticipated that 3,000 requests would be made of the pre-1992 books and journals placed in storage when, in fact, during the first year of storage, more than four times that many requests were made. Academic libraries in Ohio use five regional depositories located in central, northeast, northwest, southeast, and southwest parts of the state to store lesser-used library materials. These high-density facilities shelve items by size, and items are retrieved by barcode.[60] The Association of Research Libraries (ARL) developed a SPEC Kit related to remote shelving services that covers descriptions of high-density and remote storage facilities used by a wide range of academic libraries, as well as service policies, service request forms, frequently asked questions, and a bibliography.[61]

Signage

ADA guidelines feature specific information <http://www.access-board.gov/adaag/html/adaag.htm#4.30> about the size, height, and other qualities of directional signs used in public places. Many beautifully designed libraries use ineffective signs to direct patrons and visitors. Carnegie Library hired MAYA Design[62] to develop a wayfinding system that featured five categories: orienting/directing, identifying, educating, and connecting. This system is based on jargon-free terms that help patrons find areas and actions and connect to needed information. Librarians can observe effective signage in nonlibrary settings and incorporate new ideas that direct users to common features, such as restrooms, water fountains, staircases, and the like.

Stand-Alone versus Shared Space

In some organizations, sharing space in a signature building may forge deeper and more profound relationships with key partners than occupying a stand-alone building. On a medical campus, adjacencies are key. Oftentimes, the library serves as the educational bridge between the basic sciences and the clinical care functions and, in some cases, is a showplace designed to attract more philanthropy. In hospital settings, libraries with consumer health components, for example, may seek space within high-traffic areas.

An interesting trend has been joint-use library buildings,[63] particularly among public institutions, notably at San Jose State University (SJSU) and College Hill Library. In the case of SJSU, the state university library in San Jose shares space with the main branch of the public library in a new facility named Dr. Martin Luther King, Jr. Library. Aspects of the new building's design "symbol[ize] the union of the university with the larger community," particularly the entrance that faces the university quad.[64] In 1994, College Hill Library in Westminster, Colorado, partnered with the public library to plan a new public/community college library that opened in 1998. Interestingly, this shared facility is managed by co-directors (the public library manager and the community college library director), and "meet[s] the needs of both communities in a way that two, smaller separate buildings would not have been able to do so."[65] Of interest to medical librarians is Dorrington's example of National Health Service libraries as joint-use facilities because they serve physicians and medical students alike.[66] ALA maintains a bibliography related to joint-use libraries for individuals interested in understanding, pursuing, and/or tracking this trend.[67]

Information Technology Infrastructure

While it is tempting to imagine a totally wireless facility, the reality is that ubiquitous network access afforded by wireless systems cannot take the place of wiring and cabling necessary to power staff functions, computer laboratories, and instruction facilities. As Sparks states, wires are needed for

> servers and storage devices for all the byproducts of our new paperless office. If the past is any indication of the future, it seems that advances in computer operating systems, software applications, and content delivery platforms require faster and faster connections, more hardware, and bigger pipes (more bandwidth).[68]

Librarians at Lyman Maynard Stowe Library at the University of Connecticut Health Center use wireless technology and a bank of laptop computers to repurpose the staff lounge to function as instructional space, as needed.[69]

Library staff at Open University in Milton Keyes, United Kingdom, planned an information technology infrastructure "to meet user needs for at least 10 years," including

> the latest unshielded twisted pair (UTP) Category 6 (Cat6) cables; providing a minimum of 100 megabits (MB) per second switched Ethernet to the desktop with multi-gigabit fiber links to the campus backbone; a 100-MB link from the backbone to the Internet; and roof-mounted cable dishes providing satellite links.[70]

Open University librarians also suggested the use of flexible service routes for cables, "raised floors or vertical risers, in wiring closets or communication rooms, and in conduit trays," and floor-mounted service outlets for power and data.[70]

Librarians can work closely with systems and information technology staff to anticipate and plan for future computing needs.

CONCLUSION

The ideas discussed in this chapter are intended to serve as one of many conversations that librarians can initiate with architects, consultants, and client groups as library renovation or construction plans take shape. Norman Cousins said:

> A library is not a shrine for the worship of books. It is not a temple where literary incense must be burned or where one's devotion to the bound book is expressed in ritual. A library, to modify the famous metaphor of Socrates, should be the delivery room for the birth of ideas—a place where history comes to life.[71]

Understanding how existing and potential users work and interact, both inside and outside the library requires observation, interaction, and involvement. Renovation and construction projects initiated in the twenty-first century should feature collaborative learning spaces that invite people in and encourage them to linger and to interact in ways never imagined before, both inside and outside the library facility. Medical librarians can help reshape teaching and learning by imagining and planning library spaces that bring new ideas to life.

APPENDIX 15.A. SUGGESTED READINGS

American Library Association. *Building Blocks for Library Space: Functional Guidelines.* Chicago, IL: American Library Association, 1995.

Arlitsch, K. "Building Instruction Labs at the University of Utah." *Research Strategies* 16, no. 3 (1999): 199-210.

Association of Academic Health Sciences Libraries. *The Library As Place: Symposium on Building and Revitalizing Health Sciences Libraries in the Digital Age.* November 5-6, 2003. Bethesda, MD. Available: <http://www.aahsl.org/building/agenda.html>. Accessed: February 15, 2007.

Atkinson, R. "Contingency and Contradiction: The Place(s) of the Library at the Dawn of the New Millennium." *Journal of the American Society for Information Science and Technology* 52, no. 1 (2001): 3-11.

Bazillion, R.J. "Planning the Academic Library of the Future." *Portal: Libraries & the Academy* 1(April 2001): 151-60.

Bazillion, R.J., and Braun, C.L. *Academic Libraries As High-Tech Gateways: A Guide to Design and Space Decisions*, 2nd ed. Chicago, IL: American Library Association, 2001.

Boss, R.W. *Information Technologies and Space Planning for Libraries and Information Centers.* Boston, MA: G. K. Hall, 1988.

Brand, S. *How Buildings Learn: What Happens After They're Built.* New York: Viking, 1994.

Brown, C.R. *Planning Library Interiors: The Selection of Furnishings for the 21st Century.* Phoenix, AZ: Oryx Press, 1995.

Brown, C.R. *Interior Design for Libraries: Drawing on Function & Appeal.* Chicago, IL: American Library Association, 2002.

Cohen, A., and Cohen, E. *Designing and Space Planning for Libraries: A Behavioral Guide.* New York: R. R. Bowker, 1979.

Crosbie, M.J. and Hickey, D.D. *When Change Is Set in Stone: An Analysis of Seven Academic Libraries Designed by Perry Dean Rogers & Partners, Architects.* Chicago, IL: Association of College and Research Libraries, 2001.

Dahlgren, A.C. *Planning the Small Library Facility*, 2nd ed. Chicago, IL: American Library Association, 1996.

Dodd, J.; Forys, J.; and Dewey, B.I. "Renovating Science Branch Libraries: Two Different Paths." *Science and Technology Libraries* 19, no. 1 (2000): 39-47.

Dowler, L., ed. *Gateways to Knowledge: The Role of Academic Libraries in Teaching, Learning, and Research.* Cambridge, MA: MIT Press, 1997.

Fraley, R.A., and Anderson, C.L. *Library Space Planning: A How-To-Do-It Manual for Assessing, Allocating, and Reorganizing Collections, Resources, and Facilities.* New York: Neal-Schuman, 1990.

Friefeld, R., and Masyr, C. *Space Planning in the Special Library.* Washington, DC: Special Libraries Association, 1991.

Hagloch, S.B. *Library Building Projects: Tips for Survival.* Englewood, CO: Libraries Unlimited, 1994.

Hawthorne, P., and Martin, R.G., eds. *Planning Additions to Academic Library Buildings: A Seamless Approach.* Chicago, IL: American Library Association, 1995.

Kaufman, J.E. *IES Lighting Handbook.* New York: Illuminating Engineering Society of North America, 1981.

Lam, L.M.C. "Meeting the Challenges of Expansion and Renovation in an Academic Medical Library." *New Library World* 107, no. 1224/1225 (2006): 238-46.

Laubier, G. *The Most Beautiful Libraries in the World.* New York: Harry N. Abrams, 2003.

Leighton, P.D., and Weber, D.C. *Planning Academic and Research Library Buildings*, 3rd ed. Chicago, IL: American Library Association, 1999.

Lippincott, Joan K. "New Library Facilities: Opportunities for Collaboration." *Resource Sharing & Information Networks* 17, no. 1/2 (2004): 147-57.

Lushington, N., and Mills, W.N. *Libraries Designed for Users: A Planning Handbook.* Hamden, CT: Library Professional Publications, 1980.

McCarthy, R.C. *Designing Better Libraries: Selecting & Working with Building Professionals*, 2nd ed. Fort Atkinson, WI: Highsmith Press Handbook Series, 1999.

Medical Library Association. *MLA DocKit #5. Descriptive Floor Plans of Library Computer Centers.* Chicago, IL: Medical Library Association, 1995.

Medical Library Association. "Standards for Hospital Libraries 2002 with 2004 Revisions." *National Network* 29 (January 2005): 11-7.

Monahan, T. "Flexible Space & Built Pedagogy: Emerging IT Embodiments." *Inventio* 4, no. 1 (2002): 1-19. Available: <http://www.torinmonahan.com/papers/Inventio.html>. Accessed: February 15, 2007.

National Clearinghouse for Educational Facilities. *Library Facilities Design—Higher Education.* Available: <http://www.edfacilities.org/rl/LibrariesHE.cfm>. Accessed: February 15, 2007.

Nitecki, DA., and Kendrick, C.L., eds. *Library Off-Site Shelving: Guide for High-Density Facilities.* Englewood, CO: Libraries Unlimited, 2001.

Powell, M. "Designing Library Space to Facilitate Learning: A Review of the UK Higher Education Sector." *Libri* 52(June 2002): 110-20.

Sannwald, W.W. *Checklist of Library Building Design Considerations*, 4th ed. Chicago, IL: American Library Association, 2001.

Shill, H.B., and Tonner, S. "Creating a Better Place: Physical Improvements in Academic Libraries, 1995-2002." *College & Research Libraries* 64(November 2003): 431-66.

The Staff of the Williamsburg Regional Library. *Library Construction from a Staff Perspective.* Jefferson, NC: McFarland & Company, 2001.

Webb, T.D., ed. *Building Libraries for the 21st Century: The Shape of Information.* Jefferson, NC: McFarland & Company, 2000.

Whole Building Design Guide. "Academic Library." Available: <http://www.wbdg.org/design/academic_library.php>. Accessed: February 15, 2007.

Woodward, J. *Countdown to a New Library: Managing the Building Project.* Chicago, IL: American Library Association, 2000.

Wright, K.C., and Davie, J.F. *Serving the Disabled: A How-To-Do-It Manual for Librarians.* New York: Neal-Schuman Publishers, 1991.

REFERENCES

1. Thomas, M.A. "Redefining Library Space: Managing the Co-Existence of Books, Computers, and Readers." *Journal of Academic Librarianship* 26 (November 2000): 408-15.

2. Lindberg, D.A.B., and Humphreys, Betsy L. "2015—The Future of Medical Libraries." *New England Journal of Medicine* 352(March 17, 2005): 1067-70.

3. Anderson, J.Q., and Rainie, L. "The Future of Internet II." Pew Internet & American Life Project. Available: <http://www.pewinternet.org/>. Accessed: February 15, 2007.

4. Friedman, T.L. *The World Is Flat: A Brief History of the 21st Century.* New York: Farrar, Straus & Giroux, 2005.

5. Detlor, B., and Lewis, V. "Academic Library Web Sites: Current Practice and Future Directions." *Journal of Academic Librarianship* 32(May 2006): 251-8.

6. Lougee, W.P. *Diffuse Libraries: Emergent Roles for the Research Library in the Digital Age.* Washington, DC: Council on Library and Information Resources, 2002. Available: <http://www.clir.org/pubs/reports/pub108/pub108.pdf>. Accessed: February 15, 2007.

7. Ludwig, L.; Shedlock, J.; Watson, L.; Dahlen, K.; and Jenkins, C. "Designing a Library: Everyone on the Same Page?" *Bulletin of the Medical Library Association* 89(April 2001): 204-11.

8. Brown, J.S. "New Learning Environments for the 21st Century: Exploring the Edge." *Change* 38 (September/October 2006): 18-24. Available: <http://www.educause.edu/screencasts/JohnSeelyBrown@TWT_CU.pdf>. Accessed: February 15, 2007.

9. Belcher, J.W. "Studio Physics at MIT." *MIT Physics Annual* (2001). Available: <http://web.mit.edu/8.02t/www/802TEAL3D/visualizations/resources/PhysicsNewsLetter.pdf>. Accessed: February 15, 2007.

10. Cooke, M.; Irby, D.M.; Sullivan, W.; and Ludmerer, K.M. "American Medical Education 100 Years After the Flexner Report." *New England Journal of Medicine* 355(September 28, 2006): 1339-44.

11. Lynch, C.. "From Automation to Transformation." *EDUCAUSE Review* 35(January/February 2000): 60-8. Available: <http://www.educause.edu/apps/er/erm00/pp060068.pdf>. Accessed: February 15, 2007.

12. Bryant, W.F.; Campbell, J.M.; Oliver, K.B.; and Roderer, N.K. "The Welch Medical Library: A New Model for the Delivery of Library Services." In: *Planning, Renovating, Expanding, and Constructing Library Facilities in Hospitals, Academic Medical Centers, and Health Organizations*, edited by Elizabeth Connor, 187-202. Binghamton, NY: The Haworth Information Press, 2005.

13. Oliver, K.B. "The Johns Hopkins Welch Medical Library As Base: Information Professionals Working in Library User Environments." In: *Library As Place: Rethinking Roles, Rethinking Space.* Washington, DC: Council on

Library and Information Resources, 2005. Available: <http://www.clir.org/pubs/reports/pub129/oliver.html>. Accessed: February 15, 2007.

14. Roderer, N.; Dugdale, S.; Wildemuth, B.; Brandt, K.; and Hurd, J. "The Library of the Future: Interweaving the Virtual and the Physical." *Proceedings of the American Society for Information Science and Technology* 39, no. 1 (2005): 492.

15. Dugdale, S. "Workplace Trends." *D-News* (February 24, 2004). Available: <http://www.degw.com/dnews/ed_4_leader_2.html>. Accessed: February 15, 2007.

16. Hinton, Andrew. "We Live Here: Games, Third Places and the Information Architecture of the Future." *Bulletin of the American Society for Information Science and Technology* 32(August/September 2006): 17-21.

17. Freeman, G.T. "The Library As Place: Changes in Learning Patterns, Collections, Technology, and Use." In: *Library As Place: Rethinking Roles, Rethinking Space*. Washington, DC: Council on Library and Information Resources, 2005. Available: <http://www.clir.org/pubs/reports/pub129/freeman.html>. Accessed: February 15, 2007.

18. Ludwig, L., and Starr, S. "Library As Place: Results of a Delphi Study." *Journal of the Medical Library Association* 93(July 2005): 315-26.

19. Bennett, S. *Redesigning Libraries for Learning*. Washington, DC: Council on Library and Information Resources, 2003. Available: <http://www.clir.org/pubs/execsum/sum122.html>. Accessed: February 15, 2007.

20. Bennett, S. "Righting the Balance." In: *Library As Place: Rethinking Roles, Rethinking Space*. Washington, DC: Council on Library and Information Resources, 2005. Available: <http://www.clir.org/pubs/reports/pub129/bennett.html>. Accessed: February 15, 2007.

21. Dahlen, K. "Re: DEGW's Collaboratory Room at CDC." Personal e-mail (January 10, 2007).

22. Luther, J.; Bills, L.; McColl, A.; et al. *Library Buildings and the Building of a Collaborative Research Collection at the Tri-College Library Consortium: Report to the Andrew W. Mellon Foundation*. Washington, DC: Council on Library and Information Resources, 2003.

23. Foss, M.M.; Buhler, A.; Rhine, L.; and Layton, B. "HSCL LibQUAL+ 2004: From Numbers and Graphs to Practical Application." *Medical Reference Services Quarterly* 25, no. 1 (Spring 2006): 1-15.

24. Wei, Y.; Thompson, B.; and Cook, C.C. "Scaling Users' Perceptions of Library Services Quality Using Item Response Theory: A LibQUAL+™ Study." *Portal: Libraries & The Academy* 5, no. 1 (2005): 93-104.

25. South Jersey Regional Library Cooperative. "Trading Spaces: Do-It-Yourself Toolkit." Available: <http://www.sjrlc.org/tradingspaces/toolkit/>. Accessed: February 15, 2007.

26. Cohen, A.; Cohen, A.; and Cohen, E. "The Visual Scan and the Design for Future-Oriented Libraries." *Public Library Quarterly* 24, no. 1 (2005): 23-32.

27. Ludwig, L.; Shedlock, J.; Watson, L.; Dahlen, K.; and Jenkins, C. "Designing a Library: Everyone on the Same Page?" *Bulletin of the Medical Library Association* 89(April 2001): 204-11.

28. Connor, E., ed. *Planning, Renovating, Expanding, and Constructing Library Facilities in Hospitals, Academic Medical Centers, and Health Organizations*. Binghamton, NY: The Haworth Information Press, 2005.

29. Hyde, M.A., and Van Hine, P. "ACOG Resource Center Happily Moves to the Basement." In: *Planning, Renovating, Expanding, and Constructing Library Facilities in Hospitals, Academic Medical Centers, and Health Organizations*, edited by Elizabeth Connor, 5-23. Binghamton, NY: The Haworth Information Press, 2005.

30. Jacobsen, E. "A Tale of Two Libraries: Overview of a Merger." In: *Planning, Renovating, Expanding, and Constructing Library Facilities in Hospitals, Academic Medical Centers, and Health Organizations*, edited by Elizabeth Connor, 61-72. Binghamton, NY: The Haworth Information Press, 2005.

31. Thomas, D. "Re: New GBMC Space." Personal e-mail (February 21, 2007).

32. Association of College & Research Libraries. *Standards for Libraries in Higher Education*. Chicago, IL: American Library Association, 2004.

33. Gluck, J.C.; Hassig, R.A.; Balogh, L.; et al. "Standards for Hospital Libraries 2002." *Journal of the Medical Library Association* 90(October 2002): 465-72.

34. JCAHO Accreditation Resources. Available: <http://www.mlanet.org/resources/index.html#jcaho>. Accessed: February 15, 2007.

35. Accreditation Council for Graduate Medical Education. *Common Program Requirements*. Available: <http://www.acgme.org/acWebsite/dutyHours/dh_dutyHoursCommonPR.pdf>. Accessed: February 15, 2007.

36. LCME. *Liaison Committee on Medical Education Accreditation Standards*. Available: <http://www.lcme.org/standard.htm>. Accessed: February 15, 2007.

37. AIA. *You and Your Architect*. Available: <http://www.aia.org/SiteObjects/files/youandyourarchitect.pdf>. Accessed: February 15, 2007.

38. Adamson, M.C., and Bunnett, BP. "Planning Library Spaces to Encourage Collaboration." *Journal of the Medical Library Association* 90(October 2002): 437-41.

39. University of Texas Health Science Center at San Antonio. *Library Planning*. Available: <http://www.library.uthscsa.edu/basics/LibraryPlanning.cfm>. Accessed: February 15, 2007.

40. Connor, E. "Library 2.0: Implications for the Future of Medical Libraries." *Medical Reference Services Quarterly* 26(supplement 1, 2007): 5-23.

41. Connor, E. "Medical Librarian 2.0." *Medical Reference Services Quarterly* 26, no. 1 (Spring 2007): 1-15.

42. Boulos, M.N.K.; Maramba, I.; and Wheeler, S. "Wikis, Blogs, and Podcasts: A New Generation of Web-based Tools for Virtual Collaborative Clinical Practice and Education." *BMC Medical Education* 6(August 15, 2006). Available: <http://www.biomedcentral.com/content/pdf/1472-6920-6-41.pdf>. Accessed: February 15, 2007.

43. Chad, K., and Miller, P. "Do Libraries Matter? The Rise of Library 2.0." Available: <http://www.talis.com/applications/news_and_events/pdfs/do_libraries_matter.pdf>. Accessed: February 15, 2007.

44. "Straight Answers from Edward Vielmetti." *American Libraries* 37(October 2006): 15.

45. Weaver, M. "Flexible Design for New Ways of Learning." *Library and Information Update* 5, no.7/8 (July/August 2006): 54-5.

46. Sutton, L. "Imagining Learning Spaces at Wayne State University's New David Adamany Undergraduate Library." *Research Strategies* 17, no. 2/3 (2000): 139-46.

47. Dahlgren, A.C. *Public Library Space Needs: A Planning Outline.* Available: <http://dpi.state.wi.us/pld/plspace.html>. Accessed February 15, 2007.

48. Madrid, E.M., and Harkey, L. "Reading and Understanding Blueprints." *Seminars in Perioperative Nursing* 8(October 1999): 183-92.

49. Cirillo, S.E., and Danford, R.E. *Library Buildings, Equipment, and the ADA: Compliance Issues and Solutions.* Chicago, IL: American Library Association, 1996.

50. Kirkpatrick, C.H., and Morgan, C.B. "How We Renovated Our Library, Physically and Electronically for Handicapped Patrons." *Computers in Libraries* 21(October 2001): 24-9.

51. Sands, J. *Sustainable Library Design.* Available: <http://www.librisdesign.org/docs/SustainableLibDesign.pdf>. Accessed: February 15, 2007.

52. Holberg, J.E. "Relational Reference: A Challenge to the Reference Fortress." In: *An Introduction to Reference Services in Academic Libraries,* edited by Elizabeth Connor, 39-46. Binghamton, NY: The Haworth Information Press, 2006.

53. Allegri, F., and Bedard, M. "Lessons Learned From Single Service Point Implementations." *Medical Reference Services Quarterly* 25, no. 2 (Summer 2006): 31-57.

54. Naismith, R. "Combining Circulation and Reference Functions at One Desk." *Journal of Access Services* 2, no. 3 (2004): 15-20.

55. Buxton, K.A., and Gover, H.R. "A National Laboratory and University Branch Campus Library Partnership: Shared Benefits and Challenges from Combined Reference Services." *Reference Librarian* 40, no. 83/84 (2003): 251-62.

56. Mozenter, F.; Sanders, B.T.; and Bellamy, C. "Cross-Training Public Service Staff in the Electronic Age: I Have to Learn to Do What?!" *Journal of Academic Librarianship* 29(November 2003): 399-404.

57. Foote, S.M. "An Architect's Perspective on Contemporary Academic Library Design." *Bulletin of the Medical Library Association* 83, no. 3 (July 1995): 351-6.

58. Amrhein, R., and Resetar, D. "Maximizing Library Storage with High-Tech Robotic Shelving." *Computers in Libraries* 23(November/December 2004): 6-8, 51-5.

59. Norton, M.J. "Maintaining Quality Document Delivery Service with Off-Site Storage Facilities." *Journal of the Medical Library Association* 93(July 2005): 394-7.

60. Ohio Library and Information Network (OhioLINK). Available: <http://www.ohiolink.edu/>. Accessed: February 15, 2007.

61. Deardorff, T.C., and Aamot, G.J. *SPEC Kit 295: Remote Shelving Services.* Washington, DC: Association of Research Libraries, 2006.

62. MAYA Design. Available: <http://www.maya.com>. Accessed: February 15, 2007.

63. Dalton, P.; Elkin, J.; and Hannaford, A. "Joint Use Libraries As Successful Strategic Alliances." *Library Trends* 54(Spring 2006): 535-48.

64. Kauppila, P., and Russell, S. "Economies of Scale in the Library World: The Dr. Martin Luther King, Jr. Library in San Jose, California." *New Library World* 104, no. 1190/1191 (2003): 255-66.

65. Sullivan, K.; Taylor, W.; Barrick, M.G.; and Stelk, R. "Building the Beginnings of a Beautiful Partnership." *Library Trends* 54, no. 4 (Spring 2006): 569-79.

66. Dorrington, L. "Health Libraries As Joint Use Libraries: Serving Medical Practitioners and Students." *Library Trends* 54, no. 4 (Spring 2006): 596-606.

67. American Library Association. *ALA Library Fact Sheet Number 20.* Available: <http://www.ala.org/ala/alalibrary/libraryfactsheet/alalibraryfactsheet20.cfm>. Accessed: February 15, 2007.

68. Sparks, R.L. "Building Infrastructure for Ubiquitous Computing." *Knowledge Quest* 34(January/February 2006): 14-7.

69. Arcari, R.D. "Library Renovation Planning." In: *Planning, Renovating, Expanding, and Constructing Library Facilities in Hospitals, Academic Medical Centers, and Health Organizations*, edited by Elizabeth Connor, 203-10. Binghamton, NY: The Haworth Information Press, 2005.

70. Willars, N.; Thomas, P.; and Hunt, M. "The Leading-Edge Library: Meeting IT and Facility Planning Challenges for Academic and Research Libraries." *American School and University* 77(June 2005): 34, 36, 39, 41.

71. Cousins, N. Quotation. Available: <http://www.quoteworld.org/quotes/3228>. Accessed: February 15, 2007.

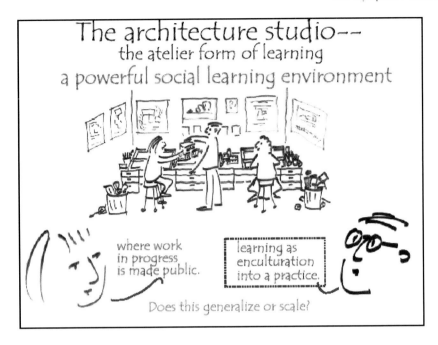

FIGURE 15.1. Architecture Atelier. *Source:* Brown, John Seely and Susan Haviland (artist of sketch). "New Learning Environments for the 21st Century: Exploring the Edge." *Change* 38 (September/October 2006): 18-24. Available: <http://www.educause.edu/screencasts/JohnSeely Brown@TWT_CU.pdf>. Accessed: February 15, 2007.

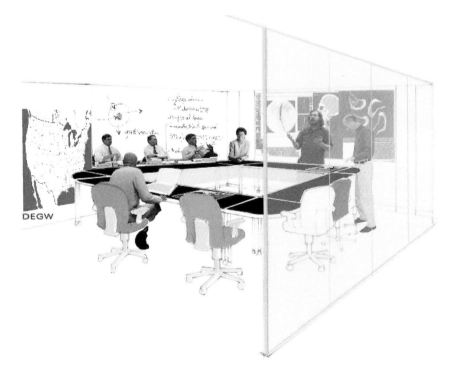

FIGURE 15.2. CDC Collaboratory Room. *Source:* DEGW North America LLC, library planning consultants, <www.degw.com>.

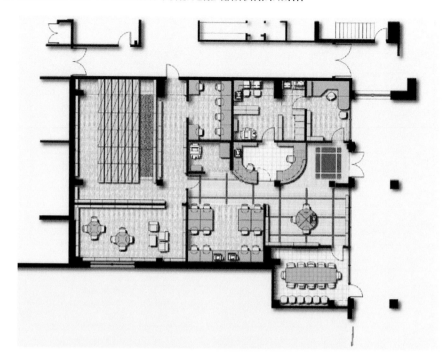

FIGURE 15.3. Greater Baltimore Medical Center Library Floor Plan. *Source:* © 2006 Cochran, Stephenson & Donkervoet, Inc.

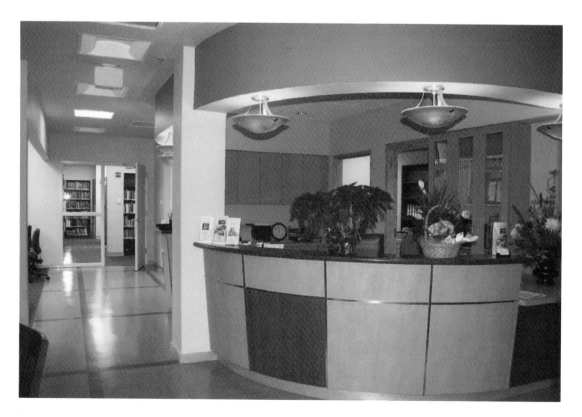

FIGURE 15.4. Greater Baltimore Medical Center Library Information Desk. *Source:* Lisa J. Swartz.

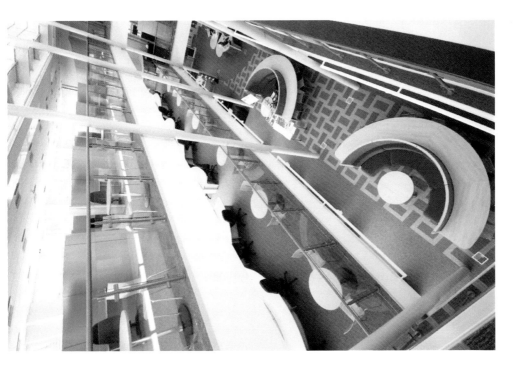

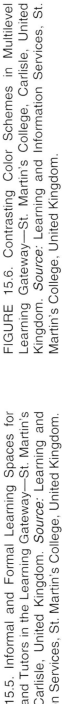

FIGURE 15.6. Contrasting Color Schemes in Multilevel Learning Gateway—St. Martin's College, Carlisle, United Kingdom. *Source:* Learning and Information Services, St. Martin's College, United Kingdom.

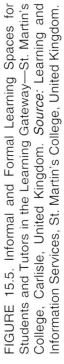

FIGURE 15.5. Informal and Formal Learning Spaces for Students and Tutors in the Learning Gateway—St. Martin's College, Carlisle, United Kingdom. *Source:* Learning and Information Services, St. Martin's College, United Kingdom.

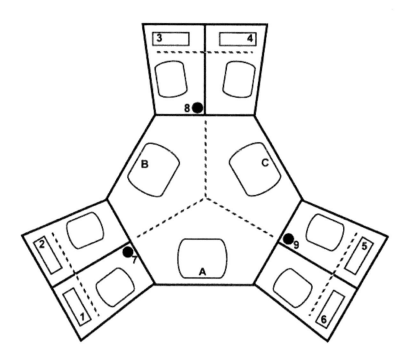

FIGURE 15.7. Collaborative Learning Table, Folsom Library—Rensselaer Research Libraries. *Source:* Collaborative Workstation, 2002, Rogers, Edwin H. (Ballston Lake, NY); Geisler, Cheryl (Troy, NY); Tobin, John M. (Albany, NY). Patent D455,911.

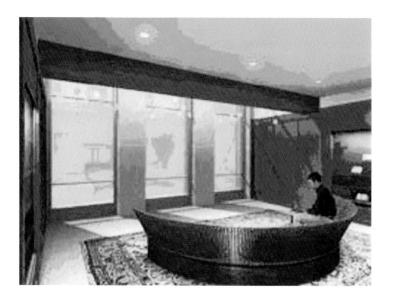

FIGURE 15.8. Astral Bench—North Carolina State University Libraries. *Source:* Artist rendering by Meyer, Scherer & Rockcastle, Ltd. (MS&R).

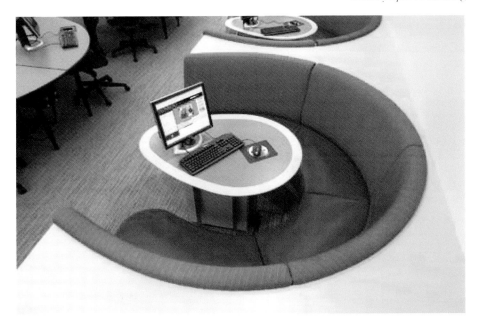

FIGURE 15.9. Example of a Computer Workstation on the First Floor of Valparaiso University's Christopher Center. *Source:* Photograph courtesy of Valparaiso University.

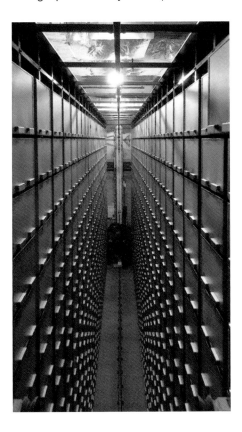

FIGURE 15.10. Robotic Publications Retriever in the Christopher Center at Valparaiso University. *Source:* Photograph courtesy of Valparaiso University.

SECTION V:
SPECIAL TOPICS

Chapter 16

Special Services Provided by Health Sciences Libraries

Brenda L. Seago

SUMMARY. Special services is a constantly changing area of dynamic services provided by health sciences librarians. In the past, special services offered by health sciences libraries might include the provision of nonbook resources such as slides, videos, CDs/DVDs, and realia. However, today's health sciences library may also provide Web-based instruction, as well as PDA services, course management systems, simulation services, audience response systems, videoconferencing, and instructional design services. Examples of newer technologies include podcasting and streaming video. This chapter focuses on the nontraditional services and the role health sciences librarians play in providing those services.

INTRODUCTION

The line between traditional and nontraditional library services is blurring. In the past, special services offered by health sciences libraries might include the provision of nonbook resources such as slides, videos, CDs/DVDs, and realia. However, today's health sciences library may also provide computer-based instruction, as well as **PDA (personal digital assistant)** services, **course management systems, simulation** services, **audience response systems,** videoconferencing, and instructional design services. Many libraries are providing these special services, but, of course, all libraries do not offer all services. Some may support only one or two, and some don't support any of these services yet. There is plenty of room for future involvement by libraries and librarians in this wide array of services.

What may be considered a special service in a library today might be fully integrated into library services in the future. New services will continue to be developed as technologies are introduced. Health sciences librarians will learn about and embrace the technologies, as well as assist with implementation and teaching of needed skills. Examples of newer technologies include **podcasting** and streaming video and will be covered later in the chapter.

The role of the librarian in the changing universe of technology depends upon a number of factors. If a librarian is enterprising and technologically adept, the opportunities to serve users and collaborate with educators, information technology (IT) specialists, instructional designers, and others will be limited only by the resources and organizational structure of the institution. The willingness of a librarian to take on new roles and responsibilities is critical in a world where old technologies are being pushed aside by new ones and will influence the fate of the institution and the individual career of the librarian.

There is no conventional rule for who evaluates, purchases, licenses, and teaches course management systems, for example. The organizational structure and institutional history determine that. The library may house the server, while the university, school, or department may license

Introduction to Health Sciences Librarianship
doi:10.1300/6041_16

the software. An information technology component of the university or hospital may manage the system, or it could be managed by technology personnel within the library. The school of medicine, for example, may pay for PDA software for students, and librarians may teach the specifics of using the software. Librarians may manage these products/services or may collaborate with other departments to manage them. Librarians need to be open to creative, but workable arrangements at their institutions.

Many times librarians work in special services without training beyond that of a graduate degree in library science. The motivation to become more venturesome and innovative can come from many sources: an interest in a specific topic; a desire to try something new (freshen the same old methods); an opportunity to teach a new skill; an ambition to be more integrated into the educational process; a need expressed by students, educators, or practitioners. Many librarians might not be comfortable working in an area that is constantly changing, and others are certainly invigorated by it. Certainly, more opportunities await the latter.

As in other areas of librarianship, ongoing education is strongly encouraged, especially in these nontraditional, emerging areas of technology. Librarians interested in exploring specialized services should find new opportunities to take short classes related to new technologies or should talk to others who are currently using these technologies. Web conferences hosted by the Medical Library Association (MLA) and other professional associations can enable librarians to become aware of, understand, and implement new technologies. Librarians shouldn't be afraid to learn something new, even if it is currently outside the scope of their current jobs.

This introduction to special services is meant to present health sciences librarians with an overview of selected services that may be offered. New services are being introduced all the time, and it is the responsibility of librarians to seek out and take advantage of these opportunities.

PERSONAL DIGITAL ASSISTANTS

PDAs, or personal digital assistants, are small wireless handheld devices that provide computing and data storage capabilities. A few years ago the major consideration was whether to buy a Palm or a Pocket PC. Recently, there has been a "convergence in the features, price and applications of the competing platforms so that the differences between them today are much less than before."[1] Now, the trend is toward smart phone technology, which combines the functionality of a PDA, cell phone, and camera. Users have the convenience of carrying one device and may ultimately save money on hardware costs.

PDAs have many applications in health care. Family physicians and specialists have been using PDAs for general medical reference, such as drug interactions, pharmacopeias, and cardiac risk.[2, 3] Other important applications of PDAs are those involving data collection and management, as in patient tracking,[4] electronic case report forms in clinical trials, patient diaries,[5] and infection surveillance.[6]

PDAs are becoming essential for use in the clinical setting. Students utilize PDAs to record the clinical procedures they observe and complete on hospital and outpatient rotations to provide documentation for accreditation (see Figure 16.1). Software such as drug databases and quick consult software are examined during rounds and at the bedside for lookups related to patient care. Many hospital information systems allow health sciences students and clinicians to download patient lists and electronic medical records directly to PDAs. All PDAs with patient information must contain proper data security and encryption to comply with **Health Insurance Portability and Accountability Act (HIPAA)** patient confidentiality standards.

The current overall adoption rate for professional use of PDAs among health care providers ranges from 45 percent to 85 percent.[7] Younger physicians, residents, and those working in

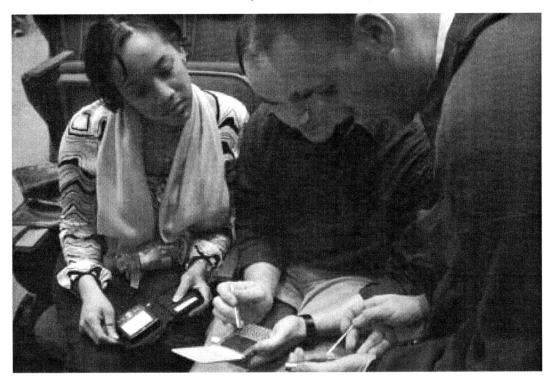

FIGURE 16.1. Students at Virginia Commonwealth University Consulting PDAs. *Source:* Photograph courtesy of Jeanne Schlesinger.

large and hospital-based practices are more likely to use a PDA than are other health professionals. Professional use in health care settings appears to be more focused on administrative tasks when compared to those related to patient care. The adoption rate is at its highest rate of increase according to a commonly accepted diffusion of innovations model.[7] The impact of PDA use on practice appears to be immediate in terms of costs and training.

Librarians continue to provide leadership in the adoption and integration of PDAs and related services. Many health sciences libraries support PDA services,[8,9] which range from basic information about PDAs, to PDA hardware comparison charts, to technical support for both Pocket PCs and Palm products. Library Web sites provide links to resources such as free software, licensed and specialty applications, medical PDA sites, online vendors for PDAs, major hardware manufacturers, and links to peripheral devices for PDAs. Libraries also provide guidelines for selecting a PDA, information about PDA requirements for students, and reporting forms for PDA technical assistance.

Librarians teach several levels of PDA classes. The beginning classes review PDA hardware and software and how to get started after a PDA is purchased. Intermediate classes cover downloading and installing programs and synchronizing the PDA to a computer. More advanced classes teach use of both productivity software and resources. Libraries sponsor PDA user groups, some of which have organized PDA symposiums and exhibits fairs. Some libraries have developed user guidelines and provide help sessions/consultations and even PDA sync stations for users. PDA services will change in the future as the PDA technology gives way to that of smart phone technology.

COURSE MANAGEMENT SYSTEMS

When an instructor develops a Web-based course or a distance education course for the first time, questions arise concerning the evaluation and choice of a learning or course management system. Sometimes called virtual learning environments, course management systems are software systems designed to provide a wide variety of virtual learning experiences. Course management systems facilitate the management of educational courses for students, especially by helping instructors and learners with course administration.[10] The system often tracks learners' progress. These virtual learning environments are often thought of as primarily tools for distance education, but they are often used to supplement the face-to-face classroom instruction. Students can log on and work anytime, anywhere.

Course management systems usually run on servers, to distribute the course to students as Internet pages. Components of these systems usually include templates for content pages, discussion forums, chat, quizzes and exercises, such as multiple-choice, true/false, and one-word answer. Instructors fill in the templates and then make them available for learners to use. New features in these systems include **blogs** and **really simple syndication (RSS).** Services generally provided include access control, provision of e-learning content, communications tools, and administration of user groups.

Librarians coordinate the implementation of course management systems by demonstrating the systems and providing training on the use of particular systems. In some cases, librarians provide technical support. In addition, librarians assist faculty in scanning lecture notes, creating digital images from slides, and uploading files.[11]

While libraries provide crucial support for coursework via course management systems, they also use these systems to provide access to library resources. Links to subject-specific resource guides, electronic reserve readings, electronic books, and databases are ways in which libraries have incorporated their resources into a course management system.

Institutions may already provide a course management product. Some of the best-known commercially available learning management systems are Blackboard; WebCT, which was acquired by Blackboard in February 2006; Desire2Learn; and ANGEL. There are also **open source** and free learning management systems, such as Moodle, Segue, Interact, CourseWork, ATutor, KEWL, and others.

Blackboard

Founded in 1997, Blackboard began as a consulting firm contracting to the nonprofit IMS Global Learning Consortium. In 1998, Blackboard LLC merged with CourseInfo LLC, a small course management software provider that originated at Cornell University. The combined company became known as Blackboard, Inc. Blackboard develops and licenses software applications and related services to over 2,200 education institutions in more than sixty countries. These institutions use Blackboard software to manage e-learning. Blackboard software enables schools to create Internet-based learning programs and communities. The company's Academic Suite connects teachers, students, parents, and administrators via the Web, enabling Internet-based assignments, class Web sites, and online collaboration with classmates. The software also assists instructors with course administration and includes a content management system for creating and managing digital course content. Blackboard's software includes transaction, community, and payment management tools that also enable students to use their college IDs for meal plans, event access, and tuition payments.[12]

Desire2Learn

Desire2Learn, Inc. is a corporation founded in 1999 that supplies enterprise software to allow users to build e-learning environments. Corporate headquarters are in Kitchener, Ontario, Canada.

Desire2Learn products include a Web-based learning platform that combines both a learning management system and a content management system, **learning object repository (LOR),** LiveRoom (chat, presentation, whiteboard technology), and a number of other tools geared toward online education. The learning platform consists of a suite of teaching and learning tools for course development, delivery, assessment, communication, and management. The LOR is a standards-based repository for storing, tagging, searching, and reusing learning objects. It allows organizations to manage and share content across multiple programs, courses, and sections.[13]

ANGEL

ANGEL (A New Global Environment for Learning) evolved from Oncourse, a course management system designed at Indiana University–Purdue University Indianapolis (IUPUI) campus and later commercially available through Cyber Learning Labs.[14] ANGEL is software that enables faculty, instructors, and teaching assistants to use the Web to enhance their courses without any knowledge of HTML. ANGEL is designed to be used in any academic discipline without imposing a particular teaching methodology on instructors and students. ANGEL can be used to make course materials such as syllabi, schedules, announcements, lecture notes, quizzes, and multimedia resources available on the Web from one location. ANGEL allows instructors to manage the administrative aspects of courses by automating repetitive tasks. The course management system also has features that allow communication between instructors and students.

Open Source Course Management Systems

Besides commercial course management systems such as Blackboard, Desire2Learn, and ANGEL, open source systems are available. Open source usually means that users have access to the source code of the software. Anyone can download and use the open source code, and, more important, users can write new features, fix bugs, improve performance, or learn how a particular problem has been solved by others. The advantage of open source solutions goes beyond cost savings. Learning management requires a degree of customization and having access to the source code lets developers make appropriate changes in the source code to adopt it to their needs.

Moodle

Moodle, a free open course management system created by Australian programmer Martin Douglamas, is a relatively inexpensive alternative to commercial e-learning platforms such as Blackboard and Desire2Learn used at universities. Moodle, which stands for Modular Object-Oriented Dynamic Learning Environment, can provide a basic collaborative environment for distance learning applications.

Moodle has many features expected from an e-learning platform, including forums, content managing, quizzes with different kinds of questions, blogs, **wikis,** database activities, surveys, chat, glossaries, peer assessment, and multilanguage support (over sixty languages currently).

Moodle is designed to help educators create online courses with opportunities for interaction. Its open source license and modular design means that many people can develop additional functionality. Moodle's interoperability features include authentication, enrollment, quizzes, resources, integration with other content management systems, and syndication using external newsfeeds. Moodle also has import features for use with other specific systems, such as importing quizzes or entire courses from Blackboard.[10]

Librarians can take the lead in the selection and use of course management systems by learning as much as possible about the various products and their features, using a course management system to provide access to library materials, and becoming a resource for others in the institution.

MANIKINS/SIMULATORS

The days of "see one, do one, teach one" are over. Changes in medical practice that limit instruction time and patient availability, the expanding options for diagnosis and management, advances in technology, and possible malpractice suits are all contributing to greater use of simulation technology in medical education. Accreditation in surgical subspecialties and proving competence using particular medical devices is also driving increased use of simulation. Most hospitals and medical centers are considering the establishment of simulation centers if they do not currently have them.

There are many new roles that librarians can play in regard to simulation. Health sciences librarians have been involved in the inventorying of simulation equipment across departments and disciplines and with the planning of new simulation centers, sometimes to be located within libraries. Simulation centers can take up much-needed space for staff, collections, and users in libraries. On the other hand, librarians can view simulation centers in libraries as an opportunity to work more closely with medical curriculum specialists, faculty, and students, as well as to bring more users into the library. Librarians have a vital role to play in assisting faculty with research related to simulation, outcomes, the reduction of medical errors, and patient safety. Libraries may not only physically house simulators, but librarians may be active in scheduling of the simulators for use in the curriculum or in requesting repair or maintenance of simulation equipment.

Simulators are used in teaching medical, dental, nursing, pharmacy, and allied health care students, as well as practicing physicians, nurses, and other health care professionals (see Figure 16.2). Many hospitals and academic medical centers are interested in utilizing simulators for training related to patient safety.[15] Simulators are currently being used extensively in the areas of laparoscopic techniques,[16] cardiovascular disease,[17] and anesthesiology.[18]

There are a number of resources available that can be used for simulation:

1. Human patient simulators are available that blink, breathe, and have a heartbeat and pulse. Human patient simulators in health care training are used as educational tools for conveying knowledge, teaching technical skills, drill training, and human factors training for single or multidisciplinary groups.
2. A simulated clinical environment, such as a simulated ICU/emergency room bay or a simulated operating room, may provide equipment for intubation, intravenous lines, suction, a crash cart, sterile technique, surgical team roles and communication, or patient safety in the operating room.
3. Virtual procedure stations are computer-controlled simulation devices that may be used for bronchoscopy, colonoscopy, or flexible sigmoidoscopy. Learners move dials or handpieces exactly as they would with a real scope, following their movements in real time on a detailed computer screen image of the lungs or colon.

4. Electronic health records enable patients to be tracked and health care providers to be alerted to patients' needs. Sample electronic health records can be used to practice clinical decision-making.
5. Performance recording utilizes video cameras and microphones with connections to wide screen monitors in conference rooms. Observers can watch a learning activity and offer feedback. Learners can watch recordings of their performance and identify opportunities for improvement.
6. Standardized patients are trained individuals who can be used in a variety of contexts to simulate a set of symptoms or problems within a health care environment or exam situation.
7. Human cadavers are used as simulators for a variety of disciplines. Plastic surgery interns might use cadavers to practice suture skills, neurosurgery residents could use cadavers to practice procedures on the head and brain, and otolaryngologists use cadavers for simulating complicated ear surgeries, for example.

Simulators will play a more important role in educating health sciences students and residents in the future before they have the opportunity to work on real patients. Health sciences librarians need to be involved at the planning stages, if possible, and be integrated into the educational team.

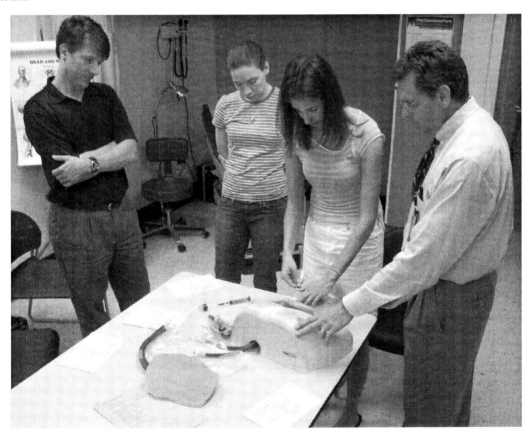

FIGURE 16.2. Instruction of Proper Central Line Placement Using Manikin. *Source:* Photograph courtesy of Dan Han.

AUDIENCE RESPONSE SYSTEMS

Audience response systems use wireless technology to interactively assess an audience's knowledge or opinions during a presentation. The audience response system (ARS) is also known as audience voting, keypad voting, audience keypads, and game show voting. In response to questions posed by the presenter, users operate wireless keypads to submit answers (see Figure 16.3). The responses are pooled and integrated with the presentation software, so presenters are able to instantly display live results for the entire audience.

Librarians have taken advantage of ARS technology in teaching informatics and information literacy[19] classes; many have become experts in the use of this technology. Libraries that have purchased portable ARS systems check them out to faculty, staff, and students for use throughout the hospital or medical center.

There are many applications for audience response systems. They include general opinion polling for presentation support, employee surveys, training, market research, learning through game shows, and parliamentary type electronic voting. The main application of audience response systems for teaching is in the classroom to make a lecture or presentation more interactive or to gauge the knowledge of a class as a lecture is presented. In this way, audience response systems can be used for formative assessment during class or for summative assessment for grading.

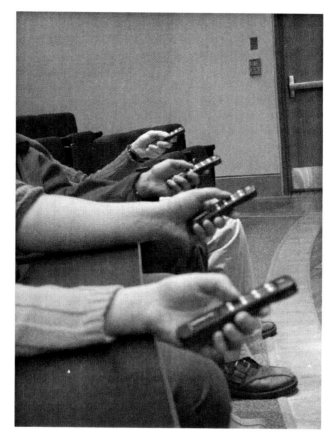

FIGURE 16.3. Audience Response System Keypads Used by Students. *Source:* Photograph courtesy of Jeanne Schlesinger.

There are two primary technologies for wireless voting: infrared and radio frequency. This refers to the methodology for data communications between a base station and its keypads. Infrared is an older and lower cost technology. Its limitations are narrow bandwidth, distance, and "line of sight." If the distance between a keypad and a base station is more than about fifty feet, using a radio technology product might be a better option. Depending on the manufacturer, most radio frequency products can support more users and can also tally the results much faster than the infrared systems. Radio frequency products come with either single-digit voting or multi-digit voting. Multi-digit capability allows the user to do things that could not be done previously with most audience response systems. For example, multi-digit voting would allow users to enter all of the choices that apply or to rank order dozens of items and actions.

The basic use of the audience response system requires four items: (1) a keypad for each participant (cellular and PDA based surveying is also possible); (2) a box used to receive the signals from the keypads; (3) a projector for display of the results; and (4) a laptop or desktop computer for the instructor.

Audience response systems can be portable or stationery. Portable systems provide more flexibility for use, but then equipment and keypads must be moved, set up, and tested in each location where the audience response system will be used. Stationery systems, on the other hand, can be used in only one location, such as a large auditorium.

Some universities require students to purchase keypads for courses in which they will be used. In many cases, students purchase keypads from their university bookstore and then register them online for each class. Another alternative is that the schools purchase the keypads, lifetime passcodes, and register the keypads online. This alternative is more expensive but provides for greater control of the keypads and recognizes the fact that not all health sciences students take semester-long classes.

Audience response systems offer a variety of software for inputting questions to be used during the lecture or presentation. Some software is specific to the system purchased, and others simply allow questions to be input using programs such as PowerPoint, Microsoft Word, Excel, and Paint. Ease of input is certainly something to consider when purchasing a system. Will faculty enter their own presentations? Will faculty need to be trained to use the software? Will staff input questions for faculty at the last minute? These are some of the questions to ask before committing to a particular system.

Most systems have a variety of customizable features, one of which enables the system to show which pads have responded. In addition, the instructor has the ability to display the correct answer as well as cumulative and question-specific response statistics. The systems also have timers so presenters can allow thirty to forty-five seconds or longer for users to respond to questions. Many systems can generate instant feedback histograms or bar charts/graphs. In addition, many systems provide detailed reports that can be generated at the conclusion of the session for presenters to review.

VIDEOCONFERENCING

Videoconferencing uses digital compression of audio and video streams in real time to conduct classes or conferences between two or more participants at different locations using computer networks to transmit the audio and video data. This can provide students and others the opportunity to learn by participating in a live two-way communication environment. Teachers and lecturers from all over the world can be brought to classes in rural areas, veterans hospitals across town, or remote campuses.

Health sciences librarians play several different roles with videoconferencing. In large hospital systems, librarians set up videoconferences between system hospitals to conduct administrative meetings and to save commuting time (see Figure 16.4). Sometimes they back up the technical person and sometimes the librarian is the one primarily responsible for the videoconference. This gives the librarians visibility and allows them to offer resources or other library services to users as well. In health sciences libraries, distance education students come to classrooms that have been linked to distant sites via videoconference.[20] Often, librarians set up the videoconferences because the facilities are housed in libraries, and because librarians possess the technical abilities to troubleshoot problems.

Most health sciences libraries that provide videoconferencing capabilities use multipoint videoconferencing and connect with either IP (Internet protocol) or ISDN (Integrated Services Digital Network) lines. IP videoconferencing has the advantage of providing higher quality images at a lower cost (if the IP infrastructure is already in place). The disadvantage of IP is that network traffic can degrade image quality. The advantage of using ISDN videoconferencing is that a dedicated line is being used; the disadvantage is that it is much more expensive than using IP.

Multipoint or simultaneous videoconferencing among three or more remote points is possible by means of a Multipoint Control Unit (MCU). This is a bridge that interconnects calls from several sources (in a similar way to the audioconference call). All parties call the MCU, or the MCU can also call the parties that are going to participate in sequence. There are MCU bridges for IP- and ISDN-based (phone line) videoconferencing. Some MCUs are pure software, and

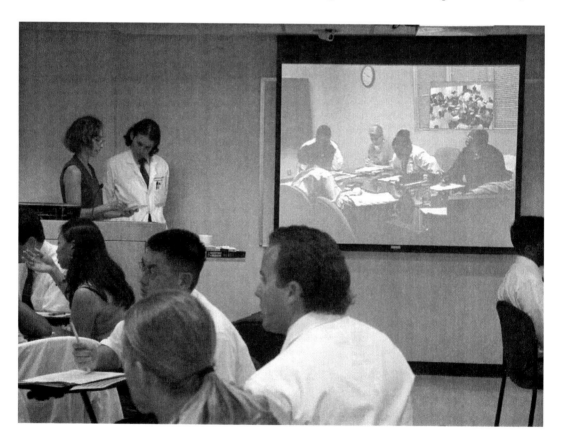

FIGURE 16.4. Team-Based Learning with Remote Medical Students via Videoconference. *Source:* Photo courtesy of JK Stringer.

others are a combination of hardware and software. An MCU is characterized according to the number of simultaneous calls it can handle, its ability to conduct transposing of data rates and protocols, and features such as Continuous Presence, in which multiple parties can be seen onscreen at once. MCUs can be stand-alone hardware devices, or they can be embedded into dedicated videoteleconferencing units.[21]

Some systems are capable of multipoint conferencing with no MCU, stand-alone, embedded, or otherwise. These use a standards-based H.323 technique known as "decentralized multipoint," where each station in a multipoint call exchanges video and audio directly with the other stations with no central "manager" or other bottleneck. The advantages of this technique are that the video and audio will generally be of higher quality because they don't have to be re-layed through a central point. Also, users can make ad hoc multipoint calls without any concern for the availability or control of an MCU. This added convenience and quality comes at the expense of some increased network bandwidth, because every station must transmit to every other station directly.

There are basically two kinds of videoteleconferencing systems:

1. *Dedicated systems* have all required components packaged into a single equipment rack, usually a console with a high-quality remote-controlled video camera. These cameras can be controlled at a distance to pan left and right, tilt up and down, and zoom. The console contains all electrical interfaces, the control computer, and the software- or hardware-based codec. Codec is short for compressor/decompressor and is any technology for compressing and decompressing data. Omnidirectional microphones are connected to the console, as well as a TV monitor with loudspeakers and/or a video projector.
2. *Desktop systems* are add-ons (hardware boards, usually) to normal personal computers (PCs), transforming them into video teleconferencing (VTC) devices. A range of different cameras and microphones can be used with the board, which contains the necessary codec and transmission interfaces. Most of the desktop systems work with the H.323 standard. Video conferences carried out via dispersed PCs are also known as e-meetings or Web conferences.

The components required for a video teleconference system include the following:

- *Video input:* video camera or Webcam
- *Video output:* computer monitor, television, or projector
- *Audio input:* microphones
- *Audio output:* usually loudspeakers associated with the display device or telephone
- *Data transfer:* analog or digital telephone network, local area network (LAN), or Internet

Other considerations include proper lighting and the number and placement of microphones in the room.

Videoconferencing, in one form or another, has been around for some time, and librarians, especially hospital librarians, can extend their roles with a little added knowledge to better serve their organizations.

INSTRUCTIONAL DESIGN

Instructional design is the development of instructional materials and learning activities to meet learner needs. Instructional design is not a technology, but a way of allowing instructors to integrate technology into their courses, which creates an advantage in terms of attracting students, faculty, and more talented staff.

Many large health sciences libraries recognize this advantage and hire instructional designers to be part of the instructional team. Instructional designers have a broad understanding of multimedia and communications technologies, familiarity with graphic design principles, and a specialized knowledge of learning theories.[22] The instructional designer advises and assists faculty and instructors in course design and content delivery. For example, the designer could assist in converting a targeted area of instruction into a more technology-based delivery system, such as a course management system. Other examples include creating a multimedia program using a variety of text, graphic, audio, or video sources; creating Web pages to allow students remote access to information; creating entire courses for delivery via the World Wide Web; or implementing conferencing software.

One frequently used instructional design methodology for training is called instructional systems design (ISD). This is a systematic approach to designing training or training materials that applies to many different learning environments. It includes analysis, design, development, implementation, and evaluation (ADDIE).[23] Using ISD, or another structured method, allows an instructor to systematically incorporate advanced educational technologies when applicable, available, and appropriate. Properly implemented instructional design ensures that specific learning goals are accomplished.

New educational technologies require new ways of designing instruction and delivering course material. Because modern learners are accustomed to advanced technology in their everyday lives, they demand the use of cutting-edge technology for information consumption and learning. Instructors must respond with something other than the same old class notes and static visuals that do not take full advantage of new technologies. To transform content delivery to meet the expectations of learners, an instructor can use instructional design to effectively incorporate innovative educational technology.

PODCASTING

A podcast is the distribution of a media file over the Internet using a syndication feed for use on a personal computer or a portable media player. The term "podcast" is derived from Apple's iPod portable media player combined with the word "broadcast" and can refer to the content of the media file or the distribution method. While iPods may be the dominant portable media player today, an iPod is not necessary for using a podcast. In general, podcasts contain audio or video files but can also contain PDF, text, or image files.

Podcasting differs from traditional download or streaming of media files because of the use of syndication, or subscription, feeds. A user subscribes to a podcast in much the same way that he or she might subscribe to a magazine. Once the subscription for a magazine is placed, the magazine is automatically delivered through the postal system. Once a podcast is subscribed to, each new episode of the podcast is delivered automatically to the user's computer. This Internet subscription feature is provided by RSS, an XML file that contains the Internet address of the media file.

Once the podcast media file is received on a computer, the user can use the media file at his or her convenience. For example, an audio file could be downloaded to a portable media player, like an iPod or other MP3 device, and the user could listen to the file while driving to work. The podcast aggregator, the software used to download and store the media, is responsible for keeping track of file names, types, and other metadata information associated with the media files. iTunes and Juice are two types of popular podcast aggregator software.

Podcast content can be wide and varied. Because of the ease of creation and publication, podcast content can be tailor-made for a specific audience. Instead of broadcasting a media message to a large, general population, podcast content can be narrowcast to a smaller, but specific, audience. For example, podcasting is used to publish and distribute health care education, patient care information, and professional continuing education to members of the health care community quickly and at low cost. Libraries use podcasting for providing monthly news updates, tours, resource guides, and other specialized content for health science students, interns, residents, and faculty. At the University of Virginia Claude Moore Library, the history of health sciences lecture series is distributed as a podcast, allowing users to listen to the lectures at their convenience.[24]

As podcasts continue to increase in number, libraries must look at these programs as possible resources to add to their collections.[25] As an emerging form of digital publishing,[26] libraries must decide whether this new medium should be cataloged and how.[27]

There are several issues coming to the forefront concerning podcasts. These issues are intellectual property and copyright, podcast preservation, podcast location, and podcast standards.[26] As podcasting matures and new uses are discovered, podcasts will be incorporated into the education, research, and patient care publication paradigm.

STREAMING VIDEO

Streaming video is any video that is delivered over the Internet. The video is not downloaded while it is being played but is received as a constant stream of compressed information. The video is played on a media player on the computer as it arrives over the network and the content is uncompressed. The rates of data connection determine the quality of the streaming video. High bandwidth and an uncongested network are needed to view the video without delays or jerkiness and to hear the audio without distortion.

Streaming video is utilized to deliver many types of information, including news clips, movie trailers, and other entertainment promotions as well as course content. Streaming video is perhaps the latest format for what was previously delivered to users as videotapes. In the past, media or audiovisual (AV) sections of health sciences libraries may have collected videocassettes, catalogued them, and either circulated them to users or kept them in a reserve collection.

The Spencer S. Eccles Health Sciences Library at the University of Utah is just one of the libraries to report that it has offered streaming media and on-demand video services since 2000. They believe the library's role is "to select, preserve, disseminate, and sometimes produce the best information sources available and make those accesible to patrons. Information collections and services must now include streaming video."[28]

CONCLUSION

The integration of innovative special services into libraries is challenging, but it provides a strong value-added component and prevents the library from being marginalized by IT departments and other service institutions. A library that is technologically innovative and well integrated into instruction helps an institution to attract better students, superior staff, and more talented faculty. And, an open attitude toward technology and a track record of innovation provides a librarian with increased opportunities for advancement.

A Day in the Life of a Special Services Librarian

Name: Nancy Lombardo, MLS
Position: Systems Librarian, Spencer S. Eccles Health Sciences Library, University of Utah

Job description: Manage the IT staff for the library and the adjoining Health Sciences Education Building (HSEB). The library manages its own network, provides public computing in both the library and the HSEB, manages the technology for more than forty classrooms in the HSEB, as well as maintains the wireless network for both buildings. Also, manage the digital video studio, teach technology classes, and act as project manager of NOVEL: the Neuro-Ophthalmology Virtual Education Library, a discipline-specific digital repository.

Sample Day

8 a.m.–12 noon
- Call neuro-ophthalmologist in Pennsylvania to discuss adding his materials to NOVEL.
- Respond to voice mail by setting up video recording session later in the week.
- Receive visit from librarian; allay fears over early daylight savings time.
- Receive help call from colleague; configure dual monitors at her workstation.
- Meet with video studio manager to discuss upcoming custom video events.
- Reschedule existing video event to accommodate nursing faculty request.
- Review performance evaluations from two of the eleven staff who are supposed to have submitted their self-assessments.
- Work with financial analyst to complete closure of National Library of Medicine (NLM) grant account.
- Order some specialized equipment for upcoming dermatology video shoot.
- Type up and send out minutes from Technical Support Team meeting last week.
- Collect names and IPs for all staff using digital asset management (DAM) server and request software upgrade for all to accommodate the latest server upgrade.
- Plan for, then meet with director to discuss report on distance education needs; also discuss staff and faculty equipment needs.
- Investigate (online) latest options for PDAs for all faculty.
- Work with reference librarian to experiment with Meebo as possible reference IM option.
- Check with technician on progress on animation for the NOVEL project.
- Meet with systems administrator to be sure that all faculty and staff are set up on the new workstation back-up program; discuss other current issues.

12:30 p.m.–5:30 p.m.
- Look for batteries for older PDAs in use for our course for the pediatric rotation of third-year medical students, as our request for funding for new devices has been denied.
- Grade assignments from twenty students taking my online information literacy course.
- Attend Outreach Team meeting.
- Attend DAM users group meeting with main campus library staff.
- Send in evaluations on presenters at recent conference where I was moderator.
- Using DAM, edit metadata on ten records in NOVEL, adding links to PowerPoint supplements to each.
- Reply to query received from NOVEL home page suggestion box, assisting user in downloading video.
- Arrange check-out of audience response system for dermatology block of second-year medical students.
- Send and receive extreme number of e-mails all day long!

REFERENCES

1. "Choosing a PDA: The Medical Library's View." Available: <http://www.med.yale.edu/library/technology/PDA/pdahardware.html>. Accessed: December 7, 2006.

2. Greiver, M.; Drummond, N.; White, D.; Weshler, J.; Moineddin, R.; and North Toronto Primary Care Research Network (Nortren). "Angina on the Palm: Randomized Controlled Pilot Trial of Palm PDA Software for Referrals for Cardiac Testing." *Canadian Family Physician* 51(March 2005): 382-3.

3. Lin, A.B. "The Top PDA Resources for Family Physicians." *Family Practice Management* 13, no. 7 (July-August 2006): 44-6.

4. Kho, A.; Henderson, L.E.; Dressler, D.D.; and Kripalani, S. "Use of Handheld Computers in Medical Education. A Systematic Review." *Journal of General Internal Medicine* 21, no. 5 (May 2006): 531-7.

5. Dale, O., and Hagen, K.B. "Despite Technical Problems Personal Digital Assistants Outperform Pen and Paper When Collecting Patient Diary Data." *Journal of Clinical Epidemiology* 60, no. 1 (January 2007): 8-17.

6. Farley, J.E.; Srinivasan, A.; Richards, A.; Song, X.; McEachen, J.; and Perl, T.M. "Handheld Computer Surveillance: Shoe-Leather Epidemiology in the 'Palm' of Your Hand." *American Journal of Infection Control* 33, no. 8 (October 2005): 444-9.

7. Garritty, C., and Eman, K.E. "Who's Using PDAs? Estimates of PDA Use by Health Care Providers: A Systematic Review of Surveys." *Journal of Medical Internet Research* 8(April-June 2006): e7.

8. Crowell, K., and Shaw-Kokot, J. "Extending the Hand of Knowledge: Promoting Mobile Technologies." *Medical Reference Services Quarterly* 22, no. 1 (Spring 2003): 1-9.

9. Morgen, E.B. "Implementing PDA Technology in a Medical Library: Experiences in a Hospital Library and an Academic Medical Center Library." *Medical Reference Services Quarterly* 22, no. 1 (Spring 2003): 11-9.

10. Cole, J. *Using Moodle: Teaching with the Popular Open Source Course Management System.* Sebastopol, CA: O'Reilly Community Press, 2005.

11. Lovett, D.G. "Library Involvement in the Implementation of a Course Management System." *Medical Reference Services Quarterly* 23, no. 1 (Spring 2004): 1-11.

12. Blackboard. Available: <http://www.blackboard.com/us/index.Bb>. Accessed: December 10, 2006.

13. Desire2Learn. Available: <http://www.desire2learn.com/products/learning_environment.asp>. Accessed: December 10, 2006.

14. Hatfield, A.J., and Brahmi, F.A. "Angel: Post-Implementation Evaluation at the Indiana University School of Medicine." *Medical Reference Services Quarterly* 23, no. 3 (Fall 2004): 1-15.

15. Hunt, E.A.; Nelson, K.L.; and Shilkofski, N.A. "Simulation in Medicine: Addressing Patient Safety and Improving the Interface Between Healthcare Providers and Medical Technology." *Biomedical Instrumentation and Technology* 40, no. 5 (September-October 2006): 399-404.

16. McDougal, E.M.; Corica, F.A.; Boker, J.R.; et al. "Construct Validity Testing of a Laparoscopic Surgical Simulator." *Journal of the American College of Surgeons* 202, no. 5 (May 2006): 779-87.

17. Hravnak, M.; Beach, M.; and Tuite, P. "Simulator Technology As a Tool for Education in Cardiac Care." *Journal of Cardiovascular Nursing* 22, no. 1 (January-February 2007): 16-24.

18. Scavone, B.M.; Sproviero, M.T.; McCarthy, R.J.; et al. "Development of an Objective Scoring System for Measurement of Resident Performance on the Human Patient Simulator." *Anesthesiology* 105, no. 2 (August 2006): 260-6.

19. Collins, L.J. "Livening Up the Classroom: Using Audience Response Systems to Promote Active Learning." *Medical Reference Services Quarterly* 26, no. 1 (Spring 2007): 81-8.

20. Kidd, R.S., and Stamatakis, M.K. "Comparison of Students' Performance in and Satisfaction with a Clinical Pharmacokinetics Course Delivered Live and by Interactive Videoconferencing." *American Journal of Pharmacy Education* 70, no. 1 (February 15, 2006): 10.

21. Barlow, J.; Peter, P.; and Barlow, L. *Smart Videoconferencing: New Habits for Virtual Meetings.* San Francisco: Berrett-Koehler, 2002.

22. Center for Education. Available: <http://ce.com/Careers/Multimedia-Instructional-Designer.htm>. Accessed: March 8, 2007.

23. Veldof, J. *Creating the One-Shot Library Workshop: A Step by Step Guide.* Chicago: American Library Association, 2006.

24. Ragon, B., and Looney, R.P. "Podcasting at the University of Virginia Claude Moore Health Sciences Library." *Medical Reference Services Quarterly* 26, no. 1 (Spring 2007): 17-26.

25. Kraft, M. "Integrating and Promoting Medical Podcasts into the Library Collection." *Medical Reference Services Quarterly* 26, no. 1 (Spring 2007): 27-35.

26. Johnson, L., and Grayden S. "Podcasts—An Emerging Form of Digital Publishing." *International Journal of Computerized Dentistry* 9, no. 3 (2006): 205-18.

27. Ellero, N.; Looney, R.; and Ragon, B. "P.O.D. Principles: Producing, Organizing, and Distributing Podcasts in Health Sciences Libraries and Education." *Medical Reference Services Quarterly* 26, Suppl. 1 (2007): 69-90.

28. Lombardo, N.T.; Dennis, S.; and Cowan, D. "Streams of Consciousness: Streaming Video in Health Sciences Libraries." *Medical Reference Services Quarterly* 26, Suppl. 1 (2007): 91-115.

Chapter 17

Health Sciences Librarianship in Rare Book and Special Collections

Stephen J. Greenberg
Patricia E. Gallagher

SUMMARY. Management of a "special" health sciences collection (rare books, archives, and supporting materials) requires different skills and training beyond the scope of the standard medical librarianship course. This chapter will discuss the problems and issues that are faced by librarians in the world of special collections, from training to the care, maintenance, and security necessary to preserve and make accessible these unique and valuable materials.

INTRODUCTION

Any discussion of rare book and special collections needs to begin with some definition of terms, and it should be noted that the term "special collections" is not without its own baggage. To a greater or lesser degree, all collections are "special"; they represent the unique organizations in which they are housed, each with its own history, institutional role, and resulting collection development and access policies. Lists have been compiled of what materials are required to create a baseline collection in a hypothetical setting, but few librarians would be satisfied with stopping there. Having said this, this chapter will be devoted to three categories that are arguably more "special" than others, while not losing track of the fact that deciding what is "special" is a local decision, to be made with due regard for local circumstances or situations. What is "special" in one collection may well be "general" or even out of scope for another.

The simplest example of a special collection is a subject collection designed to support a particular activity or interest at the home institution. The most common examples in the health sciences setting would be an enhanced collection in a particular medical specialty to support the research activities of the host institution. This is as much a collection development question as anything else and often requires little more than an awareness among staff and patrons that such a special focus exists. However, when the focus demands the selection of materials that might normally be seen as out of scope, or which cannot easily be catalogued within the usual classification or subject heading schema, then there are decisions to be made.

When there is a rare book collection in the institution, special acquisition of secondary source material is required for scholars to make the most effective use of the rare materials. The supporting material will normally fall into two categories: reference sources in the history of medicine (journals, biographies, surveys, and histories of medicine by specialty, by time period, by geographic location) and reference sources in the history of the book, which will include another list of journals, monographs, and reference works, including dictionaries in languages not usually seen in medical libraries (classical and medieval Latin, for example, as well as ancient

Introduction to Health Sciences Librarianship
Published by The Haworth Press, Taylor & Francis Group, 2008. All rights reserved.
doi:10.1300/6041_17

Greek). Online access will probably be needed for specialized databases of bibliographic information and scanned facsimiles of famous and/or variant editions, as well as to databases of general historical interest (like newspaper **backfiles** or photographic collections).

Housing this subject collection can be problematic. The convenience of the patron (and the reference staff!) is best served if the subject collection is physically close to the materials it supports and is browsable. Of course, the local shelving situation may make this impossible or at least impractical. At the very least, the OPAC should call attention to the existence of the subject collection and make it simple for patrons and staff to identify locations and bring secondary and primary source material together.

Rare book collections present many more challenges to library staff. What comprises a "rare book" is complex. A useful working definition of a rare book is one whose age, relative scarcity, fragility, and/or historical importance makes it a candidate for some sort of enhanced care, though "the definition of 'a rare book' is a favourite parlour game among bibliophiles. Paul Angle's 'important, desirable and hard to get' has been often and deservedly quoted: Robert H. Taylor's impromptu 'a book I want badly and can't find,' is here quoted for the first time."[1]

Not surprisingly, different institutions

A pamphlet from 1778 by Benjamin Rush laying down rules to keep the Continental Army healthy during the American Revolution. *Source:* Image courtesy of the National Library of Medicine.

draw their collection lines in different places. The **National Library of Medicine**'s **(NLM)** History of Medicine Division (HMD) holds monographs from before 1914, journals from before 1870, motion pictures produced before 1971, all manuscript materials (both old and modern), a prints and photographs collection, and a selection of secondary and reference sources.[2] Historical Collections at the New York Academy of Medicine Library consists of pre-1800 materials plus secondary sources.[3] Special Collections at the University of Wisconsin at Madison consists of material from 1492 to 1923,[4] while the Lane Medical Library at Stanford University has an 1850 cutoff.[5] There are, of course, always exceptions to collection policies based solely on dates. NLM recently transferred all of its 16 mm film collection, regardless of production date, to its History of Medicine Division, largely because of the difficulty in maintaining hardware. However, the films will remain in the HMD purview even after they have been reformatted and the originals placed in long-term off-site storage.

Items may be transferred to a library's special collections for all sorts of reasons. An item can be seen as requiring special handling due to controversial subject matter or instant celebrity. An example of the former would be the notorious Pernkopf anatomy texts,[6] whose illustrations are widely believed to be derived from the dissection of concentration camp prisoners. As for the latter, many libraries have transferred their copies of Watson and Crick's groundbreaking DNA article[7] to special collections, as it is very brief and easily razored out. The whole notion of transferring single issues of long journal runs to special collections based on protecting particularly important articles is controversial and will be discussed in more detail later in this chapter.

Modern manuscript collections—collections of papers by a noted individual or organization—create their own issues.[8] Special collection librarian practices are not the same as good archival management procedures, something that many well-meaning librarians learn to their dismay when they suddenly find themselves responsible for large institutional or personal collections (see Figure 17.1). Some institutions define "archives" as papers generated by their own organizations, while **"manuscripts"** are the papers of other organizations. It is also possible to distinguish between "natural" collections (the materials accumulated by chance or design by a person or organization over time) and "artificial" collections (when historians and archivists set out after the fact to gather materials documenting a person, organization, or event). In Canada and the United Kingdom, an artificial collection is referred to as a **fonds**.[9]

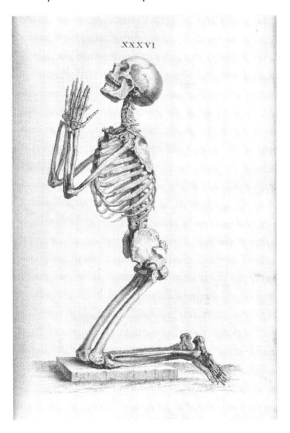

Illustration from William Cheselden (1688-1752), *Osteographia,* or *The Anatomy of the Bones,* London, 1733. *Source:* Image courtesy of the National Library of Medicine.

COLLECTION POLICIES

Collection Scope

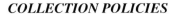

All special collection materials should relate to the overall scope of the library as a whole. If a donor carrying a Gutenberg Bible under one arm and a Shakespeare First Folio under the other arrived in the special collections reading room of a medical library, the proper (though painful!) course would be to refuse the gift (although offering the donor a comfortable chair and a cup of coffee while making frantic phone calls to colleagues in more appropriate repositories has its place as well).

The level of collection specificity will vary as well. Libraries serving medical schools or research universities will have a different scope than those supporting local hospitals or community health centers. Institutions with large programs in medical specialties (orthopedics, perhaps, or cardiology) might wish to develop special collections that support these programs. In this, collection development in special collections is no different from a proper collection development policy for the library as a whole, with the only caveat being that the library must be able to properly house and service the special collection. It is of little use to have a choice selection of rare and valuable books if they are locked up in a vault, uncatalogued, unknown, and inaccessible.

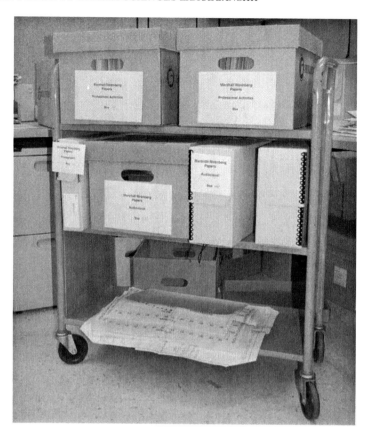

FIGURE 17.1. Part of Nobel Prize–winner Marshal Nirenberg's papers being processed at NLM. Note the acid-free archival boxes. *Source:* Image courtesy of the National Library of Medicine.

Decisions concerning levels access and bibliographic control are also pertinent in the case of archival collections. All other factors remaining equal, archival collections of primarily local interest belong in the community in which they were produced. This is equally true of institutional records and the papers of local celebrities. Oral histories and the papers of local organizations not formally connected to the library may also belong in the local setting, as do the records of famous (or infamous!) historical persons. Again, all of this assumes that the library has the institutional support to make such materials available to scholars and researchers. The papers of a Nobel laureate are not misplaced in the archives of a smaller institution, particularly if that is where the prize-winning research was done. However, the responsibility to both preserve these materials and make them available is paramount; if there is no proper support, the archivist has a professional duty to suggest that the materials be sent elsewhere.

These days, archivists and librarians accepting certain types of collection material may also have legal responsibilities under the **Health Insurance Portability and Accountability Act (HIPAA),** enacted by the United States Congress in 1996. This complex issue will be discussed in more detail later.

The acquisition of rare and valuable materials raises questions of ethical behavior not usually faced by the regular library purchasing department. Items costing thousands or even tens of thousands of dollars call for safeguards against fraud from all sides. The Rare Book and Manuscript Section of the Association of College and Research Libraries (RBMS/ACRL),[10] a divi-

sion of the American Library Association (ALA), offers excellent guidelines for the ethical behavior of both librarians and dealers. The Society of American Archivists (SAA)[11] offers
similar support. There is no space here to discuss these issues in detail, but, in the rare book
world, two important steps are to know the reputation of the dealer (membership in the Antiquarian Booksellers Association of America[12] or its European counterparts is a good start) and
to know the provenance of what is being purchased.[13, 14] Previously undocumented copies of
Vesalius rarely pop up in garage sales. It is also imperative that there be no question of conflict
of interest in relationships with dealers.

Donations

For archivists, a proper **deed of gift** is essential. The essence of good archival practice is the
ability to arrange, describe, and, when necessary, discard (**weeding,** though accurate, can sound
a little cold). It is vital that donors understand this, and that a proper deed of gift exists that allows the archivist to do a professional job. Donors may wish to impose access restrictions on all
or part of their collections; it is the archivist's job to strike a balance between the private and personal concerns of the donor and the institutional responsibility to make research materials accessible. Again, SAA offers guidelines in such matters.

As can be easily guessed, relationships with donors can be complex, and there may be factors
far outside normal library or archival considerations that will affect what is accepted and what is
not. A clearly worded and publicly available collection development policy can serve as a shield
against the most egregious attempts to place inappropriate materials in special collections, but
all archivists and librarians will face the day when the requirements of their institution's development office or some other irresistible force will prevail over good library practice. There are
worse things.

Friends Groups

Closely related to donor relations is the possibility of a "Friends of the Library" group. Such a
group can be a valuable adjunct to many library activities, but it is vital that the special collections staff create the agenda for the Friends group, and not the other way around. Fundraising
should be closely coordinated with the institution's development office. Exhibitions are a traditional way to bring in new friends and entice prospective donors, as well as helping staff learn
more about the collection in their keeping.

Access Policies

Once the collections have been obtained, policies must be put in place to monitor who should
have access to the materials and under what conditions. In most situations, the core users will be
the faculty, staff, and students of the host institution. This does not mean that an incoming freshman should be given unquestioned access to rare materials when a reprint would do as well. In
the liberal arts world, picture a student assigned *Hamlet* for a freshman literature survey requesting a First Folio for an initial read-through. It does mean, however, that reference and access
staff must be aware of the uses to which materials in their care will be put.

Policies for visiting scholars or any potential users without formal connections to the host institution will echo those of the larger entity. However, there can be anomalies here, stemming
from the core responsibility to make available materials that may in fact be unavailable elsewhere. Even elite Ivy League collections, which sometimes close their general collection doors
to all except their own populations, may open their special collections to visiting scholars from
afar who have come to study unique books or manuscripts.[15]

Is there such a thing as an inappropriate user in special collections? Honest opinions can vary, but in the broadest sense, the answer must be a resounding "No!" These are libraries, not museums, and it is the librarian's job to balance the requirements of **preservation** *and* access. The potential First Folio reader mentioned previously should be shown the book in question and given a proper explanation as to why a surrogate would be a better choice. Library professionals who find themselves in the situation where there is nothing to show a researcher (no original, no facsimile, no microform or scan), have failed in their essential responsibilities to both collection and user. A library is not a "look, don't touch" institution.

HIPAA

As alluded to earlier, HIPAA is a vexing issue. Originally designed to protect the privacy of medical records when patients transfer information from one health care provider to another, the law has had unanticipated effects on archival collections of medical information. Are patient records covered forever if the death date of the patient cannot be determined? Many repositories have original records from the American Civil War. Would those Civil War records be covered under HIPAA? What about motion pictures of unidentified but recognizable patients undergoing psychosurgery sixty years ago, where the publication status of the film (much less the possibility of determining informed consent) is unknown? Finally, not all medical library collections are housed in HIPAA "covered entities." NLM and the New York Academy of Medicine, for example, do not provide direct patient care, and therefore are not covered by HIPAA. What would be the status of collections transferred from covered entities to one of these two repositories? In the absence of direct guidance or case law, such questions (and many more) cannot be answered.

REFERENCE AREAS

Facilities

The public facilities required for a special collections reading room do not vary greatly from the ideal reading room for any library collection. The need for good lighting, comfortable chairs (ergonomic, if possible), convenient location of electrical outlets, and Internet connectivity are hardly unique to special collections. Book cradles and book weights to support fragile volumes are vital. There should be at least a few oversize tables for patrons using folio or **elephantine** volumes, or for those using boxed archival collections which have a way of spreading out when in use. Since it is customary (and appropriate!) to ask patrons not to bring briefcases, coats, and such items into special collections reading rooms, lockers should be provided.

Security

Reading room security is a complex and often touchy issue. Security tapes, labels, bookplates, and such electronic devices are inappropriate for use in rare books, as they use glues that are acidic or chemically unstable. It is technically possible to make very small metallic security tapes encapsulated in archivally acceptable polyester sleeves, electrostatically welded shut (no glue!), and dropped unobtrusively in the gutters of all but the most fragile books, from where they could be removed if necessary by a librarian with tweezers. This would not solve all security problems, but it would certainly help. At this writing, however, no such tapes are commercially available. This does *not* mean, however, that security gates have no place in a special col-

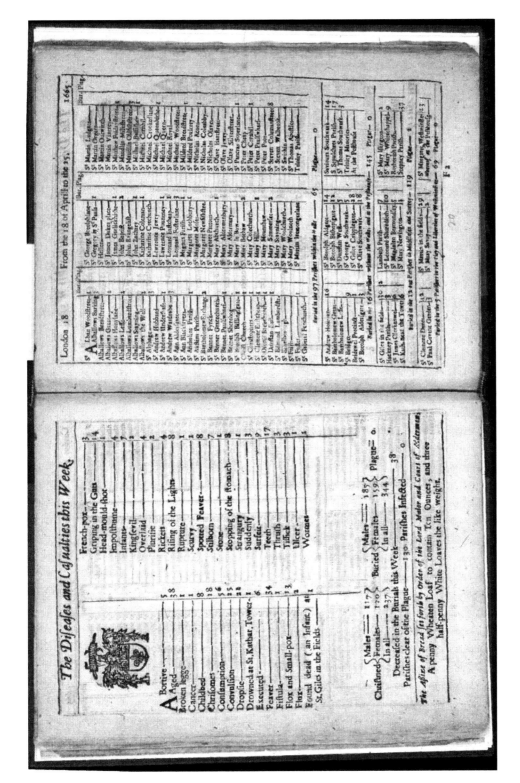

A chart showing deaths from plague and other causes in London, April 1665. *Source:* Image courtesy of the National Library of Medicine.

lection reading room. First of all, modern reference books *will* have security tapes, and (more cynically) patrons are usually unaware that the rarest books are the least likely to have electronic security tapes. To archivists, dealing with masses of unbound papers, such issues are exponentially more difficult.

Security cameras are a useful addition to any reading room, but they are far from the perfect solution for every problem. Modern technology has made available small and unobtrusive cameras with almost unlimited digital archiving and time-stamp searching, but some of these marvels miss the point. Security should not be invisible. Deterrence is to be preferred over recovery. Patrons should be aware that they are being watched. Aside from actual legal responsibilities to make electronic surveillance known to patrons, the usefulness of electronic devices is greatly enhanced by their being obvious. Signage announcing their presence is useful, but even better is a video monitor at the reading room entrance, situated so patrons see it as they enter. Signs are often unread; flickering screens are much harder to ignore. However, the best electronic system is merely an adjunct to a live person sitting at a reference desk with good sight lines over the reading room. The National Maritime Library in Greenwich, England, goes a step further with an invigilator perched on a chair that would seem to have been borrowed from a lifeguard.

Standard library security measures, such as a library card with photograph and a formal registration process, will be deterrents. The special collections patron should not be anonymous in the librarian's eyes, and the patron should be aware of this as well. Above all things, the patron should understand that the protection of the collection is a vital concern of the librarian and not just a barrier to prevent use of important material.

There is nothing wrong with preserving the air of a special space with a supplementary registration procedure. This is the proper time to make patrons aware of additional rules governing the use of collection materials: checking bags and briefcases, pencils only, no self-service photocopying, no hand-held scanners or cameras without prior arrangements—whatever is helpful and appropriate in the local circumstances. At one level, the rules are less important than the clear notion that the rules are logically, uniformly, but realistically applied. Most patrons can be convinced to use a yellow #2 pencil instead of their elegant fountain pens, but few will put up with rules that seem to vary with the weather or the mood of the presiding staff member.

Special Uses

Special collections reading rooms are often very attractive and elegant public spaces and, as such, are in great demand for meetings, receptions, and parties. There are reading rooms with kitchenettes attached, and at least one with a working (gas) fireplace installed at the behest of a very savvy curator anxious to market her collection by promoting its space. There are also horror stories about attending receptions with chafing dishes heated with Sterno® in areas protected with chemical fire suppression systems. In fact, within the limits of common sense, there is little to say against such events. They do promote the collections, and work against the ivory tower, snobby stereotypes that are so destructive to the proper integration of special collections with their host libraries and larger institutional homes. To paraphrase Lucius Cary (1610-1643), when it is not necessary to be different, it is necessary not to be different.[16]

There will be occasions to be different—plenty of them. Patrons will soon notice the lack of self-service photocopiers and the restrictions on scanning. Policies on such matters should be clearly posted and consistently applied. If staffing and budget considerations allow, photocopying and scanning by staff (for a fee!) should be made available. Excellent digital scanners using face-up cradles are widely available and give high-quality results as either hard copy or digital files. Photography raises other issues because of the complexity of the hardware involved. If the host library does not offer a photographic service with the equipment and expertise to handle a rare book, it might be possible to arrange for a local professional photographer to come to the library by appointment, so that photographs can be made under the supervision of special collections staff. If a patron can demonstrate the necessary photographic competency, special permission can be arranged, on a case-by-case basis, for a supervised session. Under no circumstances should the collection be endangered; truculent patrons can be mollified with reminders that the collection must be protected for their future use.

Copyright and permissions policies must be well thought out and reflect local conditions. Much of the material will be in the public domain and therefore not covered by copyright, but institutions can and do make various claims of reproduction rights. These two sets of rights are often confused, but they are not difficult to understand. An original sixteenth-century printed book cannot be covered by copyright, although a modern edited version of its text might be. However, a library is well within its rights to request a usage fee for a published reproduction from its copy.

REFERENCE SERVICES

The heart of any public services operations is its reference capability. Given the uniqueness of the materials in their charge, special collections reference librarians should be prepared to go further than their general collection colleagues. After all, if your collection has the sole extant copy of a significant work, your responsibilities to the public will be increased. It is not necessary to cross the line between reference and research, but the line will require revision from time to time. Archivists, being more used to handling unique materials, are predisposed to a good understanding of this situation.

Interlibrary loan requests will arrive for the most remarkable materials, as though the requesting library actually expected the lending library to drop a sixteenth-century book into a padded envelope and mail it off. Usually, the requesting librarians are doing their best to satisfy their patron, and, after all, it never hurts to ask. It is increasingly possible to provide some sort of surrogate, but the loaning of original materials is usually restricted to their use in exhibits. Scholars who need to consult long lists of original material do not need a Tarot deck to know that there is travel in their future. Fortunately, all but the most inexperienced researchers are well aware of this.

EDUCATION AND TRAINING

Ideally, reference librarians in history of the health sciences collections will have training in both their subject and in the handling of rare books. The former is the easier to obtain; there are many excellent books on the subject, and many medical schools and graduate history programs offer courses that can likely be audited by staff. Rare book expertise is harder to obtain, since hands-on experience is vital. It is one thing to read about **mezzotints** or **incunabula** or **Baskerville type** or **crushed morocco** bindings, and quite another to hold such things in your hands. Virtually no degree-granting programs offer a major in such matters, but there are alternatives. Best known and longest established is Rare Book School, originally housed at Columbia University School of Library Service, but since 1992 operating on the campus of the University of Virginia at Charlottesville.[17] Rare Book School offers an ever-growing list of nonmatriculated courses in all areas of rare book librarianship, mostly in Charlottesville but also through extension courses. There are also smaller regional programs that are well worth investigating.[18]

REFERENCE SOURCES

There is no space here to give a long list of reference sources that should be available to the history of medicine reference librarian, but a few easily available items should be mentioned. No reference desk should be without at least one copy of "Garrison and Morton"—more correctly, *Morton's Medical Bibliography.*[19] Recent articles in the history of medicine are included in NLM's PubMed® database,[20] and the continuing retrospective conversion of older *Index Medicus®* citations means that the coverage of PubMed now reaches back to the early 1950s. NLM maintains Medical Subject Headings (MeSH®) in the history of medicine, and PubMed searchers can further narrow their aim by using the History of Medicine subset on the PubMed limits menu.

Two other NLM resources worth noting briefly are IndexCat®, the online version of the *Index-Catalogue of the Library of the Surgeon-General's Office, U.S. Army* (sixty-one volumes in five series, 1880-1961),[21] the most comprehensive online source for pre–*Index Medicus* material and much else (see Figure 17.2), and an online *Directory of History Collections.*[22] All of these sources are free. It is appropriate to mention here the free list of "History of the Health Sciences World Wide Web Links,"[23] hosted by the History of the Health Science Section of the Medical Library Association (MLA) and maintained by the chapter authors (see Figure 17.3).

TECHNICAL SERVICES

The technical services challenges of maintaining a history of medicine collection can appear daunting, but they need not be so. Cataloging standards are available from the Rare Book and Manuscript Section of ACRL (*DCRB—Descriptive Cataloging of Rare Books*),[24] and librarians using the NLM classification system[25] and MeSH[26] will find the categories they need or can request to have them added. Bigger challenges will be finding foreign language expertise (Latin and Greek in particular), and finding online public access catalogs or integrated library systems that display foreign language diacritics and non-Roman alphabets in a satisfactory **format.** Dis-

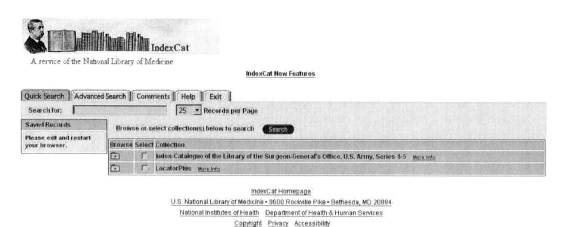

FIGURE 17.2. NLM's IndexCat® Home Page <http://www.indexcat.nlm.nih.gov>. IndexCat is the online version of the *Index-Catalogue of the Library of the Surgeon-General's Office, U.S. Army.* *Source:* Image courtesy of the National Library of Medicine.

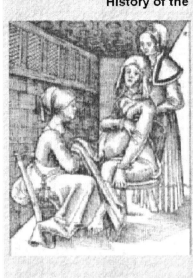

History of the Health Sciences World Wide Web Links

Organizations in the History of the Health Sciences

History of the Health Sciences Libraries and Archives

History of the Health Sciences Educational Programs

Organizations and Museums with History of the Health Sciences Interests

Important Figures in Health Sciences - Their Lives & Works

Databases

Links Pages

Oaths, Prayers and Symbols

For Children

The History of Diseases

Bibliographies/Chronologies/Histories

Listservs

Newsgroups

FIGURE 17.3. The MLA History of the Health Sciences Section Web Links Page <http://www.mla-hhss.org/histlink.htm>. *Source:* Image courtesy of the authors.

playing copy-specific information such as binding details, association copies, or structural anomalies seems to be too big a task for some systems.

Archival and manuscript collections are not "catalogued"; they are "arranged and described"[27]—and weeded, as necessary. Both SAA[28] and NLM can provide technical support in such matters, and coursework in preparing online finding aids (Encoded Archival Description or EAD) is widely available.[29] The level of bibliographic control required (container, folder, item) will be decided locally and will be determined by a number of factors: collection importance, monetary value (and subsequent security concerns), and staff hours available. Since archival collections usually have some sort of backlog of unprocessed materials, decisions must be made about the level of bibliographic control required before a collection can be made available for scholarly use. The situation with unprocessed manuscripts is more complicated than with an uncatalogued book. Put simply, can one justify handing over an uncounted box of loose papers to a relative stranger? On the other hand, how long must a patron wait for a new collection to be processed?

STORAGE AND STACK SECURITY

Storage

The storage and security of special collections used to be a highly specialized business. It is now less so, not because rare book standards have relaxed, but because general book stack conditions have improved. The temperature and humidity conditions of today are far better in most stack situations than they were ten or fifteen years ago, due to better HVAC (heating, ventilation, and air-conditioning) systems, better monitoring hardware, and a better overall awareness of the importance of stack environment. There is much discussion over the "best" temperature and humidity for stack areas, but any set of conditions will be a compromise when dealing with old paper, **vellum,** and a variety of leathers prepared in arcane and archaic ways. Rag paper likes no higher than 70°F and a relative humidity of between 30 percent and 50 percent,[30] but that's rather dry for a limp (i.e., unsupported) vellum binding (see Figure 17.4). Dry vellum will curl and warp, trying to push itself right off the shelf.[31] Sometimes all that can be done is to monitor conditions. Almost any reasonable and stable conditions are better than great swings in temperature and humidity.

Stack Security

Stack security is little different from reading room security. Locks and keys have their place, particularly high-tech keycards that can monitor and restrict access in a myriad of ways. There are also palm print recognition and retinal scanning devices if your budget runs to such luxuries. Cameras are helpful, and so is a well-thought-out set of procedures for opening, closing, and generally securing collection materials. However, the procedures should not be so complicated that staff ignore them. Big strong vaults, favored by some institutions,[32] are useless if they require several senior staff to open or close them. Too often they might simply be left unlocked. There is no security system so sophisticated that it cannot be nullified by staff who cannot be bothered with a cumbersome set of security procedures when they head for home on a chilly and damp November night.

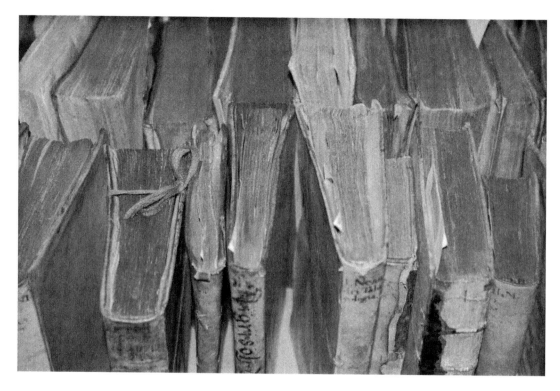

FIGURE 17.4. Seventeenth-Century Vellum Bindings. These books will be housed in custom-made acid-free boxes. *Source:* Image courtesy of the National Library of Medicine.

Fire safety presents yet another security issue. There are many ways of protecting a collection from fire: sprinklers (wet pipe/dry pipe), carbon dioxide, or Halon™ in older facilities; high-tech fire suppression gases or even reduced oxygen levels in newer ones. However, there is no single best system. Local conditions will largely dictate what is practical and what is not. What is more important than technology is integration. Does the special collection space have a separate system of smoke detectors or fire suppression, or is there a common system? Is there a disaster plan in place? Do people know what to do? Fire and disaster drills may seem very third grade (perhaps less so post-9/11), but they will save lives and rare collection materials. Readers may make their own choices, but anyone who has seen films of the 1992 fire at Windsor Castle, where members of the British Royal Family can been seen passing priceless heirlooms out the windows, will have a new appreciation of the word "priorities."

Off-Site Storage

Storage space (and the lack of it!) haunts us all. There is no reason to avoid compact shelving if the structure of the building will take the load. Modern motorized shelving can easily be set so as not to crush odd-sized protruding volumes. If need be, off-site storage (preferably in high-density stacks) can be used, particularly for such items as cataloging backlogs and unprocessed archival collections that will not be cleared up soon. Courier services can be established easily enough, but it is extremely important to have any public catalog specify (repeatedly!) that the library holds materials that are stored off-site, and prior requests need to be made for retrieval. For materials requiring long-term storage at low temperature (microfilm masters or fragile photographic and motion picture film), there are facilities such as Iron Mountain Information Protection and Storage.[33] All of this needs to be done under the supervision of trained preservation/conservation staff. Some institutions can afford their own in-house staff, while others hire their expertise as needed from outside. Not every institution needs its own preservation laboratory, but it is necessary to know where to turn for help, whether it is for the repair of a single binding or the assessment of an entire collection.

Sources for Advice

All this may seem daunting, but a librarian need not be alone. Resources available through the Rare Book and Manuscript Section of ACRL, the Society of American Archivists, and the History of the Health Sciences Section of MLA have been mentioned previously in this chapter. In addition, the history of medicine special collections librarian should be familiar with two other professional organizations: Archivists and Librarians in the History of the Health Sciences (ALHHS)[34] and the American Association for the History of Medicine (AAHM).[35] Other organizations and LISTSERVs can be found on the MLA History of the Health Sciences links page mentioned earlier.

CONCLUSION

Special collections librarianship is a challenging subset of what all librarians do. It has its difficulties and even frustrations, but they pale beside the look on a patron's face when a librarian places a long-sought-after volume or collection of unique papers down on a reading room table.

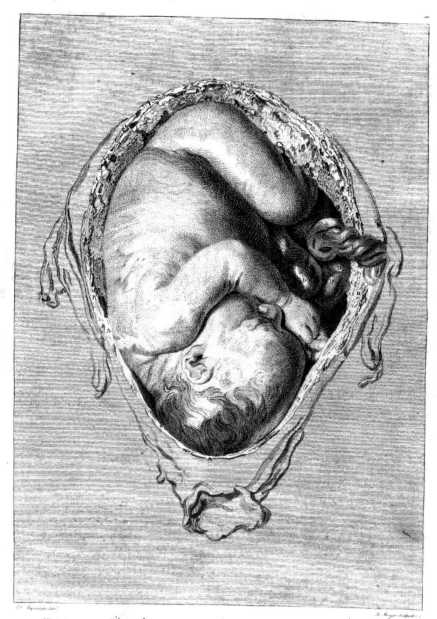

Illustration from William Hunter (1718-1783), *The Anatomy of the Human Gravid Uterus Exhibited in Figures,* Birmingham, England, 1774. *Source:* Image courtesy of the National Library of Medicine.

REFERENCES

1. Carter, J. *ABC for Book Collectors*, 7th edition, with corrections, additions, and an introduction by Nicholas Barker. New Castle, DE: Oak Knoll, 1998.

2. History of Medicine Division. National Library of Medicine. Available: <http://www.nlm.nih.gov/hmd /especiallyfor/firsttimevisitors.html#overview>. Accessed: February 1, 2007.

3. Historical Collections. The New York Academy of Medicine Library. Available: <http://nyam.org/initia-tives/im-hist.shtml>. Accessed: February 1, 2007.

4. Correspondence with Micaela Sullivan-Fowler, December 11, 2006. Ebling Library, University of Madison-Wisconsin. Available: <http://ebling.library.wisc.edu/historical/index.cfm>. Accessed: February 1, 2007.

5. Correspondence with Heidi Heilemann, December 11, 2006. Special Collections and Archives, Lane Medical Library, Stanford University. Available: <http://irt-lanelocal.stanford.edu/stage/services/collections/special .html>. Accessed: February 1, 2007.

6. Pernkopf, E. *Topographische Anatomie des Menschen, Lehrbuch und Atlas der Regionär-Stratigraphischen Präparation.* Berlin: Urban & Schwarzenberg, 1943. For a discussion of the ethical implications of this book within the context of the library, see Atlas, M.C. "Ethics and Access to Teaching Materials in the Medical Library: The Case of the Pernkopf Atlas." *Bull Med Libr Assoc* 89, no. 1 (January 2001): 51-8.

7. Watson, J.D., and Crick, F.H. "Molecular Structure of Nucleic Acids; a Structure for Deoxyribose Nucleic Acid." *Nature* 171, no. 4356 (April 25, 1953): 737-8.

8. National Library of Medicine. History of Medicine Division. Archives and Manuscripts. "What Are Manu-scripts?" Available: <http://www.nlm.nih.gov/hmd/collections/archives/index.html#A1>. Accessed: February 2, 2007.

9. Society of American Archivists. "A Glossary of Archival and Records Terminology." Available: <http://www .archivists.org/glossary/term_details.asp?DefinitionKey=756>. Accessed: February 2, 2007.

10. Rare Books and Manuscripts Section. Association of College and Research Libraries: A Division of the American Library Association. Available: <http://www.rbms.info/>. Accessed: January 30, 2007.

11. Society of American Archivists. Available: <http://www.archivists.org/>. Accessed: January 30, 2007.

12. Antiquarian Booksellers' Association of America. Available: <http://www.abaa.org/books/abaa/abaapages/ index.html>. Accessed: January 30, 2007.

13. Overmier, J.A., and Sentz, L . "Medical Rare Book Provenance." *Bull Med Libr Assoc* 75, no. 1 (January 1987): 14-8

14. Annan, G.L. "Collecting for the History of Medicine." *Bull Med Libr Assoc* 58, no. 3 (July 1970): 330-5.

15. For example, compare the access policies of Harvard's Countway Library (Countway Library Privileges and Services. Available: <http://www.countway.med.harvard.edu/countway/privileges.shtml>. Accessed: February 1, 2007), to their Center for the History of Medicine, which is "open to scholars and researchers from around the globe." (Center for the History of Medicine. Available: <http://www.countway.med.harvard.edu/countway/chm_ visiting_researchers.shtml>. Accessed: February 1, 2007).

16. Cary, Lucius (Viscount Falkland). "A Speech Concerning Episcopacy." *A Discourse of Infallibility* (1660), p. 3. The original quote is, "When it is not necessary to change, it is necessary not to change"—a popular definition of political conservatism.

17. Rare Book School at the University of Virginia. Available: <http://www.virginia.edu/oldbooks/>. Accessed: January 30, 2007.

18. The Rare Book School Web page provides some information about regional programs. Available: <http:// www.virginia.edu/oldbooks/related/>. Accessed: February 1, 2007.

19. Norman, J., ed. *Morton's Medical Bibliography: An Annotated Check-List of Texts Illustrating the History of Medicine,* 5th ed. Aldershot, England: Scolar Press, 1991. The text is generally referred to as "Garrison and Mor-ton," an acknowledgment of the work done by both Fielding H. Garrison, editor of the first (1943) edition, and Leslie T. Morton, who worked with Garrison beginning with the second edition (1954).

20. PubMed. Available: <http://www.pubmed.gov>. Accessed: January 30, 2007.

21. IndexCat. Available: <http://www.indexcat.nlm.nih.gov>. Accessed: January 30, 2007.

22. "Directory of History of Medicine Collections." Available: <http://www.nlm.nih.gov/hmd/directory/ directory home.html>. Accessed: January 30, 2007.

23. "History of the Health Sciences Web Links Page." Available: <http://www.mla-hhss.org/histlink.htm>. Ac-cessed: January 30, 2007.

24. *Descriptive Cataloging of Rare Books*, 2nd edition. The Library Corporation, 1991. Available: <http:// www.itsmarc.com/crs/rare0170.htm>. Accessed: January 30, 2007.

25. "NLM Classification 2006." Available: <http://wwwcf.nlm.nih.gov/class/>. Accessed: January 30, 2007.

26. "Medical Subject Headings." Available: <http://www.nlm.nih.gov/mesh/>. Accessed: January 30, 2007.

27. Roe, K.D. *Arranging and Describing Archives and Manuscripts*. (Archival Fundamentals Series II). Chi-cago, IL: Society of American Archivists, 2005.

28. Society of American Archivists. "Directory of Archival Education." Available: <http://www.archivists.org/prof-education/edd-index.asp>. Accessed: February 1, 2007.

29. MLANET Continuing Education Clearinghouse. *First Do No Harm: Archival Materials in Health Sciences Libraries.* Available: <http://www.mlanet.org/education/cech/index.php3?mode=cdisplay&id=744>. Accessed: February 1, 2007.

30. Ogden, Sherelyn. *Temperature, Relative Humidity, Light, and Air Quality: Basic Guidelines for Preservation.* Northeast Document Conservation Center. Available: <http://www.nedcc.org/resources/leaflets/2The_Environment/01BasicGuidelines.php>. Accessed: February 2, 2007.

31. Ogden, Sherelyn. *Storage Methods and Handling Practices.* Northeast Document Conservation Center. Available: <http://www.nedcc.org/resources/leaflets/4Storage_and_Handling/01StorageMethods.php>. Accessed: February 2, 2007.

32. Some examples of libraries with vaults include the Pierpont Morgan Library in New York City, the Cullman Library at the Smithsonian Institution, and The New York Academy of Medicine Library.

33. Iron Mountain Information Storage and Protection. Available: <http://www.ironmountain.com/index.asp>. Accessed: February 2, 2007.

34. Archivists and Librarians in the History of the Health Sciences. Available: <http://www.alhhs.org/>. Accessed: February 1, 2007.

35. American Association for the History of Medicine. Available: <http://www.histmed.org/>. Accessed: February 1, 2007.

Chapter 18

Consumer Health Information

Catherine Arnott Smith

SUMMARY. This chapter focuses on resources, users, sources, and service development in the domain of consumer health information. It is appropriate for librarians in different settings, including academic medical centers, hospitals, public libraries, and free-standing information centers.

INTRODUCTION

Consumer health information, frequently abbreviated as **CHI,** has been defined as "any information that enables individuals to understand their health and make health-related decisions for themselves and their families."[1] The Medical Library Association's (MLA) Policy Statement on Consumer Health Information and Patient Education makes it clear that librarians have important roles to play in both CHI and patient education domains.[2] However, there is an important distinction between the two. While these two domains overlap in practice, Lawrence notes that "one principle of the process of education is that the educator has specific objectives determined in advance for the pupil to meet as a result of the interaction."[3] One reason for education is to impart a successful change in behavior. For example, a nurse patient educator will instruct a postsurgical patient in the care of an incision, so that the patient can effectively care for himself or herself once he or she has left the hospital. While CHI provision may *facilitate* the acquisition and the maintenance of that new skill, the changing of an individual's behavior is not its primary purpose. Lawrence comments, too, that there is a difference in the "locus of control" between CHI provision and patient education; with CHI services, the information seeker—whether that person is the patient or a friend or family member—remains central to the process; the locus of control is that person's, not the health care professional's. The control question is central to understanding the librarian's/information professional's role: helping individuals keep that control by keeping themselves informed.

One more definition is important. That concerns the term **consumer.** Although *consumer* and *patient* can be, and frequently are, used interchangeably in conversation, the two are not synonymous. Instead, the former term includes the latter. *Consumer* means not only the *patient*, but also the patient's family, friends, and members of the general public. The origins of *consumer* are, fundamentally, economic; a consumer is the opposite of a producer. The word was first used in this sense in a Sears Roebuck catalog published in 1897: "One who purchases goods or pays for services; a customer, purchaser."[4] However, *consumer* in the health care context did not come into widespread use until the 1930s, when an employee health insurance plan was created that prefigured the health maintenance organizations (HMOs) of today.[5] Subscribers to this early Kaiser Permanente plan were referred to as "consumers" because they were purchasing services

Introduction to Health Sciences Librarianship
doi:10.1300/6041_18

in advance of actually requiring health care. Thus, the idea of empowerment, of economic choice, is embedded in the very word.

Just as the class of "consumers" includes not only patients but the generally well, the rationale for CHI provision incorporates benefits for both kinds of people. Patients can benefit through CHI because they can

- understand what's wrong;
- gain a realistic sense of their prognosis;
- get the maximum benefit from consultations with their health care providers;
- understand medical tests, procedures, and their likely outcomes;
- be active partners in taking care of themselves;
- learn more about available resources and sources of help, including support groups and health care providers;
- be reassured and strengthened in their coping skills;
- help others to better understand their diagnosis;
- be validated and legitimized in their seeking help and support; and
- learn how to prevent future illness.[6]

Consumer health is inherently a political activity. Angela Theriot, the founder of the Planetree Health Network (discussed later in this chapter), developed her grassroots CHI movement as part of her "humanizing, personalizing, and demystifying" the delivery of health care services by the purposive application of information to the problem.[7] Notkin, a physician advocate for consumer health libraries, noted additionally that CHI "amplifies the essential medical information that cannot be given by a physician because of time burdens" since "the library gives [consumers] the opportunity to become better informed in a less threatening environment and to ask more pertinent questions of their physician."[8]

For the general audience of consumers, as opposed to people with health problems, typical advantages conferred by CHI include the fact that consumers with access to information can

- make more knowledgeable choices;
- discuss medical conditions or treatments more intelligently;
- educate themselves about good health care practices; and
- learn about the health care system.[9]

CHI IN LIBRARIES

The creation myth of consumer health generally claims the late 1960s to early 1970s as the dawn of CHI in libraries. While demand from the general public had been demonstrably present in hospital, academic medical centers, and public libraries for decades, Baker and colleagues' groundbreaking study of Michigan public libraries, published in 1998, revealed how difficult it would be for this library type to meet the need. While 94 percent of respondents stated they provided reference services in the library, 41 percent found their collections in CHI "less than adequate," 40 percent "adequate," and only 18 percent to be exceeding specifications.[10] "Who is responsible," asked Catherine Alloway, "for providing consumer health information?"[11]

Lynda Baker and Virginia Manbeck, in their comprehensive text, stress the importance of seeing libraries as only one system in a network of interacting systems of health information.[1] Consumers' own sources since the early 1980s have included not only the public library[12] but physicians,[12, 13] pharmacies,[12] friends,[12, 13] bookstores, radio, and TV,[12, 13, 14, 15] the Internet,[16, 17] telephone information services, cable TV, and family.[13] This chapter, of necessity, focuses on dedicated CHI provision by libraries. Other providers of CHI that are all possible collaborative partners with libraries include

- members of the community;
- leaders of affinity groups (e.g., religious, cultural, ethnic, linguistic, educational);
- **gatekeepers,** or "information intermediaries";
- lay health advisors;
- social service agencies;
- physicians, dentists, chiropractors, nurses, visiting nurse services, other health or auxiliary health professionals and associations of professionals;
- pharmacies;
- health-related agencies;
- support service agencies focusing on special populations;
- hospice services;
- funeral homes;
- homeless shelters;
- service providers targeting particular groups, for example, teenagers, elders, new mothers, new immigrants, refugees; and, finally,
- community networks that tie any and all of these entities together.[1]

The consumer receives health information through various communication and media outlets, including, of course, the Internet and the World Wide Web. American researchers Tu and Hargreaves found in 2003 that 11 percent of American adults looked for health information online, but 23 percent sought it specifically from books and magazines.[15]

Focusing on libraries and information centers, the principal venues for CHI are public libraries' journal collections; specialized collections in public libraries; hospital libraries, which may consider hospital staff or patients to be their primary clientele, but can serve nonaffiliated consumers with everything from simple reference service to book circulation to interlibrary loan; and specialist libraries in academic medical centers, which have historically played a significant role in provision of CHI, education of other librarians for CHI, or both. In December 2006, the National Network of Libraries of Medicine listed 899 member libraries offering consumer health services to the public; 553 are hospital libraries, 151 academic libraries, 141 public libraries, and 54 other types.[18] Examples of each of these CHI library settings are described next.

CHI Collections in Public Libraries

Baker and Manbeck cite several advantages of the public library setting, including easy accessibility and a diverse subject coverage that permits one-stop shopping for related materials; the explicit educational function of the public library in the community it serves; and the fact that as a *public* library, it will always be open to everybody. However, the necessarily generalist emphasis of the public library means that cooperation within and across library types is always essential.

Example. The Consumer Health Information Service of the Toronto Public Library was one of the earliest examples of successful collaboration for not only enhanced but dedicated CHI service in a public setting. Founded as a pilot project in the fall of 1991, based in a concept of "informed choice . . . [as] one of the fundamental values for health," this service was begun as a partnership of the University of Toronto (the Centre for Health Promotion and the Faculty of Information Studies); the Consumers' Association of Canada; the Toronto Reference Library; and Toronto General Hospital.[19] Today it is funded by the Ontario Ministry of Health and Long-Term Care and the Canadian Health Network. The CHI service is located on the third floor of the

A Day in the Life of a Consumer Health Librarian

Name: Susan Murray
Position: Manager, Consumer Health Information Service, Toronto Public Library *and* Project Manager, Complementary and Alternative Health Affiliate for the Canadian Health Network

Job description: Responsible for overall management of the Consumer Health Information Service (CHIS), a provincial service that assists consumers in becoming more informed about their health; also responsible for managing the work of the Complementary and Alternative Health Affiliate of the Canadian Health Network <http://www.canadian-health-network.ca>, a nationally funded bilingual network of existing Internet-based health information; funded externally, so responsible for negotiation of contracts and preparing reports for the CHIS's provincial and federal grants.

Sample Day

10:00 a.m.–12 noon
- Meet with Children's Mental Health Programming Group (Toronto Public Library).
- I am coordinating two high-profile programs at the library in May: the first is a lecture by André Picard, the *Globe & Mail* Health Reporter, and Gordon Floyd, the Executive Director of Children's Mental Health Ontario; the second is a film screening with panel discussion.

Noon–1:00 p.m.
- Prepare feedback for Canadian Health Network (CHN) third quarterly report in advance of 1 p.m. teleconference.
- Update CHIS staff on Children's Mental Health programs.

1:00 p.m.–1:30 p.m.
- Teleconference with CHN project officer.

1:30 p.m.–2:00 p.m.
- Prepare box of CHN promotional materials to send for trade conference (EPIC—Ethical, Progressive, Intelligent Consumer) in Vancouver on March 16-18 and arrange to send by courier.

2:00 p.m.–5:00 p.m.
- Meet with Marketing & Communications Manager to discuss developing new CHIS promotional materials.

5:00 p.m.–8:00 p.m.
- Check/respond to e-mail requests.
- Coordinate evaluations (prepared by CHIS librarians) of Web sites for four organizations attending a CHN network contributors' meeting in Vancouver on March 19.
- Request back-up CHN presentation if there are problems accessing the Internet at the EPIC Conference.
- Throughout the day when I have a spare minute, work on finalizing CHN banner ad to be placed on <www.canadianhealth.ca> and CHN print ad for EPIC Conference Directory.

Summary statement: This somewhat hectic day captures my trifold managerial responsibilities to the Toronto Public Library, CHIS, and the Canadian Health Network. Much multitasking is necessary to coordinate programs, make arrangements for conferences and advertising, and keep the day-to-day work going on the various projects.

Toronto Reference Library. Its services include walk-in and telephone reference service and referrals to appropriate agencies, organizations, and collections; its resources, available for in-library use only, include not only typical library materials, but also clipping files, resource guides, and databases. The Consumer Health Information Service is available at <http://www.tpl.toronto.on.ca/uni_chi_resources.jsp>.

Academic Libraries

Academic libraries, particularly **academic medical center (AMC)** libraries, were identified by the conveners of the "Librarian's Role" conference, held at Wayne State University's library school in 1979, as an important factor in CHI delivery, but only as joiners and supporters of CHI initiatives directed by public libraries. Dealing with the public in 1979 placed an additional stress on already overstressed people. "Medical reference librarians are less accustomed to handling the types of questions frequently asked by the public, and they feel unable to devote sufficient time to answer needs adequately, even if appropriate materials are not available."[20] In 2000, Hollander found the situation changed—or maybe not. Of 148 AMC libraries identified through MLA membership, 98.4 percent of public AMCs (and 71.4 percent of private AMCs) gave the general public access and services, including not only reference but mediated searching; however, only 15 percent were actively promoting such services. Private AMCs were more likely than public ones to treat their consumer collections as separate collections, that is, place them in an identifiable location signaling certain materials as more appropriate for laypeople than practitioners. Less than half of these libraries (44.4 percent private, 36.5 percent public) had such a collection in the first place. Typical contents, where these collections existed, were books, electronic resources, and pamphlets; serials and audiovisuals were less common.

In some respects, as shown by Hollander's data, the questions of access and services remain unresolved in AMC libraries. More than 80 percent of private AMCs surveyed do not circulate to the public; even in public AMCs only 35.1 percent check out materials, and two-thirds of those circulate only books.[21]

Example. A prototype of CHI services in a public AMC library, developed with NLM support, is the Consumer Health Information Center at SUNY Upstate Medical University in Syracuse, New York. This center, dedicated in April 1996, was funded through the Paul A. Swerdlow Endowment, named in memory of a man who died of leukemia and whose parents formed the advocacy group Families Against Cancer Terror (FACT).[22] The SUNY Research Center has also donated to a permanent endowment fund supporting new purchases for the center. Located in a separate space inside the medical library, this center is staffed by a two-person team, one nurse educator and one medical librarian. The population served includes university hospital staff, patients, and family members, as well as the general public. Services include circulation of books, videos, CD-ROMS, and anatomical models; the collection also holds newsletters, pamphlets, and journals. Library users can request literature searches and are given photocopies of relevant articles to answer their questions. The shortage of parking in this urban location means that business is primarily virtual as opposed to walk-in. For this reason, the center has a busy Web presence, with a site that features streaming videos, an online health library of licensed content, full-text consumer health books from NetLibrary, and online pathfinders. Reference requests can be made via Web or via phone. The Consumer Health Information Center is online at <http://www.upstate.edu/library/healthinfo>.

Hospital Libraries

Eakin and colleagues pointed out that the provision of CHI services in hospitals relates directly to the degree of patient education done by that institution.[20] The origins in hospital-based patient care means that these CHI services often have a purposely limited "public," which can be a targeted population for marketing dollars. Prominent medical informaticist Masys sees the CHI's educational function as "enhanc[ing] the market visibility of a health care institution" and "attractive to health systems administrators even in a time of fiscal austerity for its potential to generate new business."[23]

Example. An example of a hospital-based CHI library in a rural/small urban center is the Clark Family Library at Mercy Hospital, one of the Affinity Health Sciences Libraries, in Oshkosh, Wisconsin. In contrast to the "grateful patient" or "grateful family" foundation story typical in consumer health, the Clark Library is the gift of a physician family that contributed three generations to Oshkosh health care. Although it is located within a hospital, its services are available to the community at large. Its collection is like that of the other CHI facilities discussed in this chapter but includes historical materials, such as the archives of Mercy Hospital and the Mercy School of Nursing. This facility includes a reading area with child-proportioned chairs and tables; private rooms for health video viewing; free photocopying of health-related information; study carrels; and a professional reading room for consultations. The Clark Family Library has three locations in local hospitals and has also partnered with the Oshkosh YMCA to create a Sports Medicine and Wellness Center, specializing in books, videos, audiobooks, and magazines with a concentration in wellness, injury prevention, and general health. The Clark Family Library can be visited online at <http://www.affinityhealth.org/page/health-library>.

Free-Standing CHI Centers

The Planetree libraries serve as exemplars of their own type. Spatz writes that the Planetree Health Resource Center's services "[sprang] from a grass-roots movement started by Angela Theriot, who endured an unpleasant hospital stay at a major United States medical center."[7] Cosgrove defines Planetree simply as "a medical library for the public."[24] In an interesting reversal of the grateful patient model, the Planetree system was born of a disgruntled former patient's desire to improve the patient's experience through means including the use of information. The first Planetree Health Resource Center was opened in 1981 in San Francisco and, renamed the Health and Healing Library, is still in service today at California Pacific Medical Center <http://www.cpmc.org/services/ihh/hhc/ihhlibrary/>; there are five other Resource Centers located in California, Texas, and Virginia.[25] As of 2006, there were eighty-three hospital affiliates of the Planetree Alliance in the United States, Canada, and the Netherlands, which still maintain an emphasis on "empowering patients through information and education."[26]

One significant contribution of the Planetree System to CHI was the Planetree Classification System, described in detail by Cosgrove[24] as a thesaurus and classification system developed to be easy for consumers to use and more intuitively understandable than the **National Library of Medicine** classification.

THE NATIONAL LIBRARY OF MEDICINE AND CHI

The National Library of Medicine (NLM) has, in theory and practice, served the general public for a very long time. Consumer health questions were being sent to NLM's predecessor, the Library of the Surgeon General's Office, as early as the World War I era ("Is there a connection between dandruff and hay fever? Are germs transmitted by postage stamps?").[27] The library began to treat consumers with new and intensified attention in 1997, after a Web-based survey revealed that one-third of PubMed users self-reported themselves to be consumers, and not the health professionals and searchers considered the "typical" MEDLINE searcher for so long.[28] Awareness of the growing consumer appetite forced evolutionary change at NLM, and the development of MedlinePlus, discussed in the next section, occurred in tandem with the library's increasing support for consumer-focused initiatives. In 1999, the Board of Regents resolved in its Policy on Consumer Health that "NLM's goal is to improve the national infrastructure that supports the public's access to electronic health information" and that its priorities therefore included not only organization and publicizing of authoritative, reputable electronic health information services, but also development of mechanisms to enable public access to health information and working with other providers to make that access most effective.[29] The partner project, linking public and AMC libraries for development of CHI expertise and collections, is the example with the widest impact (see Ruffin et al.[30] for details). This project is discussed later under CHI Service Evaluation.

MedlinePlus

MedlinePlus (see Figure 18.1) began in October 1998 as a small Web site with only twenty health topics; the topics were chosen based on the frequency of their occurrence in search logs of NLM's home page. These logs revealed that 90 percent of the search terms described specific diseases and conditions. The most frequently sought topics included diabetes, hypertension, cancer, and asthma. By the end of 1998, there were a total of forty-four English-language topics; tremendous link collecting occurred during the next two years. Spanish resources were added beginning in 2002. NLM began adding licensed resources to MedlinePlus in April 2000; the

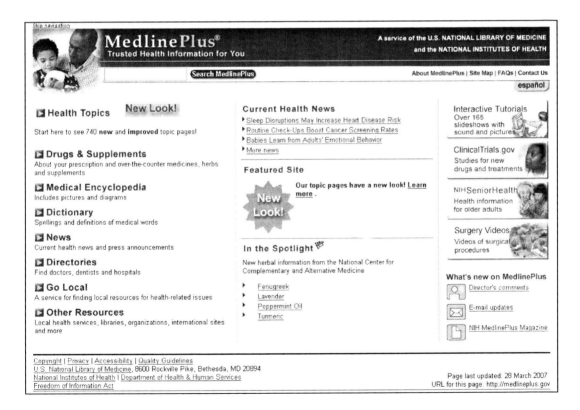

FIGURE 18.1. MedlinePlus Home Page

first was *A.D.A.M. Medical Encyclopedia* (licensed from A.D.A.M., Inc.). It was followed by the *U.S. Pharmacopeia,* a high-quality source of consumer-level drug information, and drug monographs from MedMaster (Thomson Micromedex, Inc., and the American Society of Health-System Pharmacists, respectively); news feeds from wire services, including Reuters Health, the Associated Press, the New York Times Syndicate, and HealthDay; the *Merriam-Webster's Medical Dictionary;* and patient education tutorials (the Patient Education Institute) and Webcasts of surgical procedures (OR-Live.com).[31]

Usage of the site increased in tandem with its resources—53,071 unique visitors between October and December 1998; eight years later, in the third quarter of 2006, 24,800,000 were logged, viewing 209,000,000 pages.[32] MedlinePlus's Go Local project, piloted in 2003 in North Carolina, was developed to give users location-specific information—"Web sites from hospitals, physicians, nursing homes, support groups, health screening providers and many others."[33] In October 2006, Nebraska became the twentieth Go Local site. Figure 18.2 shows the MedlinePlus Go Local sites as of March 2007.

MedlinePlus has received positive attention in the press, including *Consumer Reports, U.S. News and World Report* ("Best of the Web" 2001), *Yahoo! Internet Life* (one of "Seven Most Trusted Sites" in Health, 2002), *PC World* ("the gold standard" for medical information on the Web, 2003), and the *Wall Street Journal* ("the first stop in any Internet health search," 2004).[34]

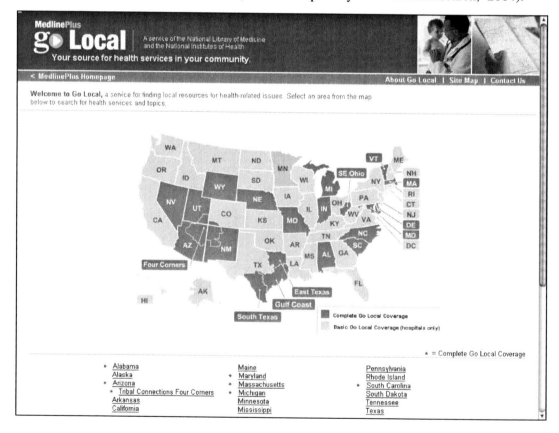

FIGURE 18.2. MedlinePlus Go Local Sites, March 2007

CHI SEEKERS

In Library Settings

The need for health information by the general population—as opposed to the patient population—seems to have been a constant from the earliest days of librarianship. Every writer appears convinced that his or her generation is more interested in health than any generation before it. Williams, a medical publisher, reported in 1934 that health books for the public were "now" a very popular subject, as opposed to "a few years ago."[35] However, in 1921, Dr. Farlow had said exactly the same thing: "A very lively interest . . . in subjects which, not so very long ago, were supposed to be the monopoly of the medical profession."[36] Gillaspy wrote in 2000 that the "occasional question thirty years ago has become a torrent of increasingly specific requests."[37] Perhaps the real phenomenon of interest, attested to by every writer from 1917 to the present, is that health information and interest in health information has been increasing exponentially for as long as anyone can remember, and that no librarian has ever felt able to keep up.

The first research study to focus on health questions in public libraries was authored by Marshall, Sewards, and Dilworth, who investigated Canadian public libraries and discovered that 8 percent of reference questions were health-related.[38] Dewdney, Marshall, and Tiamiyu followed up on this study to compare legal and health questions in public libraries. Of respondents, 70 percent reported that 5 percent to 10 percent of all reference questions dealt with one or the other subject.[39] The first U.S. study in a public library setting was Baker and colleagues' survey of Michigan libraries; these authors found a difference between main libraries, where health questions appeared "often," and branches, where they were heard only "seldom."[10]

In General

Several studies have examined the need for health information *not* specific to a library setting. Since every member of the general public is a potential CHI seeker, these data are also important to understand. Moeller and Deeney in 1982 polled a mixed public audience in pharmacies, public libraries, and junior/senior high school classes, as well as parents of elementary school children. With a response rate of 27 percent, these researchers learned that 72 percent of those polled had needed health information in the past year. However, 38 percent were unable to find it. This was particularly true of the parents polled, 69 percent of whom did not have their questions answered.[12]

The findings of Tu and Hargreaves, cited previously in the discussion of health information sources, are particularly interesting because this study, unlike Moeller and Deeney's, occurred post-Web. These authors conducted a very large random telephone survey and found that 62 percent of the U.S. adults polled (a response rate of 59 percent from 60,000 households) reported that they did not seek health information from any source at all—from a range of possible choices including books/magazines and the Internet.[15] As Khalil points out, there are "pockets" of individuals who actively do *not* pursue information about a diagnosed condition.[40]

Web Information Seekers

The long-running telephone poll research of the Pew Internet and American Life Project <http://www.pewinternet.org> has been publishing health information-specific reports periodically since the year 2000. Market researchers had been interested in health information seekers almost from the beginning of the Web. The Pew initiative, however, has been significant as the first and (at this writing) the longest-running *nonprofit* research study producing actual data about Web-based behavior, including health-specific behaviors. Since Internet-enabled health information seekers are either active or potential users of CHI services, whether those services are virtually based or offered in person, understanding these information seekers is also important to understanding the motives of CHI seekers anywhere, as well as the possible range and impact of CHI provision by libraries.

There have been three focused Pew studies of health and information-seeking, published in 2002, 2004, and 2006, each reflecting data collection in the previous year. The most current of these reports found the percentage of Internet users interested in health information to have been very stable over the past four years; 64 percent had looked for information about a specific disease or problem (66 percent in 2004; 63 percent in 2002); 7 percent, a figure which extrapolates to 10 million American adults, looked for health information on a typical day in August 2006, which makes this Internet activity as frequent an occurrence as paying bills online or reading blogs.[14]

Some recent studies suggest, however, that the use of general search engines for health searches has been declining over time; Jansen and Spink's longitudinal analysis of six major U.S. and European search engines' query logs from 1997 to 2002 shows that health subjects have actually *declined* as a topic.[41] This may reflect the increasing popularity of Google as a favored portal, since Google (like Yahoo) has never been subjected to external study of this kind. But it may also be a symptom of the advancing sophistication and preference for subject-specific health Web sites over general search engines as information resources.

Why Seek CHI?

The introduction to this chapter touched on some advantages for CHI provision that have been tested in research studies and cited by library and information professionals for decades as support for their advocacy of CHI. Baker and Pettigrew remind us, however, that there are competing beliefs about health information, and that theories of information-seeking have to take account of these conflicts. "If information is such a good thing," these researchers ask, "(1) Why do some people seem not to need it? (2) Why do they prefer to obtain it from noninstitutional or nonprofessional sources?"[42] Fox found, for example, that only 15 percent of searchers for health information checked the source of the information they found.[14]

Both the nondesire for health information and the nonpreference for quality resources are factors that must be confronted by librarians and information professionals in the CHI domain. The latter issue is the focus of the information literacy movement. The former issue—people who simply do not seek or actively avoid CHI—has been explored by nursing researchers since the late 1980s with the theory-building work of psychologist Suzanne Miller. Miller developed an instrument called the Miller Behavioral Style Scale (MBSS) that distinguishes between two types of people. *Monitors* are information seekers; *blunters* are information-avoiders.[43] (An alternate metaphor was voiced by Pinder, who used the terms *seeker, weaver,* and *avoider* to describe people wanting as much information as possible; people who were selective about what they wanted; and blunters.[44])

These categories and labels describe individual coping styles, each of which needs to be respected by CHI providers. The sensitive librarian can do outreach, educate members of the public, and otherwise market his or her services to people who may be unaware that CHI resources exist. However, a respectful CHI professional must recognize the existence of people who, even when shown useful health information, may decline to use it.

Nonusers of information services in all domains, not only health, are a difficult population to identify—let alone study. The research picture is further complicated by the fact that information-seeking in health has tended to focus on specific subgroups of a population, or on people who have specific conditions; for example, see Detlefsen[45] and Leydon et al.[46] The literature of CHI has focused on services to Latinos, African Americans, and Asians as particular groups by ethnicity, as well as services to the elderly and the "underserved" (see Collection Development for Special Populations, later in this chapter).

Who Seeks CHI?

In 1997, writing for a generalist library readership, Moeller categorized "consumers" into six essential types: the worried well, the chronically ill, adolescents, pregnant women, family members, and the "health-conscious."[47] Unfortunately, knowing more about health information seekers is made difficult by the ethical concerns and legal regulations of privacy in this domain. The best study to date of CHI seekers in general was done by Pifalo and colleagues in 1997.[48] These researchers wanted to find out what clients of the Delaware Academy of Medicine Library CHI service did with the information. They found that their respondents were overwhelmingly white, female, and college-educated; the Pew study of 2006 found similar results.

Tu and Hargreaves' large survey saw an increased likelihood of CHI seeking in *any* medium, from books to the Internet, when the consumer had more years of education. Women, the young, and higher-income respondents were more likely than men, the elderly, or lower-income people to seek CHI in any medium at all. Interestingly, Tu and Hargreaves found that race and ethnicity had no significant effect on health information-seeking; even the presence of a chronic medical condition had only a small effect.[15]

While few researchers have studied—or, in fact, are even able to study in a distributed virtual environment—the salient personal characteristics of CHI seekers online, what we do know about Internet health information seekers may relate to information-seeking and use of CHI in multiple venues. The typical Internet CHI seeker is younger than sixty-five, a college graduate, more likely to be female, and has health problems, but is more likely to be looking for information to help someone else than for herself; she also has health insurance.[14] In other words, the American Internet CHI seeker of 2006 resembles the CHI service user in Delaware in 1997.

What CHI Seekers Want

Developers of CHI services typically assess their current library collections and their potential customer base to determine what information is sought and what gaps need to be bridged in the existing collections. Moeller described five common types of information resources:

- drugs and diseases;
- coping;
- health care and medical ethics;
- prevention and wellness; and
- "normal bodily functions."[47]

Eakin and colleagues found in 1980 a pattern of questions that has held constant in the literature ever since. Half of all questions in both an AMC library and a science/technology branch of the public library were about specific diseases or procedures; 23 percent involved specific book titles; 15 percent were definitional; and 11 percent dealt with directory-type information, for example, physician names and addresses.[20] The largest American study, by Baker and colleagues, found very similar results almost twenty years later.[10]

Sullivan, Schoppman, and Redman found more research questions from the general public (26 percent) followed by ready reference (13 percent).[49] Specific topics of interest have been researched also. Compare those listed by Moeller and Deeney in 1982—in descending order of popularity:

- Cancer
- Heart disease
- Mental disease
- Childhood disease
- Arthritis
- Alcohol
- Drug abuse
- Hypertension
- Diabetes
- Stroke
- "Other" (sexually transmitted diseases; eye and ear; allergies; self-help; stress; dental; first aid)[12]

—to the "most frequently sought topics" by consumers at MedlinePlus, according to Naomi Miller, Manager of Consumer Health Information at NLM:

- Diabetes
- Shingles
- Prostate
- Hypertension
- Asthma
- Lupus
- Fibromyalgia
- Multiple sclerosis
- Cancer
- Viagra
- Zoloft
- St. John's Wort.[32]

From the MedlinePlus data, the preference for information about specific diseases, drugs, and treatments apparently extends into the virtual environment of CHI. Marilyn White examined question-asking behavior on a colon cancer LISTSERV™ and, of the 200 questions, found that 43 percent were about diagnosis, 36 percent about treatment, and 33 percent were about medications.[50] The most recent Pew study, similarly, revealed that 64 percent of CHI seekers were in need of information about a specific disease or problem; 51 percent a treatment or procedure; 37 percent prescription drugs; but diet and nutrition, as well as exercise/fitness, exceeded prescriptions as a topic of interest. All these percentages have remained relatively stable since the Pew study began asking these questions in 2002.[14]

CHALLENGES IN CHI PROVISION

Medical questions are problematic for all types of librarians and information professionals. The historical attitude among librarians in generalist public settings was expressed nicely by the late William Katz, author of the long-running reference services text used widely in North American library science degree programs. In the very first edition of the text, published in 1982, Katz wrote:

At one time, reference librarians hesitated to answer any type of medical question. . . . A few librarians still believe medical reference questions should not be answered, or only in a non-committal way, such as sending the person to the card catalog or popular index or the shelf with the medical books. No other help is given, because the librarian fears possible complications.[51]

Academic medical center librarians in particular felt themselves unaccustomed to the kinds of questions asked by the public.[52] Public librarians and health sciences librarians have both experienced anxiety over CHI because for both kinds of practitioners it means a change in the boundaries of their professional domains. On the one hand, the public library's traditional user base has been vocal in its demand for many years; this much is clear in the literature. On the other hand, there is an accurate professional perception that a different, and a more specialized, knowledge base helps librarians handle this kind of demand. The dilemma of the twenty-first-century librarian is that CHI practice—no matter where it is based—requires a health sciences librarian's knowledge of information resources, particularly information retrieval, and a public librarian's skills at dealing with a wide range of possible publics.

John Berry, future editor of *Library Journal,* editorialized in 1978 about "medical information taboos" that were discussed at a New York MLA regional chapter meeting. Participants' fears about medical information provision to the general public included the librarians' being placed "in legal jeopardy" and being accused of "practicing medicine without a license" or "malpractice." Most serious were concerns that "most citizens [are] insufficiently educated or knowledgeable to properly handle full disclosure of information about their illnesses [and that] most librarians [are] incompetent to provide the kinds of medical or legal information most often requested."[53]

Professional dialogue about the ethical dimensions of CHI began to occur in tandem with the CHI advocacy, CHI empowerment thinking of the 1970s and 1980s. In fact, it is clear that such conversations had to occur for professional attitudes to change, which had to happen if librarians were to retain any role in provision of health information to the general public. In 1978, an MLA panel met to discuss "ethical and legal issues in the dissemination of health information to the healthcare consumer,"[20] and the Wayne State University conference, "The Librarian's Role," followed the next year. Also in 1979, the San Francisco Public Library System held a two-day workshop; proceedings were published as *The Ethics and Problems of Medical Reference Services in Public Libraries.* Speakers included Rochelle Schmaltz of Kaiser Permanente's Patient Education Division (and later of Planetree) and other librarians representing the Palo Alto VA hospital and UC-Berkeley and public Berkeley libraries. Attendees came from 138 public, academic, and special libraries in the Bay Area; 50 percent when polled stated that their institutions had a formal written medical reference policy, while the other half had informal guidelines. Two-thirds referred "difficult medical questions" to other sources.[54]

As Sandra Wood wrote in 1991, although the core ethical problems are similar within the CHI domain and outside it, "access to information; quality of service; confidentiality; neutrality and intellectual freedom" are particularly problematic in CHI.[55] Here are some typical challenges mentioned in the CHI literature.

Access

One access problem for consumers is the highly technical nature of the information due to the assumed audience for health information. This manifests itself both in a specialized vocabulary and in the relative difficulty of obtaining health care literature once outside a health care professional-focused library. CHI responses to these known issues include work on patient- and consumer-friendly literature as well as development of patient- and consumer-friendly pathfinders and information packages. In the meantime, however, these twin problems of semantic gap and resource limitations can make good CHI reference service difficult.

Quality

Public librarians faced with medical questions, and health sciences librarians faced with questions from the public, not only wrestle with problems of access to material, but also with finding high-quality answers. Dewdney, Marshall, and Tiamiyu comment that medical information has this issue in common with legal information, another potential minefield for reference and information services; in both domains, currency is usually critical for the information to be at all useful.[39] Medical information that is wrong, old, or both can be actively dangerous; both librarian and library user are, on some level, aware of this, which adds tension to the interaction.

Developers of CHI services who want to bring quality information to the public attempt to face this problem head-on by having consumer-focused collections with a consumer readership in mind. However, as Baker and Manbeck point out, this places real-world librarians in a stressful situation "because of the limited budgets with which librarians have to work. . . . Should librarians purchase more quality material, such as standard medical texts that provide authoritative information, or should they purchase more popular materials that meet the demands of healthcare consumers?"[1] Another stressor arises from the fact that consumer health questions, like many health questions asked by clinicians, arise in high-pressure, high-need, even patient care situations; answers must be found quickly.[55]

Confidentiality

In a special issue of *RQ* published in 1991, Dewdney and colleagues point out that medical questions in any library setting are likely to be personal questions; in fact, the library user generally has to give up some personal information in order to get an answer that fits the need. The questions "tend to arise from highly personal problems that the user may not wish to disclose to the librarian . . . or . . . which the librarian may not wish to hear."[39]

This has several pitfalls. One is that the librarian runs the risk of being perceived as a counselor instead of an information provider. This opposes the librarian's professional commitment to information neutrality (see later). A second problem is that librarians who have this kind of personal contact over personal questions may experience a conflict. Do they provide extended, in-depth service to the needy person immediately in front of them, or give quicker, perhaps more superficial service to that person and the ten thus-far-unknown library users waiting behind the person in line at the desk, on the phone, or in a queue on the library's reference chat service? Finally, it cannot be forgotten that the answer to a medical question may be an entirely accurate answer and still constitute very bad news to the recipient. This bad news can be upsetting to people on both sides of the reference transaction. The ethical principle of confidentiality is sorely tested here, but must be strongly held—not only despite, but because of, these potential pitfalls.

Intellectual Freedom

Statements about the quality, or lack of quality, of information resources for the needs of a health-hungry public sometimes mask a debate over the politics of that information. How to handle complementary and alternative medicine in a CHI collection? The equation of "consumer" with "alternative" has been raised periodically whenever the provision of health information to the public is discussed. Dr. Farlow, in his 1921 address to MLA, commented that "the various sects of irregular medicine add to the impression that one doctor is as good as another and thus tend to weaken the confidence of politicians in educated physicians" and for this reason considered it "confusing" for libraries to stock multiple medical viewpoints.[36] Elsesser and Epstein in an early collection development piece commented that librarians had to decide between "the mainstream of medical practice or . . . the whole gamut of medical opinions."[56] A fundamental plank of the Library Bill of Rights is, "Materials should not be proscribed or removed because of partisan or doctrinal disapproval."[57] However, Curry and Smith found considerable gaps between librarians' and health care professionals' opinions on the presence of complementary and alternative medicine in an AMC collection.[58]

Neutrality

Librarians providing health information must at all times be aware that they are librarians and not health care professionals, a distinction embedded in the very basic understanding that consumer health information providers are not educators. "The role of health sciences librarians is not educate or advise, but rather to serve as a natural resource for consumer health information."[59] Kay, a psychoanalyst assessing the consumer health movement in the early 1980s, felt that achieving neutrality is not as easy as it looks; even when the librarian wants to be perceived as neutral, the library user may not agree. The library user may perceive the librarian as a friendly person in a friendly, supportive place; in fact, much of library marketing is directed to achieve this very result. But for the librarian, this affinity may have the importance of an emotional bond, and patient–library users in particular "pose special intellectual and emotional problems."[60] Finally, librarianship of the twenty-first century challenges its practitioners to be advocates for their communities as well as their profession, even while maintaining a value-neutral perspective on the information with which they support their advocacy. The tension between the personal and the professional is one that CHI providers struggle with to this day.

Balance

As Wood cautioned readers in 1991, professional ethics is situational, "and seldom as coherent as various documents on the issue would have you think."[55] Rothstein, in a stirring piece, "Ethics and the Role of the Medical Librarian: Healthcare Information and the New Consumer," argues that some ethical values need to be balanced against each other and sometimes traded off. For example, the medical value of "beneficence," giving the patient the best medical care according to the patient's best interests, may outweigh the equally important value of patient autonomy, of self-determination, and of desire for information in a particular case.[61] Values do compete, and perhaps the best advice to the caring and ethically conscious provider of CHI is to be aware of competing stresses in each CHI situation, construct a workplace environment that permits free discussion of these stresses, and work toward an informed solution.

Guidelines specifically developed for the provision of CHI can be found at the CAPHIS (Consumer and Patient Health Information Section of the MLA) Web site <http://caphis .mlanet.org>, and for health information in general public library settings, the RUSA (Reference and User Services Association) guidelines promulgated by ALA can be helpful.[62]

A 1984 Upstate New York conference on consumer health in the public library articulated these guidelines for CHI provision, which are still current today:

1. Do not interpret medical information.
2. Do not give medical advice or provide medical opinion.
3. Do not recommend a method or procedure of treatment.
4. Do not recommend a drug or alternate drug.
5. Do not provide a diagnosis.
6. Do not recommend a particular practitioner.
7. *Do* describe your role, its limitations, and the limitations of medical information.[63]

The advice of Kay, a psychoanalyst, for librarians dealing with health questions was to see each encounter as a "teachable moment"; to direct library users to people or agencies that could help; to direct them to "literature which could help [patrons] formulate and ask their physicians questions superior to their own" or that simply helps them talk to their physicians better; and, finally, to encourage library users to develop a basic understanding of health, disease, and the whole process of knowledge transfer in health care.[60] Eisenstein and Faust stress that "the librarian is the conduit to the source of information, not the source itself."[64]

Health Literacy

"Health literacy" is defined as "the degree to which individuals have the capacity to obtain, process, and understand basic health information and services needed to make appropriate health decisions."[65] Health illiteracy is perceived as more and more of a problem as health information becomes widely disseminated to consumers via the World Wide Web. Empowering consumers to make their own decisions about care and treatment has a prerequisite: They need to be armed with the information literacy skills to find and understand resources.[66] In fact, there is evidence that these skills may be the foundation for health status itself; poor health literacy has been called "a stronger predictor of a person's health than age, income, employment status, education level, and race."[67]

Health literacy is itself a slippery thing to study because, as Schillinger and colleagues point out, "it is possible that health literacy is simply a marker for other factors, such as health-seeking behavior or psychological makeup."[68] For example, while Schillinger found that health literacy was independently associated with glycemic control among diabetic patients, Rothman and colleagues at Vanderbilt University suggested that it was not health literacy alone, but a direct correlation between health literacy and knowledge of diabetes self-care that explained Schillinger's findings.[69] Baker and colleagues mention an additional assessment difficulty; patients studied may be experiencing global communication problems of which health literacy is simply a visible feature.[1] Whether health literacy is a cause or an effect, there is ample evidence that health literacy is related to patient adherence to treatment (see, e.g., Powers and Bosworth,[70] Roter,[71] Rost and Roter,[72] Crane,[73] Aspden, Wolcott, Bootman, and Cronenwett[74]). The Institute of Medicine's in-depth report, *Health Literacy: A Prescription to End Confusion,* details the costs of low health literacy, including nonadherence to medication schedules, missed appointments, and failure to follow instructions.[75]

Parker and Kreps state that library staff are as likely as health professionals and health providers to need health literacy training, in order to understand the challenges faced by their clients.[76] Librarians interested in CHI provision, regardless of their setting, need to understand the effect of low literacy on the adequacy of their collections. The Institute of Medicine report found more than 300 published studies documenting the extreme gap between patient health education materials and the reading ability of most U.S. adults.[75] For example, the average reading level for the health education material was grades ten to twelve in one study, but that of the patients needing the material, grades six to eight.[77]

PROVIDING FOR CHI SERVICES

Genesis

Why do dedicated CHI sites develop? The literature generally credits activist librarians and other professionals, activist patients, and/or dawning institutional awareness that CHI is much in demand. As the history of the Planetree Centers illustrates, patient demand may express itself as grassroots political consumerism—a response to what some patients see as the dehumanizing process of a modern health care system. In some cases, this occurs spontaneously when potential clients express a need. As one hospital librarian put it, "Hospital administrators are beginning to realize that there is a community need for accurate, timely information which their institutions can fill." The main impetus behind the Health Information Center at West Suburban Hospital, Oak Park, Illinois, was "the frustration experienced by the medical library staff when lay health information was requested by inpatients" and nurses were unable to find good patient education content.[64] In a public library setting, development of CHI services often begins as part of a larger movement to publicize the library's services to the existing clientele to a *new* clientele,[78] or in the service of a new library facility or new collections. For example, Moeller and Deeney describe a public library task force, charged with collecting evidence of CHI needs for a new collection.[12] Mitchell and colleagues recognized a lack of Internet access in their public library customer base coupled with the problem of outdated collections.[79] Nurses who built the Blum Family Patient and Family Learning Center in Boston described the initiative as a response to both health care trends and patient demand.[80]

Planning

Numerous authors describe certain features as absolutely essential before development of a CHI facility can even begin. The first is ongoing institutional support; administrator champions are absolutely "critical" for the success of a project.[64, 80] Phillips and Zorn stress that physician support and understanding is equally important in a hospital setting, where the hospital library and any CHI services provided are just one of multiple systems and services the patient perceives in the institution.[81] The second critical element is funding. Friends groups are often key drivers of new funding approaches; Halsted and colleagues report support from a local foundation.[82] Gillaspy outlines the basic stages of CHI service development that recur throughout the literature.[37]

Identifying the Target Audience and Its Needs

A common strategy is to conduct a needs assessment survey of the designated population, even if it is not a new population. Eakin and colleagues,[20] Richetelle,[83] and Marshall, Sewards, and Dilworth[38] all offer examples of needs assessment in the name of CHI service-building. Moeller and Deeney, in a public library setting, sent a questionnaire to potential clients in multiple and overlapping communities outside the library.[12] Hospital librarians who determine their primary clientele to be patients have the advantage of a known and therefore a marketable client base; Tarby and Hogan used their survey to identify gaps and barriers in information provision to their patients, as well as problem areas perceived by others. From the results of this survey, these hospital librarians developed a core list of more than 100 CHI topics on which to base their service development.[84] One conclusion of a needs assessment may be that patients' families are another target population.[80] Phillips and Zorn surveyed both physicians and consumers, including physicians specifically to address skeptical hospital staff and convince them of the value of the CHI service.[81]

Establishing Common Philosophy, Mission, and Vision to Guide the Service

Pittman and colleagues' Blum Center project took three years to happen, two-thirds of which were spent in foundational activities, including developing a mission and vision plan.[80] Fitting the CHI service to the supporting institution's mission is equally important, since it guarantees that objectives are aligned; it is not an accident that the Planetree information centers relate directly to the Planetree Model of Care, with a distinct emphasis on "educating patients and making them active partners in the care process."[85] One must also allow for the possibility that one's existing mission may be changed by the discovery process inherent in CHI assessment. Tarby and Hogan describe their library's mission as expanding through re-envisioning patients, and not clinicians, as the primary focus, in the wake of their needs assessment survey.[84]

Determining the Scope of the Service

Some key issues to resolve in the early stages: Will there be materials for children and/or young adults? If so, where will these materials be located? Will there be vertical files, brochures, audiovisual resources available? How about circulation? For example, will some materials be available for in-library use only? Will the CHI library offer mediated search services? Telephone reference? Reference by other media?[37]

Planning the Physical Facility

Pittman and colleagues were an interdisciplinary team of three nurses and a health sciences librarian. They offer the most complete description found in the literature of the design issues for a CHI library. Five teams made up of relevant professionals took responsibility for different aspects of Pittman and colleagues' facility; the "construction team . . . tapped into the embedded knowledge of architects, designers, and craftsman to create a library that reflects the long history of the hospital."[80] Design of CHI service facilities requires thinking about not only furniture (seven wheelchair-accessible terminals; a welcoming reference desk, in Pittman's case) but also spaces (a private media room to facilitate private watching of health education videos).

Determining Baseline Staffing

Hospital-based CHI services, as distinct from those in public or AMC libraries, are staffed by people with a range of different interests and qualifications; they might be volunteers, nurses, health sciences librarians, or some combination of the three.[84] Eisenstein and Faust wrote in 1986 of the strong need for a professional librarian on staff,[64] but facilities that can afford staffing by nurses and librarians are able to address patient education/counseling and information needs in one center.

Determining Automation/Technical Services Requirements and Needs

Physical accommodation of Internet terminals as "furniture" has already been mentioned; in hospital settings, it is important to address, early and often, the impact of the institution's network security policies on CHI terminals and on laptops. Pittman and colleagues describe an information systems team made up of cross-institutional representatives of nursing, clinical support systems, hospital information systems and telemedicine departments. This team was responsible for determining hardware and software configurations for the CHI facility's printers and workstations—both those intended for the public and those designated for staff.[80]

Tarby and Hogan used the results of their pilot CHI study in their redesign of library services, having found through their institutional survey that "practitioners were still thinking in terms of a traditional library and physical access to resources rather than considering database linkages, faxes, and electronic communications."[84] As is so often the case, a focus on information technology (IT) within the organization can teach a great deal about information in all formats and how it is handled within that organization.

Developing Policies and Procedures

It is also important to develop and articulate policies and procedures that support the mission and the staffing levels that have been determined. Concerns about staff liability should be addressed early, since this has repeatedly been cited as an obstacle for public and health sciences librarians alike. Work on policies generally incorporates a discussion of disclaimers—whether printed on bookplates, signs, or fliers and displayed on Web sites—that clearly inform the library user of the services and the limitations of the facility and staff. Generally, a disclaimer includes a statement that the information provided is not intended to replace consultation with a health care professional. Examples of common CHI disclaimers for use in library books, on Web sites, and on signage can be found at the CAPHIS Web site <http://caphis.mlanet.org/resources/ disclaimers.html>.

Planning for Special Populations

Planning CHI facilities for particular kinds of people is well documented in the library literature, and these efforts can serve as models not just for "special" groups but for good, targeted facility development in general.

Poor access to health information has been called a contributing factor to health disparities in ethnic minority low-income communities. Ruffin and colleagues' evaluation of NLM-funded projects found that nine of fifty-three projects specifically addressed services for racial and ethnic minorities; seven addressed senior citizens.[30] Two ethnic groups have received particular attention—Latinos[86-88] and African Americans.[89] Detlefsen[45] and Broering and colleagues have also written about the elderly.[90, 91] Detlefsen comments that while senior citizens (the "young-old," sixty-five to seventy-nine, and the "old-old" of eighty years and older) have been found to have health literacy problems, they are not necessarily uninterested in health information; their preferred sources range from health care providers and family members to mass media and the Internet.[45] Finally, Halsted and colleagues described an Asian CHI effort in Texas.[82]

Hartel and Mehling's article, "Consumer Health Services and Collections for Hispanics," remains an important review of considerations of this specific group. This piece could be used as a template for any collection and service-building initiatives in CHI, but particularly for those focusing on specific populations. The authors suggest identifying these resources:

- Helpful organizations representing not only consumers but health care practitioners that specialize in the particular group
- ALA documents written by ALA task forces, committees, etc., typically made up of librarian practitioners with expertise in serving the population
- Challenges and factors that are unique to, or particularly present in, the group's members[86]

Typical CHI Services

Commonly described CHI services include mediated searching, reference assistance, physician referral,[92] consumer-oriented bibliographic instruction and/or workshops,[79] telephone reference service, interlibrary loan and document delivery,[10] lecture series, support groups,[93] provision of information packets to patients,[94] health information "kiosks" at various locations in the community,[82] and developing and maintaining useful Web sites to reach a remote audience while publicizing the service to those less remote who may not know what CHI is and what it does.[78] CHI facilities in public AMC libraries were more likely than private AMC libraries (65 percent versus 20 percent) to circulate materials to the public, and 61 percent versus 14 percent circulated only books. Although every AMC library surveyed by Hollander provided ready reference services in person and virtually all did by phone (93 percent versus 97 percent), fewer included in-depth research services (83 percent versus 58 percent). Mediated searching revealed the greatest gap between public and private CHI services in these libraries, with 90 percent of public but only 59 percent of private libraries providing this kind of assistance.[21]

Collection Development for CHI

The core of CHI services remains the consumer-friendly collection, which has occupied the attention of librarians in every setting where consumer health information is provided, largely because it has to differ from collections of both public and medical libraries. Core principles of collection development continue to apply in CHI collections, with a few key differences that will be discussed in this section.

E. G. Wigmore first wrote about "health books for public libraries" for *Library Journal* on May 1, 1933.[95] Bibliographies for medical reference work with the public focused largely on useful reference sources (then, as today, dictionaries; encyclopedias; directories; and texts on medical subjects thought appropriate for the layman, such as public health, nutrition, hospitals and pharmacology).[96] By 1978, however, John Cormier could write, also for *Library Journal*, that he felt "more justified in giving the layman the latest medical texts" and published a list of twenty-five medical books for public libraries, each a medical text in a particular specialty, plus a medical dictionary (*Stedman's*) and the *Physician's Desk Reference*.[97]

A classic guide to collection development for consumers, which still reads well today, was written by Lionelle Elsesser and Howard Epstein. Their advice was to move beyond the "cookbook" approach of the earlier era and try instead to match the target population's own specific needs to the collection. The stages of collection development identified include these:

- Developing written goals and objectives
- Determining access policies—users, level of service, types of materials
- Defining content of the collection
- Identifying needs of the target population and frequent causes of hospitalization—using such sources as demographics from the census; health care literature; other community resources; and polling health care providers
- Using selection tools[98]

In addition to these suggestions, Hartel and Mehling add that librarians need to agree on selection criteria.[86]

Hollander's extensive survey of CHI sites in AMC libraries found the typical CHI collection of 2000 to consist of books, electronic resources, and pamphlets, with less focus on serials and audiovisual materials.[21] For example, Pifalo and colleagues describe their service at the Delaware Academy of Medicine as offering "700 consumer-oriented books, 20 consumer-oriented journals, a referral and clipping file" and access to a consumer database.[48] Pittman and colleagues' hospital-based CHI service features not only books, pamphlets, brochures, and periodicals, but also videos, audiotapes, and software.[80]

Baker and Manbeck discussed the ways in which CHI collection development differs from the process in other kinds of libraries. The generic collection development policy that exists in a public library, for example, cannot effectively address health information that changes regularly; plus, a threat of litigation is going to be present in health information provision that is not a factor in other situations. These authors caution that a collection development policy tailored to fit the particular mission, target population, and needs of CHI can help address these problems before they arise.[1] Elsesser and Epstein also wrote that a health information collection should not ever be considered a "finished work," but instead a "work in progress."[56] This was particularly true because of the heightened need for evaluation and re-evaluation of materials in CHI; Eakin and colleagues pointed out, long before the World Wide Web presented even more problems, that there was no reviewing mechanism for CHI texts with which a librarian collection developer could assess quality.[20]

Hartel and Mehling[86] suggest the following criteria, which are familiar across library types and collections, but need to be applied in CHI settings with a CHI focus:

- *Availability* (i.e., ordered easily; accessible on Web)
- *Audience* ("generally written for consumers")

These authors comment that given the broad definition of *consumer,* a "varied" educational level needs to be assumed, and that the suitability of particular resources for particular age groups or reading levels needs to be part of the decision. Baker and Manbeck add that precisely because low literacy has been linked to poor health outcomes, reading level is even more important in a CHI collection than in other places.[1]

- *Timeliness* (for Web-based resources this means that links are live; for print, that the information is current and publication dates contemporary)[1]

The outdated demographics of medical books in many public libraries has incentivized numerous CHI efforts over the years.[79]

Baker and Manbeck point out that traditional selection tools in CHI are a mix of materials focused on patient education, and those focused on library resources.[1] Cosgrove writes that in the consumer advocate Planetree System, title recommendations from both patients and practitioners are used as input into selection decisions, as well as data showing library user interest in particular topics.[24]

It is common practice for librarians to become familiar with publishers' catalogs and Web sites; in dealing with consumers, it also pays to get to know publishers of patient education pamphlets. These companies often produce posters of human anatomy, plastic models of organs and people, mannequins for learning CPR, and gadgets for illustrating disease processes. For example, the Consumer Health Information Center at SUNY-Upstate in Syracuse displays anatomical models produced by HealthEdCo <http://www.healthedco.com/> in its CHI center as well as online. Examples of organ systems available as models—which circulate outside the library—include the colon, respiratory organs and heart, and a see-through artery.

Voluntary health associations, such as the American Cancer Society, Resolve (for infertility patients), and the American Diabetes Association, focus on particular diagnoses or related conditions. These groups not only raise research money and sponsor activities to raise awareness about affected people, but they also serve as clearinghouses and publishers of information. They may have resources not provided by the mainstream medical publishers precisely because these organizations focus on specialized kinds of consumers. Voluntary health associations have informative Web sites to which CHI service users can be directed via pathfinders and Web bookmarks. They also frequently produce regular newsletters, brochures, and glossy magazines aimed at their niche readership. For example, the American Cancer Society categorizes books on its Web site as suitable for physicians/health care professionals or for patients; the American Diabetes Association has an entire store online, and at Resolve's Web site, you can find advertised not only books, magazines, booklets, and fact sheets for infertility patients, but also resources for family and friends of people affected by the disease. MedlinePlus can direct the alert librarian to dozens of such voluntary associations for every health topic listed there, and the site should be the first stop for those seeking to augment a CHI collection or to build one from the grassroots up.

Another important source of CHI materials is the professional specialty organization, which serves, among other things, as a professional education/networking/contact point for people working in the field. These organizations often publish educational materials for their patients which are suitable for CHI work as well. For example, ACOG (the American College of Obstetricians and Gynecologists) and the American Academy of Pediatrics both feature online bookstores with brochures, bookmarks, and posters for consumers.

Indexes and Databases for CHI

While MEDLINE indexes sixteen consumer health titles as of this writing, CINAHL (*Cumulative Index to Nursing and Allied Health Literature*) may be a better consumer-friendly resource for CHI because of its patient-centered literature, including patient education materials, and less technical reading level. The Health and Wellness database produced by the Gale Group includes complementary and alternative medicine (CAM)–specific resources. For CAM resources specifically, the British Library's long-running bibliographic database Allied and Alternative Medicine and MANTIS, produced by Action Potential, Inc., are good commercial products.

Publishers in CHI

Consumer health has been such a major growth area for medical publishers that virtually every major player in the field now produces a consumer sideline. *Literary Market Place,* an annual classic of all things publishing, lists publishers by subject area and is a good first resource. *Books In Print,* from Bowker, will also help identify series and popular titles for which particular publishers show a strength or a preference. Both these products are available in digital format by subscription, as well as in print.

Important Journals for CHI

Journals are the selector's principal ally when it comes to finding reviews. Sources for CHI reviews include *Library Journal,* which reviews both CH texts and serials, including CAM topics; the *Journal of the Medical Library Association,* primarily a research and practice journal but with an occasional CH title reviewed; and the eminently practical *Journal of Consumer Health on the Internet* and *Medical Reference Services Quarterly.* The literature of medical informatics devotes increasing attention to consumer health issues; the free online, MEDLINE-indexed, peer-reviewed *Journal of Medical Internet Research* is a particularly good resource for librarians interested in their Internet-using current or future clientele. Finally, just as patient education resources are often core elements of CHI collections, so is the literature of patient education, such as *Patient Education and Counseling,* a rich resource to help in understanding consumers.

Core Lists of Titles

The Toronto Consumer Health Information Service (CHIS) Web site provides an excellent list of collections for CHI, including recommended titles and journals in their collection, at <http://www.tpl.toronto.on.ca/uni_chi_index.jsp>. The Collection Development Section of MLA is another good resource <http://colldev.mlanet.org/about/index.html>, as is, naturally, CAPHIS <http://caphis.mlanet.org/>. Developers of collections in CHI can take advantage of the authoritative list originally developed for medical libraries, the famous Brandon/Hill list (see Chapter 3, "Journal Collection Development," and Chapter 4, "Monographic and Digital Resource Collection Development").

Collection Development for Special Populations

Tailoring CHI to a particular community requires, of course, that the communications and the dominant culture of that community be understood. Needs assessment can inform the collection development librarian of gaps and strengths alike. Being culturally competent requires keeping current with research and publications that focus on your community of interest. For example, Gollop's groundbreaking study of elderly African-American women found that while not all of these women used their public library as a source of health information, those who did use it for this purpose tended to be magazine readers. This might suggest that magazines focusing on African-American health, and specific health issues, might be popular with this audience.[89] Hartel and Mehling's report that 50 percent of Latinos experience literacy problems suggests that a CHI librarian collecting for this population should pay attention to low literacy as well as Spanish-language resources.[86] Halsted and colleagues' Asian-language initiative translated health information brochures into Mandarin Chinese and Vietnamese because data showed these to be the predominant languages in the Asian population in Houston.[82]

Promotion and Marketing

Baker and Manbeck describe four categories of promotion: advertising, personal selling, sales promotion, and public relations.[1] This chapter has described CHI services as embedded in a network of competing and collaborating information sources. In marketing, the trick is to perceive the flow of information between the librarian and the public as occurring in all of these categories. Chapter 9, "Marketing, Public Relations, and Communication," of this text addresses marketing by medical libraries in general; specific CHI marketing materials mentioned in Ruffin and colleagues' evaluation study include "bookmarks, information prescription pads, fliers, posters, displays, videos and screen sweeps."[30] Suggestions in the literature include participating in health fairs[78]; holding a press conference and sending out press releases[80, 82, 84]; presentation of posters at professional meetings[82]; sending CHI librarians to speak to community groups[82]; advertising via in-house fliers and systemwide e-mails[80]; designing and strategically placing brochures[80, 84]; presentations to organization staff and professional groups[84]; and, of course, building and maintaining a dedicated Web space, which can serve simultaneously as information resource and publicity.[78, 80, 82] Smith and colleagues, at Iowa City Public Library, even created their own TV health information training program for local cable and exhibited at their county 4-H and Future Farmers of America fairs.[78]

CHI SERVICE EVALUATION

Friedman and Wyatt, in the classic medical informatics text on evaluation, write that "the term . . . describes a wide range of data collection activities designed to answer questions."[99] The specific questions, and thus the objectives of a specific evaluation, will ideally have been determined during the long-range goal-setting process for the CHI facility.

Two evaluation studies of particular relevance to CHI services have been published; these can serve as models for any CHI service wishing to evaluate itself. The first was by Wood and colleagues[100] and looked at outcomes from NLM's pilot partner project. Ruffin and colleagues reviewed outcomes of fifty-three electronic resource grants, also from NLM.[30]

The partner project began in the spring of 1998, coincident with the launch of MedlinePlus, NLM's consumer health Web site, and the addition of twelve consumer health titles to MEDLINE[101]; as of November 2006, there were sixteen.[102] The pilot concluded in June 1999. Partners included forty-one public libraries, eight resource libraries, and three RMLs (Regional

Medical Libraries) from nine states in the Northeast and the District of Columbia. Most of the public libraries involved did not have a health information center when the pilot began; in fact, most reported no prior focus on health information, even though the librarians perceived it as one of their library users' highest subject areas of interest. One disappointing finding from an evaluation of the pilot project was that MedlinePlus usage by the librarians involved did not increase, although since library user usage was not monitored, it was impossible to state whether library user usage increased.

Ruffin and colleagues' evaluation describes fifty-three projects funded through NLM's succeeding electronic resource initiatives in 1999 and 2000. The focus of all of these projects was "improving electronic access to health information for a variety of groups, including consumers, underserved and minority populations, public health workers, public libraries, and community-based and faith-based organizations."[30] Collaboration across library types was addressed through the funding approach; single institutions could request up to $10,000, and formal institutional collaborators, $40,000.

Data arising from an evaluation can be used productively to modify an existing activity or to measure the success of an activity that has ended. Tarby and Hogan were able to use the results from their evaluation of cancer-specific CHI delivery in a hospital to document the CHI's impact on quality of the patient's hospital stay. This generated support for a longer-term, more widespread CHI program.[84] Smith and colleagues' questionnaire method asked attendees of a public library–based CHI workshop to report how their use of the Internet as a health information resource changed after they took the workshop.[78]

Surveys are a common means of assessing library user opinions and needs in libraries. Ruffin and colleagues report that of the fifty-one NLM grantees employing a structured, systematic evaluation method, surveys were the most common method used (in thirty-six projects). These surveys were administered across the spectrum of the individual projects, from evaluations of training sessions to pre- and post-tests measuring information acquired during a consumer workshop. Questionnaires were used by nine projects; six sought feedback online. Statistics of Web traffic were also obtained (in ten projects) and usage of reference desk services or a hospital library were also outcome measures in three projects.[30]

COLLABORATION

The fifty-three projects described by Ruffin and colleagues were funded in thirty-four states and the District of Columbia; eleven funded proposals came from single institutions, and forty-two from collaborators. Thirty-eight of the fifty-three worked directly with the general public, and twenty-nine focused on public librarians as a professional group. The grant monies covered activities from librarian training (forty-five projects) to Web site development (thirty-eight).[30]

Consumer health information practice, no matter where it is located, is inherently multitype in nature because the consumer is multitype in nature; the consumer is everywhere. Ruffin and colleagues point out that the increased collaboration between libraries and other entities—community organizations, representatives of ethnic groups, and so on—was one very definite and positive outcome of NLM's funding for electronic resources.[30] Four types of collaboration for CHI can be discerned as enduring and successful, albeit challenging, in the literature.

Academic Medical Center Libraries and Public Libraries

J. W. Farlow in 1921 commented on the distaste of public librarians for medical information: "The public library knows little, and consequently cares little, about medical books."[36] By 1982, Eakin and colleagues were recommending that AMC libraries join public libraries in their CHI efforts; that medical libraries should train, provide backup reference service, and educate public librarians; but should not *lead* these efforts, because, in these authors' opinion, AMC and hospital librarians are "presently inexperienced in, and their libraries are ill-suited for, extensive services to the nonmedical public."[20] Catherine Alloway agreed plaintively in 1989 that "neither public nor health sciences libraries can bear the full brunt" of health information need, and that "it is time to shift responsibility to an enterprising group and away from one specific type of library to another."[11]

It is a strong testimony to librarians' responsiveness to need that these early and enduring professional biases were overcome. Ruffin and colleagues wrote,[30] and Pifalo and colleagues agreed,[48] that the Title I grants funded by the Library Services and Construction Act engendered a "handful" of early collaborations between libraries in the late 1970s. CHIPS (Consumer Health Information Program and Services/Salud y Beienestar), described by Goodchild and colleagues, was one such collaboration.[87] Some other examples of public-AMC collaboration for CHI services are described in Georgia (public libraries and the University of Alabama)[79] and Texas (Dallas Public and Texas Women's University).[103]

Some AMC libraries have even further extended their reach and included a health education center and a library school as partners,[79] as well as library councils and public university libraries. NOAH (New York Online Access to Health), one of the longest-running CHI Web sites in existence, was a product of the New York partnership described by Voge.[88] A landmark study of the challenges facing public libraries, and the potential of AMC libraries to help, is that of Wessel, Wozar, and Epstein.[104] These authors conducted a needs assessment of Pittsburgh area public librarians and evaluated responses of participants post–consumer health training by academic librarians. Based on survey responses, this health information instruction had a positive impact on the public librarians and, these authors argue, on the communities served by those public libraries.

Consortia

Library consortia have been formed in consumer health practice, just as they have in non–health sciences library settings, to maximize sharing of resources among multitype libraries with common missions. Examples of CHI consortia include CHIPIG (Consumer Health Information Providers Group) <http://www.chipig.ca/>. CHIPIG was formed in Toronto in 1998 and includes libraries from public, academic, hospital, government, and nonprofit settings. The Pennsylvania Association of Consumer Health Librarians, consisting of twelve hospital libraries, was able to collectively develop a Web site and obtain vendor discounts for CHI materials through consortial buying power. LOON (Libraries Online/Outreach North) <http://www.ourkingdom.com/>, a New Hampshire/Vermont consortium, established public access Internet stations, a pediatric literacy outreach program, and a women's health collection.[105]

Librarians and Other Professionals

Collaboration across professional lines also appears necessary for CHI work. The community health information networks of the 1970s described by Gartenfeld[106] relied on a holistic understanding of health information as a participatory act involving multiple disciplines. Pittman and colleagues' Blum Family Center, in Boston, articulated this effort in multidisciplinary teams, featuring not only nurses and librarians but representatives of clinical information systems in their design; an equally pluralistic Steering Committee oversaw the teams.[80] Halsted's advisory committee for the Consumer Health Information for Asians (CHIA) project was made up of representatives from numerous city and state agencies, all either health professionals or librarians.[82] Smith and colleagues describe participation of health professionals (both doctors and nurses) in their public library CHI program.[78]

Librarians and Community Partners

Defined formally in the field as "outreach," the ability of libraries and staff to connect with their communities is perhaps the most challenging and yet the most vital test for library-based CHI providers. Community partners can help to alleviate barriers to effective outreach, which include the lack of computer training,[107, 108] attendance problems,[106, 109, 110] and, of course, health illiteracy.[108] The inclusion of neighborhood leaders, for example, from community organizations and from houses of worship, can ensure that the CHI services are responsive to the community's real needs[106, 109, 110]; assist with planning[111]; and generate community support and site "champions" for long-term success of the project.[82]

RESOURCES FOR CONSUMER HEALTH INFORMATION PRACTICE

The ephemeral nature of the World Wide Web ensures that any print resource listing URLs is likely to be incorrect within a few months. For this reason, the list of resources provided here is not intended to be comprehensive. The omission of any particular resource should not be taken as a statement about that resource's quality. Instead, the author has listed here those "meta"-resources that have been important in consumer health information practice for years and that serve as guides and jumping-off places for the interested reader. This is particularly true in the case of the Web sites; there are literally thousands of good consumer health information sites referred to by CHI practitioners, each one fulfilling a specific need on the part of a particular population. The meta-resource MedlinePlus is the gateway to most of them!

Education for CHI

The Medical Library Association (MLA) offers a continuing education program focused on Consumer Health Information Specialization (CHIS). This program is open to allied health professionals as well as librarians. More information can be found at the MLA Web site at <http://www.mlanet.org>.

Professional Associations

Within MLA, CAPHIS has been the driving force behind consumer health information services for years. Its Web site <http://caphis.mlanet.org> is a significant information resource of its own; its LISTSERV™ offers support, information exchange, and engenders advocacy in CHI practice.

Meta-Resources

- Books
  Baker, L.M., and Manbeck, V. *Consumer Health Information for Public Librarians.* Metuchen, NJ: Scarecrow Press, 2002.
  Barclay, D.A. and Halsted, D.D. *The Medical Library Association Consumer Health Reference Service Handbook.* New York: Neal-Schuman, 2001.
  Rees, A., ed. *Consumer Health Information Source Book.* 7th ed. Westport, CT: Greenwood Press, 2003.

- Journals
  Journal of Consumer Health on the Internet

- Web Sites
  MedlinePlus: <http://www.medlineplus.gov>

REFERENCES

1. Baker, L.M., and Manbeck, V. *Consumer Health Information for Public Librarians.* Metuchen, NJ: Scarecrow Press, 2002.

2. CAPHIS Task Force, Medical Library Association. "The Librarian's Role in the Provision of Consumer Health Information and Patient Education." *Bulletin of the Medical Library Association* 84(April 1996): 238-9.

3. Lawrence, V. "Consumer Health Information Sources: A Growing Area in Hospital Libraries." *National Network* 23(October 1998): 1.

4. "Consumer." *OED Online.* 2nd ed., 1989.

5. Hendricks, R.L. *A Model for National Health Care: The History of Kaiser Permanente.* New Brunswick, NJ: Rutgers University Press, 1993.

6. Coulter, A.; Entwisle, V.; and Gilbert, D. "Sharing Decisions with Patients: Is the Information Good Enough?" *BMJ; British Medical Journal* (January 30, 1999): 318-22.

7. Spatz, M.A. "Providing Consumer Health Information in the Rural Setting: Planetree Health Resource Center's Approach." *Bulletin of the Medical Library Association* 88(October 2000): 382-8.

8. Notkin, H. "How a Consumer Health Library Can Help Streamline Your Practice." *Western Journal of Medicine* 161(August 1994): 184-5.

9. White, P.J. "Evidence-Based Medicine for Consumers: A Role for the Cochrane Collaboration." *Journal of the Medical Library Association* 90(April 2002): 218-22.

10. Baker, L.M.; Spang, L.; and Gogolowski, C. "The Provision of Consumer Health Information by Michigan Public Librarians." *Public Libraries* 37(July/August 1998): 250-5.

11. Alloway, C. "Issues in Consumer Health Information Services." *RQ* 23(Winter 1983): 143-9.

12. Moeller, K.A., and Deeney, K.E. "Documenting the Need for Consumer Health Information: Results of a Community Survey." *Bulletin of the Medical Library Association* 70(April 1982): 236-9.

13. Huntington, P.; Nicholas, D.; Williams, P.; and Gunter, B. "Characterising the Health Information Consumer: An Examination of Digital Television Users." *Libri* 52(March 2002): 16-27.

14. Somers, A. *Promoting Health: Consumer Education and National Policy.* Germantown, MD: Aspen, 1976.

15. Smith, F.A. "Health Information During a Week of Television." *New England Journal of Medicine* 286 (March 9, 1972): 516-20.

16. Fox, S. "Online Health Search 2006: Most Internet Users Start at a Search Engine When Looking for Health Information Online. Very Few Check the Source and Date of the Information They Find." *Pew/Internet Report* (October 29, 2006). Available: <http://www.pewinternet.org/PPF/r/190/report_display.asp>. Accessed: February 14, 2007.

17. Tu, H.T., and Hargreaves, J.L. *Seeking Health Care Information: Most Consumers Still on the Sidelines.* Center for Studying Health Change Report No. 61 (Summer 2003). Available: <http://www.hschange.org/CONTENT/537/>. Accessed: February 14, 2007.

18. National Network of Libraries of Medicine. *Members Directory.* Available: <http://nnlm.gov/members/>. Accessed: March 9, 2007.

19. Consumer Health Information Service, Toronto Public Library. "Goals and Partners" (November 21, 2006). Available: <http://www.tpl.toronto.on.ca/uni_chi_more.jsp>. Accessed: December 22, 2006.

20. Eakin, D.; Jackson, S.J.; and Hannigan, G. "Consumer Health Information: Libraries As Partners." *Bulletin of the Medical Library Association* 68(April 1980): 220-9.

21. Hollander, S.M. "Providing Health Information to the General Public: A Survey of Current Practices in Academic Health Sciences Libraries." *Bulletin of the Medical Library Association* 84(January 2000): 11-6.

22. "The Health Information Center (HIC): A New Consumer Health Information Service." *SUNY Upstate Medical University Library Synapse* 3(Winter/Spring 1997): 6-7. Available: <http://www.upstate.edu/library/synapse/syn-3-1and2-winterspring97.shtml>. Accessed: March 9, 2007.

23. Masys, D.R. "The Informatics of Health-Care Reform." *Bulletin of the Medical Library Association* 84(January 1996): 11-6.

24. Cosgrove, T.L. "Planetree Health Information Service: Public Access to the Information People Want." *Bulletin of the Medical Library Association* 82(January 1994): 57-63.

25. Planetree Health System. "Planetree Commemorates 25 Years of Consumer Health Libraries at Annual Conference" (November 9, 2006). Available: <http://www.emediawire.com/releases/2006/11/emw474587.htm>. Accessed: December 22, 2006.

26. Planetree Health System. "Planetree Components." Available: <http://www.planetree.org/about/components.htm>. Accessed: December 22, 2006.

27. Miles, W.D. *A History of the National Library of Medicine: The Nation's Treasury of Medical Knowledge.* Bethesda, MD: National Library of Medicine, 1982.

28. National Library of Medicine. "Online Usage Statistics Smashed; Free MEDLINE Rewrites NLM Record Book." *NLM Newsline* 53(January-March 1998): 1-2.

29. Board of Regents, National Library of Medicine. *Board of Regents Policy on Consumer Health* (May 6, 1999). Available: <http://www.nlm.nih.gov/pubs/plan/lrp06/briefing/panel2/consumerhealth.html>. Accessed: March 9, 2007.

30. Ruffin, A.B.; Cogdill, K.; Kutty, L.; and Hudson-Ochillo, M. "Access to Electronic Health Information for the Public: Analysis of Fifty-Three Funded Projects." *Library Trends* 53(Winter 2005): 434-52.

31. National Library of Medicine. "MedlinePlus Milestones" (December 1, 2006). Available: <http://www.nlm.nih.gov medlineplus/milestones.html>. Accessed: December 22, 2006.

32. National Library of Medicine. "MedlinePlus Statistics" (November 7, 2006). Available: <http://www.nlm.nih.gov/medlineplus/usestatistics.html#topicsyear>. Accessed: December 22, 2006.

33. National Library of Medicine. "'Go Local'—A Project of MedlinePlus" (December 11, 2006). Available: <http://www.nlm.nih.gov/medlineplus/golocal.html>. Accessed: December 22, 2006.

34. National Library of Medicine. "MedlinePlus in the News" (January 10, 2007). Available: <http://www.nlm.nih.gov/medlineplus/recognition.html>. Accessed: February 13, 2007.

35. Williams, R. "Changing Fashions and Habits in Medical Literature." *Bulletin of the Medical Library Association* 70(April 1934): 93-100.

36. Farlow, J.W. "The Relation of the Large Medical Library to the Community." *Bulletin of the Medical Library Association* 32(July 1921): 2-4.

37. Gillaspy, M.L. "Starting a Consumer Health Information Service in a Public Library." *Public Library Quarterly* 18, no. 3/4 (2000): 5-19.

38. Marshall, J.G.; Sewards, C.; and Dilworth, E.L. "Health Information Services in Ontario Public Libraries." *Canadian Library Journal* 48(February 1991): 37-44.

39. Dewdney, P.; Marshall, J.G.; and Tiamiyu, A. "A Comparison of Legal and Health Information Services in Public Libraries." *RQ* 31(Winter 1991): 185-96.

40. Khalil, F.E.M. "Consumer Health Information: A Brief Critique on Information Needs and Information-Seeking Behaviors." *Malaysian Journal of Library and Information Science* 6(December 2001): 83-99.

41. Jansen, P., and Spink, A. "How Are We Searching the World Wide Web? A Comparison of Nine Search Engine Transaction Logs." *Information Processing & Management* 42(January 2006): 248-63.

42. Baker, L.M., and Pettigrew, K.E. "Theories for Practitioners: Two Frameworks for Studying Consumer Health Information-Seeking Behavior." *Bulletin of the Medical Library Association* 87(October 1999): 444-50.

43. Miller, S.M. "Monitoring and Blunting: Validation of a Questionnaire to Assess Styles of Information-Seeking Under Threat." *Journal of Personality and Social Psychology* 52(February 1987): 345-53.

44. Pinder, R. *Management of Chronic Illness.* Basingstoke, England: Macmillan, 1990.

45. Detlefsen, E.G., "Where Am I to Go? Use of the Internet for Consumer Health Information in Two Vulnerable Communities." *Library Trends* 53(Fall 2004): 283-300.

46. Leydon, G.M.; Boulton, M.; Moynihan, C.; et al. "Cancer Patients' Information Seeking Behaviour: In Depth Interview Study." *BMJ; British Medical Journal* 320(April 2000): 909-13.

47. Moeller, K.A. "Consumer Health Libraries: A New Diagnosis." *Library Journal* 122(July 1997): 36-8.

48. Pifalo, V.; Hollander, S.; Henderson, C.L.; DeSalvo, P.; and Gill, G.P. "The Impact of Consumer Health Information Provision by Libraries: The Delaware Experience." *Bulletin of the Medical Library Association* 85(January 1997): 16-22.

49. Sullivan, W.; Schoppmann, L.; and Redman, P.M. "Analysis of the Use of Reference Services in an Academic Health Sciences Library." *Medical Reference Services Quarterly* 13(Spring 1994): 35-55.

50. White, M.D. "Questioning Behavior on an Electronic List." *Library Quarterly* 70(July 2000): 302-34.

51. Katz, W.A. *Introduction to Reference Work,* 1st ed. New York: McGraw-Hill, 1982.

52. Dahlen, K.H. "The Status of Health Information Delivery in the United States: The Role of Libraries in the Complex Health Care Environment." *Library Trends* 42(Summer 1983): 152-79.

53. Berry, J. "Medical Information Taboos [Editorial]." *Library Journal* (January 1, 1978): 7.

54. Powers, A., ed. *The Ethics and Problems of Medical Reference Service in Public Libraries: Summary and Addenda to the September 1979 Bay Area Reference Center Workshop* (ERIC Document 188586). San Francisco, CA: San Francisco Public Library, 1979.

55. Wood, M.S. "Public Service Ethics in Health Sciences Libraries." *Library Trends* 40(Fall 1991): 244-57.

56. Elsesser, L., and Epstein, H. "Beyond the Core Bibliography: A Guide to Developing a Consumer Health Library." *Promoting Health* 4(May/June 1983): 4-6.

57. Office of Intellectual Freedom, American Library Association. "Library Bill of Rights" (June 18, 1948). Available: <http://www.ala.org/ala/oif/statementspols/statementsif/librarybillrights.htm>. Accessed: December 22, 2006.

58. Curry, A., and Smith, T. "Information on Alternative Medicine: A Collection Management Issue." *Bulletin of the Medical Library Association* 86(January 1998): 48-53.

59. Knowles, J.H. "Responsibility for Health." *Science* 198(December 16, 1997): 1103.

60. Kay, P. "Public Access to Health Information: A Psychoanalyst's View." *RQ* (Winter 1983): 407-10.

61. Rothstein, J.A. "Ethics and the Role of the Medical Librarian: Healthcare Information and the New Consumer." *Bulletin of the Medical Library Association* 81(July 1993): 253-8.

62. Reference and User Services Association, American Library Association. "Guidelines for Medical, Legal, and Business Responses." Available: <http://www.ala.org/ala/rusa/rusaprotools/referenceguide/guidelinesmedical.htm. 2001>. Accessed: February 13, 2007.

63. Bain, C.A. *Health Information from the Public Library: A Report on Two Pilot Projects.* Albany, NY: State Education Department, 1984.

64. Eisenstein, E.R., and Faust, J.B. "The Consumer Health Library in the Hospital Setting." *Medical Reference Services Quarterly* 5 (Fall 1986): 63-74.

65. Selden, C.R.; Zorn, M.; Ratzan, S.; et al., eds. *Health Literacy, January 1990 Through 1999* (Current Bibliographies in Medicine) (NLM Pub. No. CBM 2000-1). Bethesda, MD: National Library of Medicine, 2000.

66. Glassman, P. "Health Literacy" (2006). Available: <http://nnlm.gov/outreach/consumers/hlthlit.html>. Accessed: February 14, 2007.

67. Ad Hoc Committee on Health Literacy for the Council on Scientific Affairs. "Report on the Council of Scientific Affairs." *JAMA; Journal of the American Medical Association* 281(February 10, 1999): 552-7.

68. Schillinger, D.; Grumbach, K.; Piette, J.; et al. "Association of Health Literacy with Diabetes Outcomes." *JAMA; Journal of the American Medical Association* 288(July 24-31, 2002): 475-82.

69. Rothman, R.; Malone, R.; Bryant, B.; Dewalt, D.; and Pignone, M. "Health Literacy and Diabetic Control." *JAMA; Journal of the American Medical Association* 288(December 4, 2002): 2687-8.

70. Powers, B.J., and Bosworth, H.B. "Revisiting Literacy and Adherence: Future Clinical and Research Directions." *Journal of General Internal Medicine* 21, no. 12 (December 2006): 1341-2.

71. Roter, D. "The Enduring and Evolving Nature of the Patient-Physician Relationship." *Patient Education and Counseling* 39(January 2000): 5-15.

72. Rost, K., and Roter, D. "Predictors of Recall of Medication Regimens and Recommendations for Lifestyle Change in Elderly Patients." *Gerontologist* 27(August 1987): 510-5.

73. Crane, J.A. "Patient Comprehension of Doctor-Patient Communication on Discharge from the Emergency Department." *Journal of Emergency Medicine* 15(January 1997): 1-7.

74. Aspden, P.; Wolcott, J.; Bootman, J.L.; and Cronenwett, L.R., eds. *Preventing Medication Errors* (Quality Chasm Series). Washington, DC: National Academies Press, 2006.

75. Nielsen-Bohlman, L.; Panzer, A.M.; and D.A. Kindig, D.A., eds. *Health Literacy: A Prescription to End Confusion.* Washington, DC: National Academies Press, 2004.

76. Parker, R., and Kreps, G.L. "Library Outreach: Overcoming Health Literacy Challenges." *Journal of the Medical Library Association* 93(suppl. October 2005): S81-5.

77. Davis, T.C.; Mayeaux, E.J.; Frederickson, D.; Bocchini, J.A., Jr.; Jackson, R.H.; and Murphy, P.W. "Reading Ability of Parents Compared with Reading Level of Pediatric Patient Education Materials." *Pediatrics* 93(March 1994): 460-8.

78. Smith, C.; Logsden, K.; and Clark, M. "Consumer Health Information Services at Iowa City Public Library." *Library Trends* 53(Winter 2005): 496-511.

79. Mitchell, W.B.; Sullivan, P.; Pung, M.K.; and Smith, L. "Expanding Access to Consumer Health Information: A Multi-Institutional Collaboration." *Georgia Library Quarterly* 39(Fall 2002): 14-21.

80. Pittman, T.J.; O'Connor, M.D.; Millar, S.; and Erickson, J. I. "Designing a State-of-the-Art Consumer Health Information Library." *JONA; Journal of Nursing Administration* 31(June 2001): 316-23.

81. Phillips, S.A., and Zorn, M.J. "Assessing Consumer Health Information Needs in a Community Hospital." *Bulletin of the Medical Library Association* 82(July 1994): 288-93.

82. Halsted, D.D.; Varman, B.; Sullivan, M.; and Nyugen, L. "Consumer Health Information for Asians (CHIA): A Collaborative Project." *Bulletin of the Medical Library Association* 90(October 2002): 400-5.

83. Richetelle, A.L. "Healthnet: Connecticut Consumer Health Information Network." *Connecticut Medicine* 54(November 1990): 632-4.

84. Tarby, W., and Hogan, K. "Hospital-Based Patient Information Services: A Model for Collaboration." *Bulletin of the Medical Library Association* 85(April 1997): 158-66.

85. Blank, A.E.; Horowitz, S.; and Matza, D. "Quality with a Human Face? The Samuels Planetree Model Hospital Unit." *Joint Commission Journal of Quality Improvement* 21(June 1995): 289-99.

86. Hartel, W.J., and Mehling, R. "Consumer Health Services and Collections for Hispanics: An Introduction." *Medical Reference Services Quarterly* 21(Spring 2002): 35-52.

87. Goodchild, E.Y.; Furman, J.A.; Addison, B.L.; and Umbarger, H.N. "The CHIPS Project: A Health Information Network to Serve the Consumer." *Bulletin of the Medical Library Association* 66(October 1978): 432-6.

88. Voge, S. "NOAH : New York Online Access to Health : Library Collaboration for Bilingual Consumer Health Information on the Internet." *Bulletin of the Medical Library Association* 86(1998): 326-34.

89. Gollop, C. "Health Information-Seeking Behavior and Older African-American Women." *Bulletin of the Medical Library Association* 85(April 1997): 141-6.

90. Broering, N.C., Chauncey, G.A., and Gomes, S.L. "Senior Health Goes Electronic: Partnership on Access to Health Senior Health Information Services." *Journal of Consumer Health on the Internet* 9, no. 2 (2005): 11-26.

91. Broering, N.C.; Chauncey, G.A.; and Gomes, S.L. "Outreach to Public Libraries, Senior Centers, and Clinics to Improve Patient and Consumer Health Care: An Update." *Journal of Consumer Health on the Internet* 10, no. 3 (2006): 1-17.

92. La Rocco, A. "The Role of the Medical-School Based Consumer Health Information Service." *Bulletin of the Medical Library Association* 82(January 1994): 46-51.

93. Spatz, M.A. "Providing Consumer Health Information in the Rural Setting: Planetree Health Resource Center's Approach." *Bulletin of the Medical Library Association* 88(October 2000): 382-8.

94. Williams, M.D.; Gish, K.W.; Giuse, N.B.; Sathe, N.A.; and Carrell, D.L." The Patient Informatics Consult Service (PICS): An Approach for A Patient-Centered Service." *Bulletin of the Medical Library Association* 89 (April 2001): 185-93.

95. Wigmore, E.G., "Health Books for Public Libraries." *Library Journal* 58(May 1, 1933): 413.

96. Stein, E.A., and Lucioli, C.E. "Books for Public Library Medical Reference Work." *Library Journal* (August 1, 1958): 2110-3.

97. Cormier, J. "Medical Books for Public Libraries." *Library Journal* (October 15, 1978): 2051.

98. Elsesser, L., and Epstein, H. "Beyond the Core Bibliography: A Guide to Developing a Consumer Health Library." *Promoting Health* (May/June 1983): 4-6.

99. Friedman, C.P., and Wyatt, J.C. *Evaluation Methods in Medical Informatics.* New York: Springer, 1997.

100. Wood, F.B.; Lyon, B.; Schell, M.B.; Kitendaugh, P.; Cid, V.H.; and Siegel, E.R. "Public Library Consumer Health Information Pilot Project: Results of a National Library of Medicine Evaluation." *Bulletin of the Medical Library Association* 88(October 2000): 314-22.

101. Miller, N.; Lacroix, E.M.; and Backus, J. "MEDLINEPlus: Building and Maintaining the National Library of Medicine's Consumer Health Web Service." *Bulletin of the Medical Library Association* 88(January 2000): 11-7.

102. National Library of Medicine. "Number of Titles Currently Indexed for Index Medicus® and PubMed®" (November 15, 2006). Available: <http://www.nlm.nih.gov/bsd/num_titles.html>. Accessed: December 22, 2006.

103. Huber, J.T., and Snyder, M. "Facilitating Access to Consumer Health Information: A Collaborative Approach to Employing Applied Research." *Medical Reference Services Quarterly* 21(Summer 2002): 39-46.

104. Wessel, C.B.; Wozar, J.; and Epstein, B. "The Role of the Academic Medical Center Library in Training Public Librarians." *Journal of the Medical Library Association* 91(July 2003): 352-60.

105. Babish, J.A. "Consumer Health Library Websites: Great Marketing Tools." *National Network* 27(January 2003): 6-7.

106. Gartenfeld, E. "The Community Health Information Network: A Model for Hospital and Public Library Cooperation." *Library Journal* 103(October 1, 1978): 1911-4.

107. Basler, T.G. "Community Outreach Partnerships." *Reference Services Review* 33, no. 1 (2005): 31-7.

108. Bowden, V.M.; Wood, F.B.; Warner, D.G.; Olney, C.A.; Olivier, E.R.; and Siegel, E.R. "Health Information Hispanic Outreach in the Texas Lower Rio Grande Valley." *Journal of the Medical Library Association* 94(April 2006): 180-9.

109. Olney, C.A. "Using Evaluation to Adapt Health Information to the Environments of Community-Based Organizations." *Journal of the Medical Library Association* 93(suppl. October 2005): S57-S67.

110. Scherrer, C.S. "Outreach to Community Organizations: The Next Consumer Health Frontier." *Journal of the Medical Library Association* 90(July 2002): 285-93.

111. Alpi, K.M., and Bibel, B.M. "Meeting the Health Information Needs of Diverse Populations." *Library Trends* 53(Fall 2004): 268-82.

Glossary

Glossary terms and definitions were provided by chapter authors. Sources of definitions, as provided by authors, are listed in brackets following definitions. Definitions taken from *ODLIS—Online Dictionary for Library and Information Science* <http://lu.com/odlis/> are simply listed as *ODLIS*.

AAHC: *See* ASSOCIATION OF ACADEMIC HEALTH CENTERS.

AAHSL: *See* ASSOCIATION OF ACADEMIC HEALTH SCIENCES LIBRARIES.

AAMC: *See* ASSOCIATION OF AMERICAN MEDICAL COLLEGES.

academic medical center (AMC): An institution that has a school of medicine, conducts research, and provides patient care.

academic medicine: Academic medicine is traditionally considered to have three roles: teaching, research, and service. These roles are changing: academic medicine still has the primary responsibility for training doctors; research remains a core role but more is being done in institutes of biotechnology and biomedicine; and most clinical service, even in academic centers, is now provided by nonacademic doctors.

Academy of Health Information Professionals (AHIP): The Medical Library Association credentialing program that recognizes a professional librarian's level of achievement in academic preparation, professional experience, and professional accomplishment.

access points: Searchable fields such as authors, editors, titles, or series, prescribed by *AACR2R* as elements by which a record may be retrieved.

ADA: *See* AMERICANS WITH DISABILITIES ACT.

advertising: Paid promotion of a product or service.

AHA: *See* AMERICAN HOSPITAL ASSOCIATION.

AHIP: *See* ACADEMY OF HEALTH INFORMATION PROFESSIONALS.

alerts: Computer flags or notations that indicate possible simple actions, such as the need for vaccination updating.

AMC: *See* ACADEMIC MEDICAL CENTER.

American Hospital Association (AHA): The major U.S. association for hospitals, health care providers and networks, and patients, headquartered in Chicago. It provides continuing education, analysis of trends and issues, and accredits hospitals through the JOINT COMMISSION ON ACCREDITATION OF HEALTHCARE ORGANIZATIONS. Although there are no specific guidelines for hospital libraries, hospitals must provide services for access to information and information management.

Introduction to Health Sciences Librarianship
© 2008 by The Haworth Press, Taylor & Francis Group. All rights reserved.
doi:10.1300/6041_19

American Osteopathic Association (AOA): The AOA is a member association representing more than 56,000 osteopathic physicians (DOs); it serves as the primary certifying body for DOs and is the accrediting agency for all osteopathic medical colleges and health care facilities. [http://www.osteopathic.org]

Americans with Disabilities Act (ADA): This act gives civil rights protection to individuals with disabilities. It affects libraries as service and facility providers and as employers.

AOA: *See* AMERICAN OSTEOPATHIC ASSOCIATION.

appeal to authority: A cognitive bias and logical fallacy that causes decision makers to act on the basis of an authority figure's views on a subject based upon views that are outside the expertise or legitimate control of that authority figure.

approval plan: A method of acquiring library materials, particularly books, in which a vendor or publisher is given a profile outlining types of books and subjects to be supplied. The library retains the option of returning unwanted books.

Ariel®: A document transmission system developed by the Research Libraries Group (RLG) that provides rapid, inexpensive, high-quality document delivery over the Internet by integrating scanning, sending, receiving, and printing functions. The user can send text and gray-scale images (illustrations, photographs, etc.) in letter, legal, and other sizes to another Ariel workstation, to an e-mail account used by an Ariel machine, or to anyone who uses MIME-compliant e-mail software and a multipage TIFF viewer. The system is used in libraries to facilitate interlibrary loan and document delivery service. [*ODLIS*]

ARL: *See* ASSOCIATION OF RESEARCH LIBRARIES.

assessment: Any measures or protocols used to determine whether the teaching and learning process is working or failing, and to find areas of potential improvement.

Associate Fellowship Program: Competitive postgraduate program sponsored by the U.S. NATIONAL LIBRARY OF MEDICINE for new library professionals who demonstrate potential for leadership in the profession. The program includes training in NLM programs and services, onsite internships at leading health sciences libraries, and opportunities to work on special projects.

Association of Academic Health Centers (AAHC): AAHC is a national, nonprofit organization that seeks to improve health and well-being through vigorous leadership of the nation's academic health centers. [http://www.aahcdc.org/about.php]

Association of Academic Health Sciences Libraries (AAHSL): AAHSL is composed of the directors of libraries of 142 accredited U.S. and Canadian medical schools belonging to the ASSOCIATION OF AMERICAN MEDICAL COLLEGES. AAHSL's goals are to promote excellence in academic health sciences libraries and to ensure that the next generation of health practitioners is trained in information-seeking skills that enhance the quality of health care delivery. AAHSL produces annual comparative statistics for member libraries, programs to develop new leaders, an annual meeting with continuing education programs, and a LISTSERV for academic health science library directors.

Association of American Medical Colleges (AAMC): AAMC is a nonprofit association of medical schools, teaching hospitals, and academic societies that seek to improve the nation's health by enhancing the effectiveness of academic medicine. Today AAMC represents 125 accredited U.S. medical schools, 17 accredited Canadian medical schools, nearly 400 major teaching hospitals, including 98 affiliated health systems and 68 Veterans Affairs medical centers, 96 academic and professional societies representing 109,000 faculty members, and the nation's 67,000 medical students and 104,000 residents. [http://www.aamc.org]

Association of Research Libraries (ARL): An association of large research libraries in the United States.

astral: Related to the stars or celestial bodies.

atelier: An artist's studio or workshop.

audience response system: Wireless technology used to assess an audience's knowledge or opinions. Handheld devices allow an instructor to instantly poll the students in a class; particularly useful in larger, hard-to-navigate classrooms, where the instructor is at a disadvantage in engaging the class in discussion.

backfile: Electronic version of back or older issues of journals.

basic sciences: Disciplines that form the foundation for the practice of medicine. In some programs, education in the basic sciences forms the first two years of a medical school program, followed by two years applying this knowledge as students learn clinical applications. Basic sciences can include anatomy, physiology, and microbiology, among other subjects.

Baskerville type: A family of type fonts cut for John Baskerville (1706-1775), an English printer and publisher. Baskerville types are highly regarded for their esthetic excellence.

behavioral sciences: The term encompasses all the disciplines that explore the activities of and interactions among organisms in the natural world. It involves the systematic analysis and investigation of human and animal behavior through controlled and naturalistic experimental observations and rigorous formulations.

behaviorism: Learning theory proposed by psychologist B. F. Skinner that all learning is "conditioned" in the learner, as a result of positive or negative reinforcement.

benchmarking: Comparing one's institution against similar institutions as a basis for improvement.

bibliographic databases: Databases of documents, usually journal articles, that can be searched, for example, by authors, titles, subject headings, and keywords.

bibliographic record: Description of a separately cataloged item which includes information that identifies it and distinguishes it from other items. For books, the bibliographic record includes title, author(s) or editors(s), edition, publisher information, and physical description, among other elements.

bioinformatics: The discipline of computers and computer tools to collect, analyze, and present biologic data (genes, cells, and proteins), to improve understanding of biologic entities, especially humans.

blog: Shortened form of Web logs, a type of publishing by individuals that consists of journal entries. A Web page that provides frequent continuing publication of Web links and/or comments on a specific topic or subject (broad or narrow in scope), often in the form of short entries arranged in reverse chronological order, the most recently added piece of information appearing first. [*ODLIS*]

born-digital: Related to materials that exist in digital formats without any print counterparts; sometimes refers to persons who were born after computers became commonplace in homes, schools, and workplaces.

branding: Building a favorable image for a product or service that differentiates it from others; placing a logo or other identifying information on library products and/or on Web pages of electronic resources made available by the library to differentiate the product/service from others.

case study: A common research method in librarianship that, while easy to conduct, often tends to be subject to multiple cognitive biases that can be controlled for better by other research methods.

case study method: A form of problem-based learning whereby a specific situation is codified into a "case," oftentimes as a medical patient or outbreak of a disease, and students are asked to develop solutions.

catalog copy: A previously created bibliographic record obtained from another source that a librarian can use or adapt instead of creating an original record.

CDSS: *See* CLINICAL DECISION SUPPORT SYSTEM.

CEO: *See* CHIEF EXECUTIVE OFFICER.

CEPH: *See* COUNCIL ON EDUCATION FOR PUBLIC HEALTH.

Charting the Future: A key report of the ASSOCIATION OF ACADEMIC HEALTH SCIENCES LIBRARIES that details how librarians' expertise and skills can be applied to managing knowledge produced by faculty, researchers, students, and staff of health sciences centers. The full name of the report is *Building on Success: Charting the Future of Knowledge Management Within the Academic Health Center.*

CHI: *See* CONSUMER HEALTH INFORMATION.

chief executive officer (CEO): A person in this position typically oversees the company's finances and strategic planning and may also serve as the chairman of the board and, sometimes, the president of an organization.

chief information officer (CIO): The individual in an organization who is responsible for the strategic use and management of information, information systems, and information technology.

CIO: *See* CHIEF INFORMATION OFFICER.

citation indexing: A concept originated by Eugene Garfield in which the references (cited articles, or citations) of an article are used to locate other articles on the same topic.

classroom control software: Software used in e-classrooms and computer labs to allow instructors greater control over student workstations.

clinical decision support system (CDSS): A computerized information system that integrates patient information with established care standards to produce prompts or alerts to clinicians about patient care decisions or actions.

clinical decision tools: Systems intended to assist physicians and other health professionals in making clinical decisions, usually at the point of care.

clinical informatics: The discipline concerned with health data on individuals or patients collected and used by many health professionals. This is the largest domain of health informatics.

clinical information system: A broad term for a fully integrated and broad-based system that incorporates many sources of information on patients.

clinical medical librarian: A librarian who attends rounds with a health care team and provides case-specific information to assist with patient care. [http://www.hls.mlanet.org/otherresources/standards2004.pdf]

clinical sciences: Disciplines that relate to diseases or conditions that a health care provider might encounter in a clinic or hospital. These can include etiology, diagnosis, treatment, and prognosis of diseases and health conditions.

clinical trials: Research studies testing safety and efficacy of new drugs or treatments and interventions. These studies are often funded by the federal government or pharmaceutical companies.

ClinicalTrials.gov: A database of the U.S. NATIONAL LIBRARY OF MEDICINE that describes federally and privately supported clinical research studies that are being conducted or are recruiting for possible human volunteers.

CME: *See* CONTINUING MEDICAL EDUCATION.

co-browsing: Simultaneous viewing of a Web page by both the client and the librarian during a virtual reference session.

cognitive biases: The variety of ways that the human mind can fail to clearly perceive a situation or to analyze it properly, thereby interfering with sound decision-making in EVIDENCE-BASED PRACTICE.

cognitivism: Learning theory that proposes that all mental processes can be understood through the application of the scientific method.

cohort studies: Studies that observe how a carefully defined population that shares a common experience or condition changes over time.

collaboratory: A physical place designed, equipped, or furnished for collaborative work or project planning.

collection development policy: Policy that guides a library's overall collection approach by defining the library's environment, its audience, the purpose of its collection, and subject areas to acquire.

COLT: *See* COUNCIL ON LIBRARY/MEDIA TECHNICIANS.

competitive intelligence: Researching and obtaining information on products, services, strategies, or organizations that might be seen as rivaling the parent organization. If two hospitals in the same region both provide similar services to the community, the end goal of obtaining competitive intelligence would be to develop services with unique advantages.

computers and technology in medicine: Early term for health and medical informatics.

confidentiality: In an electronic information system, defined as the ability of a system to allow only those people who are authorized to have access to certain information.

connectivism: Learning theory proposed by George Siemens in 2004 that learning occurs as a part of the formation of networks, and that this learning can exist both within and outside of the human condition.

consortium (consortia): A combined organization of libraries or library directors, formed to provide joint services that benefit the entire group. Consortia have been formed to share strengths in collection development, develop joint purchasing power, and exchange resources developed, such as informatics curriculum or database training materials.

constructivism: Learning theory that proposes that learning is a construction, built upon by the perceptions and experiences of the learner.

consumer: Originally an economic term, in modern times, it means not only patients but family, friends, and members of the general public, particularly those who need health information.

consumer health information (CHI): An umbrella term encompassing the continuum extending from the specific information needs of patients to the broader provision of health information for the layperson. [http://www.hls.mlanet.org/otherresources/standards2004.pdf]

continuing medical education (CME): Educational activities which serve to maintain, develop, or increase the knowledge, skills, and professional performance and relationships that a physician uses to provide services for patients, the public, or the profession. The content of CME is that body of knowledge and skills generally recognized and accepted by the profession as within the basic medical sciences, the discipline of clinical medicine, and the provision of health care to the public. [http://www.accme.org/index.cfm/fa/Policy.policy/Policy_id/16f1c 694-d03b-4241-bd1a-44b2d072dc5e.cfm]

controlled thesaurus: A thesaurus with a preselected, or "controlled," list of terms; for example, MESH is a controlled thesaurus.

COTH: *See* COUNCIL OF TEACHING HOSPITALS AND HEALTH SYSTEMS.

Council of Teaching Hospitals and Health Systems (COTH): The AAMC's COTH is composed of approximately 400 major teaching hospitals and health systems, including 64 Veterans Affairs medical centers. COTH was established in 1965 to provide representation and services related to the special needs, concerns, and opportunities facing major teaching hospitals in the United States and Canada. It serves as the principal source of hospital and health system input into overall AAMC policy and direction. [http://www.aamc.org/members/coth]

Council on Education for Public Health (CEPH): An independent agency recognized by the U.S. Department of Education to accredit schools of public health and graduate public health programs outside schools of public health. [http://ceph.org]

Council on Library/Media Technicians (COLT): An international organization that works to address the issues and concerns of library and media support staff personnel. [http://colt .ucr.edu]

COUNTER (Counting Online Usage of NeTworked Electronic Resources): International initiative to define and achieve consistency with the usage measurement for electronic information resources.

course management systems: Software systems designed to provide a wide variety of virtual learning experiences.

course-based instruction: Library instruction that is provided as part of a regular course or program of the school.

courseware: Any content management system specialized for course development and instruction. Commercial courseware products include ANGEL, Blackboard, and WebCT.

crushed morocco: A particular way of preparing goatskin ("morocco leather") for bookbinding that gives an especially luxurious texture.

curriculum-integrated programming: Library instruction that is consistently integrated into the requisite curriculum of the school.

deed of gift: An agreement transferring title to property without an exchange of monetary compensation. [Society of American Archivists]

Delphi study: A study that describes topics of consensus by experts about future trends. The process usually occurs in several steps. First, experts may describe future scenarios. Next, consensus is reached on several likely scenarios. Then, all participants may be asked to rate the likelihood of the scenarios, as well as the desirability of the scenarios actually occurring.

descriptor: Subject heading; a term or terms used to describe the topic of a work.

development: In a fundraising context, this is the identification, cultivation, stewardship, and recognition of donors. Donations can be requested from individuals, businesses, charitable foundations, or governmental agencies. Libraries make use of endowments, Friends of the Library groups, direct mail such as for annual giving campaigns, personal contacts, gifts-in-kind, and similar techniques in development work.

diagnosis-related group (DRG): This is a system to classify hospital cases into one of approximately 500 groups (DRGs) expected to have similar hospital resource use, developed for Medicare as part of the prospective payment system. DRGs are assigned by a "grouper" program based on *International Classification of Diseases (ICD)* diagnoses, procedures, age, sex, and the presence of complications or comorbidities. DRGs have been used since 1983 to determine how much Medicare pays the hospital.

Digital Millennium Copyright Act (DCMA): This 1998 U.S. law criminalizes production and dissemination of technology whose primary purpose is to circumvent measures taken to protect copyright, not merely infringement of copyright itself, and heightens the penalties for copyright infringement on the Internet. The DMCA amended Title 17 of the U.S. Code to extend the reach of copyright, while limiting the liability of online providers for copyright infringement by their users.

diversity plan: Specific goals, action plans, and evaluation methods that define, measure, increase, or sustain diversity.

DOCLINE®: The NATIONAL LIBRARY OF MEDICINE's automated INTERLIBRARY LOAN request routing and referral system. [http://www.nlm.nih.gov/pubs/factsheets/docline.html]

downsizing: Reduction in size, usually in reference to a reduction in number of employees.

EBL: *See* EVIDENCE-BASED LIBRARIANSHIP.

EBLIP: *See* EVIDENCE-BASED LIBRARIANSHIP.

EBM: *See* EVIDENCE-BASED MEDICINE.

EBM Specific Search Method: A form of bibliographic database searching in EVIDENCE-BASED MEDICINE intended to retrieve a limited number of references with a high probability of having great relevance to the EBM question posed by a clinician.

EBP: *See* EVIDENCE-BASED PRACTICE.

EFTS: *See* ELECTRONIC FUND TRANSFER SYSTEM.

e-health: Dealing with finding and using information about health by professionals and consumers; often, but not always, associated with computers or information technology.

EHR: *See* ELECTRONIC HEALTH RECORD.

Electronic Fund Transfer System (EFTS): A transaction-based electronic billing system developed by the University of Connecticut Health Center for INTERLIBRARY LOAN and document delivery charges. The NATIONAL LIBRARY OF MEDICINE participates in the EFTS for billing DOCLINE libraries for NLM-supplied documents. EFTS reduces the need to create invoices and to process reimbursement checks for interlibrary loans between participants. EFTS also provides monthly detailed transaction reports, and the ability to handle differential charges, to vary charges to members of special groups, and to handle non-DOCLINE transactions.

electronic health record (EHR): A secure, real-time, point-of-care, patient-centric information resource for clinicians. The EHR aids clinicians' decision-making by providing access to patient health record information where and when they need it and by incorporating evidence-based decision support. The EHR automates and streamlines the clinician's workflow, closing loops in communication and response that result in delays or gaps in care. The EHR also supports the collection of data for uses other than direct clinical care, such as billing, quality management, outcomes reporting, resource planning, and public health disease surveillance and reporting. [http://www.himss.org/content/files/EHRAttributes.pdf]

electronic medical record (EMR): An EMR is a medical record in digital format. In health informatics, an EMR is considered to be one of several types of electronic health records, but confusion between the two terms still exists.

elephantine: The largest of all book formats; the most famous example of an elephantine is *The Birds of America,* by John James Audobon. Many early anatomy books were printed in very large formats, so that the illustrations were nearly life sized.

embargo: Period of time when access may be restricted to the most current digital content.

emergency preparedness: As used here, preparation of plans and documents to assist a library in case of disaster or emergency events. These could include situations caused by natural events, such as earthquakes or hurricanes, epidemics, manmade disasters like bioterrorism, or even the loss of electricity. Emergency preparedness plans are devised to allow clients of the library to continue to access information and critical library services.

EMR: *See* ELECTRONIC MEDICAL RECORD.

end user: The client who accesses library resources directly rather than having the librarian serve as a mediator between the client and the resource; a term often used in reference to a client who does his or her own database searching.

environmental scanning: Using techniques to become aware of major trends, driving forces, and changes in the library's constituent communities, as well as in the library profession.

ephemera: Any printed or handwritten item normally discarded after its intended use, such as calendars, postcards, posters, and pamphlets.

evidence-based librarianship (EBL): A practice-oriented process for integrating the best available scientifically generated evidence into making important decisions. EBL is sometimes known as evidence-based library and information practice (EBLIP).

evidence-based medicine (EBM): EBM is the "conscientious, explicit, and judicious use of current best evidence in making decisions about the care of individual patients" that integrates "individual clinical expertise with the best available external clinical evidence from systematic research." [Sackett, D. L., et al., "Evidence-Based Medicine: What It Is and What It Isn't." *BMJ* 312(1996): 71-2]

evidence-based practice (EBP): EBP refers to a sequential process employed by professionals to reach informed decisions. The EBP process involves formulating answerable questions, searching for relevant answers in the knowledge base, and then critically appraising any available evidence to make a decision.

expert opinion: In the LEVELS OF EVIDENCE, the lowest level of evidence for making a decision.

failure modes and effects analysis (FMEA): A systematic, proactive method for evaluating a process to identify where and how it might fail, and to assess the relative impact of different failures in order to identify the parts of the process that are most in need of change. [http://www.ihi.org/ihi/workspace/tools/fmea/]

federal overhead (facilities and administration): Costs that are incurred by a grantee for common or joint objectives and that, therefore, cannot be identified specifically with a particular project or program. Examples include costs such as lab space, utilities, libraries, and general administration. [http://www.hms.harvard.edu/spa/glossary.htm]

field: 1. An area identified by a MARC TAG that contains a certain type of information. 2. A component of a database record.

filtering information/literature: Process whereby the librarian uses professional judgment and critical appraisal skills to evaluate literature (information) retrieved from a search and eliminates that which is least useful before presenting the retrieval to the client.

FISA: *See* FOREIGN INTELLIGENCE SECURITY ACT.

fixed field: Field of fixed length that contains coded information describing an item.

Flexner Report: Published in 1910 under the aegis of the Carnegie Foundation and written by the professional educator Abraham Flexner, this book-length study of medical education in the United States and Canada has influenced many aspects of the present-day American medical profession. The report (also called Carnegie Foundation Bulletin Number Four) called on American medical schools to enact higher admission and graduation standards, and to adhere strictly to the protocols of mainstream science in their teaching and research.

FMEA: *See* FAILURE MODES AND EFFECTS ANALYSIS.

focus groups: In market research, a group of people gathered together to share their thoughts and opinions.

fonds: The entire body of records of an organization, family, or individual that has been created and accumulated as the result of an organic process, reflecting the functions of the creator. [Society of American Archivists]

Foreign Intelligence Security Act (FISA): Legislation under which FBI agents may obtain library records and library staff may not notify the affected clients.

format: The shape or size of a book; used to indicate the number of times a single printed sheet is folded to form constituent leaves. Strictly speaking, only hand press books have a format, since they were printed from single sheets of paper. However, the term is loosely used for books printed on mechanical presses and continuous rolls of paper. [Carter, J. *ABC for Book Collectors,* 7th ed. New Castle, DE: Oak Knoll, 1998.]

formative assessment: Sometimes called "assessment for learning," an examination of the educational process itself, the type and form of the instruction offered, and the experiences of the students, both in the classroom and online, to determine how learning occurred and whether the educational experience can be improved.

Freeshare: A cross-regional DOCLINE Library Group whose members agree to fill DOCLINE requests free of charge on a reciprocal basis. [http://nnlm.gov/rsdd/freeshare/]

FTE: *See* FULL-TIME EQUIVALENT.

full-time equivalent (FTE): A term used to normalize personnel numbers whereby a full-time employee (frequently considered to be working 40 hours/week) = 1.0, and a half-time employee = 0.5. The number of FTEs is used to define an authorized user group, such as the total of full-time and part-time faculty or students, or number of full-time employees.

gaming engines: Programming software and tools that are used for the creation of online video games.

gatekeeper: A person who acts as an information intermediary for others.

genomics: The study of genes using information technology and biological computing techniques. One aspect of bioinformatics.

Go Local: Locally developed services to connect health topic pages in MEDLINEPLUS to information about area health services, providers, and support groups.

groupthink: A form of cognitive bias characterized by stereotyping those outside of a group and maintaining an illusion of unanimity by silencing dissenters within the group.

health informatics: Applications of advanced computer and communications technologies to health care and specifically to information in health care. Emphasis can be on computer technology or health information. Health informatics has four domains: bioinformatics, imaging, clinical informatics, and public health informatics.

Health Insurance Portability and Accountability Act (HIPAA): Passed in 1996, Title I of this law protects health insurance coverage for workers and their families when they change or lose their jobs; Title II of HIPAA, the Administrative Simplification (AS) provisions, requires the establishment of national standards for electronic health care transactions and national identifiers for providers, health insurance plans, and employers.

health maintenance organization (HMO): An HMO is a type of managed care organization (MCO) that provides a form of health insurance coverage in the United States that is fulfilled through hospitals, doctors, and other providers with which the HMO has a contract. Unlike traditional indemnity insurance, care provided in an HMO generally follows a set of care guidelines provided through the HMO's network of providers. Under this model, providers contract with an HMO to receive more patients and in return usually agree to provide services at a discount. This arrangement allows the HMO to charge a lower monthly premium, which is an advantage over indemnity insurance, provided that its members are willing to abide by the additional restrictions.

health records system: A more broadly based system of computer applications that includes hospital and clinical patient-specific information.

health services research: Studies conducted with access to and consumption of health care services that focus on utilization, costs, quality, delivery, organization, financing, and outcomes.

Hill-Burton Act: This act, also known as the Hospital Survey and Construction Act, is a U.S. federal law passed in 1946. This act responded to the first of President Truman's proposals and was designed to provide federal grants and guaranteed loans to improve the physical plans of the nation's hospital system. Money was designated to the states to achieve 4.5 beds per 1,000 people.

HIPAA: *See* HEALTH INSURANCE PORTABILITY AND ACCOUNTABILITY ACT.

hiring freeze: Prohibition against hiring that prevents filling vacant positions or adding new staff positions; generally not long term.

HL7 (Health Level 7): A set of North American communication standards that allow multiple computer applications to pass data (communicate) across applications.

HMO: *See* HEALTH MAINTENANCE ORGANIZATION.

house officers: In the United States, this term is generally used to refer to residents. In the United Kingdom, a senior house officer (SHO) is a physician undergoing specialist training in the National Health Service.

ILL: *See* INTERLIBRARY LOAN.

ILS: *See* INTEGRATED LIBRARY SYSTEM.

imaging informatics: The discipline of understanding biologic processes at the organ and tissue level. Almost always concerned with images or pictures taken by trained technicians and managed by health professionals such as radiologists and pathologists.

IMLS: *See* INSTITUTE OF MUSEUM AND LIBRARY SERVICES.

impact factor: Measurement for determining how often articles are cited in a specific journal.

incunabula: Books printed in Western Europe with metal movable type from about 1450 (the invention of the process traditionally ascribed to Guttenberg) through 1500. Incunabula is plural; the singular is "incunabulum"; the word "incunable" is also used. The term refers to "the infancy of printing." It has also been used to denote the first printed books from any geographic area. There will be lunar incunabula when the first printing press is set up on the moon.

indicators: Qualitative and quantitative measures that help assess progress toward an outcome where direct causal links are not obvious or changes in behavior or performance are difficult to measure directly. Also, fixed-position elements in variable fields that provide indexing or system information.

information button (or Infobutton): A button in the electronic record system that, when clicked from within a patient's record, retrieves knowledge-based information relevant to that patient.

information fluency: Integrated approach to learning information skills blending "traditional" library-oriented information skills training, computer literacy instruction, and critical thinking skills.

information literacy: A minimally acceptable set of skills that enable one to locate, use, and synthesize information in a meaningful way.

Information Rx: A free program offered by the NATIONAL LIBRARY OF MEDICINE and the American College of Physicians Foundation to assist physicians in referring their patients to MEDLINEPLUS [http://nnlm.gov/hip/infoRx/]; a program adopted by others, as well, to write prescriptions for health information that may be filled by health sciences librarians.

information specialist in context (ISIC): Originally labeled an "informationist," an expert in the information and evidence base of a particular domain. Emphasis is on in-depth knowledge of both the subject matter and information science so that the practitioner can operate as a full team member and problem solver in a clinical, biomedical research, health policy, public health, or other information-intensive context. [http://www.mlanet.org/members/pdf/isic_final_report_feb06.pdf]

informationist: Also called an "informaticist," an emerging type of specialist who has a solid understanding of the clinical environment and a clear conceptual understanding of information linked to practical skills in its management. This person usually plays a central role in the practice of EVIDENCE-BASED MEDICINE.

Institute of Museum and Library Services (IMLS): IMLS is the primary source of federal support for the nation's 122,000 libraries and 17,500 museums. The institute's mission is to create strong libraries and museums that connect people to information and ideas. The institute works at the national level and in coordination with state and local organizations to sustain heritage, culture, and knowledge; enhance learning and innovation; and support professional development.

institutional repository (IR): A collection of scholarly publications and teaching materials created by authors of an institution that the institution has made available electronically, usually on its Web site.

institutional review board (IRB): Sometimes called an investigational review board or an ethical review board. An independent group composed of health care professionals and community representatives who have the responsibility and authority to review and approve all studies involving human subjects in a particular community or facility. The IRB's main responsibility is to protect research participants (human volunteers). [http://www.clinicalstudyresults.org/glossary/]

integrated library system (ILS): An automated library system consisting of several functional modules sharing a common bibliographic database. Commonly used modules include acquisitions, cataloging, circulation, reserves, serials, and an ONLINE PUBLIC ACCESS CATALOG.

intellectual property: A term often used to refer generically to property rights created through intellectual and/or discovery efforts of a creator that are generally protected under patent, trademark, copyright, trade secret, trade dress, or other law. [http://www.techtransfer.umich.edu/index/glossary.html]

interactive whiteboard: An electronic projection screen that is linked to the instructor's workstation, with pressure-sensitive touch points for inputs, and the ability to record any drawings or markings made on the screen.

interlibrary loan (ILL): The borrowing and lending of materials (books, journals, and media) between libraries; most ILLs in health sciences libraries involve transmission of nonreturnable copies of journal articles. ILL occurs within the parameters of copyright laws.

intranet: A network operating like the World Wide Web but having access restricted to a limited group of authorized users (such as employees of a company). [*Merriam-Webster's Online Dictionary*]

invisible college: Term first coined in the 1970s to refer to social networks of researchers and experts working on similar topics who communicated with one another and sometimes collaborated in person, by mail, or over the telephone. Today many invisible colleges are technology enabled by blogs, collaboration software, interactive video, and more.

IP (Internet protocol) address: A unique numeric identifier for a computer or other network device. Often thought of as the equivalent of a street address for a computer or other network device on the Internet.

IP (Internet protocol) recognition: A mechanism to ensure that licensed content is provided only to particular users at the institution that has purchased access to the content; involves a process whereby the licensee provides to the vendor the authorized IP addresses so that the vendor can permit viewing of its Web site content specifically to those having authorized IP addresses. An institution is usually assigned a range of IP addresses for its computers.

IR: *See* INSTITUTIONAL REPOSITORY.

IRB: *See* INSTITUTIONAL REVIEW BOARD.

ISIC: *See* INFORMATION SPECIALIST IN CONTEXT.

JCAHO: *See* JOINT COMMISSION ON ACCREDITATION OF HEALTHCARE ORGANIZATIONS.

Jiffy bag: A mailing envelope that contains protection for the enclosed item in the form of bubble wrap or loose fibers between outer and inner layers.

Joint Commission on Accreditation of Healthcare Organizations (Joint Commission, formerly JCAHO): An independent, not-for-profit organization that evaluates and accredits nearly 15,000 health care organizations and programs in the United States. It is the nation's predominant standards-setting and accrediting body in health care. [http://www.jointcommission.org/AboutUs/joint_commission_facts.htm]

KBI: *See* KNOWLEDGE-BASED INFORMATION.

knowledge management: Tools and techniques that assist in the discovery, creation, collection, documentation, organization, sharing, and dissemination of knowledge, which is often regarded as an institution's most valuable asset. INSTITUTIONAL REPOSITORIES are examples of library-supported tools that assist in management of an organization's knowledge.

knowledge-based information (KBI): The type of information that is found in textbooks, journal articles, clinical guidelines, and other external resources (as opposed to the type of information found in raw data).

LATCH (*literature attached to chart*): Pertinent health information attached to patients' medical charts in the form of photocopied journal articles or textbook information provided by the librarian.

LCME: *See* LIAISON COMMITTEE ON MEDICAL EDUCATION.

learning object repository (LOR): A place to store content, assets, and resources as well as their metadata record.

lesson plan: An outline for instruction, often including a title for the lesson, projected time frame and lesson objectives, materials and facilities needed, and evaluation.

Levels of Evidence: Employed by EVIDENCE-BASED PRACTICE in some professions to distinguish between varying qualities of evidence when making a decision. The Levels of Evidence for EBM can be found at <http://www.cebm.net/levels_of_evidence.asp>, and the EBL Levels of Evidence can be found in the Fall 2002 issue of *Hypothesis* at <http://research.mlanet.org/>.

Liaison Committee on Medical Education (LCME): Accreditation by LCME is required for schools to receive federal grants for medical education and to participate in federal loan programs. Most state boards of licensure require that U.S. medical schools be accredited by LCME, as a condition for licensure of their graduates. Eligibility of U.S. students to take the United States Medical Licensing Examination (USMLE) requires LCME accreditation of their school. Graduates of LCME-accredited schools are eligible for residency programs accredited by the Accreditation Council for Graduate Medical Education (ACGME). [http://www.lcme.org]

library as place: Term used to describe the physical library facility. Also the name of key studies, documents, and conferences by the Council on Library and Information Resources, NATIONAL LIBRARY OF MEDICINE, and ASSOCIATION OF ACADEMIC HEALTH SCIENCES LIBRARIES, focusing on how libraries can be envisioned as education, cultural, and social centers.

license: A contract; a binding, legally enforceable agreement between two or more parties.

license agreement: A formal written contract between a library and a vendor for the lease of one or more proprietary (copyrighted) bibliographic databases or online resources, usually for a fixed period of time in exchange for payment of an annual subscription fee or per-search charge. [*ODLIS*]

life-cycle replacement: Regular updating of hardware, software, and other technology support, for example, replacing desktop computers on a three-year cycle.

Lister Hill National Center for Biomedical Communication: A division of the U.S. NATIONAL LIBRARY OF MEDICINE; responsible for research and development in high-quality imagery, medical language processing, high-speed access to biomedical information, intelligent database systems, multimedia visualization, knowledge management, data mining and machine-assisted indexing, and producing ClinicalTrials.gov.

Loansome Doc®: A utility whereby a PUBMED or NLM Gateway user can request document delivery through a DOCLINE-participating library with which he or she has preregistered.

long-range planning: Planning on a five-year, or longer, basis.

LOR: *See* LEARNING OBJECT REPOSITORY.

magnet hospital: A hospital that has been recognized by the American Nurses Credentialing Center's Magnet Recognition Program® for providing nursing excellence.

manuscript: 1. A handwritten document. 2. An unpublished document. 3. An author's draft of a book, article, or other work submitted for publication. [Society of American Archivists]

MARC tag: Numerical designation between 001 and 999 that indicates the type of information carried in a field. For example, tag 245 is used for title, tag 650 for topical subject, and tag 440 for series title.

marketing: Techniques used to attract and draw consumers to a product or service.

Match Day: Occurring in March each year, this event links the preferences of applicants for residency positions with the preferences of residency programs for applicants.

matrix management: An organizational structure in which project managers and functional managers share responsibility for assigning priorities and for directing work. Sometimes used to describe "flat" organizations, which are ones in which many subordinates report to one manager.

mediated searching: Searching of a database done by a trained intermediary, for example, a librarian, for the end user.

Medicaid: This is the U.S. health insurance program for individuals and families with low incomes and resources. It is jointly funded by the states and federal government and is managed by the states. Among the groups of people served by Medicaid are eligible low-income parents, children, seniors, and people with disabilities. Medicaid is the largest source of funding for medical and health-related services for people with limited income.

medical informatics: Applications of advanced computer and communications technologies to health care and specifically to information in medicine and medical care; a more specific term than "health informatics," it concentrates on the medical aspects of health care, that is, physicians and disease.

Medical Library Association (MLA): MLA, the major professional organization supporting health sciences librarianship, is a nonprofit, educational organization, comprising health sciences information professionals with more than 4,500 members worldwide. Through its programs and services, MLA provides lifelong educational opportunities, supports a knowledge base of health information research, and works with a global network of partners to promote the importance of quality information for improved health to the health care community and the public.

medical records systems: Also called a hospital information system, it is a computer-based system that integrates different electronic services in a hospital (e.g., pharmacy, laboratories, nursing) to support patient care.

Medical Subject Headings (MeSH): Controlled vocabulary used to index and search health sciences databases, including journal articles, monographs, and other publications. MeSH is developed by the NATIONAL LIBRARY OF MEDICINE and used by most health sciences libraries. It is similar in concept to the Library of Congress subject headings but is specific to the health sciences.

Medicare: Medicare is the name given to a health insurance program administered by the U.S. government, covering people who are either age 65 and over, or who meet other special criteria. It was originally signed into law on July 30, 1965, by President Lyndon B. Johnson as amendments to Social Security legislation.

MEDLIB-L: An e-mail discussion list that provides a forum for MEDICAL LIBRARY ASSOCIATION members and other health sciences information professionals to discuss important issues about administrating their libraries and developing their careers. [http://www.mlanet.org/discussion/medlibl.html]

MEDLINE®: A bibliographic database from the NATIONAL LIBRARY OF MEDICINE covering medicine, nursing, dentistry, veterinary medicine, the health care system, and preclinical sciences.

MedlinePlus®: The NATIONAL LIBRARY OF MEDICINE's Web site for consumer health information. [http://www.nlm.nih.gov/pubs/factsheets/medlineplus.html]

MeSH: *See* MEDICAL SUBJECT HEADINGS.

metadata: Data that describe attributes of a resource; typically, the data support a number of functions: location, discovery, documentation, evaluation, selection, and others. [http://www.vraweb.org/metadata.html]

mezzotint: Invented in the seventeenth century, a process for producing fine-quality book illustrations and prints. In mezzotint, a metal plate (traditionally copper) is roughened all over with a special tool. The image is then placed on the plate by smoothing the roughened surface. The smooth portions of the plate do not hold ink and print as white. The roughened areas hold ink and therefore print black. No early process yields the subtlety of line, tone, and texture available through mezzotint. However, both the plates and the prints are exceedingly fragile, making them a preservation challenge for the special collections librarian.

Millennials: The generation of learners born between 1982 and 2001.

"Mirror me": A simple method whereby students follow the specific examples used by the instructor, typically as part of a demonstration of online resources or Web sites.

MLA: *See* MEDICAL LIBRARY ASSOCIATION.

MLANET: The Web page for the Medical Library Association, available at <http://www.mlanet.org>.

narrative reviews: Summaries of a subject that lack a systematic approach and a methodological rigor, so they tend to offer biased, dated, and sometimes even erroneous advice; not considered to be as useful as systematic reviews.

National Board of Medical Examiners (NBME): NBME is an independent, not-for-profit organization that provides high-quality examinations for the health professions. [http://www.nbme.org/index.html]

National Center for Biotechnology Information (NCBI): Division of the NATIONAL LIBRARY OF MEDICINE that is responsible for providing Web access to the MEDLINE database through PUBMED, genome-sequencing data in GenBank, and other biotechnology information.

National Institutes of Health (NIH): The NIH, a part of the U.S. Department of Health and Human Services, is the primary federal agency for conducting and supporting medical research. Composed of twenty-seven institutes and centers, the NIH provides leadership and financial support to researchers in every state and throughout the world. [http://www.nih.gov]

National Library of Medicine (NLM): The largest health sciences library in the world, located on the campus of the NATIONAL INSTITUTES OF HEALTH in Bethesda, Maryland. NLM provides leadership, products, and support for health sciences libraries and librarians, researchers, health practitioners, and the public. NLM produces PUBMED, MEDLINEPLUS, PUBMED CENTRAL, and many other Web products that benefit health providers and consumers worldwide. [http://www.nlm.nih.gov/pubs/factsheets/nlm.html]

National Network of Libraries of Medicine (NN/LM®): NN/LM is a network of medical libraries administered by the NATIONAL LIBRARY OF MEDICINE and divided into eight regions. [http://www.nlm.nih.gov/pubs/factsheets/nnlm.html]

National Residency Matching Program (NRMP): NRMP, a not-for-profit corporation, was created in 1952 to provide a fair and impartial process for applying to, and obtaining, residency positions, results, matching fourth-year medical students to residency programs, are revealed on MATCH DAY. [http://www.nrmp.org]

NBME: *See* NATIONAL BOARD OF MEDICAL EXAMINERS.

NCBI: *See* NATIONAL CENTER FOR BIOTECHNOLOGY INFORMATION.

NCLEX-RN (National Council Licensure Examination—Registered Nurse): A licensing examination for registered nurses. It is required by each state in the United States and must be passed before a nurse can be licensed to practice in that state.

need for cognitive closure: A personality trait that prompts wanting to make a decision quickly. This trait is helpful in circumstances requiring quick decisions, whereas it becomes a detriment to group decision-making processes in situations requiring a more deliberative approach.

NIH: *See* NATIONAL INSTITUTES OF HEALTH.

NLM: *See* NATIONAL LIBRARY OF MEDICINE.

NN/LM®: *See* NATIONAL NETWORK OF LIBRARIES OF MEDICINE.

NRMP: *See* NATIONAL RESIDENCY MATCHING PROGRAM.

Objective Structured Clinical Examination (OSCE): An examination often used in medicine to test skills such as communication, clinical examination, medical procedures, prescribing, and interpretation of results. It normally consists of several short (5-10 minutes) stations, and each is examined on a one-to-one basis with either real or simulated patients (actors).

OCLC (Online Computer Library Center): The largest bibliographic utility in the world, providing cataloging and acquisitions services, serials and circulation control, INTERLIBRARY LOAN support, and access to online databases. [*ODLIS*]

one-shot: Short, course-based library instruction, usually focused on a particular assignment that the students need to complete using library resources.

OPAC (online public access catalog): A computerized online catalog of the materials held in the library, made available to library users for direct searching.

open access: Concept that information should be available at no cost to either readers or their institutions. The information can be read, downloaded, copied, distributed, or printed. Creators of the information still hold other intellectual property rights. Health sciences libraries often support open access for research and health care information that results from publicly funded research studies.

open source: Refers to source code of software that is available to the general public through relaxed or nonexistent intellectual property restrictions; it is generally available free of charge or for a nominal fee. [*Wikipedia*]

operations research: The application of mathematical modeling, statistical techniques, and similar tools to problems involving the operation of real-life systems, to provide solutions or obtain efficiencies.

OSCE: *See* OBJECTIVE STRUCTURED CLINICAL EXAMINATION.

outcomes: Things that occur as a result of having conducted a program. They can be intended/unintended, positive/detrimental, relevant/nonrelevant, and so on. [staff.cce.cornell.edu/administration/program/documents/glossary.htm]

PACS (picture archiving and communication system): Usually part of a hospital information system that stores, indexes, and retrieves images of individual patients. Most hospitals have their own PACS.

patient health education (PHE): Provision of information to help inpatients or outpatients, or their family members, understand and cope with the condition for which they are receiving medical care. This education assists patients and/or their families in taking an active role in health care decision-making. [http://www.hls.mlanet.org/otherresources/standards2004.pdf]

PDA: *See* PERSONAL DIGITAL ASSISTANT.

personal digital assistant (PDA): Small wireless handheld device that provides computing and data storage capabilities.

pedagogy (pedagogies): The practical application of education and the science of teaching.

personal health records: An electronic health records system that allows patients access to their files and encourages them to enter data on themselves and their families.

PHE: *See* PATIENT HEALTH EDUCATION.

Planetree: A nonprofit membership organization working with hospitals and health centers to develop and implement patient-centered care in healing environments. The Planetree classification system groups subject matter into ten categories. [http://www.planetree.org/about/welcome.htm]

Platform for Change: Original education policy statement of the MEDICAL LIBRARY ASSOCIATION, detailing knowledge, skills, and competencies needed by health information professionals.

Platform for Lifelong Learning and Professional Success: Revision of the *Platform for Change,* being drafted by the MEDICAL LIBRARY ASSOCIATION.

podcast(ing): Distribution of a media file over the Internet using a syndication feed.

positive outcome bias: The tendency to publish only successful programs or to report only the positive aspects of programs while ignoring the less successful elements.

postdoc: An MD or PhD scientist who received additional training in an established investigator's laboratory prior to launching an independent career.

presentation skills: Techniques used to engage an audience, including the use of voice, eye contact, and gestures.

preservation: A process or series of actions that seek to maintain the physical information package or its intellectual content.

primacy effects: A cognitive bias that can interfere with sound decision-making in EVIDENCE-BASED LIBRARIANSHIP when information gathered early in the process exerts disproportionate influence.

primary care: In medicine, a term used for a health care provider who acts as a first point of consultation for all patients. Generally, primary care physicians are based in the community, as opposed to the hospital. Alternative names for the field are "general practice" and "family medicine," although the terms are not synonymous.

privacy: The ability of an individual to control the data that are collected on him or her, who has access to the data, how the data are stored and used, to whom the data are passed, and who maintains the data.

Privacy Rule: In 1996, the Medical Information Privacy rule was issued as part of the HEALTH INSURANCE PORTABILITY AND ACCOUNTABILITY ACT to protect the privacy and confidentiality of individuals' personal health information and to give patients increased access to their medical records.

problem-based learning (PBL): A student-centered learning model that engages students with open-ended problems, typically working in small groups and with minimal intervention by the instructor.

profession: Defined by a body of knowledge, specialized training, professional organizations, continuing education, services to clients, ethical standards for delivering those services, and research to help members perform their duties. Under this definition, health sciences librarianship is a profession.

proteomics: The study of proteins using information technology and biological computing techniques. It is one aspect of bioinformatics.

proxy server: An application program that operates between a client and server on a computer network, usually installed as a firewall to provide security or to increase speed of access by performing some of the housekeeping tasks that would normally be handled by the server itself, such as checking authentication or validating user requests. [*ODLIS*]

public access: Similar to open access. Concept that the public should have access to information that has been produced from publicly funded research activities.

public health informatics: The discipline concerned with the collection, analysis, and presentation of data based on populations and societies.

public relations: Communicating with the public about a product or service.

PubMed®: A search utility hosted by the NATIONAL LIBRARY OF MEDICINE that includes access to MEDLINE, a database of citations to literature from the clinical and preclinical sciences.

PubMed Central: A free digital archive of biomedical and life sciences journal literature produced by the NATIONAL LIBRARY OF MEDICINE and the NATIONAL INSTITUTES OF HEALTH.

qualifiers: Subheadings; terms appended to descriptors to further refine them.

qualitative research studies: A family of research methods, such as focus groups, interviews, and participant observation, used to answer exploratory types of EVIDENCE-BASED LIBRARIANSHIP questions.

radio frequency identification (RFID): A generic term for technologies that use radio waves as a means of identifying and tracking the location of objects.

radiology information system (RIS): Another name for a PACS (PICTURE ARCHIVING AND COMMUNICATION SYSTEM); used to store, index, and retrieve hospital collections of images taken of individual patients.

randomized controlled trial: A high-ranking research method in the LEVELS OF EVIDENCE; enrolls all members in a single population that then typically becomes randomized into a control group and an intervention (or "study") group. The control group usually receives the normal treatment whereas the intervention group receives an experimental treatment.

RCA: *See* ROOT CAUSE ANALYSIS.

really simple syndication (RSS): A syndication format that was developed by Netscape in 1999 and became very popular for aggregating updates to blogs and the news sites. [http://www.pcmag.com/encyclopedia_term/0,2542,t=RSS&i=50680,00.asp]

recency effects: A cognitive bias that can interfere with sound decision-making in EVIDENCE-BASED LIBRARIANSHIP when information gathered more recently in the process exerts disproportionate influence.

repurposing: Related to space planning, this is the use of existing space to serve a function other than the one for which it was originally intended.

residents: Physicians who have recently completed medical school and are in training.

return on investment (ROI): End result usually measured in terms of profit or cost savings, but can also be measured in terms of an objective achieved.

RFID: *See* RADIO FREQUENCY IDENTIFICATION.

RIS: *See* RADIOLOGY INFORMATION SYSTEM.

ROI: *See* RETURN ON INVESTMENT.

root cause analysis (RCA): A process for identifying the basic or causal factors that underlie variation in performance, including the occurrence or possible occurrence of a sentinel event.

round-robin searching: A group learning technique whereby students compare and contrast different resources by running the same series of searches through a progressive list of databases.

RSS: *See* REALLY SIMPLE SYNDICATION.

satellite clinic: An off-site, ambulatory facility affiliated with a hospital.

screencast: Any brief movie of computer activity with a narrative voiceover, typically demonstrating the features of an online resource or Web site.

secondary care: Services provided by medical specialists who generally do not have first contact with patients (e.g., cardiologist, urologists, dermatologists).

security: In a computer system, deals with how robust the application is in relation to protecting its data from external tampering or access from unauthorized people or systems.

signage: The use of various signs featuring letters, numbers, and/or symbols to label, direct, and identify.

simulation: A technique used to imitate real patient experiences.

SIS: *See* SPECIALIZED INFORMATION SERVICES.

social contract for health-related research: The NATIONAL INSTITUTES OF HEALTH became the primary federal agency responsible for implementing the social contract for health-related research proposed in Vannevar Bush's *Science—The Endless Frontier*. Bush believed that there must be a stream of new scientific knowledge to turn the wheels of private and public enterprise, and plenty of men and women trained in science and technology, for upon them depend both the creation of new knowledge and its applications to practical purposes.

social informatics: This emerging multidisciplinary field focuses upon the underlying assumptions made when introducing information technology and tracking the social consequences, both positive and negative, resulting from information technology.

Specialized Information Services (SIS): Division of the U.S. NATIONAL LIBRARY OF MEDICINE that provides information and resources on toxicology, chemistry, environmental health, HIV/AIDS, and health disparities.

standing order or **continuation:** An order with a vendor or publisher for nonperiodical serials that will continue until either the title is inactive or canceled by the library. These types of publications are generally published on an irregular basis.

storytelling: A prevalent cognitive bias in decision-making in EVIDENCE-BASED LIBRARIANSHIP that causes a person to lend greater importance to a compelling anecdote disproportionate or even contrary to the entire array of evidence reviewed.

strategic plan: Sometimes used interchangeably with long-range planning. A strategic plan consists of an organization's mission and future direction, near-term and long-term performance targets, and strategy. Involves creating an action plan based on clear end results (desired outcomes) and accurate assessment of current reality (an environmental scan).

student-centered learning: Pedagogy that emphasizes the student as an active participant who builds upon his or her own knowledge.

subfield: Contains data, identified by a subfield code, that is used to further define the information within a variable field.

subject-centered learning: As proposed by Parker J. Palmer, a pedagogy that emphasizes putting the educational subject "in the middle" of the learning experience.

subscription agents: Third parties who serve as intermediaries between librarians and publishers or vendors.

summative assessment: Sometimes called "assessment of learning," in that it is intended to address whether the student learned the material or not.

SUSHI (Standardized Usage Statistics Harvesting Initiative): Protocol aimed at automatically integrating statistical use data into electronic repositories.

systematic reviews: Scientifically conducted literature searches coupled to rigorous reviews and syntheses of all relevant evidence to answer focused clinical questions at the highest LEVELS OF EVIDENCE in EVIDENCE-BASED PRACTICE.

TACO: *Ta*ble of *co*ntents distribution service that involves the librarian supplying journal contents listings to clients as a means of alerting them to new articles.

Taft-Hartley Act: Officially known as the Labor-Management Relations Act, this U.S. federal law greatly restricts the activities and power of labor unions and is still largely in effect. The law amended the National Labor Relations Act (NLRA; also known as the Wagner Act) passed by Congress in 1935.

teacher-centered learning: Pedagogy that emphasizes information or knowledge being transferred in a direct method from the instructor to the student, whether by lecture, course notes, or textbook.

teaching hospital: A hospital that provides medical training to medical students and residents. Medical students typically spend three years in a teaching hospital doing clinical training, after completing their preclinical training in the medical school of a university.

teaching library: A library that actively advances the objectives of the parent organization, including education, research, community service, and patient care.

telehealth: A broader term than telemedicine; encompasses telemedicine as well as educational uses of telecommunications technology.

telemedicine: The use of telecommunications technology for medical diagnoses and patient care, and as a medium for delivering medical services to sites that are at a distance from the provider.

10:90 gap: This term refers to the fact that 10 percent of global spending for health research is allocated to the health problems of 90 percent of the population.

tertiary care: Specialized consultative care, usually on referral from primary or secondary medical care personnel, by specialists working in a center that has personnel and facilities for special investigation and treatment. Specialist cancer care, neurosurgery (brain surgery), burns care, and plastic surgery are examples of tertiary care services.

textwords: Words searchable in a database, usually in the author, title, abstract, or subject fields.

Think-Pair-Share: A classroom-based group learning technique whereby students are asked to think about a question briefly, partner with a neighbor or desk mate to discuss, and then share their thoughts with the class.

Toxline: A Web database service of the NATIONAL LIBRARY OF MEDICINE providing bibliographic information on pharmacology and toxicology.

TOXNET: A collection of toxicology services from SPECIALIZED INFORMATION SERVICES in the NATIONAL LIBRARY OF MEDICINE. The TOXNET databases include TOXLINE, a database of bibliographic information; HSDB, the Hazardous Substances Data Bank; Gene-Tox, containing information about genetic toxicology; and CCRIS, the Chemical Carcinogenesis Research Information System. [http://sis.nlm.nih.gov/Tox/ToxMain.html]

translational research: Activities focused on demonstrating that information from new discoveries in genetics, bioengineering, neuroscience, and molecular and structural biology can have practical benefits, thereby "translating" the science into new and effective medical practices and products.

turnover: Employee terminations, both voluntary and involuntary; sometimes expressed as a rate or ratio of the number of terminations divided by the average number of employees during a time period, usually an annual figure.

UMLS: *See* UNIFIED MEDICAL LANGUAGE SYSTEM.

Unified Medical Language System (UMLS®): A program that takes existing health vocabularies and maps them together. UMLS enables computerized health information systems to pass information back and forth (communicate).

USA PATRIOT Act: Uniting and Strengthening America by Providing Appropriate Tools Required to Intercept and Obstruct Terrorism Act, passed in 2001; legislation that amended previously passed statutes and affects FBI access to library records.

user-centered design: A process of involving users of a product or service in the design, development, and use of the product or service.

USMLE (United States Medical Licensure Examination): A multipart professional exam that medical students are required to complete before being authorized to practice medicine in the United States. It consists of three steps; all three must be passed before a physician is eligible to apply for a license to practice medicine.

variable fields: Fields containing data that vary in length and content, identified by MARC TAGS and containing subfields.

vellum: A fine-grained animal skin specially prepared for writing upon or for binding books. To the purist, vellum implies calfskin; however, it is often made from sheepskin or kidskin. [*Merriam-Webster's Dictionary*]

virtual private network (VPN): A private network that is configured within a public network (a carrier's network or the Internet) in order to take advantage of the economies of scale and management facilities of large networks. Encrypting data that travel between a remote user and the corporate LAN over the Internet is very popular. It is much more economical than using private, leased lines or making long-distance data calls via modem. Today, in fact, many people think that "VPN" and "encrypted connections over the Internet" are synonymous. [http://www.pcmag.com/encyclopedia_term/0,2542,t=VPN&i=54123,00.asp]

virtual reference: Reference services requested and provided over the Internet, usually via e-mail, instant messaging ("chat"), or Web-based submission forms, and usually answered by librarians in the reference department of a library, or sometimes by the participants in a collaborative reference system serving more than one institution. [*ODLIS*]

vodcasting: Shorthand for "video podcasting," or the syndication of video content via RSS or Atom feeds.

VPN: *See* VIRTUAL PRIVATE NETWORK.

Webinar: Interactive live Web conference. The term combines "Web" and "seminar."

Web usability testing: A method of evaluating Web sites in which users are asked to perform specific tasks while their actions are recorded and observed.

weeding: The process of identifying and withdrawing library materials from the collection due to age, condition, lack of use, need for shelf space, or other factors. Sometimes referred to as deselection or deacquisition.

white coat ceremony (WCC): A relatively new (1993) ritual for incoming medical students practiced in more than 100 American medical schools, as well as internationally. It is also beginning to be practiced in pharmacy and other health schools. Involves donning a white laboratory coat, a symbol of the medical profession. [Huber, S. J. "The White Coat Ceremony: A Contemporary Medical Ritual." *Journal of Medical Ethics* 29(2003): 364-6.]

WiFi: A wireless local area network that uses high-frequency radio waves.

Wiki: A Web application that allows users to add content to a collaborative hypertext Web resource (coauthoring), as in an Internet forum, and permits others to edit that content (open editing). [*ODLIS*]

Index

AACP Core Journals List, 79
AACR2R, 131, 132t, 140
AAHC. *See* Association of Academic Health Centers
AAHSL. *See* Association of Academic Health Sciences Libraries
AAMC. *See* Association of American Medical Colleges
Abridged Index Medicus, 79, 183
Academic health sciences libraries, 14-15
 and consumer health information, 433
 composite library, 14-15, 149
 facility management, 329-331
 and health sciences environment, 301-302
 management of, 301-340
 personnel management, 315, 318-329
 roles of library administrators, 302-315
Academic medical center (AMC) libraries. *See* Academic health sciences libraries
Academic medicine
 challenges, 52-54
 drivers of, 54-55
 future of, 51-57
 medical schools, 42-44
 organization of, 40-44
 scenarios, 55-57
 teaching hospitals, 41-42
Academic Search Premier, 191
Academy of Health Information Professionals (AHIP), 10, 326, 344. *See also* Medical Library Association
Access issues, 147-159
 access services department, 148-149
 borrowing, 150
 for consumer health information, 441
 for disabled, 157, 380
 electronic access, 76, 152-154
 in hospital libraries, 349
 library hours, 150
 network access, 156-157
 physical access, 149-152
 public access, 149-150
 security, 150-151
 in special collections, 417-418
Accreditation Council for Graduate Medical Education (ACGME), 376-377
Accreditation Council for Pharmacy Education standards (library and education), 220

ACGME. *See* Accreditation Council for Graduate Medical Education
ACP Journal Club, 79, 191, 244
Acquisitions, 98
ACRL. *See* Association of College and Research Libraries
ADA. *See* American Dental Association
ADA. *See* Americans with Disabilities Act
Advisory groups. *See* Library committees
AGRICOLA, 188
AHA. *See* American Hospital Association
AHA Guide to the Healthcare Field, 342, 344
AHIP. *See* Academy of Health Information Professionals
AIM-TWX, 183
ALA. *See* American Library Association
Alerting systems, 278
American Dental Association (ADA) accreditation standards, 220-221
American Hospital Association (AHA), 16
American Library Association (ALA)
 ethics position statement, 172-173
 and library education, 6
American Medical Informatics Association (AMIA)
 informatics training, 289
American Nurses Association (ANA)
 Scope and Standards of Nursing Informatics Practice, 220
American Osteopathic Association (AOA), 42, 345
Americans with Disabilities Act (ADA), 157, 330, 359, 380
ANA. *See* American Nurses Association
ANGEL, 401
AOA. *See* American Osteopathic Association
Appeal to authority, 263
Approval plans, 98-99, 100-101
Archives
 electronic journals, 92-94
 policies, 91
Ariel®, 155, 361
ARL. *See* Association of Research Libraries
Assessment. *See* Evaluation
Association of Academic Health Centers (AAHC), 302
Association of Academic Health Sciences Libraries (AAHSL), 7, 9
 Annual Statistics, 9, 310
 Assessment and Statistics Committee, 310
 composite library, 14-15, 149

Association of Academic Health Sciences Libraries
  (continued)
  and legislation, 39
  planning resources, 375
  professional development, 325
Association of American Medical Colleges (AAMC),
  41, 42. *See also* Council of Teaching
  Hospitals and Health Systems (COTH);
  Liaison Committee on Medical Education
  (LCME)
  Medical School Objectives Project, 219-220
Association of College and Research Libraries (ACRL)
  information literacy standards, 218-219
  Rare Book and Manuscript Section, 425
  Standards for Librarians in Higher Education, 376
Association of Research Libraries (ARL)
  statistics, 310
Associations, professional
  informatics, 292
  library, 9-10, 11t, 39-40, 162, 325, 363, 454
Audience response systems, 233, 397, 404-405
Automatic indexing programs, 287

Backfiles, 78, 112, 329, 351, 414
Basic sciences, 12
Behavioral research, 33, 49
Behaviorism, 222
Benchmarking, 364-365. *See also* Evaluation
  journals, 89-92
Bibliographic databases, 180-181
Bibliographic record, 128, 129, 130, 137. *See also*
  MARC record
Binding, 120
Bioinformatics, 275-276
Biomedical research, 33, 49, 50t. *See also* Health
  sciences research
BioOne, 91
BIOSIS, 188
  in collection development, 74, 80
Blackboard, 400
Blogs, 235, 362
BMJ Clinical Evidence, 191, 244, 291
BOAI Forum, 89
Board certification, 47t
Books. *See* Monographs
Boolean logic, 194
Booth and Brice's Critical Appraisal Checklist, 263
Borrowing privileges, 150
Branding, 202-203, 354
Brandon/Hill Selected Lists, 79, 101
Budgeting. *See* Fiscal management

CA SEARCH® (*Chemical Abstracts*), 188
  in collection development, 80
Case study, 261
Case study method, 223

Catalog copy, 130-131
Catalog records, 129
Cataloging practices, 131-139. *See also* Information
  organization
  classification, 134-135
  descriptive cataloging, 131
  subject assignment, 132-134
Cataloging-In-Publication (CIP), 129, 139t
CDSS. *See* Clinical decision support system
CEO. *See* Chief executive officer
CEPH. *See* Council on Education for Public Health
CHI. *See* Consumer health information
Chief executive officer (CEO), 302, 342
Chief information officer (CIO), 302
CINAHL® (*Cumulative Index to Nursing and Allied
  Health Literature*), 74, 76, 187-188, 191, 233,
  347
  in collection development, 74, 76, 80
  controlled vocabulary, 128
CIO. *See* Chief information officer
Circulation services. *See* Access issues
Citation indexing, 189
Classroom control software, 232-233
Clinical decision support system (CDSS), 277, 279
Clinical decision tools, 118
Clinical informatics, 277-281
Clinical information systems, 171, 277-278
Clinical medical librarian, 171, 354
Clinical research, 50
Clinical sciences, 12
ClinicalTrials.gov, 20
CLOCKSS, 94
CME. *See* Continuing medical education
Cochrane Collaboration, 191
Cochrane Library, 244, 249
Code of Ethics for Health Sciences Librarianship,
  6, 173-175
Cognitive biases, 254, 255t-256t
Cognitivism, 222
Collaborative learning environments, 372
Collection development
  for consumer health information, 448-50
  in hospital libraries, 349, 351-352
  for minorities, 451
Collection development, digital resources and
  monographs, 97-126
  and acquisitions, 98
  and book vendors, 101-102
  budget, 103
  digital resource selection, 109-119
  monograph selection, 100-108
  needs assessment, 99-100
  overview, 98-100
  policies, 102-108
  preservation, 119-122
  selection criteria, 109-113
  staffing for, 98-99

Collection development, journals, 69-96
  benchmarking, 89-92
  budget/costs, 76-77, 89-90
  consortia, 83
  copyright, 85-87
  core lists, 78-79
  digital archives, 92-94
  electronic journals, 75-85
  evaluation, 89-92
  journal quality, 11-14
  journal recommendation forms, 72f, 73f
  legal aspects, 84
  online licensing/vendor relations, 82-85
  open access, 87-89
  policies, 70
  selection, 70-81
COLT. *See* Council on Library/Media Technicians
Communication, 201-216
Community partnerships, 454
Compact storage. *See* Storage
Computerized health records, 277-281
Confidentiality, 288-289, 442
CONFU, 86
Connectivism, 223
CONSER, 130, 141
Consortia
  and consumer health information, 453
  and journal licensing, 78, 83, 91
Constructivism, 222-223
Consumer health information (CHI), 25, 348, 429-458
  challenges, 440-444
  collaborations, 452-454
  collection development for, 102
  defined, 429-430
  evaluation of services, 451-452
  information seekers, 437-440
  in libraries, 430-431, 433-434
  National Library of Medicine involvement,
      434-436
  policies, 108
  resources, 454-455
  services, 444-451
Content preservation, 121-122
Continuing medical education (CME), 345, 355. *See
      also* Medical education
Controlled thesaurus, 128, 194
CONTU, 86
Copyright, 85-87
Cost-benefit analysis. *See also* Evaluation; Fiscal
      management
  in collection development, 89-90, 118-119
COTH. *See* Council of Teaching Hospitals and Health
      Systems
Council of Teaching Hospitals and Health Systems
      (COTH), 41, 118-119
Council on Education for Public Health (CEPH), 312
Council on Library/Media Technicians (COLT),
      325-326

COUNTER (Counting Online Usage of NeTworked
      Electronic Resources), 78, 118
Course management systems, 156, 157t, 234-235, 397,
      400-402
Course reserves, 156
Course-based instruction, 227-228
Courseware. *See* Course management systems
Current Contents, 189
Curriculum-integrated programming, 228-229

DARE, 244
Data collection. *See* Evaluation
Database retrieval, 196-197
Database searching, 193-197
Databases, 181-182, 187-190. *See also specific
      databases*
  for consumer health information, 450
  full-text, 191-192
Day in the Life of . . .
  academic health sciences library associate director,
      322
  academic health sciences library director, 303
  collection development librarian, 117
  consumer health librarian, 432
  education librarian, 230
  hospital librarian, 350
  reference librarian, 170
  special services librarian, 410
Departmental liaisons, 171-172
Descriptive cataloging, 131
Descriptor, 128
Desire2Learn, 401
Diagnosis-related groups (DRGs), 36
DIALOG, 182, 184
Digital archives, 92-94
Digital Millennium Copyright Act (DMCA), 40
Digital resources
  assessment strategies, 113-114
  categories, 115, 116t
  criteria, 109-113
  evaluation, 118-119
  selection and evaluation, 109-119
Directory of Open Access Journals, 88
Disabled access, 157
Disaster planning, 27, 307-308, 360
Dispersed care, 34
Diversity, 319-320
DOCLINE®, 155, 348, 365
DoctorEvidence, 191
Document delivery. *See* Interlibrary loan
Donations, 417
Doody's Core Titles, 101
DRGs. *See* Diagnosis-related groups
DynaMed, 181, 191

EBL. *See* Evidence-based librarianship
EBL Levels of Evidence. *See* Levels of Evidence
EBL process, 256-264
EBLIP. *See* Evidence-based librarianship
EBM. *See* Evidence-based medicine
EBM Specific Search Method, 246, 247-251
    EBM diagnosis searches, 249-250
    EBM prognosis searches, 250
    EBM therapy searches, 250-251
EBP. *See* Evidence-based practice
EBSCO*host*, 91, 182
Education services. *See* Information literacy
EFTS. *See* Electronic Fund Transfer System
e-health, 273
EHR. *See* Electronic health record
Electronic access, 152-154
Electronic Fund Transfer System (EFTS), 365
Electronic health record (EHR), 278, 353
Electronic health records systems, 277, 279-280
Electronic journals. *See also* Electronic resources
    archiving, 92-94
    and consortia, 83
    legal aspects, 84
    licensing/negotiation, 82-85
    selection criteria, 75-81
Electronic medical record (EMR), 51
Electronic resources. *See also* Electronic journals
    categories, 116t
    content analysis, 118
    evaluation of, 118-119
Elsevier, 74, 191
EMBASE (*Excerpta Medica*), 188
    in collection development, 80
Emergency preparedness. *See* Disaster planning
EMR. *See* Electronic medical record
End users, 192
EndNote, 197
Environmental scanning, 90
Ephemera, policies, 108
Ethics
    and consumer health information, 442-444
    and hospital libraries, 358-359
    information, 172-175
    and rare books, 416-417
Evaluation. *See also* Benchmarking
    of consumer health information services, 451-452
    of electronic resources, 99, 113-114, 118
    in hospital libraries, 363-365
    of journals, 89-92
    of search results, 197
Evidence Based Medicine, 244
Evidence-based databases, 191
Evidence-based librarianship (EBL), 252-265
    defined, 252-253
    EBL process, 253-254, 256-264
    future, 265
    levels of evidence, 243-244, 260t, 260-262
    obstacles, 254-256

Evidence-based medicine (EBM), 163, 191. *See also*
    EBM Specific Search Method
    defined, 242-244
    levels of evidence, 243-244
    role of librarians, 242-252
Evidence-based practice (EBP), 24, 241-269
Expert opinion, 261

Facilities management, 329-331
Faculty of 1000, 74
FDA Web site, 188
Federal legislation (U.S.), 58-62
Filtering information/literature, 162
FISA. *See* Foreign Intelligence Security Act
Fiscal management
    in academic health sciences libraries, 313-315,
        316-317
    for collection development, 99, 103, 112-113
    of electronic journals, 76-77
    of electronic resources, 118-119
    in hospitals, 365
    for marketing, 214-215
    policies, 103
Fixed field, 135
Flexner Report, 32-33
Focus groups, 212, 372
Foreign Intelligence Security Act (FISA), 358
Formative assessment, 236
Freeshare, 365
Friends groups, 214, 417
FTE. *See* Full-time equivalent
Full-text databases, 191
Full-time equivalent (FTE), 76, 112, 321, 343, 376
Funding. *See* Fiscal management

Gifts, policies, 106
Go Local, 25, 436, 436f. *See also* MedlinePlus®
Google Scholar, 191
Government documents, policies, 107
Gray literature, 259
Groupthink, 264

Health care. *See also* Modern health care system
    costs, 34-36, 38
    right versus privilege, 31-32
Health care environment, 31-65
Health care legislation (U.S.), 37-40, 58-62
    and professional library associations, 39-40
Health informatics, 271-296
    associations, 292
    bioinformatics, 275-276
    clinical informatics, 277-281
    data, 273-274
    defined, 272

Health informatics *(continued)*
 education, 289
 future, 290
 and health sciences librarians, 290-291
 history, 272-273
 imaging informatics, 276
 information retrieval, 286-288
 journals, 292-293
 privacy, confidentiality, and security, 288-289
 public health informatics, 281-282
 standards/vocabulary, 283-286
 training, 289
Health information
 data, 273-274
 formats, 274-275
Health Insurance Portability and Accountability Act
  (HIPAA), 40, 51, 288, 356, 398, 416, 418
Health literacy, 444
Health maintenance organizations (HMOs), 34
Health records systems. *See* Electronic health records
  systems
Health sciences librarians. *See also* Health sciences
  librarianship
 role in clinical settings, 357
 role in evidence-based medicine, 242-252
 role in informatics, 290-291
Health sciences librarianship. *See also* Health sciences
  libraries
 competencies/skills, 7t
 consumer health, 25
 defined, 3-4, 5t
 duties, 8t
 education for, 6
 emergency preparedness, 27
 evidence-based practice, 24
 and health sciences research, 26
 knowledge base, 6
 knowledge management, 26
 library as place, 22-24
 maximizing resources, 25-26
 nature of work, 6-7
 profession of, 4-10
 professional organizations, 9-10, 11t
 recruitment, 9
 salaries, 7, 9
 scholarly communication, 24-25
 teaching library, 24
 technology, 20-22
 trends, 20-27
 values, 4, 6
Health sciences libraries, 10-17. *See also* Academic
  health sciences libraries; Health sciences
  librarianship; Hospital libraries
 academic health sciences libraries, 14-15
 and administrative support, 14
 clients, 12-14
 collections, 10
 and community services, 14

Health sciences libraries *(continued)*
 and education, 12-13
 facilities, 11-12
 hospital libraries, 16-17
 and patient care, 13
 promotion of, 204-212
 and research, 13-14
 special health sciences libraries, 17
 special services, 397-412
 types of health sciences libraries, 14-17
Health sciences research, 26, 48-51. *See also*
  Biomedical research
 financing, 48
 regulation, 51
 training, 48-49
Health services research, 31, 50
Hill-Burton Act, 37
HIPAA. *See* Health Insurance Portability and
  Accountability Act
Hiring process, 323-324
Historical materials, policies, 107
HL7 (Health Level 7), 283
HMO. *See* Health maintenance organizations
Hospital libraries, 16-17, 341-367
 accreditation, 16
 collection development, 349-352
 consumer health information, 433-434
 evaluation, 363-365
 fiscal management, 365
 legal/ethical issues, 358-359
 library users, 345-346
 marketing, 353-354
 networking, 352-353
 professional development, 360-361
 reporting structure, 342-343
 roles, 354-357
 security, 362-363
 services, 346-349
 space planning, 348, 376
 staffing, 343-344
 standards/accreditation, 344-345
 strategic planning, 360
 technology, 361-362
 time management, 359-360
House officers, 47
Human resources. *See* Personnel management

ILL. *See* Interlibrary loan
ILS. *See* Integrated library system
Imaging informatics, 276
IMLS. *See* Institute of Museum and Library Services
Immersive learning, 371
Impact factors, 74, 80, 172
Index Medicus, 182, 183, 246, 422
IndexCat, 422f
Indicators, 137
InfoPOEMs, 79, 181, 191

Information access, 147-159
Information button (or Infobutton), 353
Information fluency, 221, 222
Information literacy, 169, 217-240
    assessment, 236-239
    definition, 217-218
    future, 239
    in hospital libraries, 348
    instruction techniques, 229, 231-236
    learning theories and pedagogies, 222-224
    and Millennials, 224-225
    program design, 227-229
    program planning, 225-227
    standards and objectives, 218-221
Information needs, health sciences
    education, 164
    patient care, 163-164
    research, 164
Information organization, 127-144
    audiovisual materials, 140
    electronic resources, 140
    future, 141-142
    history, 127-128
    rules and standards, 128
Information requests
    offline reference, 166
    real-time requests, 165-166
Information retrieval, 179-199
    databases, 181-191
    evaluation, 193-197
    and informatics, 286-288
    mediated search process, 193-197
    search services, 192
Information Rx, 347
Information seeking
    consumer health information, 437-430
    health professionals, 163-164
Information services, 161-178
    ethics, 172-175
    health sciences information needs, 163-164
    in hospital libraries, 347-348
    in special collections, 421
Information specialist in context (ISIC), 319, 355
Information systems department. *See* Information
    technology department
Information technology. *See also* Information
    technology department; Technology
    legislation, 40
    and space planning, 383
Information technology department
    and electronic journal licensing, 82-83
    relationship of library with, 302, 349, 356, 361-362,
    397-398
Informational/factual questions, 169
Informationist, 162-163, 244, 355
    role, 246-247
Institute for Scientific Information, 74, 189
Institute of Museum and Library Services (IMLS), 39

Institutional repository (IR), 172
    policies, 107
Institutional review board (IRB), 49, 356
Instructional design, 407-408
Integrated library system (ILS), 34, 129-130
    in hospital libraries, 346-347
Intellectual freedom, 442-443
Interlibrary loan (ILL), 155-156, 348-349
    and journal selection, 71
International Classification of Diseases (ICD), 284
Internet, 21
    consumer health information, 437-440
Intranet, 349
IP (Internet protocol) authentication, 153
IP (Internet protocol) recognition, 362
IR. *See* Institutional repository
IRB. *See* Institutional review board
ISI. *See* Institute for Scientific Information
ISIC. *See* Information specialist in context

JCAHO. *See* Joint Commission on Accreditation of
    Healthcare Organizations
Joint Commission on Accreditation of Healthcare
    Organizations (Joint Commission), 16, 312,
    341, 344, 376
Journal Citation Reports®, 80, 189, 190t
Journal Use Reports, 92
Journals. *See* Collection development, journals
JSTOR, 91, 93, 94

KBI. *See* Knowledge-based information
Knowledge management, 6, 26
Knowledge-based information (KBI), 341, 344-345

LATCH (literature attached to chart), 171, 354
LC. *See* Library of Congress
LCME. *See* Liaison Committee on Medical Education
Learning contracts, 320
Learning object repository (LOR)
Learning theories, 222-223
Legal issues
    and electronic journals, 84
    and hospital libraries, 358-359
Lesson plan, 229, 231
Levels of Evidence, 243-244, 260-262
Liaison Committee on Medical Education (LCME), 15,
    42, 312, 375-376
LibQUAL+, 372
Librarian-user interaction, 164-166, 352-353
Libraries. *See also* Academic health sciences libraries;
        Health sciences libraries; Hospital libraries;
        Library space planning
    building maintenance, 329-330
    consultants, 377

Libraries *(continued)*
  furniture, 381
  handouts, 204, 206
  in-person events, 207-209
  newsletters, 204, 205t
  promotion via Web site, 211f
  promotional items, 206
  safety and security, 330
  signage, 382
  standards, 376-377
  use policies, 330
  virtual world, 209-212
Library administrators, roles of, 302-315
  advocacy, 313
  assessment/evaluation, 309-312
  fiscal responsibilities, 313-315
  leadership, 304-305
  management, 302, 304
  management styles, 305-306
  managing change, 305
  marketing, 312-313
  planning, 306-307
  vision/mission, 308-309
Library as place, 22-24, 358, 372
Library collaboration, 452-454
Library committees, 343
  for journal selection, 70-71
  for monograph collection development, 103
  policies for collection development, 103
Library hours, 150
Library of Congress
  classification, 128, 134
  subject headings, 128, 129
Library security. *See* Security
Library space planning, 329, 358, 369-393
  consumer health information programs, 446
  consultant/architect, 377
  in hospital libraries, 376
  and Library 2.0, 378-379
  predesign planning, 374
  site visits and research, 374-376
  standards, 376-377
  and strategic planning, 377-378
  trends, 370-373
Library 2.0
  and space planning, 378-379
Library users, health sciences
  administration, 14
  basic sciences, 12
  clinical sciences, 12
  community, 14
  consumers, 445, 447, 451
  education, 12-13, 164
  in hospitals, 345-346
  patient care, 13, 163-164
  research, 13-14, 164
License agreements, 351
  for electronic journals, 82-85

Lister Hill National Center for Biomedical
    Communication, 18
Loansome Doc®, 156, 184, 348
LocatorPlus, 130, 134, 137, 139f
LOCKSS, 93
LOR. *See* Learning object repository

Magnet hospitals, 345
Management
  of academic health sciences libraries, 301-340
  of hospital libraries, 341-367
Manikins. *See* Simulators
MARC format, 129
MARC record, 130, 134, 135, 137, 138t, 139t
MARC tags, 134, 137
Marketing, 201-216
  branding, 202-203
  and collection development, 99-100
  for consumer health information, 451
  funding, 214-215
  in hospital libraries, 353-354
  and libraries, 203, 204
  role of library administrator, 312-313
Marketing mix, 202, 202t
Match Day, 47
Maximizing resources, 25-26
MDConsult, 76, 181, 191
Mediated searching, 169, 192, 193-197
Medicaid, 36, 38
Medical education, 44-47
  curriculum, 45-46
  graduate, 46-47
  in nineteenth century, 32-33
  undergraduate, 44-46
Medical informatics. *See* Health informatics
Medical Library Association (MLA), 6, 9-10, 325, 361.
    See also Academy of Health Information
    Professionals
  CAPHIS, 454
  Code of Ethics for Health Sciences Librarianship,
    6, 173-175
  *Competencies and Skills for Health Sciences
    Librarianship,* 7t
  continuing education courses, 184, 252, 307, 325,
    454
  DocKit, 70
  Educational Policy Statement, 344
  and "The Future of Librarians in the Workforce,"
    323
  History of the Health Sciences Section, 422, 423f,
    425
  Hospital Libraries Section, 16
  and legislation, 39
  Platform for Change, 6
  *Platform for Lifelong Learning and Professional
    Success,* 6

Medical Library Association *(continued)*
  Standards for Hospital Libraries, 342, 356, 376
  Vital Pathways Project, 345
Medical records systems, 272
Medical schools, 42-44. *See also* Medical education
  faculty, 43-44
  faculty practice organizations, 44
  financing, 42-43
Medical Subject Headings (MeSH), 18, 128, 129,
      132-134, 151, 182, 186, 191, 283-284, 422
  tree structure categories, 133t, 186, 187, 196
Medicare, 36, 38-39
MEDLARS®, 182, 183
MEDLIB-L, 356
MEDLINE®, 18, 115, 181, 182-187, 191, 232, 233,
      244, 246, 274
  in collection development, 74, 80, 109
  in EBM searching, 248, 249-251
  fields, 184-185
  free versus fee-based, 115
  full text, 186-187
  history, 182-184
  and PubMed®, 187
  record, 185t
  use of MeSH, 186
  vendors, 184
MedlinePlus®, 18, 20, 276, 347, 435-436, 435t, 440,
      454. *See also* Go Local
MeSH. *See* Medical Subject Headings
Metadata, 130
Micromedex, 188
Millennials, 167, 224-225
miniMEDLINE, 184
"Mirror me," 233
Mission statement, 324-325
MLA. *See* Medical Library Association
MLANET, 9-10
Modern health care system, 33-40
  and federal role (U.S.), 36-40
  costs, 34-36
  health care spending, 35f
  history, 32-33
  levels of care, 33-34
  origins, 32
  providers of care, 36
Monographs
  content preservation, 121
  policies, 102-106, 107
  repair, 120
  resources for selection, 100-108
  security, 121
  weeding, 122
Moodle, 401-402

Narrative reviews, 244-245
National Board of Medical Examiners (NBME), 46

National Center for Biotechnology Information
      (NCBI), 18, 184
National health information policy, 39-40
National Institutes of Health (NIH), 17-18, 33
  and research funding, 48, 49
National Library of Medicine (NLM), 4, 17-20. *See
      also* Loansome Doc®; LocatorPlus;
      MEDLINE®; Medical Subject Headings;
      National Network of Libraries of Medicine;
      NLM classification; PubMed; PubMed
      Central; TOXNET
  Associate Fellowship Program, 20, 325
  consumer health information services, 434-436
  databases, 187
  electronic resources, 20
  funding, 39
  history, 17-18
  History of Medicine Division, 414
  informatics training, 289
  long-range plan, 305
  mission, 18
  online tutorials, 236
  organization, 18-19
  regions, 19f
  resources, 20
National Network of Libraries of Medicine
      (NN/LM®), 16, 17, 19, 19t, 155, 183, 361
National Residency Matching Program (NRMP), 47
NBME. *See* National Board of Medical Examiners
NCBI. *See* National Center for Biotechnology
      Information
NCLEX-RN (National Council Licensure Examination
      for Registered Nursing), 105
Need for cognitive closure, 264
Network access, 156-157
Networking. *See* Librarian-user interaction
New technologies. *See* Technology *and individual
      technologies*
NIH. *See* National Institutes of Health
NLM. *See* National Library of Medicine
NLM classification, 104, 128, 134-135, 136t, 137t,
      346, 434
NLM Gateway, 184
NLM/AAHSL Leadership Fellows Program, 325
NN/LM®. *See* National Network of Libraries of
      Medicine
Nonprint material, policies, 106
NRMP. *See* National Residency Matching Program

Objective Structured Clinical Examination (OSCE), 46
OCLC (Online Computer Library Center), 129,
      130-131, 141, 348. *See also* WorldCat
Odyssey, 155
Online journals. *See* Electronic journals
Online public access catalog, 129, 140, 151, 154-155
OPAC. *See* Online public access catalog
Open access, 87-89. *See also* PubMed Central

Open source software, 401
Open WorldCat. *See* WorldCat
Organization of information. *See* Information organization
Organizational structure
   in academic health sciences libraries, 320-321
   in hospital libraries, 342-343
OSCE. *See* Objective Structured Clinical Examination
Out-of-print books, policies, 108
Ovid, 115, 182, 184

PACS (picture archiving and communication system), 276
PaperChase, 184
Patient health education (PHE), 346
Patron recommendations. *See* User recommendations/ feedback
PDAs. *See* Personal digital assistants
Pedagogies, 223-224
Performance evaluation, 326-327
Personal digital assistants (PDAs), 349, 397, 398-399
Personal filing systems, 197
Personal health records, 278
Personnel management
   in academic health sciences libraries, 315, 318-329
   hiring, 323-325
   organizational structure, 320-321
   personnel records, 328-329
   recognition, motivation, retention, 327-328
   regulations, 315, 318
   staff development, 325-327
   staffing needs assessment, 318-320
Pew Internet and American Life Project, 437-438
PHE. *See* Patient health education
Physicians Desk Reference, 188
PICO format, 251
Planetree
   classification, 346, 434
   consumer health information services, 434
Planning, 306-308
Platform for Change, 6
Platform for Lifelong Learning and Professional Success, 6
Podcasting, 235, 362, 397, 408-409
Popular reading, policies, 108
Portico, 94
Positive outcome bias, 261
Presentation skills, 231
Preservation
   binding, 120
   collection development policies, 105
   collection security, 121
   content preservation, 121-122
   repair/conservation, 120-121
   weeding, 122
Primacy effects, 259-260
Primary care, 33
Primary literature, 180

Privacy, 288-289
Privacy Rule, 51
Problem-based learning (PBL), 46, 223
ProCite®, 197
Professional development, 325-326, 360-361
Professional organizations. *See* Associations, professional
Promotion. *See* Marketing
ProQuest®, 188
Proxy server, 153-154, 351
PsycINFO®, 188
   in collection development, 80
Public health informatics, 281-282
Public libraries
   collaboration, 452-453
   consumer health information, 431, 433
Public relations, 201-216
PubMed®, 18, 20, 115, 182, 184, 347, 422, 434
   in EBM searching, 244, 246, 247f, 248-251, 248f
   legislation, 40
   and MEDLINE®, 187
PubMed Central, 10, 20, 40, 88, 93, 186-187
   and journal archiving, 91, 93

Qualifiers, 134
Quality of health information, 442

Radio frequency identification (RFID), 150
Radiology information system (RIS), 276
Rare Book School, 421
Rare books, 414
Recency effects, 260
Recruitment, 321, 323-324, 335-337
Reference interview, 167-168
Reference Manager, 197
Reference services. *See* Information services
Regionalized care, 34
Remote storage facilities. *See* Storage
Repurposing space, 329
Residency, 47
Retention of older materials, policies, 104-105
Return on investment (ROI), 354
RFID. *See* Radio frequency identification
RIS. *See* Radiology information system
RLIN (Research Libraries Information Network), 129
ROI. *See* Return on investment
Round-robin searching, 233-234
RSS (really simple syndication), 235, 362, 408

Satellite clinics, 351
Scholarly communication, 24-25
ScholarlyStats, 92
SCHOLCOMM Discussion List, 89
Science Citation Index, 74, 189, 195
   in collection development, 74, 80

Scopus, 74, 191
Screencast, 235
Search services, 192-197
    end-user searching, 192
    evaluation, 197
    mediated searches, 192
    search process, 193-197
Secondary care, 33-34
Secondary literature, 180-181
Security, 288-289
    of collection, 121
    data, 288-289
    of facility, 150-151, 330
    in hospital libraries, 362-362
    policies, 103
    in special collections, 418-420
Semantic Net, 285t
Shared space, 282-283
Shelving, 371
Signage, 382
Simulators, 397, 402-403
Single-service desks, 168-169, 381
SIS. *See* Specialized Information Services
SNOMED®, 284-286
Social Science Citation Index, 189
Society of American Archivists, 425
SPARC Open Access Forum, 89
Special collections, 413-428
    education for, 421
    policies, 415-418
    reference areas and services, 418, 420-421
    reference sources, 422
    stack security, 424-425
    storage, 423-424
    technical services, 422-423
Special Libraries Association, 325, 344
Specialized Information Services (SIS), 18
Staff development, 325-327
Staffing
    in academic health sciences libraries, 315-329
    for collection development, 98-99
    for consumer health information services, 446
    in hospital libraries, 343-344
Standing order (continuation), policies, 105-106
Statistics. *See* Evaluation
Storage
    compact storage, 381-382, 425
    remote facilities, 152
    in special collections, 423-424, 425
Storytelling, 261
Strategic planning, 306
    in hospital libraries, 360
    library planning, 377-378
Streaming video, 409
Student-centered learning, 223
Subject-centered learning, 223-224
Subscription agents, 77, 80
Summative assessment, 236

Surveys, 213
SUSHI (Standardized Usage Statistics Harvesting
    Initiative), 78
Systematic reviews, 244-245

TACOs, 169, 171, 354
Taft-Hartley Act, 38
Teacher-centered learning, 223
Teaching hospitals, 32, 41-42, 341
Teaching library, 24
Technical services
    in hospital libraries, 346-347
    in special collections, 422-423
Technology, 20-22, 162-163
    in hospital libraries, 361-362
    implications for health sciences libraries, 22t
    planning, 307
Telehealth, 280
Telemedicine, 280-281
10:90 gap, 54
Tertiary care, 34
Tertiary literature, 181
Think-Pair-Share, 232
Thomson Corporation, 74, 92, 184, 188, 189
Toxline, 20
TOXNET, 20, 188
Translational research, 26, 50

Ulrich's Serials Analysis System, 92
UMLS. *See* Unified Medical Language System
Unified Medical Language System (UMLS®), 284-286
Update services, 169, 171
UpToDate®, 181, 191
U.S. NLM *See* National Library of Medicine
USA PATRIOT Act, 40, 358
User education. *See* Information literacy
User recommendations/feedback
    collection development policies, 104
    for collection development, 71, 74, 113, 119
    in marketing, 214
User-centered design, 214
USMLE (United States Medical Licensure
    Examination), 105

Variable fields, 135
Venn diagrams, 195t
Videoconferencing, 405-407
Virtual private network (VPN), 154, 351
Virtual reference, 167, 347
Virtual world, 209-212
Visualization, 373
Vodcasting, 235
VPN. *See* Virtual private network

Web of Science®, 188, 189, 197
Web searching, 191
Web sites, 346, 355
   history of medicine, 422
   as promotional tools, 209-212
Web usability testing, 213-214
Weeding, 122, 351-352, 417
White coat ceremony (WCC), 304
WiFi, 157
Wikis, 235-236, 362
Wireless access, 156-157
WorldCat, 79, 92